Disorders|Differences of Sex Development

Editors
John M. Hutson
Department of Urology
The Royal Children's Hospital
Melbourne
VIC
Australia

Murdoch Children's Research Institute
Melbourne
VIC
Australia

Sonia R. Grover
Department of Gynaecology
The Royal Children's Hospital
Melbourne
VIC
Australia

Murdoch Children's Research Institute
Melbourne
VIC
Australia

Michele A. O'Connell
Department of Endocrinology
and Diabetes
The Royal Children's Hospital
Melbourne
VIC
Australia

Murdoch Children's Research Institute
Melbourne
VIC
Australia

Aurore Bouty
Department of Urology
The Royal Children's Hospital
Melbourne
VIC
Australia

Murdoch Children's Research Institute
Melbourne
VIC
Australia

Chloe A. Hanna
Department of Gynaecology
The Royal Children's Hospital
Melbourne
VIC
Australia

Murdoch Children's Research Institute
Melbourne
VIC
Australia

ISBN 978-981-13-7863-8 ISBN 978-981-13-7864-5 (eBook)
https://doi.org/10.1007/978-981-13-7864-5

This Springer imprint is published by the registered company Springer Nature Singapore Pte Ltd.
The registered company address is: 152 Beach Road, #21-01/04 Gateway East, Singapore 189721, Singapore

Preface for the Second Edition

This new edition necessitated a change in editors, with Prof. Garry Warne retiring. This provided me with an opportunity to invite Dr. Michele A. O'Connell to supervise the medical chapters and Dr. Aurore Bouty to help me revise the genetics, embryology and surgical chapters. Also, I invited Ms. Chloe A. Hanna, our DSD team coordinator, to join the editorial board, as she has the ear of all the patients and their parents, and her contributions highlight this.

Although the first edition was only published in 2012, there have been significant changes in DSD management and, hence, the need for a new edition. This new edition commences with a new chapter about the language and the background and socio-political changes that engulfed DSD management. Many of these new ways of thinking come from the patients themselves, as the number of adults with DSD increases, and social changes allow this once-forbidden topic to be discussed in the media. The chapter on the genetics of DSD has been completely rewritten to highlight the rapid advances in understanding what genes are involved in genital development. The chapters on normal and abnormal embryology and the hormones regulating sex development have been revised to keep pace with the changing terminology. All the chapters on the main diagnoses have been rewritten by Dr. O'Connell following the retirement of our colleague, Prof. Garry Warne.

We added a small new chapter on 'The Foetus', as prenatal diagnosis is becoming much more common. Chapters on medical, surgical and gynaecological and psychological management have been updated, and some old chapters have been amalgamated to simplify the flow. The previous chapter on 'The Family' has been rewritten to emphasise the importance of psychosocial counselling and support. We have kept the chapter on outcomes from our own centre, as despite the fact that although the follow-up studies are now a bit dated, they represent a potential benchmark and were the best published results worldwide at the time. These can be compared with the new chapter on outcomes elsewhere in the developed as well as in the developing world, courtesy of our colleagues in Chittagong, Bangladesh. Finally, the guide for parents on CAIS has been retained and updated, as it is still sought after by families.

We hope this new edition will continue to educate and inspire the next generation of clinicians to continually strive to improve the lot in life for children with DSD.

Melbourne, Australia
December 2018

John M. Hutson

Acknowledgements for the Second Edition

We thank all our current and previous patients who were born with a DSD for helping us learn how to improve their management. We have not quite achieved yet an adult expert DSD centre to enable DSD patients to transition to the adult world with expert lifelong care, but it is within sight. However, we now have our own paediatric DSD team with monthly meetings across three centres in two countries, which is a major advance.

As the senior member of the editorial team, I would like to thank my coeditors for bringing this new edition to fruition so successfully. Finally, we all thank Ms. Shirley D'Cruz for patiently and extremely competently using her secretarial skill to turn this dream into a reality, yet again!

Contents

About the Editors

John M. Hutson is the Chair of Paediatric Surgery at the University of Melbourne, and one of the consultant Paediatric Urologists at The Royal Children's Hospital and Joint Group Leader for the Surgical Research Group at Murdoch Children's Research Institute.

Professor Hutson has three doctorates (MD, UMelb; MD, Monash; DSc, UMelb) in the area of sexual development and has studied the mechanism of testicular descent for many years. He has developed special expertise and interest in understanding the causes of (and new treatments for) intractable constipation in children. He is the author of numerous papers and books for teaching medical students, as well as monographs on testicular descent, kidney and urogenital malformations and DSD.

Sonia R. Grover is Director of the Department of Gynaecology at RCH. She is a member of the multidisciplinary team at RCH providing care for patients with DSD. Prof. Grover has been involved in research, teaching, supervision of research students and publishing, which has included work on long-term outcomes of women with DSDs, MRKH and CAH and those who have had genitoplasties. Her work also involves supporting the development of adolescent gynaecology services around Australia and overseas, in her role in the International Federation of Paediatric and Adolescent Gynaecology (FIGIJ).

Michele A. O'Connell trained as a Paediatrician in Ireland, before moving to Australia in 2005 to undertake subspecialty training and doctoral research in Paediatric Endocrinology at the Royal Children's Hospital, Melbourne. Since the retirement of Prof Garry Warne, Michele has been the co-ordinating Paediatric Endocrinologist on the RCH multidisciplinary DSD team. She has served as a member and is current co-chair of the Australasian Paediatric Endocrine Group DSD subcommittee. Together with colleagues at RCH and MCRI, she has supervised undergraduate and postgraduate research and has ongoing research collaborations across the fields of DSD, transgender health and paediatric diabetes.

Aurore Bouty is a Paediatric Urologist at the Royal Children's Hospital, Melbourne. She trained as a Paediatric Surgeon in France and subsequently migrated to Australia in 2015 to further specialise in Paediatric Urology. Since then she has benefited from the experience of Professor John Hutson in the management of children born with DSD. Her research interest resides in the Genetics of DSD, and she is currently a PhD student in Andrew Sinclair's Reproductive Development team at Murdoch Children's Research Institute.

Chloe A. Hanna completed a B.Sc. in Biomedical Science at the RMIT University followed by a Master of Genetic Counselling in 2014 at the University of Melbourne, completing a thesis exploring the psychosocial needs of women with DSD. Chloe previously worked in the disability sector for over 15 years. In 2016, Chloe established the role of Clinical Coordinator for individuals with DSD at the Royal Children's Hospital and currently provides direct support to individuals, families and the broader community throughout Australia. Chloe's key interest is to enhance the multidisciplinary approach to DSD healthcare including psychosocial support pathways.

1 Introduction: Changing Landscapes

Sonia R. Grover, Chloe A. Hanna, and Michele A. O'Connell

What's in a name? *A rose by any other* ***name*** *would smell as sweet.*

Ref Romeo and Juliet. Shakespeare

To open a book with an uncertainty regarding what term and title to use sounds like a poor start. Yet, to put this uncertainty and challenge upfront highlights exactly the issues that this book wishes to tackle.

The cluster of conditions collected under the expression Disorders|Divergences|Differences of Sex Development (DSD), Conditions Associated with Reproductive Development (CARD), Intersex and Variations in Sex Characteristics (VSC) consist of those associated with atypical genetic, phenotypic or hormonal makeup.

Where possible, each individual condition has its own specific or diagnostic term, which attempts to describe the difference or variation in a recognisable, defined way. This serves to enable advancement and achievement of understanding and optimal health care—so that we can share knowledge and experience, and thereby, we are all speaking the same language.

The challenge lies in the 'umbrella' expression or terminology. It is this expression which is fraught with difficulties, as two of the key umbrella expressions (DSD and intersex) are not directly interchangeable, and an individual who may have a condition that falls under a medical DSD classification (e.g. Turner syndrome) may identify with one term but not the other, or indeed neither.

There are also challenges in deciding which conditions or variations should be included and excluded under a given umbrella expression, as well as what care is required to provide optimal outcomes for affected babies, infants, young people and adults.

S. R. Grover (✉)
Department of Gynaecology, The Royal Children's Hospital, Melbourne, VIC, Australia

Murdoch Children's Research Institute, Melbourne, VIC, Australia

Department of Paediatrics, University of Melbourne, Melbourne, VIC, Australia
e-mail: Sonia.grover@rch.org.au

C. A. Hanna
Department of Gynaecology, The Royal Children's Hospital, Melbourne, VIC, Australia

Murdoch Children's Research Institute, Melbourne, VIC, Australia
e-mail: chloe.hanna@rch.org.au

M. A. O'Connell
Department of Endocrinology and Diabetes, The Royal Children's Hospital, Melbourne, VIC, Australia

Murdoch Children's Research Institute, Melbourne, VIC, Australia
e-mail: Michele.Oconnell@rch.org.au

J. M. Hutson et al. (eds.), *Disorders|Differences of Sex Development*,
https://doi.org/10.1007/978-981-13-7864-5_1

Definitions and meanings change over time. Given that this book is about sex development, a simple example relates to colours and dichotomous sex stereotypes. From the mid-1900s, colours have been increasingly used to denote gender, with girls/females being linked to pink and often clothed in pink (with the stereotypical presumption that they have a preference for this colour), whereas boys/males have been linked to the colour blue (Del Giudice 2012). Prior to this, the gender coding of pink and blue was inconsistent and not used in such a gender-dimorphic manner to masculinity and femininity (Paoletti 1997).

The origins of our words are clearly very old, and thus, it is not surprising that the meanings and significance change. English dictionaries tell us that the word 'sex' came from *sexe* (from middle French, 1382), which comes from the Latin *sexus* (gender), derived from *seco, secare* ('divide, cut') in the concept of 'half' of the race. 'Sex' tends to refer to biological differences, and historically, there was male sex and other, or male and a second sex.

In contrast, the expression 'gender' comes from *gendre* (old French), which is derived from Latin *genus* (gender) birth, family, nation. 'Gender' tends to refer to cultural or social aspects of sex.

Historically, the concept of a people who do not fit the dichotomous male/female sex and gender extends well back into Mesopotamian mythology. Inscribed upon a stone tablet from the second millennium BC (Sumer—pre Babylon), there is a myth about the creation of a type of human who is neither man nor woman. The goddess Ninmah fashions a being with 'no male organ and no female organ', for whom there is a position in society—'to stand before the king.' In an Akkadian myth, the goddess of birth establishes a third category of people, which includes demons who steal infants, women who are unable to give birth and priestesses who are prohibited from bearing children (Murray and Roscoe 1997).

In India's three ancient spiritual traditions—Hinduism (Wilhelm 2004), Jainism (Zwilling and Sweet 1996) and Buddhism (Jackson 1996), there is also reference to a third gender. In the Buddhist Vinaya (codified around the second century BC), there were four main categories: male, female, people of dual sexual nature and people of various sexual natures (Jackson 1996; Gyatso 2003).

A 'third sex' known as Hijra (in Hindi हिजड़, in Urdu ہجڑ) exists in India, Pakistan and Bangladesh. These people are mostly men dressed as women, although they are not trying to pass as female. Less than 10% are thought to have a DSD. Although this population has been held up as an example that these societies tolerate non-dichotomous sexuality, it is worth noting that the Hijra hold a very low social status, with a very defined function in society. They appear at weddings and births to bring good luck; refusing their presence will bring bad luck (Khan et al. 2009).

Sexuality is defined as *how* people experience the erotic and express themselves as sexual beings. Again, this has changed over time. In ancient Egypt and Greece, homosexuality was well described and accepted, with evidence from the tomb of Niankhkhnum and Khnumhotep, as well as in Homer's The Iliad. In Persia (1500s–1700s), homosexuality was well accepted in public (with the existence of erotic poems, and male prostitution houses that paid taxes). During the Renaissance, in northern Italy, same-sex love was widespread, although authorities were prosecuting individuals. In the mid-1800s, in European culture, homosexuality was a crime and considered an abnormality that required treatment. Nowadays, in many places, homosexuality is recognised and accepted, including having all the relevant legal rights (many of which were previously denied). The Royal College of Psychiatry considered 'Sexual orientation biological in nature' in 2014, and homosexuality was removed from DSM in 1973 (Bayer 1981). But there are many countries today where sadly homosexuality is still not tolerated or is considered an abnormality. As a general principle, broader societal awareness and acknowledgement of diversity is very important in ensuring its acceptance.

1.1.2 Recent History of DSD

From a more recent historical perspective, a number of important developments that have impacted significantly on the clinical management of individuals with DSD occurred in the 1980s and 1990s.

Patient advocacy groups were first established in the late 1980s and early 1990s and became vocal, establishing a 'contested collaboration' (Kessler 1998; Davis 2015). Some patient advocacy groups took a high-profile approach (Intersex Society of North America (now named Accord Alliance), Organisation Intersex International), appearing at conferences and challenging the attending clinicians. Important limitations in clinical care such as a lack of robust outcome studies and insufficient psychological support were thus increasingly brought to the attention of the clinicians. Unfortunately, in many countries, the ongoing lack of funding for comprehensive prospective patient databases to support high-quality research means that longitudinally acquired data on medium- and long-term outcomes are still relatively limited.

In the late 1990s, John Colapinto publicised the long-term outcome of the life of David Reimer following a disastrous surgical accident, whereby he suffered irreparable damage to his penis when cauterising equipment malfunctioned during a circumcision at the age of 8 months in Canada in 1966 (Colapinto 1997, 2000, 2001). At the age of 22 months, David Reimer's parents were advised to raise 'John' (one of twin boys) as 'Joan' following the recommendations of Dr. John Money, a renowned psychologist at the time, based at John Hopkins University. Money's theory of gender identity development, which was then increasingly popular, claimed that gender was a societal construct that was malleable; hence, nurture rather than nature determined gender identity (Money 1985). Thus, appropriate nurturing and 'corrective'/feminising surgery (orchidectomy and feminising genitoplasty) were recommended to reinforce the gender role. As children, David (Joan) and his twin brother were not told that they were both born boys; nor did they know the story of David's surgeries. Money regularly presented this 'John/Joan' case as a success story in academic settings, which led to both dissemination of and increased support for the theory, hence potentially influencing medical/surgical decisions in the management of children with DSD where sex of rearing was uncertain in infancy. Sadly, this was despite there reportedly being evidence when David (Joan) was as young as 6 years old that he was increasingly unhappy with his female sex assignment (Diamond and Sigmundson 1997). He went on to have pubertal induction with oestrogen, but on learning his personal history as an adolescent, he transitioned to living as a male with the name David. In allowing his story to be told publically in the late 1990s, a number of issues relating to his care were highlighted, not only in relation to apparent inaccuracies in Dr. Money's theory and reporting of the case, but also in relation to the importance of open disclosure and optimal information sharing in clinical settings and decision-making. While David's path arose from an acquired injury rather than a congenital DSD, there were many similarities and implications for care pathways in DSD, which is why it is included here.

Furthermore, in the 1990s, there were several publications regarding gender change from female to male in classical CAH (Warne 1992; Meyer-Bahlburg et al. 1996). These cases additionally highlighted that future gender identity was beyond the control of managing clinicians and emphasised the need for awareness amongst all parties (family and clinicians) that, while sex assignment can occur at birth, gender cannot be known by anyone other than a given individual.

From the early 2000s, along with the increasing recognition of the role of patient advocacy and a desire to review management strategies and long-term outcomes, these events culminated in the 2005 Chicago meeting, the changed definition and terminology, as well as recommendations in relation to management of various conditions (Hughes et al. 2006). Management guidelines continue to be revised and evolve as knowledge also improves (Ahmed et al. 2016; Lee et al. 2016; Cools et al. 2018). While the terminology remains contentious, since the introduction of the medical DSD classification system, there has been a significant increase in DSD-related scientific publications and DSD-specific international meetings and conferences, all of which will serve to further advance knowledge in the field. In tandem with this, our understanding of the underlying genetic variants that may be associated with different DSD has also increased exponentially. These will be discussed further in Chap. 2.

1.1.3 Clinical Definition of DSD

If the challenge regarding definitions is now extended to the clinical definition of DSD, further problems arise. There are a number of diagnoses for which there is ongoing debate as to whether they belong under the DSD umbrella. In particular, this applies to structural anomalies such as bladder exstrophy and cloacal anomalies. Hypospadias, in its more severe forms, is increasingly recognised as a DSD, with specific genetic testing allowing recognition of variations in hormone production and androgen receptor sensitivity. But should the less severe forms of hypospadias be considered a DSD? In line with the decision to stay with the terminology of 'DSD' that arose at the Chicago meeting, this book will encompass those conditions that were accepted at that consensus meeting (Table 1.1).

Table 1.1 Summary of new terminology

Title	Previous terminology
Disorders of sex development	Intersex
46,XY DSD	Male pseudohermaphrodite Under-virilised male Under-masculinised male
46,XX DSD	Female pseudohermaphrodite Virilised female Masculinised female
Ovo-testicular DSD	True hermaphrodite
46,XY complete gonadal dysgenesis	XY female XY sex reversal
46,XX testicular DSD	XX male XX sex reversal

Adapted from Hughes et al. (2007)

1.1.4 Incidence of DSD

The incidence of DSD is clearly influenced by which definition is used. A few incidences of the common forms of DSD are shown in Table 1.2. Many estimates of the relative proportion of the different diagnoses have used the selection criteria as ambiguous genitalia. Few papers have used the Chicago definition. A study at The Royal Children's Hospital in Melbourne attempted to utilise the Chicago definition but limited the cohort to children aged up to 10 years. This means that adolescents presenting with lack of pubertal development and girls with primary amenorrhoea were not identified in this cohort (Table 1.2).

Beyond acknowledging the challenges in terminology, definitions and incidence of these conditions, this discussion is not the primary purpose of this book. This book aims to explore the challenges of providing optimal care in situations where outcomes are often uncertain.

1.1.5 Clinical Care: Historical Perspective and Changes Over Time

History has a place to play here, as what is known in medical and psychological spheres has changed over time, and thus, what care is possible has changed rapidly in recent decades. This is important, as a comparison of care provided 30 or 40 years ago will reflect significantly different knowledge.

The first report of a female with congenital adrenal hyperplasia (CAH) is thought to be from 1865 (De Crecchio 1865). Although the association between altered function of the adrenal gland and excessive sex steroid production ('adrenogenital syndrome') was understood in the early twentieth century, it was not until 1950 that the successful use of cortisone as a therapeutic intervention to alleviate excess ACTH stimulation was first reported. The endocrine basis of congenital adrenal hyperplasia (CAH) was only discovered in 1953 by Lawson Wilkins, an endocrinologist in Baltimore (Wilkins 1965). Further advances in

Table 1.2 Diagnostic breakdown of reported DSD cohorts

Authors	Country	Cohort size	Study population	Common diagnoses
Parisi et al. (2007)	United States	250	Children with DSD assessed by hospital gender team (excluding Klinefelter, Turner and multiple congenital abnormality patients)	CAH 14% AIS 10% MGD 8%
Thyen et al. (2006)	Germany	80	Infants with ambiguous genitalia	CAH 18% AIS 16% MGD 9%
Al Agha et al. (2001)	Australia	51	Infants with ambiguous genitalia	CAH 31% AIS 10% MGD 6%
Bhullar et al. (2011)	Melbourne	199	All children aged 0–10 years identified with DSD using consensus statement	Perineal hypospadias 34% CAH 22% Exstrophy 14%
Joshi et al. (2006)	India	109	Infants with ambiguous genitalia	CAH 28% AIS 15% 5ARD 12%

CAH congenital adrenal hyperplasia, *AIS* androgen insensitivity syndrome, *MGD* mixed gonadal dysgenesis, *5ARD* 5α-reductase deficiency

genetics and classification of different enzyme deficiencies followed in the 1960s. Synthetic glucocorticoid and mineralocorticoid medications have been available since the 1950s; however, these medications are still not readily accessible in some parts of the world. Thus, even survival for a child with salt-losing 21-hydroxylase deficiency congenital adrenal hyperplasia (CAH) is a relatively recent expectation, and even today in some parts of the world, the mortality of affected children, particularly boys with severe salt-wasting CAH, remains high (see Chap. 22). In some parts of the world, the essential hormonal treatment is available only on the black market, thus compromising health and increasing mortality and morbidity.

Vaginal agenesis was recognised in ancient Greek times with endeavours to create a vagina dating back to 460 BC by Hippocrates (Goldwyn 1977). Today, there are a number of different techniques of creating a vagina, including approaches that require no surgery, yet we still do not know which approach results in the best long-term outcomes (McQuillan and Grover 2014a, b).

The capacity to provide hormone replacement therapy for people with non-functioning ovaries or testes to allow the development of secondary sexual characteristics and, importantly, provide the necessary protection for bone and cardiovascular health became available only in the last few decades.

Children with bladder and cloacal exstrophy still die in many parts of the world due to lack of access to the necessary complex surgery.

The first surgery for CAH was undertaken in the late 1950s. Open disclosure to patients and their families began in the Royal Children's Hospital and some other places in the 1980s, although in many places, this may not be still happening. Previously, this full disclosure and explanation regarding the underlying diagnosis and previous interventions (if relevant) was not given, in the misguided belief that knowing might be more painful or difficult. Clearly, evidence and experience have shown that this approach was not appropriate.

Over the last decade, psychosocial support for DSD has been recognised to be an essential aspect of medical care. Testimony from cohorts of adults who have been treated as infants and children without these supports and resources has highlighted their importance.

Therefore, over time, evolution in medical understanding and interventions have allowed gradual improvements in the understanding of, and care across, a number of diagnoses. However, there have been many areas where proposed therapeutic interventions have been subsequently shown over time not to result in the desired outcome. Surgical interventions in particular have been the subject of increased debate and with increased recognition of the potential for adverse outcomes in this regard, approaches have changed in recent years and continue to evolve (Hrabovszky and Hutson 2002). The practice of early genital surgery and sex assignment has shifted in recent decades. For example, in the late twentieth and early twenty-first centuries, in boys with partial androgen insensitivity syndrome (PAIS), where a female sex of rearing was assigned based on genital appearance at birth and predictions of little further virilisation of appearance in puberty, interventions such as removal of testes in childhood were commonly undertaken. It is now recognised that this intervention can lead to harm and many affected individuals who had such surgery in childhood are deeply unhappy that this occurred. Prior to 1990, 35% of those with 46,XY DSD diagnosed as PAIS, variations of gonadal development or androgen biosynthesis were assigned male, compared to 68% after 1999 (Kolesinska et al. 2014). Various factors contribute to this trend, including shifting cultural and societal views, improved surgical reconstruction techniques and better understanding about the potential fertility, oncogenic risk and adult gender identity in this cohort. Gender dysphoria is not uncommon in individuals with PAIS, but this is regardless of sex assigned and not convincingly influenced by such surgery. While malignancy risk is higher in intra-abdominal gonads in those with PAIS, this risk is low pre-puberty; hence, removal of gonads is now recognised to be more appropriately considered at an age when the individual can be involved in this decision for themselves (see Chap. 7). Deferring such surgery also allows for potential effects of endogenous hormone production in puberty and an individual's own gender identity to be established.

In contrast, those conditions where there are gonads with Y genetic material but the gonads are non-functioning (i.e. with no fertility potential and no hormone production), there can be a malignancy risk of up to 30%, even in childhood. Hence, removal of these gonads is considered important to prevent cancer.

Other surgeries performed in individuals with DSD are also the subject of much debate. Feminising genitoplasty for girls with CAH is a case in point, with opinions on this intervention ranging from support in those with significant virilisation (Prader stage 3+) due to the high incidence of satisfaction with outcomes (e.g. RCH follow-up studies (Lean et al. 2005, 2007; Crawford et al. 2009)) to opinions that it should not be performed in infancy (Creighton et al. 2001) but rather deferred until the girl herself is old enough to be involved in the decision.

1.1.6 Human Rights and DSD: Where to from Here?

Internationally, in recent years, human rights agencies and UN treaty bodies, agencies and special rapporteurs have increasingly called on Member States to strengthen protections for the human rights of people born with variations in sex characteristics (e.g. San Francisco 2005, Germany 2012, Switzerland 2012). In 2013, the UN Human Rights Council called upon all states to repeal laws allowing 'intrusive and irreversible treatments for children with intersex variations'. Such interventions included genital surgery and involuntary sterilisation without the free and informed consent of the person concerned (UNHRC 2013). In 2016, a group of UN and international human rights experts published a statement on Intersex Awareness Day (26 October) that sought for governments to prohibit medical procedures on intersex infants, children and adolescents without 'the full, free and informed consent of the person concerned (http://www.ohchr.org/EN/NewsEvents/Pages/DisplayNews.aspx?NewsID=20739&LangID=E).

It is clear therefore that there is growing impetus for change in this space in recent years. Rulings such as those from the UN where people with intersex variations who have experienced so-called 'normalising' surgery or treatment have been recognised as 'victims of abuses and mistreatment', and where medical interventions have been labelled 'harmful practices,' may understandably be confronting for clinicians and surgeons who have offered such interventions with best intentions for optimal outcomes. Nonetheless, although not universal, suboptimal historical outcomes cannot be ignored and the lived experience of affected individuals has both changed practices and greatly increased awareness of the need to continually scrutinise all interventions undertaken. However, it remains the case today that the life-course and outcomes of a given individual with some DSD (such as PAIS or androgen biosynthetic variations) can be very difficult to predict in infancy or childhood, and decisions that may result in future regret are, and will likely remain, difficult to fully eliminate. It should be noted that this may indeed be the case whether a decision to intervene or to defer intervention is made. Deferring intervention, particularly where outcomes in relation to this are unknown (and should not automatically be presumed to be better), is as much a decision as opting to intervene.

How best to progress to ensure ongoing improvement to maximising optimal outcomes for affected individuals not surprisingly remains the subject of much debate. Clinically, there has been a significant shift over the last decade towards optimising care through management in specialised multidisciplinary teams, using a clinical ethics framework (see Chap. 15 for detailed discussion). A clinical ethics framework incorporates key concerns from the human rights field, but framed in a way that gives room for nuanced considerations of the circumstances of each individual child. Human rights discourse has a tendency to be black-and-white, implying that one approach is always the right thing for every individual. It works best for civil and political rights, which can reasonably be seen to transcend individual difference. In contrast, the principle-based approach of clinical ethics aims to better acknowledge the complexity of seeking to promote each individual's well-being in their specific circumstances. There are multiple aspects of a person's well-being, and the clinical ethics framework allows for structured ethical consideration of these in decision-making for each individual.

Many individual DSD or variations are very uncommon, hence infrequently encountered even in large tertiary clinical centres. This, along with the many uncertainties in outcomes, means that decisions in relation to care are often highly complex and need to be taken in the context of current knowledge, with open discussion of the uncertainties and controversies in approaches, while being individualised for a given child and family's unique circumstances.

Approaches to these difficult issues vary internationally. In 2015, Malta became the first country to institute a legal ban to prohibit deferrable interventions or surgery. Groups in other countries are also seeking legal frameworks. For example, in March 2017, Australian and Aotearoa/New Zealand intersex organisations and independent advocates issued a joint consensus statement (Darlington Statement 2017) calling for the criminalisation of deferrable medical interventions and the development of human rights-based lifetime standards of care. This statement also declared, however, that the Family Court system (in Australia) has 'failed to adequately consider the human rights and autonomy of children born with variations of sex characteristics'; hence, oversight in this setting is not thought to be optimal (nor likely feasible). An alternative put forward in place of the Court was an 'independent effective human rights-based oversight mechanism/s consisting of human rights experts, clinicians and intersex-led community organisations'.

Deferring decisions about surgery until an age when an individual may develop the capacity to be involved in decisions relating to their own care fits in with rights-based considerations such as autonomy and bodily integrity. However, the effects of deferring such decisions on the overall well-being of the child and future adult are not known. There are currently no data to support the hypothesis that such a management plan will invariably have preferable outcomes to interventions performed earlier, with informed parental consent on the child's behalf. As surgical practices and techniques have evolved (albeit to varying extents internationally), regulating to put a blanket ban on all surgery in infancy on the basis of sub-optimal outcomes using historical evidence from outdated surgical practices, is argued to not be a sound approach.

There is, however, some agreed ethical ground. Perhaps one of the most notable advances in recent decades is much greater involvement of parents of young children and older children themselves in decision-making. As part of best practice, clinicians discuss with parents and older children both what is known and not known about the child's particular condition and introduce some of the existing controversies in relation to potential management. Awareness of and openness to change over time (e.g., in future, gender identity relative to assigned sex in infancy) are increasingly promoted. Parents' and adolescents' decision-making and consent to any intervention is arguably much better informed than it has been in the past.

We do not presume to give final answers to these difficult issues in this book, but rather raise them to highlight the many changes that are occurring in the current context in which children and adolescents with DSD are managed. Like all ethical issues, good ethics depends on good facts. Recent and ongoing scientific advances such as the generation of international/multicentre registries (e.g. iDSD, iCAH and the DSD Translational Research Network) and ongoing strides in our understanding of the genetics relating to DSD will increasingly allow the collection of higher quality prospectively acquired data in very specific conditions, to optimally inform progress in this regard. Good ethics also depends on sustained reflection and deliberation on the values underpinning decision-making, recognition of pluralism about values in our communities and awareness of the limits of one's own perspective. So we can expect good ethics to lead to further debate and further change over time.

References

Ahmed SF, Achermann JC, Arlt W, et al. Society for Endocrinology UK guidance on the initial evaluation of an infant or an adolescent with a suspected disorder of sex development (Revised 2015). Clin Endocrinol. 2016;84(5):771–88.

Al-Agha AE, Thomsett MJ, Batch JA. The child of uncertain sex: 17 years of experience. J Paediatr Child Health. 2001;37(4):348–51.

Bayer R. Homosexuality and American psychiatry: the politics of diagnosis. New York, NY: Basic Books; 1981.

Bennecke E, De Vries A. European research project 'dsd-LIFE'. Guildford: University of Surrey; 2016.

Bhullar K, Grover S, Hutson J, Warne G, Loughlin E, Hewitt J. Spectrum of Disorders in Sex Development in Children aged 0–10 years. J Pediatr Adolesc Gynecol. 2011;24(2):e50.

Colapinto J. The true story of John/Joan. Rolling Stone, vol. 775. New York: Straight Arrow Publishers; 1997. p. 54–97.

Colapinto J. The boy who was turned into a girl. Horizon. BBC; 2000.

Colapinto J. As nature made him: the boy who was raised as a girl. New York; 2001.

Cools M, Nordenstrom A, Robeva R, et al. Caring for individuals with a difference of sex development (DSD): a consensus statement. Nat Rev Endocrinol. 2018;14(7):415–29.

Crawford JM, Warne G, Grover S, et al. Results from a pediatric surgical centre justify early intervention in disorders of sex development. J Pediatr Surg. 2009;44(2):413–6.

Creighton SM, Minto CL, Steele SJ. Objective cosmetic and anatomical outcomes at adolescence of feminising surgery for ambiguous genitalia done in childhood. Lancet. 2001;358(9276):124–5.

Davis G. Contesting intersex: the dubious diagnosis. New York: University Press; 2015.

De Crecchio, L. (1865). Sopra un caso di apparenzi virili in una donna.

Del Giudice M. The twentieth century reversal of pink-blue gender coding: a scientific urban legend? Arch Sex Behav. 2012;41(6):1321–3.

Diamond M, Sigmundson HK. Sex reassignment at birth. Long-term review and clinical implications. Arch Pediatr Adolesc Med. 1997;151(3):298–304.

Goldwyn RM. History of attempts to form a vagina. Plast Reconstr Surg. 1977;59(3):319–29.

Gyatso J. One plus one makes three: Buddhist gender, monasticism, and the law of the non-excluded middle. Hist Relig. 2003;43(2):89–115.

Hrabovszky Z, Hutson JM. Surgical treatment of intersex abnormalities: a review. Surgery. 2002; 131(1):92–104.

Hughes IA, Houk C, Ahmed SF, et al. Consensus statement on management of intersex disorders. Arch Dis Child. 2006;91(7):554–63.

Jackson PA. Non-normative Sex/Gender categories in the Theravada Buddhist Scriptures. Aust Humanit Rev. 1996;hdl:1885/41884.

Juan E. Méndez, Report of the Special Rapporteur on torture and other cruel, inhuman or degrading treatment or punishment, UN Doc A/HRC/22/53 (1 February 2013). At http://daccess-ods.un.org/access.nsf/Get?Open&DS=A/HRC/22/53&Lang=E (accessed 14 May 2020).

Jones T, Hart B, Carpenter M. Intersex: stories and statistics. Cambridge: Open Book Publishers; 2016.

Joshi RR, Rao S, Desai M. Etiology and clinical profile of ambiguous genitalia an overview of 10 years experience. Indian Pediatr. 2006;43(11):974–9.

Kessler SJ. Lessons from the intersexed. New Brunswick, NJ: Rutgers University Press; 1998.

Khan SI, Hussain MI, Parveen S, et al. Living on the extreme margin: social exclusion of the transgender population (hijra) in Bangladesh. J Health Popul Nutr. 2009;27(4):441–51.

Kolesinska Z, Ahmed SF, Niedziela M, et al. Changes over time in sex assignment for disorders of sex development. Pediatrics. 2014;134(3):e710–5.

Lean WL, Deshpande A, Hutson J, et al. Cosmetic and anatomic outcomes after feminizing surgery for ambiguous genitalia. J Pediatr Surg. 2005;40(12):1856–60.

Lean WL, Hutson JM, Deshpande AV, et al. Clitoroplasty: past, present and future. Pediatr Surg Int. 2007;23(4):289–93.

Lee PA, Nordenstrom A, Houk CP, et al. Global disorders of sex development update since 2006: perceptions, approach and care. Horm Res Paediatr. 2016;85(3):158–80.

Lundberg T. Knowing bodies: making sense of intersex/DSD a decade post consensus. PhD thesis, Faculty of Social Science University of Oslo; 2017.

Lundberg T, Hegarty P, Roen K. Making sense of 'intersex' and 'DSD': how laypeople understand and use terminology. Psychol Sex. 2018;9(2):161–73.

McQuillan SK, Grover SR. Systematic review of sexual function and satisfaction following the management of vaginal agenesis. Int Urogynecol J. 2014a;25(10):1313–20.

McQuillan SK, Grover SR. Dilation and surgical management in vaginal agenesis: a systematic review. Int Urogynecol J. 2014b;25(3):299–311.

Meyer-Bahlburg HF, Gruen RS, New MI, et al. Gender change from female to male in classical congenital adrenal hyperplasia. Horm Behav. 1996;30(4):319–32.

Money J. Gender: history, theory and usage of the term in sexology and its relationship to nature/nurture. J Sex Marital Ther. 1985;11(2):71–9.

Mortimer R. Supports for parents of children with differences of sex development. MDRP Thesis, University of Melbourne; 2017.

Murray SO, Roscoe W. Islamic homosexualities: culture, history and literature. New York: New York University Press; 1997.

Paoletti JB. The gendering of infants and toddlers clothing in America. In: Martinez KA, Ames KL, editors. The material culture of gender/The gender of material culture. Hanover, NH: University Press of New England; 1997. p. 27–35.

Parisi MA, Ramsdell LA, Burns MW, et al. A Gender Assessment Team: experience with 250 patients over a period of 25 years. Genet Med. 2007;9(6):348–57.

Darlington Statement. Joint consensus statement from the intersex community retreat in Darlinghurst. Darlington Statement; 2017 https://ihra.org.au/darlington-statement/.

Thyen U, Lanz K, Holterhus PM, et al. Epidemiology and initial management of ambiguous genitalia at birth in Germany. Horm Res. 2006;66(4):195–203.

Warne G. Jackie: a girl in crisis. Matern Child Health. 1992;17:359–69.

Wilhelm AD. Tritiya Prakriti (People of the Third Sex): Understanding Homosexuality, Transgender Identity and Intersex conditions through Hinduism. XLibris Corporation; 2004.

Wilkins L. The diagnosis and treatment of endocrine disorders in childhood and adolescence. Springfield, IL: Charles C. Thomas; 1965.

Zwilling L, Sweet MJ. "Like a city ablaze": the third sex and the creation of sexuality in Jain religious literature. J Hist Sex. 1996;6(3):359–84.

2 The Molecular Basis of Sex Determination and Differentiation: Implications for Understanding DSD

Aurore Bouty, Katie Ayers, and Andrew Sinclair

Sexual reproduction in mammals requires two sexes characterised by specific genetic and anatomical features. The phenotypic sex of an individual is largely driven by the type of gonad that develops in the embryo, a process itself determined by sex chromosome complement. Human males and females both have 22 pairs of autosomes and differ only in their sex chromosome complement. Typically, females have two X chromosomes (46,XX), while males have one X and one Y (46,XY). From the initial bi-potential gonad, a cascade of genes allows differentiation into a testis or an ovary, a process known as sex determination. Once gonads have developed and differentiated, they start producing sex-specific hormones, which, in turn, determine the development of secondary sexual characteristics, including the differentiation of the external genitalia (Eggers et al. 2014).

A. Bouty (✉)
Department of Urology, The Royal Children's Hospital, Melbourne, VIC, Australia

Murdoch Children's Research Institute, Melbourne, VIC, Australia
e-mail: aurore.bouty@rch.org.au

K. Ayers · A. Sinclair
Murdoch Children's Research Institute, Melbourne, VIC, Australia

Department of Paediatrics, University of Melbourne, Melbourne, VIC, Australia
e-mail: Katie.ayers@mcri.edu.au; Andrew.sinclair@mcri.edu.au

Disruption to the genetic network underlying these pathways can lead to DSD, a group of congenital conditions where chromosomal, gonadal or anatomical sex is atypical (Hughes et al. 2006). Studies in both humans and mice have identified a number of genes that play critical roles in internal and external genitalia development (Eggers and Sinclair 2012). In this chapter, we will review some of the key genes and genetic pathways involved in gonad and genital development and demonstrate how defects in these genes result in DSD. For a summary of genes involved in human DSD, see Table 2.1. Disruption of the sex chromosome complement can also lead to DSD but is out of the scope of this review.

2.1 Formation of the Bi-potential Gonad

In mammals, testes and ovaries arise from bilateral bi-potential gonads, which derive from the genital ridge. A number of genes have been shown to be critical for the development of these undifferentiated gonads.

In mice, *Gata4* (GATA-binding factor 4) is the earliest expressed gene specific for the genital ridge development (Piprek et al. 2016). In mice, loss of *Gata4* expression leads to the absence of genital ridges (Hu et al. 2013). The Homeobox protein *Emx2* and Lim/homeobox protein *Lhx9* are

J. M. Hutson et al. (eds.), *Disorders|Differences of Sex Development*,
https://doi.org/10.1007/978-981-13-7864-5_2

Table 2.1 Genes known to be involved in DSD

		Gene	Locus	OMIM	Associated DSD	Inheritance
46,XX DSD						
	Disorders of ovarian development					
		BMP15	Xp11.22	300247	Ovarian dysgenesis	AD
		FOXL2	3q22.3	608996	POI alone or with blepharophimosis, ptosis and epicanthus inversus syndrome	AD
		NR5A1	9q33.3	184757	POI	AD
		RSPO1	1p34.3	609595	46,XX OT DSD with palmoplantar hyperkeratosis	AR
		SOX3	Xq27.1	313430	46,XX T or OT DSD—gain of function	XL: dup
		SOX9	17q24.3	608106	46,XX T DSD—duplication	AD: dup
		SRY	Yp11.2	480000	46,XX T DSD—gain of function	Translocation
		WNT4	1p36.12	603490	46,XX T DSD	AR
		WT1	11p13	607102	Frasier and Denys-Drash syndrome	AD
		HSD17B4	5q23.1	233400	Perrault syndrome (with ovarian dysgenesis in 46,XX)	AR
		FSHR	2p16.3	136435	Ovarian dysgenesis	AR
	Androgen excess					
		NR0B1	Xp21.2	300473	CAH	XLR
		ARX	Xp21.3	300215	X-linked lissencephaly with ambiguous genitalia	XL
		CYP11A1	15q24.1	118485	CAH	AR
		CYP11B1	8q24.3	610613	CAH (11-beta-hydroxylase deficiency)	AR
		CYP17A1	10q24.32	609300	17, 20-lyase deficiency	AR
		CYP19A1	15q21.2	107910	Aromatase deficiency	AR
		CYP21A2	6p21.33	613815	CAH (21-hydroxylase deficiency)	AR
		HSD3B2	1p12	613890	CAH (3-beta-hydroxysteroid dehydrogenase deficiency)	AR
		NR3C1	5q31.3	138040	46,XX hyperandrogenism	AD
		POR	7q11.23	124015	Cytochrome P450 oxydoreductase deficiency	AR
		STAR	8p11.23	600617	CAH (cholesterol desmolase deficiency)	AR
	Other (Müllerian agenesis)					
		WNT4	1p36.12	603490	MRKH	AD
		HOXA13	7p15.2	142959	Hand-foot-uterus syndrome, MRKH	AD
46, XY DSD						
	Disorders of testicular development					
		CBX2	17q25.3	602770	CGD	AR
		DHH	12q13.12	605423	PGD or CGD	AR, AD
		DMRT1	9p24.3	602424	CGD	AD: deletion
		DMRT2	9p24.3	604935	CGD	AD: deletion
		GATA4	8p23.1	600576	GD	AD
		NR0B1	Xp21.2	300473	GD—gain of function	XL: dup
		NR5A1	9q33.3	184757	Various forms of 46,XY DSD	AD
		MAP3K1	5q11.2	600982	GD	AD
		SOX9	17q24.3	608106	GD and campomelic dysplasia	AD
		SRY	Yp11.2	480000	46,XY ovarian DSD	AD
		TSPYL1	6q22.1	604714	Sudden infant death syndrome with dysgenesis of the testes syndrome	AR
		WNT4	1p36.12	603490	46,XY OT DSD or CGD—duplication	AD: dup
		WT1	11p13	607102	Frasier and Denys-Drash syndrome	AD
		ZFPM2	8q23.1	603693	GD	AD
		FGFR2	10q26.13	176943	GD with cranioynostosis. Apert syndrome	AD
	Disorders of androgen synthesis or action					
		AKR1C2	10p15.1	600450	Various forms of 46,XY DSD	AR
		AKR1C4	10p15.1	600451	Various forms of 46,XY DSD	AR

Table 2.1 (continued)

		Gene	Locus	OMIM	Associated DSD	Inheritance
		AMH	19p13.3	600957	PMDS	AR
		AMHR2	12q13.13	600956	PMDS	AR
		AR	Xq12	313700	CAIS, PAIS	XL
		ARX	Xp21.3	300215	X-linked lissencephaly with ambiguous genitalia	XL
		ATRX	Xq21.1	300032	46,XY DSD associated with alpha-thalassaemia X-linked intellectual disability syndrome	XL
		CDKN1C	11p15.4	600856	Genital anomalies associated with Beckwith-Wiedemann and IMAGE syndrome	AD
		CYB5A	18q22.3	613218	various forms of 46,XY DSD	AR
		CYP11A1	15q24.1	118485	46,XY DSD with adrenal insufficiency	AR
		CYP17A1	10q24.32	609300	17, 20-lyase deficiency	AR
		HSD17B3	9q22.32	605573	17-beta-hydroxysteroid dehydrogenase III deficiency	AR
		HSD3B2	1p12	613890	3-beta-hydroxysteroid dehydrogenase deficiency	AR
		LHCGR	2p16.3	152790	Leydig cell hypoplasia, precocious puberty	AR
		POR	7q11.23	124015	Cytochrome P450 oxidoreductase deficiency	AR
		SRD5A2	2p23.1	607306	Steroid 5-alpha-reductase deficiency	AR
		STAR	8p11.23	600617	CAH (cholesterol desmolase deficiency)	AR
		BBS9	7p14.3	615986	Bardet-Biedl syndrome	AR
		CHD7	8q12.2	608892	CHH or KS, CHARGE syndrome	AD
		FGF8	10q24.32	612702	CHH or KS	AD
		FGFR1	8p11.23	147950	CHH or KS	AD
		FSHB	11p14.1	136530	CHH	AD
		GNRH1	8p21.2	152760	CHH	AR
		GNRHR	4q13.2	138850	CHH	AR
		HESX1	3p14.3	601802	KS or CPHD	AD
		KAL1	Xp22.31	300836	CHH or KS	XL
		KISS1R	19p13.3	604161	CHH or KS	AD
		LEP	7q32.1	164160	CHH with obesity	AR
		LHX3	9q34.3	600577	CPHD	AR
		PROK2	3p13	607002	CHH or KS	AD
		PROKR2	20p12.3	607123	CHH or KS	AD
		PROP1	5q35.3	601538	CPHD	AR
		TAC3	12q13.3	162330	CHH	AR
		WDR11	10q26.12	606417	CHH or KS	AD
	Other (isolated hypospadias, cryptorchidism)					
		AR	Xq12	313700	Isolated hypospadias	XL
		CYP11A1	15q24.1	118485	Isolated hypospadias	AD
		HSD3B2	1p12	613890	Isolated hypospadias	AD
		SRD5A2	2p23.1	607306	Isolated hypospadias	AD
		ATF3	1q32.3	603148	Isolated hypospadias	AD
		HOXA13	7p15.2	142959	Guttmacher syndrome	AD
		INSL3	19p13.11	146738	Cryptorchidism	AD
		MAMLD1	Xq28	300120	Hypospadias	XL
		RXFP2	13q13.1	606655	Cryptorchidism	AD

also involved in the early development of the bipotential gonad. Mice deficient in *Emx2* lack gonads, kidneys and genital tracts (Pellegrini et al. 1997). In humans, a microdeletion encompassing *EMX2* has been found in a patient with 46,XY DSD (Piard et al. 2014). *Lhx9*-null mice also fail to develop gonads, and deficient XY mice develop as female (Birk et al. 2000). However, variants in this gene have yet to be associated with DSD in humans. Lhx9 regulates the expression of the orphan nuclear receptor *Nr5a1*, also known as steroidogenic factor 1 (SF1), a transcription factor that is expressed in both gonads and adrenal glands. *Nr5a1*-null mice lack both gonads and adrenal glands (Luo et al. 1994; Val et al. 2003). Another player, the Wilms tumour protein homolog (WT1) protein, in particular, the –KTS isoform, is necessary for early bi-potential gonad development and *Wt1*-null mice fail to develop gonads and kidneys, which is lethal (Kreidberg et al. 1993). In mice, *Cbx2* is also involved in early gonad formation, and mice deficient in *Cbx2* display delayed gonad development and male-to-female sex reversal (Eggers et al. 2014). Finally Insulin-like growth factors (IGFs) are involved in the regulation of genital ridge formation (Pitetti et al. 2013). All these genes are evolutionarily conserved among vertebrates. In mice null for *Gata-4*, the genital ridges do not form at all, suggesting that *Gata-4* is required for initiation of bi-potential gonad formation. However, in mice null for *Sf1*, *Wt1*, *Emx2* and *Lhx9*, the bi-potential gonads form but quickly degenerate, suggesting that these genes are involved in maintenance and further development (Piprek et al. 2016). Homeodomain proteins such as HOXA9, HOXA10, HOXA11 and HOXA13 are thought to be responsible for the precise determination of the site of genital ridge formation. Other homeobox genes such as Sine Oculis Homeobox Homologs (*Six1* and *Six4*), pre-B-cell leukemia Homeobox 1 (*Pbx1*) or Podocyte Expressed 1 (*Pod1*) are implicated in the regulation of genital ridge formation, and development in mice is reviewed in Piprek et al. (2016). Finally, it is interesting to note that many of these bi-potential gonad genes continue to play a later role in the gonads, in particular, during testis sex determination.

2.2 Testis Determination and Development

2.2.1 SRY

Attempts to identify the exact sequence responsible for male development, referred to as testis-determining factor (TDF), focussed on males with a 46,XX karyotype. In 90% of these males, translocation of a small piece of the Y chromosome is observed, and molecular studies finally identified the translocated gene responsible, denoting it the *SRY* (sex-determining region of the Y) gene (Sinclair et al. 1990). Further evidence of the key sex-determining role of *SRY* came from the identification of causative variants in this gene in 46,XY phenotypic females (Berta et al. 1990). Final proof that *SRY* is critical for male development was demonstrated using transgenic mouse studies, which showed that expression of *Sry* alone is sufficient for XX mice to develop testis and become males (Koopman et al. 1991). Therefore, in both mice and humans, *Sry* is necessary and sufficient to induce testis development (Eggers et al. 2014). More recently, *SRY* has been demonstrated to determine Sertoli cell fate in mice by repressing the ovarian pathway and activating testicular differentiation genes (Li et al. 2014).

2.2.2 SOX (SRY Box) Transcription Factors

SOX9 is a member of the SRY-related HMG box protein family of transcription factors. In mice, *Sox9* is the immediate downstream target of *Sry*, and its expression is activated when *Sry* levels reach a critical threshold. Although *Sox9* is expressed in the genital ridge of both male and female mouse embryos, it becomes sexually dimorphic after *Sry* expression peaks, with a considerable increase in XY compared to XX gonads. Conditional gonad-specific knockout of Sox9 in XY mouse embryos leads to the development of ovaries, while ectopic overexpression in XX embryonic mouse gonads results in testicular development (Eggers et al. 2014). An upstream region of *Sox9*, known as the testis-specific enhancer core element (TESCO), is required for upregulation of mouse *Sox9* expression (Sekido and Lovell-Badge 2008). Another region upstream of SOX9 in humans, known as RevSex, has been involved in various forms of DSD (Kim et al. 2015; Sreenivasan et al. 2017). However, this region remains to be defined in detail.

Many of the downstream targets of SOX9 have been characterised. In mice, *Sox9* initiates expression of anti-Müllerian hormone (*Amh*) and cerebellin 4 (*Cbln4)*. Another downstream target of Sox9 in mice is fibroblast growth factor 9 (*Fgf9*), which acts through its receptor FGFR2 for the development of Sertoli cells and through a feedback loop to upregulate Sox9 (Bagheri-Fam et al. 2008, 2017). In humans, patients with deletion of chromosome 10q26.13, which includes the *FGFR2* locus, demonstrate atypical sexual differentiation (Bagheri-Fam et al. 2008).

Sox9 seems to be regulated by nuclear receptor subfamily 0 group B member 1 (Nr0b1), also known as *Dax1* (Ludbrook et al. 2012*)*. However, both the contribution and the precise function of *DAX1* in testis development remain unclear, as it is considered both a pro-testis (Meeks et al. 2003) and an anti-testis gene (Swain et al. 1998). Several studies in both mice and human suggest that *DAX1* acts within a narrow window and that both the activity and concentration of NR0B1 are critical (Ludbrook and Harley 2004).

Studies in mice have demonstrated a certain level of redundancy among members of the *SOX* gene family. In humans, *SOX8* has recently been identified in patients with 46,XY DSD (Portnoi et al. 2018). In mice, *Sox10* is thought to be sufficient to drive testis development when overexpressed/duplicated but is not required for testis determination when other members of the Sox family are present (Polanco et al. 2010). Likewise, *Sox3* is not normally expressed in the developing gonads in mice or humans. However, a transgenic mouse line with ectopic overexpression of *Sox3* showed XX female-to-male sex reversal. Sex reversal is also seen in 46,XX patients with a *SOX3* duplication (Sutton et al. 2011). This supports the notion that other *Sox* genes can functionally replace *SRY* or *SOX9* and drive testis differentiation.

2.3 Regulators of Sry Expression

2.3.1 GATA Genes and ZFPM2

GATA4 and *GATA6* belong to the *GATA* family of zinc finger transcription factors that recognise a GATA factor present in the promoter of many genes. Padua et al. demonstrated that these genes are necessary for normal testis development, as conditional double-mutant mice lacked normal steroidogenic function in the testes (Padua et al. 2015). In mice, expression of *Gata4* becomes sexually dimorphic with high expression in the Sertoli cells, where it acts with zinc finger protein, FOG Family Member 2 (*Zfpm2*), as a dimer that is required for *Sry* regulation (Manuylov et al. 2011). *Zfpm2* expression is directly controlled by *Six1* and *Six4*, which may be functionally redundant (Fujimoto et al. 2013).

2.3.2 NR5A1 Gene encodes Steroidogenic Factor 1 (SF1)

In mice, the *Nr5a1* gene has been identified as another target of *Six1* and *Six4*, which seem responsible for the control of gonad precursor cell formation and determination of gonadal size (Kawakami et al. 2000). SF1 together with SRY is also required for proper expression of SOX9 in the developing testis (Park et al. 2005).

2.3.3 WT1

The WT1 protein exhibits alternative splicing, and a specific isoform, Wt1 +KTS, has an important function in very early testis development, as mice lacking *Wt1 +KTS* undergo male-to-female sex reversal as a result of failure to upregulate *Sry* expression (Hammes et al. 2001). In humans, causative variants in the *WT1* gene have been associated with numerous cases of syndromic or isolated DSD (Hastie 2017). In particular, variants in *WT1* are responsible for Frasier syndrome, which includes a male-to-female sex reversal (Barbaux et al. 1997), Denys-Drash syndrome, where patients present with atypical genitalia (Pelletier et al. 1991) and WAGR syndrome (Wilms tumour, aniridia, genitourinary malformations and mental retardation) (Le Caignec et al. 2007).

2.3.4 Mitogen-Activated Protein Kinase Pathway

Using a forward genetic screen in mice, Bogani et al. demonstrated that mitogen-activated protein kinase kinase kinase 4 (MAP3K4, also known as

MEKK4) was necessary for normal expression of *Sry* during testis development (Bogani et al. 2009). They subsequently showed that *Gadd45γ* was required to promote *Map3k4*-mediated activation of p38 MAPK signalling for testis determination in mice (Warr et al. 2012). More recently, the same team has found that *Map2k6* and more moderately *Map2k3* had functions in mouse sex determination through positive effects on *Sry* (Warr et al. 2016). Interestingly, while *MAP3K1* does not appear to be required for normal testis determination in mice (Warr et al. 2011), numerous variants in this gene have been reported in 46,XY DSD with gonadal dysgenesis (Pearlman et al. 2010) (Loke et al. 2014).

2.4 The Hedgehog Signalling Pathway

Hedgehog is an important morphogen that controls patterning and differentiation of numerous organs during embryogenesis. Desert Hedgehog (*Dhh*) is the sole HH member expressed in the developing XY mouse gonad. Differentiated Sertoli cells secrete DHH, which subsequently binds to its receptor protein patched homologue 1 (*Ptch1*) on pre-Leydig cells and activates the hedgehog signalling pathway in these cells, resulting in their differentiation. Null mice for *Dhh* have disrupted testis cords and lack mature Leydig cells (Clark et al. 2000). Hedgehog acyl transferase (HHAT) also plays a role in proper testis cord formation and the differentiation of foetal Leydig cells in both humans and mice (Callier et al. 2014).

2.5 DMRT1

Although the primary sex-determining gene in several non-mammalian vertebrates such as the chicken is present on the sex chromosomes (Lambeth et al. 2014), Doublesex and Mab-3-related Transcription Factor 1 (*Dmrt1*) have evolved to become dispensable in mammals (Raymond et al. 2000). It plays an important role, however, in maintaining Sertoli cells in postnatal mouse testis by blocking testicular retinoic acid signalling from activating genes involved in female sex determination (Matson et al. 2011; Minkina et al. 2014). It is one of the downstream targets of GATA4 (Zaytouni et al. 2011), and disruptions to this gene have been implicated in human DSD (Marsudi et al. 2018). Loss of *DMRT1* gene was seen in a Mos 45,XY,-9[8]/46,XY,r(9)[29]/47,XY,+idic r(9)×2[1]/46,XY,idic r(9)[1]/46,XY[1] female presenting with short stature (11, p.28). Partial deletion of *DMRT1* causes 46,XY ovotesticular disorder of sexual development (Ledig et al. 2012).

2.6 Epigenetic Regulation of Testis Determination

Epigenetic modifications including modification of histones such as methylation can alter gene expression. Studies in mice have shown that the H3K9 demethylase Jmjd1a positively controls *Sry* expression by regulating H3K9me2 marks (Kuroki et al. 2013). In humans, this gene is increasingly reported in various cancers but not DSD.

2.7 Ovarian Differentiation

While numerous genes and pathways have been implicated in testis differentiation and development, much less is known about ovarian differentiation. Initially, It was thought to be a 'default' pathway in the absence of SRY. However, a number of specific genes and genetic pathways have now been implicated in ovarian development, and several of these cause DSD in humans when disrupted.

2.7.1 Forkhead Box L2 (Foxl2)

Foxl2 is a member of the forkhead box gene family of evolutionarily conserved transcription factors. It is one of the earliest upregulated genes in the developing ovary, suggesting a role in early ovary differentiation, the importance of which may differ between species (Baron et al. 2005). For instance, sex reversal is observed in goats with homozygous loss of FOXL2 (Gustin et al. 2016) but not in mice (Schmidt et al. 2004). In mice, it appears to play a major role in postnatal maintenance of the ovary (Uhlenhaut et al. 2009).

In mice, genes regulating testis development are upregulated shortly before birth and follicle activation is impaired in postnatal stages (Garcia-Ortiz et al. 2009). In humans, heterozygous loss-of-function mutations in *FOXL2* cause autosomal-dominant blepharophimosis-ptosis-epicanthus inversus syndrome (BPES, OMIM #110100) (Crisponi et al. 2001). There are two forms of the syndrome; type 1, with associated premature ovarian insufficiency and type 2, without it (Meduri et al. 2010). Variants in *FOXL2* have also been associated with isolated premature ovarian insufficiency without BPES.

A recent study in 79 patients with 46,XX *SRY*-negative testicular or ovotesticular DSD with virilisation found two new heterozygous frameshift variants in the orphan nuclear receptor *NR2F2*, encoding the transcription factor chicken ovalbumin upstream promoter transcription factor 2 (COUP-TF2) (Bashamboo et al. 2018). Although, in mice, *Coup-Tf2* negatively regulates the expression of the pro-testis *Sox9* gene, virilisation and testis development were not reported in *Coup-Tf2*$^{+/-}$ XX female mice (Rastetter et al. 2014). This indicates that nuclear receptors might have divergent functions in mouse and human biology (Bashamboo et al. 2018).

2.7.2 Wnt4, Rspo1 and β-catenin

Two components of the Wnt signalling pathway, Wnt4 and Rspo1, play major roles in ovarian development. Both function through the activation of β-catenin, which, in turn, regulates a variety of genes important for ovarian development. β-Catenin and Wnt4 antagonise the pro-testis genes *Sox9* and *Fgf9* (Chassot et al. 2014). Foxl2 expression is also partially dependent on RSPO1, β-catenin and Wnt4, as deletion of both Foxl2 and Wnt4 or Rspo1 and Foxl2 results in a more severe phenotype than the single knockout models. Gonads in these mice develop as ovotestes, indicating a partial sex-reversal (Chassot et al. 2014). Additionally, while Rspo1 null mice exhibit a decreased number of germ cells, null Wnt4 mice have an initial normal number of germ cells that suffer from massive apoptosis. Therefore, it seems that Rspo1 stimulates germ cell proliferation, while Wnt4 is required for germ cell survival (Chassot et al. 2014). In humans, overexpression of *WNT4* has been associated with 46,XY sex reversal (Jordan et al. 2001). Additionally, heterozygous loss-of-function variants in *WNT4* have been reported in 46,XX patients with virilisation (Biason-Lauber et al. 2004; Philibert et al. 2008). Loss-of-function variants in *RSPO1* have been associated with a recessive syndrome including 46,XX testicular or ovotesticular DSD, palmoplantar hyperkeratosis and predisposition to squamous cell carcinoma of the skin (Parma et al. 2006; Tomaselli et al. 2008; Naasse et al. 2017).

2.8 Internal Genital Tract Development

As further detailed in the embryology chapter, mammalian male and female internal genital tracts derive from the paramesonephric and mesonephric ducts. Differentiation into these tracts is triggered by the differentiation of the bi-potential gonad into ovary or testis, according to the genetic sex of the individual. Numerous genes have been involved in the development of the female reproductive tract, in both mice and humans. The Mayer–Rokitansky–Küster–Hauser syndrome (MRKH) is a syndrome where the Müllerian tract development is incomplete, resulting in aplasia of the upper third of the vagina and uterus. Most studies of this condition have demonstrated recurrent changes in chromosomal regions 1q21.1 (Cheroki et al. 2008; Ledig et al. 2011), 16p11.2 (Nik-Zainal et al. 2011; Sandbacka et al. 2013), 17q12 (Cheroki et al. 2008; Bernardini et al. 2009; Ledig et al. 2011; Nik-Zainal et al. 2011; Sandbacka et al. 2013) and 22q11.21 (Cheroki et al. 2006, 2008; Ledig et al. 2011; Nik-Zainal et al. 2011). Most likely involved genes in these regions are *RBM8A* for 1q21.1, *TBX6* for 16q11.2 and *LHX1* and *HNF1B* for 17q12. Patients presenting with MRKH combined with hyperandrogenism have exhibited variants in WNT4 (Biason-Lauber et al. 2004, 2007; Philibert et al. 2008, 2010). For a complete description of candidate genes, refer to the review from Ledig et al. (Ledig and Wieacker 2018).

Table 2.2 Hypospadias candidate genes (48)

Humans		Animal models	Expression studies
SHH	HOXA4	DHH	PTCH1
GLI1	HOXB6	Wnt5a	Frizzled
GLI2	MAP3K1	Ctnnb1	
GLI3	CHD7	Hoxa13	
FGF8	NR5A1	Hoxd13	
FGF10	MAMLD1	EfnB2	
FGFR2	BMP4	EphB2	BMP2
ESR1	BMP7	EphB3	
ESR2	WT1	FKBP52/FKBP4	
WTAP	AKR1C3		
DGKK	HSD3B2		
HSD3B1	CYP11A1		CTGF
HSD17B3	CYP19A1		CYR61
ATF3	SRD5A2		GADD45B
BNC2	AR		ZEB1
MID1	VAMP7		
32		9	7

2.9 External Genitalia Development

As further detailed in the embryology chapter, after gonad differentiation and hormone production, the external genitalia will usually differentiate into female or male structures. From a genetic standpoint, differentiation of the genital tubercle and closure of the urethral plate to form the male penis and penile urethra are of particular interest. Several studies in both humans and mice have been carried out, and a recent review of the literature determined 48 candidate genes involved in the development of the penis and potentially responsible for hypospadias (Bouty et al. 2015). For a summary of these findings, see Table 2.2.

2.10 Genetics and DSD

Genetic variants are thought to underlie most DSD, and a wide variety of genetic changes have been implicated in DSD. As described above, 46,XY DSD can be caused by variants in a number of genes involved in both early gonad development and testis differentiation. Failure in gonadal development can cause complete gonadal dysgenesis or streak gonads, whereas failure in those genes involved in testis differentiation can cause the development of ovarian tissue or ovo-testis, as the ovarian pathway is no longer repressed. Some genes cause DSD in a dominant manner (i.e. SOX9 and MAP3K1), whereas others require both alleles to be affected (i.e. DHH). Large chromosomal deletions or duplications can also cause DSD. In particular, in 46,XX DSD, duplication of SOX3 or SOX9 or its regulatory regions can cause testicular development in the absence of a Y chromosome and *SRY*. Another well-studied phenotype of 46,XX DSD is premature ovarian insufficiency (POI, OMIM #311360). Apart from chromosomal abnormalities, such as 45,X Turner syndrome, this heterogeneous condition can result from variants in genes affecting the development of the ovary, DNA division and repair, follicle development and hormonal signalling, metabolism and immune regulation. For a thorough description of genes involved in this diagnosis, see review from Tucker et al. (Tucker et al. 2016). An up-to-date list of causative genes for POI is presented in Table 2.3. POI can occur prior to pubertal changes, part way through the development of secondary sexual characteristics or may present as an early menopause.

Table 2.3 Candidate genes for premature ovarian insufficiency (POI)

Gene	Inheritance	Phenotype
AARS2	AR	Leukodystrophy + POI
AFF2	XLD (susceptiblity)	POI
AIRE	AR	Autoimmune polyglandular syndrome, type 1 + POI
ATM	AR	Ataxia telangiecstasia + POI
BLM	AR	Bloom syndrome + POI
BMP15	XLD	POI
BMPR1B	AR	Acromesomelic chondrodysplasia + POI
C10ORF2	AR	Perrault syndrome + POI
CLPP	AR	Perrault syndrome + POI
CSB-PGBD3	AD	POI
CYP17A1	AR	POI
CYP19A1	AR	POI, foetal masculinization
DMC1	AR	POI
EIF2B2	AR	Ovarioleukodystrophy + POI
EIF2B4	AR	Ovarioleukodystrophy + POI
EIF2B5	AR	Ovarioleukodystrophy + POI
EIF4ENIF1	AD	POI
FANCA	AR	Fanconi anaemia + POI
FANCC	AR	Fanconi anaemia + POI
FANCG	AR	Fanconi anaemia + POI
FANCM	AR	POI
FIGLA	AR	POI
FOXL2	AD	BPES type 1 + POI
FMR1	XLD (premutation)	POI
FSHR	AR	POI
GALT	AR	Galactosaemia + POI
GDF9	AR	POI
HARS2	AR	Perrault syndrome + POI
HAX1	AR	POI
HFM1	AR	POI
HSD17B4	AR	Perrault syndrome + POI
LARS2	AR	Perrault syndrome + POI
LMNA	AD	Cardiomyopathy + POI
MCM8	AR	POI
MCM9	AR	POI
MSH4	AR	POI
NANOS3	AR	POI
NBN	AR	Nijmegen breakage syndrome + POI, infertility
NOBOX	AD	POI
NOG	AD	Proximal symphalangism + POI
NR5A1	AR	POI (DSD in males)
NUP107	AR	POI (XX gonadal dysgenesis)
PGRMC1	AD	POI
PMM2	AR	Congenital disorder of glycosylation + POI
POF1B	XLR	POI
POLG	AR, AD	Progressive external opthalmoplegia and parkinonism + POI
POLR2C	AD	POI
PSMC3IP	AR	POI, XX ovarian dysgenesis
RCBTB1	AR	POI, retinal dystrophy, intellectual disability

(continued)

Table 2.3 (continued)

Gene	Inheritance	Phenotype
RECQL4	AR	Rothmund-Thomson syndrome + POI
SGO2	AR	POI
SOHLH1	AR	POI
STAG3	AR	POI
STAR	AR	Congenital lipoid adrenal hyperplasia + POI
SYCE1	AR	POI
TRIM37	AR	POI, Mulibrey nanism disorder
WRN	AR	Werner syndrome + POI

Early identification of the molecular cause of a DSD can help clinicians in their management and treatment of the patient and counselling of the family. Many molecular biology techniques have been utilised to improve diagnostic rates, especially in 46,XY DSD (Croft et al. 2016; Eggers et al. 2016). Different genetic changes require different techniques for their identification, that is, identification of large genetic duplications or deletions requires microarray analysis, MLPA or whole-genome sequencing, as generally these changes will not be detected using exome or gene-specific sequencing. On the other hand, smaller changes such as single-nucleotide variants or small deletions require gene-specific sequencing, often in the form of massively parallel sequencing, with either a targeted approach or whole-exome sequencing (Baxter et al. 2015; Dong et al. 2016; Eggers et al. 2016; Fan et al. 2017, Kim et al. 2017; Ozen et al. 2017). Even though the genes considered to be 'known diagnostic genes' were different in all of these studies, the overall diagnostic rate in 46,XY DSD varied from 28% to 43% pathogenic or likely pathogenic variants, with approximately 15% variants of unknown significance. It is likely that many other causes of DSD are a result of defects in non-coding regulatory regions (Baetens et al. 2017).

The Victorian Clinical Genetics Services (VCGS) provides diagnostic tests for at least 68 diagnostic genes in DSD and that are identified using a targeted panel that is available internationally (Eggers et al. 2016).

2.11 Conclusion

Sex determination and differentiation in mammals are driven by a complex interplay of genes that are required for the development of bipotential gonads, differentiation of testes or ovaries, all of which ultimately result in male or female secondary sexual characteristics. Figure 2.1 summarises the molecular basis of this phenomenon. Disruption in any step of this cascade can cause DSD. However, despite all progress that has been made since the discovery of SRY 28 years ago (Koopman et al. 2016) we are still far from having a comprehensive understanding of sex determination and many more genes, and regulation pathways remain to be uncovered. This is particularly the case in humans where currently more than 50% of patients with DSD still receive no genetic diagnosis.

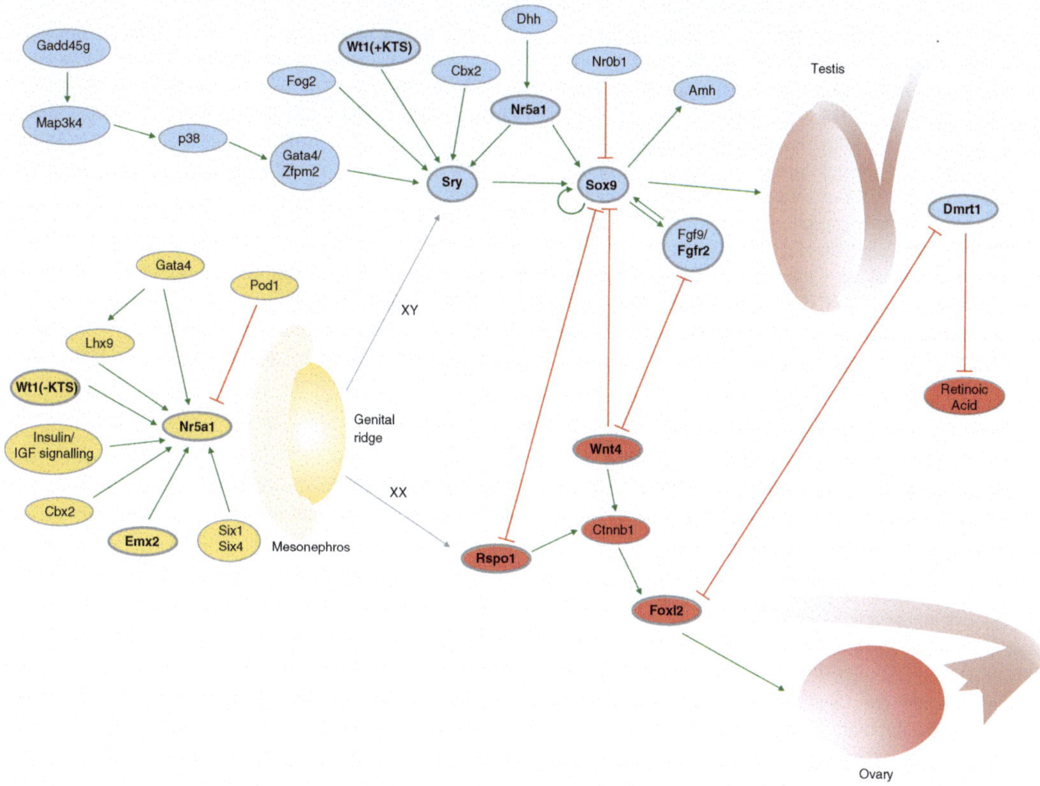

Fig. 2.1 Sex determination and differentiation pathways in mice. Those genes highlighted in bold have been implicated in human sex development and DSD as well

References

Baetens D, Mendonca BB, Verdin H, et al. Non-coding variation in disorders of sex development. Clin Genet. 2017;91(2):163–72.

Bagheri-Fam S, Sim H, Bernard P, et al. Loss of Fgfr2 leads to partial XY sex reversal. Dev Biol. 2008;314(1):71–83.

Bagheri-Fam S, Bird AD, Zhao L, et al. Testis determination requires a specific FGFR2 isoform to repress FOXL2. Endocrinology. 2017;158(11):3832–43.

Barbaux S, Niaudet P, Gubler MC, et al. Donor splice-site mutations in WT1 are responsible for Frasier syndrome. Nat Genet. 1997;17(4):467–70.

Baron D, Batista F, Chaffaux S, et al. Foxl2 gene and the development of the ovary: a story about goat, mouse, fish and woman. Reprod Nutr Dev. 2005;45(3):377–82.

Bashamboo A, Eozenou C, Jorgensen A, et al. Loss of function of the nuclear receptor NR2F2, encoding COUP-TF2, causes testis development and cardiac defects in 46,XX children. Am J Hum Genet. 2018;102(3):487–93.

Baxter RM, Arboleda VA, Lee H, et al. Exome sequencing for the diagnosis of 46,XY disorders of sex development. J Clin Endocrinol Metab. 2015;100(2):E333–44.

Bernardini L, Gimelli S, Gervasini C, et al. Recurrent microdeletion at 17q12 as a cause of Mayer-Rokitansky-Kuster-Hauser (MRKH) syndrome: two case reports. Orphanet J Rare Dis. 2009;4:25.

Berta P, Hawkins JR, Sinclair AH, et al. Genetic evidence equating SRY and the testis-determining factor. Nature. 1990;348(6300):448–50.

Biason-Lauber A, Konrad D, Navratil F, et al. A WNT4 mutation associated with Mullerian-duct regression and virilization in a 46,XX woman. N Engl J Med. 2004;351(8):792–8.

Biason-Lauber A, De Filippo G, Konrad D, et al. WNT4 deficiency—a clinical phenotype distinct from the classic Mayer-Rokitansky-Kuster-Hauser syndrome: a case report. Hum Reprod. 2007;22(1):224–9.

Birk OS, Casiano DE, Wassif CA, et al. The LIM homeobox gene Lhx9 is essential for mouse gonad formation. Nature. 2000;403(6772):909–13.

Bogani D, Siggers P, Brixey R, et al. Loss of mitogen-activated protein kinase kinase kinase 4 (MAP 3K4)

reveals a requirement for MAPK signalling in mouse sex determination. PLoS Biol. 2009;7(9):e1000196.

Bouty A, Ayers KL, Pask A, Heloury Y, Sinclair AH. The genetic and environmental factors underlying hypospadias. Sex Dev. 2015;9(5):239–59.

Callier P, Calvel P, Matevossian A, et al. Loss of function mutation in the palmitoyl-transferase HHAT leads to syndromic 46,XY disorder of sex development by impeding Hedgehog protein palmitoylation and signaling. PLoS Genet. 2014;10(5):e1004340.

Chassot AA, Gillot I, Chaboissier MC. R-spondin1, WNT4, and the CTNNB1 signaling pathway: strict control over ovarian differentiation. Reproduction. 2014;148(6):R97–110.

Cheroki C, Krepischi-Santos AC, Rosenberg C, et al. Report of a del22q11 in a patient with Mayer-Rokitansky-Kuster-Hauser (MRKH) anomaly and exclusion of WNT-4, RAR-gamma, and RXR-alpha as major genes determining MRKH anomaly in a study of 25 affected women. Am J Med Genet A. 2006;140(12):1339–42.

Cheroki C, Krepischi-Santos AC, Szuhai K, et al. Genomic imbalances associated with mullerian aplasia. J Med Genet. 2008;45(4):228–32.

Clark AM, Garland KK, Russell LD. Desert hedgehog (Dhh) gene is required in the mouse testis for formation of adult-type Leydig cells and normal development of peritubular cells and seminiferous tubules. Biol Reprod. 2000;63(6):1825–38.

Crisponi L, Deiana M, Loi A, et al. The putative forkhead transcription factor FOXL2 is mutated in blepharophimosis/ptosis/epicanthus inversus syndrome. Nat Genet. 2001;27(2):159–66.

Croft B, Ayers K, Sinclair A, et al. Review disorders of sex development: the evolving role of genomics in diagnosis and gene discovery. Birth Defects Res C Embryo Today. 2016;108(4):337–50.

Dong Y, Yi Y, Yao H, et al. Targeted next-generation sequencing identification of mutations in patients with disorders of sex development. BMC Med Genet. 2016;17:23.

Eggers S, Sinclair A. Mammalian sex determination-insights from humans and mice. Chromosome Res. 2012;20(1):215–38.

Eggers S, Ohnesorg T, Sinclair A. Genetic regulation of mammalian gonad development. Nat Rev Endocrinol. 2014;10(11):673–83.

Eggers S, Sadedin S, van den Bergen JA, et al. Disorders of sex development: insights from targeted gene sequencing of a large international patient cohort. Genome Biol. 2016;17(1):243.

Fan Y, Zhang X, Wang L, et al. Diagnostic Application of Targeted Next-Generation Sequencing of 80 Genes Associated with Disorders of Sexual Development. Sci Rep. 2017;7:44536.

Fujimoto Y, Tanaka SS, Yamaguchi YL, et al. Homeoproteins Six1 and Six4 regulate male sex determination and mouse gonadal development. Dev Cell. 2013;26(4):416–30.

Garcia-Ortiz JE, Pelosi E, Omari S, et al. Foxl2 functions in sex determination and histogenesis throughout mouse ovary development. BMC Dev Biol. 2009;9:36.

Gustin SE, Hogg K, Stringer JM, et al. WNT/beta-catenin and p27/FOXL2 differentially regulate supporting cell proliferation in the developing ovary. Dev Biol. 2016;412(2):250–60.

Hammes A, Guo JK, Lutsch G, et al. Two splice variants of the Wilms' tumor 1 gene have distinct functions during sex determination and nephron formation. Cell. 2001;106(3):319–29.

Hastie ND. Wilms' tumour 1 (WT1) in development, homeostasis and disease. Development. 2017;144(16):2862–72.

Hu YC, Okumura LM, Page DC. Gata4 is required for formation of the genital ridge in mice. PLoS Genet. 2013;9(7):e1003629.

Hughes IA, Houk C, Ahmed SF, et al. Consensus statement on management of intersex disorders. Arch Dis Child. 2006;91(7):554–63.

Jordan BK, Mohammed M, Ching ST, et al. Up-regulation of WNT-4 signaling and dosage-sensitive sex reversal in humans. Am J Hum Genet. 2001;68(5):1102–9.

Kawakami K, Sato S, Ozaki H, et al. Six family genes—structure and function as transcription factors and their roles in development. Bioessays. 2000;22(7):616–26.

Kim GJ, Sock E, Buchberger A, et al. Copy number variation of two separate regulatory regions upstream of SOX9 causes isolated 46,XY or 46,XX disorder of sex development. J Med Genet. 2015;52(4):240–7.

Kim JH, Kang E, Heo SH, et al. Diagnostic yield of targeted gene panel sequencing to identify the genetic etiology of disorders of sex development. Mol Cell Endocrinol. 2017;444:19–25.

Koopman P, Gubbay J, Vivian N, et al. Male development of chromosomally female mice transgenic for Sry. Nature. 1991;351(6322):117–21.

Koopman P, Sinclair A, Lovell-Badge R. Of sex and determination: marking 25 years of Randy, the sex-reversed mouse. Development. 2016;143(10):1633–7.

Kreidberg JA, Sariola H, Loring JM, et al. WT-1 is required for early kidney development. Cell. 1993;74(4):679–91.

Kuroki S, Matoba S, Akiyoshi M, et al. Epigenetic regulation of mouse sex determination by the histone demethylase Jmjd1a. Science (New York, NY). 2013;341(6150):1106–9.

Lambeth LS, Raymond CS, Roeszler KN, et al. Overexpression of DMRT1 induces the male pathway in embryonic chicken gonads. Dev Biol. 2014;389(2):160–72.

Le Caignec C, Delnatte C, Vermeesch JR, et al. Complete sex reversal in a WAGR syndrome patient. Am J Med Genet A. 2007;143a(22):2692–5.

Ledig S, Wieacker P. Clinical and genetic aspects of Mayer-Rokitansky-Kuster-Hauser syndrome. Med Genet. 2018;30(1):3–11.

Ledig S, Schippert C, Strick R, et al. Recurrent aberrations identified by array-CGH in patients with Mayer-Rokitansky-Kuster-Hauser syndrome. Fertil Steril. 2011;95(5):1589–94.

Ledig S, Hiort O, Wunsch L, et al. Partial deletion of DMRT1 causes 46,XY ovotesticular disorder of sexual development. Eur J Endocrinol. 2012;167(1):119–24.

Li Y, Zheng M, Lau YF. The sex-determining factors SRY and SOX9 regulate similar target genes and promote testis cord formation during testicular differentiation. Cell Rep. 2014;8(3):723–33.

Loke J, Pearlman A, Radi O, et al. Mutations in MAP 3K1 tilt the balance from SOX9/FGF9 to WNT/beta-catenin signaling. Hum Mol Genet. 2014;23(4):1073–83.

Ludbrook LM, Harley VR. Sex determination: a 'window' of DAX1 activity. Trends Endocrinol Metab. 2004;15(3):116–21.

Ludbrook LM, Bernard P, Bagheri-Fam S, et al. Excess DAX1 leads to XY ovotesticular disorder of sex development (DSD) in mice by inhibiting steroidogenic factor-1 (SF1) activation of the testis enhancer of SRY-box-9 (Sox9). Endocrinology. 2012;153(4):1948–58.

Luo X, Ikeda Y, Parker KL. A cell-specific nuclear receptor is essential for adrenal and gonadal development and sexual differentiation. Cell. 1994;77(4):481–90.

Manuylov NL, Zhou B, Ma Q, et al. Conditional ablation of Gata4 and Fog2 genes in mice reveals their distinct roles in mammalian sexual differentiation. Dev Biol. 2011;353(2):229–41.

Marsudi BA, Kartapradja H, Paramayuda C, et al. Loss of DMRT1 gene in a Mos 45,XY,-9[8]/46,XY,r(9)[29]/47,XY,+idic r(9)x 2[1]/46,XY,idic r(9)[1]/46,XY[1] female presenting with short stature. Mol Cytogenet. 2018;11:28.

Matson CK, Murphy MW, Sarver AL, et al. DMRT1 prevents female reprogramming in the postnatal mammalian testis. Nature. 2011;476(7358):101–4.

Meduri G, Bachelot A, Duflos C, et al. FOXL2 mutations lead to different ovarian phenotypes in BPES patients: case report. Hum Reprod. 2010;25(1):235–43.

Meeks JJ, Weiss J, Jameson JL. Dax1 is required for testis determination. Nat Genet. 2003;34(1):32–3.

Minkina A, Matson CK, Lindeman RE, et al. DMRT1 protects male gonadal cells from retinoid-dependent sexual transdifferentiation. Dev Cell. 2014;29(5):511–20.

Naasse Y, Bakhchane A, Charoute H, et al. A novel homozygous missense mutation in the FU-CRD2 domain of the R-spondin1 gene associated with familial 46,XX DSD. Sex Dev. 2017;11(5–6):269–74.

Nik-Zainal S, Strick R, Storer M, et al. High incidence of recurrent copy number variants in patients with isolated and syndromic Mullerian aplasia. J Med Genet. 2011;48(3):197–204.

Ozen S, Onay H, Atik T, et al. Rapid molecular genetic diagnosis with next-generation sequencing in 46,XY disorders of sex development cases: efficiency and cost assessment. Horm Res Paediatr. 2017;87(2):81–7.

Padua MB, Jiang T, Morse DA, et al. Combined loss of the GATA4 and GATA6 transcription factors in male mice disrupts testicular development and confers adrenal-like function in the testes. Endocrinology. 2015;156(5):1873–86.

Park SY, Meeks JJ, Raverot G, et al. Nuclear receptors Sf1 and Dax1 function cooperatively to mediate somatic cell differentiation during testis development. Development. 2005;132(10):2415–23.

Parma P, Radi O, Vidal V, et al. R-spondin1 is essential in sex determination, skin differentiation and malignancy. Nat Genet. 2006;38(11):1304–9.

Pearlman A, Loke J, Le Caignec C, et al. Mutations in MAP 3K1 cause 46,XY disorders of sex development and implicate a common signal transduction pathway in human testis determination. Am J Hum Genet. 2010;87(6):898–904.

Pellegrini M, Pantano S, Lucchini F, et al. Emx2 developmental expression in the primordia of the reproductive and excretory systems. Anat Embryol. 1997;196(6):427–33.

Pelletier J, Bruening W, Kashtan CE, et al. Germline mutations in the Wilms' tumor suppressor gene are associated with abnormal urogenital development in Denys-Drash syndrome. Cell. 1991;67(2):437–47.

Philibert P, Biason-Lauber A, Rouzier R, et al. Identification and functional analysis of a new WNT4 gene mutation among 28 adolescent girls with primary amenorrhea and mullerian duct abnormalities: a French collaborative study. J Clin Endocrinol Metab. 2008;93(3):895–900.

Philibert P, Leprieur E, Zenaty D, et al. Steroidogenic factor-1 (SF-1) gene mutation as a frequent cause of primary amenorrhea in 46,XY female adolescents with low testosterone concentration. Reprod Biol Endocrinol. 2010;8:28.

Piard J, Mignot B, Arbez-Gindre F, et al. Severe sex differentiation disorder in a boy with a 3.8 Mb 10q25.3-q26.12 microdeletion encompassing EMX2. Am J Med Genet A. 2014;164a(10):2618–22.

Piprek RP, Kloc M, Kubiak JZ. Early development of the gonads: origin and differentiation of the somatic cells of the genital ridges. Results Probl Cell Differ. 2016;58:1–22.

Pitetti JL, Calvel P, Romero Y, et al. Insulin and IGF1 receptors are essential for XX and XY gonadal differentiation and adrenal development in mice. PLoS Genet. 2013;9(1):e1003160.

Polanco JC, Wilhelm D, Davidson TL, et al. Sox10 gain-of-function causes XX sex reversal in mice: implications for human 22q-linked disorders of sex development. Hum Mol Genet. 2010;19(3):506–16.

Portnoi MF, Dumargne MC, Rojo S, et al. Mutations involving the SRY-related gene SOX8 are associated with a spectrum of human reproductive anomalies. Hum Mol Genet. 2018;27(7):1228–40.

Rastetter RH, Bernard P, Palmer JS, et al. Marker genes identify three somatic cell types in the fetal mouse ovary. Dev Biol. 2014;394(2):242–52.

Raymond CS, Murphy MW, O'Sullivan MG, et al. Dmrt1, a gene related to worm and fly sexual regulators, is required for mammalian testis differentiation. Genes Dev. 2000;14(20):2587–95.

Sandbacka M, Laivuori H, Freitas E, et al. TBX6, LHX1 and copy number variations in the complex genetics of Mullerian aplasia. Orphanet J Rare Dis. 2013;8:125.

Schmidt D, Ovitt CE, Anlag K, et al. The murine winged-helix transcription factor Foxl2 is required for granulosa cell differentiation and ovary maintenance. Development. 2004;131(4):933–42.

Sekido R, Lovell-Badge R. Sex determination involves synergistic action of SRY and SF1 on a specific Sox9 enhancer. Nature. 2008;453(7197):930–4.

Sinclair AH, Berta P, Palmer MS, et al. A gene from the human sex-determining region encodes a protein with homology to a conserved DNA-binding motif. Nature. 1990;346(6281):240–4.

Sreenivasan R, Gordon CT, Benko S, et al. Altered SOX9 genital tubercle enhancer region in hypospadias. J Steroid Biochem Mol Biol. 2017;170:28–38.

Sutton E, Hughes J, White S, et al. Identification of SOX3 as an XX male sex reversal gene in mice and humans. J Clin Investig. 2011;121(1):328–41.

Swain A, Narvaez V, Burgoyne P, et al. Dax1 antagonizes Sry action in mammalian sex determination. Nature. 1998;391(6669):761–7.

Tomaselli S, Megiorni F, De Bernardo C, et al. Syndromic true hermaphroditism due to an R-spondin1 (RSPO1) homozygous mutation. Hum Mutat. 2008;29(2):220–6.

Tucker EJ, Grover SR, Bachelot A, et al. Premature ovarian insufficiency: new perspectives on genetic cause and phenotypic spectrum. Endocr Rev. 2016;37(6):609–35.

Uhlenhaut NH, Jakob S, Anlag K, et al. Somatic sex reprogramming of adult ovaries to testes by FOXL2 ablation. Cell. 2009;139(6):1130–42.

Val P, Lefrancois-Martinez AM, Veyssiere G, et al. SF-1 a key player in the development and differentiation of steroidogenic tissues. Nucl Recept. 2003;1(1):8.

Warr N, Bogani D, Siggers P, et al. Minor abnormalities of testis development in mice lacking the gene encoding the MAPK signalling component, MAP 3K1. PLoS One. 2011;6(5):e19572.

Warr N, Carre GA, Siggers P, et al. Gadd45gamma and Map 3k4 interactions regulate mouse testis determination via p38 MAPK-mediated control of Sry expression. Dev Cell. 2012;23(5):1020–31.

Warr N, Siggers P, Carre GA, et al. Genetic analyses reveal functions for MAP 2K3 and MAP 2K6 in mouse testis determination. Biol Reprod. 2016;94(5):103.

Zaytouni T, Efimenko EE, Tevosian SG. GATA transcription factors in the developing reproductive system. Adv Genet. 2011;76:93–134.

Embryology of the Human Genital Tract

3

John M. Hutson and Aurore Bouty

3.1 The Urogenital Ridge

The genital tract is derived initially from the intermediate mesoderm of the urogenital ridge, which projects from the posterior wall of the primitive cavity that will eventually form the thorax and abdomen. The urogenital ridge contains the developing kidney, which includes at first the pronephros, then the mesonephros and, finally, the metanephros (Hutson 2008). In addition, the developing gonad forms anterior to the mesonephros and its duct, the mesonephric (Wolffian) duct. The mesonephros develops at approximately 4 weeks of gestation after the pronephros begins to degenerate. It also undergoes regression at approximately 7–8 weeks, which is the time that the gonad begins to develop into an ovary or testis. The mesonephric duct persists from the pronephric duct and was originally named by Wolff. The paramesonephric or Müllerian duct develops as an evagination of the peritoneum adjacent to the gonad and migrates to the cloaca following the Wolffian duct (Fig. 3.1a–c).

The germ cells develop in the extra-embryonic tissues surrounding the yolk sac. Between 3 and 5 weeks of development, they migrate around the yolk sac through the caudal umbilical stalk and into the urogenital ridge (Fig. 3.1d, e). Once they arrive in the developing gonad, they stimulate the development of the ovary or testis. In the developing ovary, the granulosa cells surround the germ cells and trigger meiotic arrest. By contrast, in the testis, the newly formed Sertoli cells, which are derived from the surface epithelium of the gonad, enclose the primordial germ cells to form the testicular cords and trigger mitotic arrest of the germ cells (Fig. 3.2a–c).

3.1.1 Wolffian and Müllerian Duct Development

At the caudal end of the Wolffian duct, the metanephric mesenchyme of the urogenital ridge stimulates the development of a ureteric bud from the Wolffian duct just before it reaches the cloaca. The ureteric bud will then stimulate the development of the definitive kidney or metanephros. When the cloaca separates into hindgut

J. M. Hutson (✉)
Department of Urology, The Royal Children's Hospital, Melbourne, VIC, Australia

Murdoch Children's Research Institute, Melbourne, VIC, Australia

Department of Paediatrics, University of Melbourne, Melbourne, VIC, Australia
e-mail: john.hutson@rch.org.au

A. Bouty
Department of Urology, The Royal Children's Hospital, Melbourne, VIC, Australia

Murdoch Children's Research Institute, Melbourne, VIC, Australia
e-mail: aurore.bouty@rch.org.au

J. M. Hutson et al. (eds.), *Disorders|Differences of Sex Development*,
https://doi.org/10.1007/978-981-13-7864-5_3

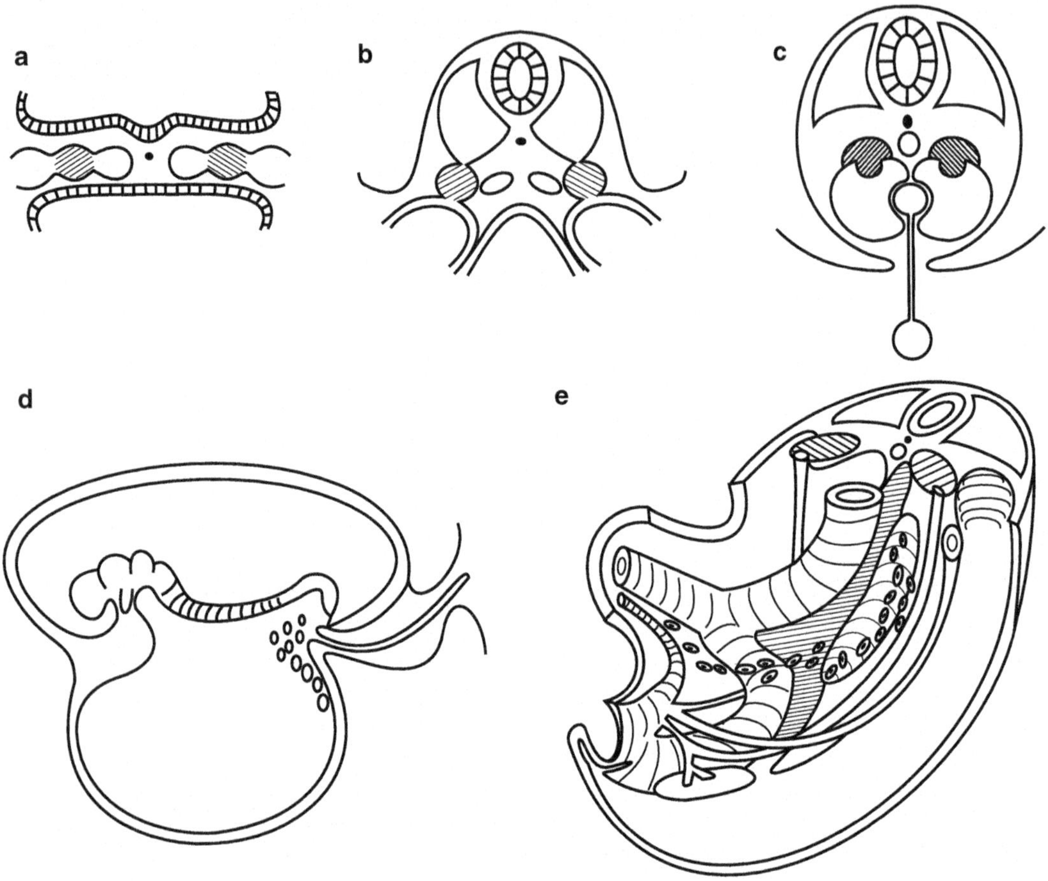

Fig. 3.1 Origin of the intermediate mesoderm in the early embryo. (**a**) Day 19. Transverse section of the trilaminar embryo showing the notochord and developing neural groove in the midline. The mesoderm forms into three segments, as it develops away from the midline: (1) the paraxial mesoderm (the future somites), (2) the intermediate mesoderm (the future urogenital tracts) and (3) the lateral plate (which forms the body wall muscles. (**b**) Day 21. The neural tube and dorsal aortas have formed, and the lateral plate mesoderm has split into parietal (somatic) and visceral layers. (**c**) Days 21–22. The embryo has now grown into a three-dimensional form. One dorsal aorta remains and the intermediate mesoderm is now proliferating and bulging into the future intraembryonic cavity (future pleura and peritoneum). (**d**) At 3 weeks, the primordial germ cells proliferate in the caudal wall of the yolk sac near the allantois. (**e**) Migration of the germ cells by amoeboid movement around the hindgut and through its dorsal mesentery to reach the retroperitoneum and then into the urogenital ridges to reach the primitive gonads, which is required for their further normal gonadal development. Migration is regulated by Steel, fibronectin and laminin, and the primordial germ cells are visible because they express c-Kit, Oct4 and alkaline phosphatase

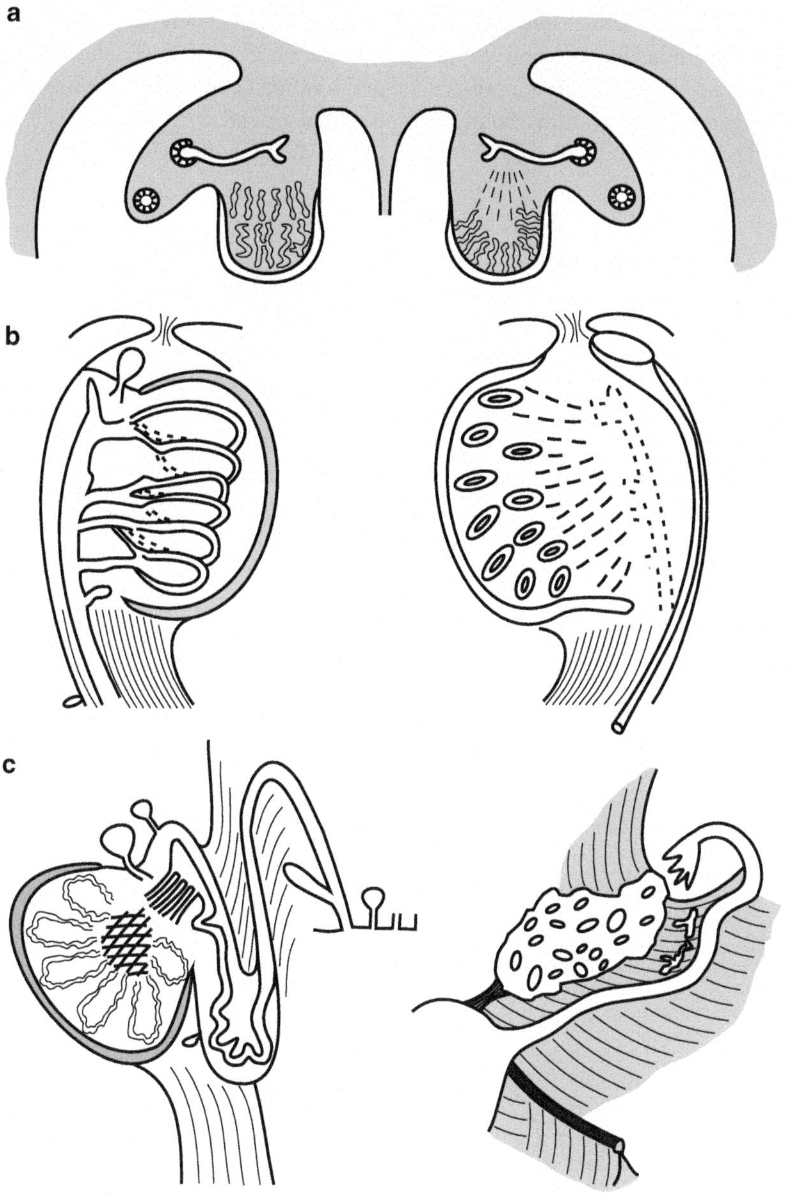

Fig. 3.2 (**a**) Transverse sections through the testis (on the right side of the embryo) and ovary (left) at 7–8 weeks. The testis is developing a tunica albuginea, a rete testis (from regressing mesonephric tubules) and primitive cords containing primordial germ cells. In the ovary, the primitive medullary cords degenerate and the germ cells are in cortical cords, with proliferating surface epithelium. (**b**) The testis (on the right side of the embryo) has developed seminiferous cords (horseshoe-shaped) connected through the rete testis to the ductuli efferentes and the mesonephric (Wolffian) duct. The ovary contains degenerated medullary cords and mesonephric tubules. The cortex has now developed primitive follicles around each germ cell. (**c**) The definitive genital ducts after testicular descent and formation of the broad ligament. The seminiferous tubules are in a horseshoe shape, connecting to the rete testis, efferent ductules and the developing epididymis. Caudally, the vas deferens has a lateral diverticulum that forms the seminal vesicle. Note cranial and caudal remnants after regression of the paramesonephric (Müllerian) ducts: appendix testis (Hydatid of Morgagni) and prostatic utricle, respectively

posteriorly and urogenital sinus anteriorly, the distal end of the Wolffian duct beyond the ureteric bud becomes incorporated into the posterior surface of the urogenital sinus to form the trigone of the bladder. The caudal ends of the Wolffian ducts and ureters enlarge as they are incorporated into the urogenital sinus, and differential growth and rotation occur so that the ureteric openings in the bladder end up being cranial to the distal end of the Wolffian duct (Fig. 3.3).

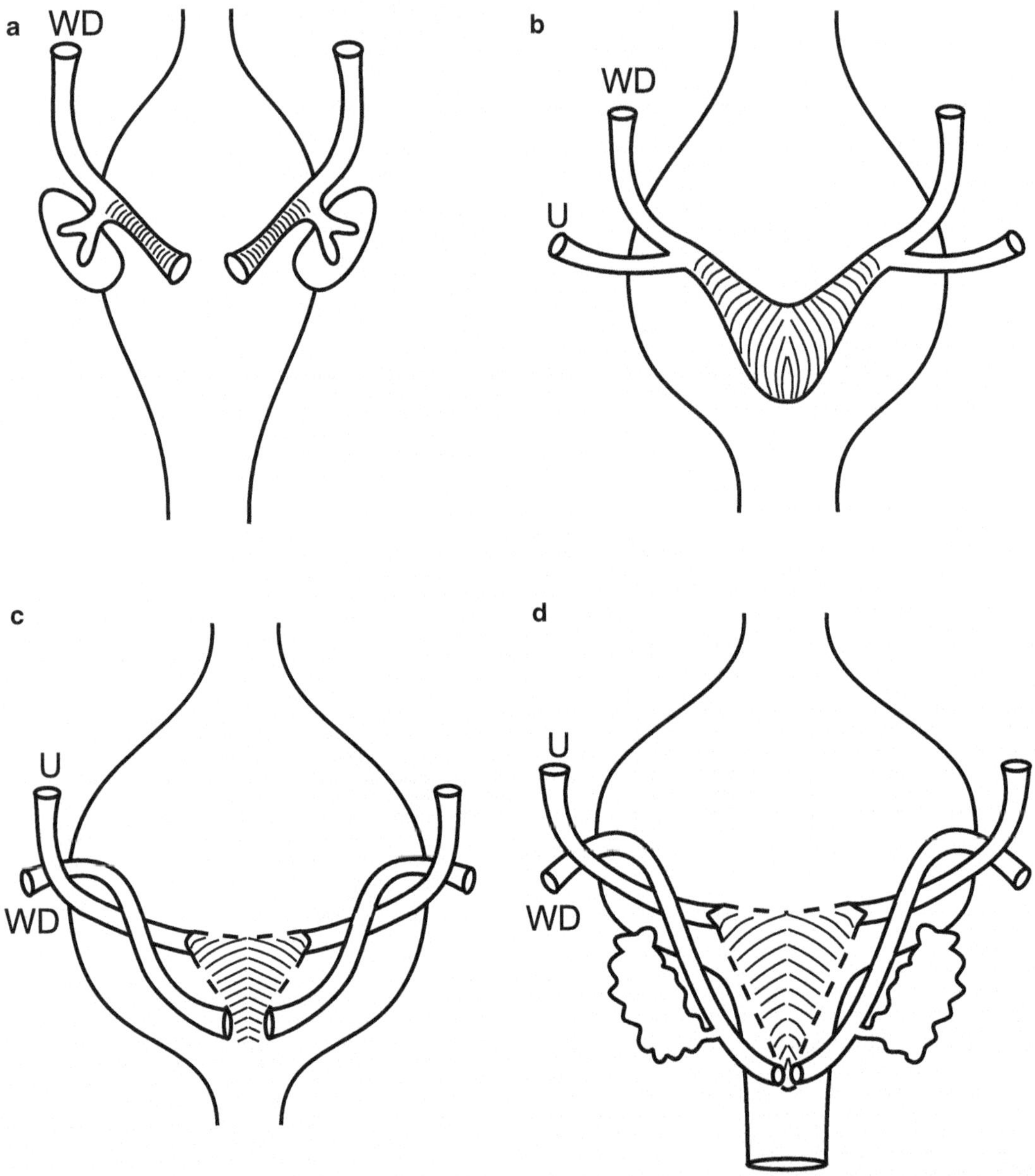

Fig. 3.3 The urogenital sinus between 6 and 8 weeks, shown from behind, to demonstrate how the mesonephric (Wolffian) duct below the ureteric bud is absorbed into the back wall of the urogenital sinus, to form the trigone of the bladder between the ureters, which migrate cranially around the lateral sides of the mesonephric ducts. (**a**) Common mesonephric ducts entering the urogenital sinus. (**b**) Common stem of mesonephric ducts being absorbed into the back wall. (**c**) Origin of the ureter rotating laterally around the mesonephric duct to acquire cranial, independent opening into the developing bladder. (**d**) Definitive anatomical arrangement with ureters opening into the bladder at lateral corners of the trigone. Ejaculatory ducts enter into the prostatic urethra at the verumontanum. Seminal vesicles develop as lateral diverticula of caudal vasa deferentia

The Müllerian ducts rotate antero-medially around the Wolffian ducts as they grow to the cloaca and fuse with each other. The distal end of the ducts contains no lumen and forms a solid uterovaginal primordium, which contacts the endodermal urogenital sinus at the Müllerian tubercle. Proliferation of the endoderm of the tubercle produces the vaginal plate, which invades the uterovaginal primordium to form the vaginal lumen by canalisation and also elongates caudally to bring the opening of the vagina to the exterior of the urogenital sinus (Figs. 3.4 and 3.5).

Anomalies of Müllerian duct development include fusion defects, such as a bicornuate uterus or uterus didelphys. Failed canalisation of the primordium leads to uterine atresia or non-cavitated uterine horns, obstructive cervical anomalies or vaginal atresia. One relatively common anomaly is obstruction of one hemivagina associated with absence of the ipsilateral kidney. This is caused by failure of the Wolffian duct to reach the cloaca, which prevents caudal migration of the ipsilateral Müllerian duct and prevents the development of a ureteric bud, leading to ipsilateral renal agenesis (Rokitansky sequence) (Fig. 3.6) (Stephens et al. 2002). Anomalies of the Müllerian tract are now classified to describe uterine, cervical and vaginal components in the ESHRE/ESGE system (Di Spiezio Sardo et al. 2015). Nevertheless, not all anomalies can be explained by failed fusion, canalisation or migration defects, and the vast majority are not associated with DSD.

3.2 Sexual Differentiation

At 7–8 weeks of development, regression of the mesonephros leaves the gonad suspended on a mesentery known as the mesogenitale. With sexual differentiation, the gonad forms primary epithelial sex cords and mesenchymal medulla. Presence of XY chromosomes triggers activation of the SRY gene, which initiates the development of a testis (as described in Chap. 2), where the primary sex cords develop into Sertoli cells (Fig. 3.2). The Sertoli cells produce anti-Müllerian hormone (AMH) (also known as Müllerian inhibiting substance, MIS), which leads to regression of the Müllerian duct (Seifer and Maclaughlin 2007). Leydig cells form outside the testicular tubules and produce testosterone, which is secreted down the Wolffian duct and stimulates it to persist and form the epididymis, vas deferens and seminal vesicles (Tong et al. 1996). Insulin-like hormone 3 (INSL3) is also produced from the Leydig cells and is important for the development of the gubernaculum (Nef and Parada 1999; Zimmerman et al. 1999).

3.2.1 Testosterone

Testosterone is a steroid formed from cholesterol and progesterone in the Leydig cells. It is secreted down the Wolffian duct in an exocrine manner, exposing the Wolffian duct to very high concentrations (Tong et al. 1996) (Fig. 3.7a). In addition, testosterone is secreted in an endocrine manner into the bloodstream where it will act on the external genitalia to cause masculinisation. Sexual differentiation begins at approximately 8 weeks of gestation with production of AMH to trigger Müllerian duct regression, along with testosterone, stimulating the Wolffian duct to persist to form the epididymis, vas deferens and seminal vesicles. The initial blood level of testosterone is probably too low to stimulate the external genital development without conversion to dihydrotestosterone (DHT) by the enzyme 5-alpha reductase type-2. Dihydrotestosterone binds about five to ten times more tightly than testosterone itself to androgen receptors in the external genitalia, thereby increasing the effective concentration of testosterone tenfold (Handelsman 2006). Some effects of testosterone in the brain may be mediated by conversion of testosterone to oestrogen through the enzyme aromatase, which is another mechanism to increase the effective concentration of androgen (Fig. 3.7b).

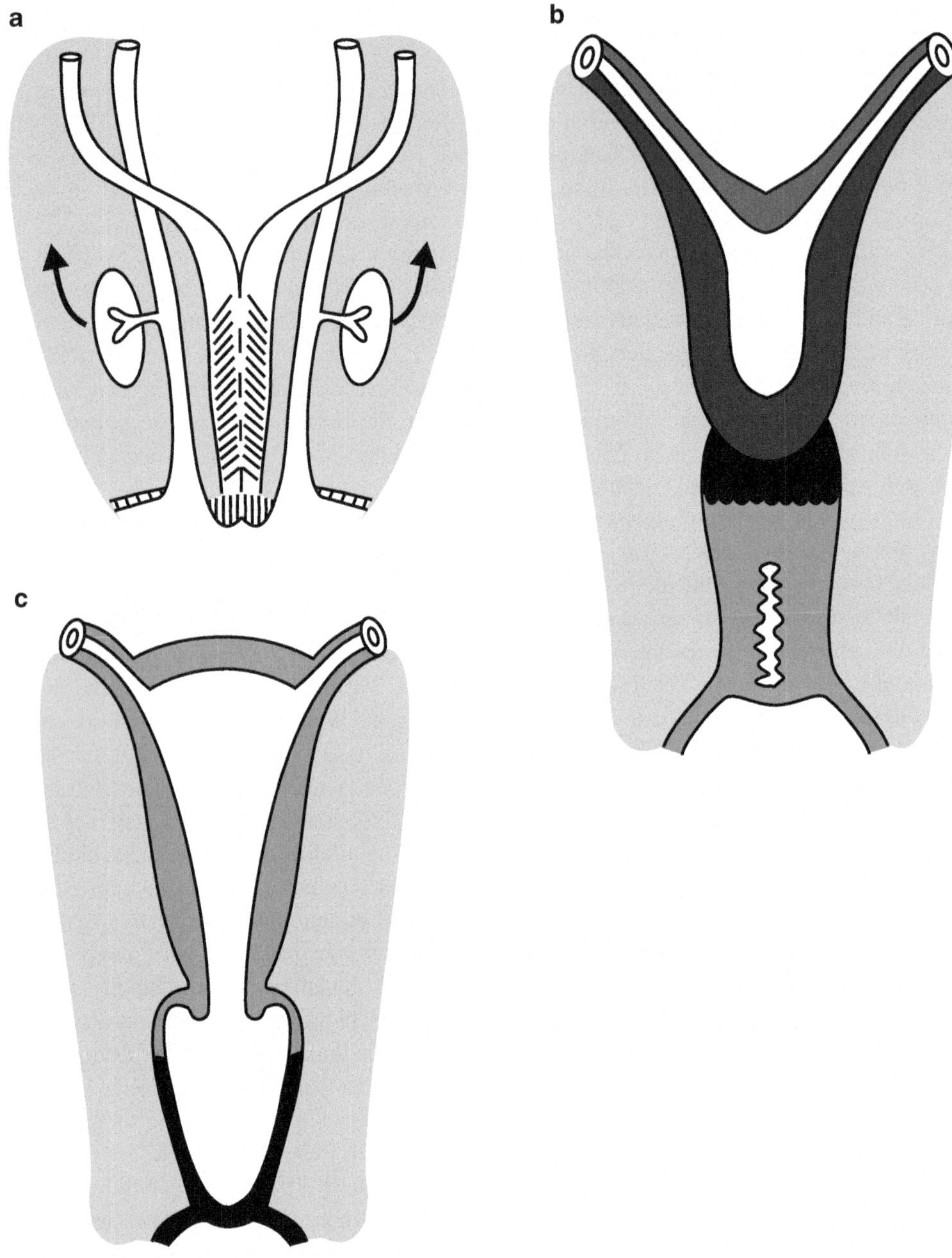

Fig. 3.4 Development of the uterus and vagina around 8–10 weeks. (**a**) Paramesonephric (Müllerian) ducts migrate to the urogenital sinus, fusing with the contralateral duct. Distal ends are solid. Contact of solid tips of paramesonephric ducts triggers proliferation of endoderm to form the sino-vaginal bulb (Müllerian tubercle). (**b**) Proliferation of the bulb cells forms the vaginal plate, which begins to breakdown centrally to form a lumen. Meanwhile, a lumen is developing in the fused Müllerian ducts to form a single uterine cavity. (**c**) Late gestation with the lumen in the uterus and cervix and vaginal vault now in continuity with the lumen within the vaginal plate to form the vagina. The hymen breaks down to become patent before term

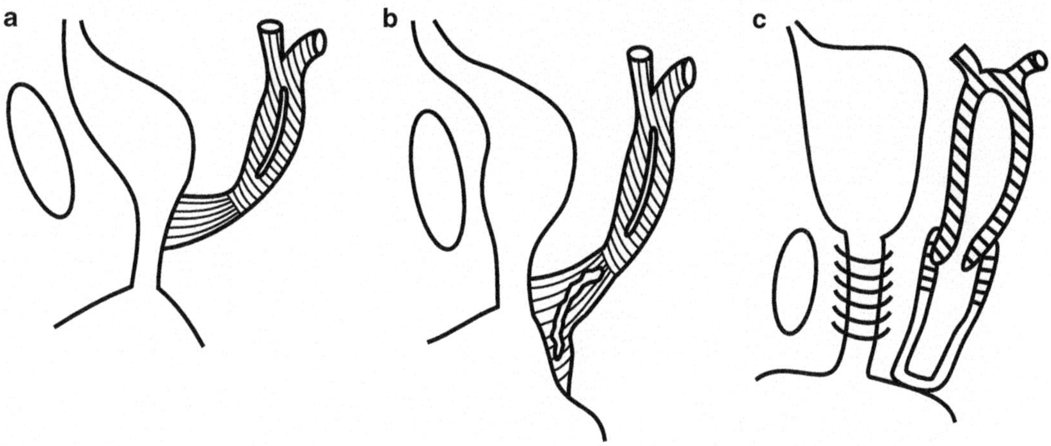

Fig. 3.5 Sagittal views of Müllerian tubercle (**a**) developing into the vaginal plate (**b**), which, by relative growth, extends caudally to open eventually through a separate opening in the urogenital sinus to form the introitus (**c**)

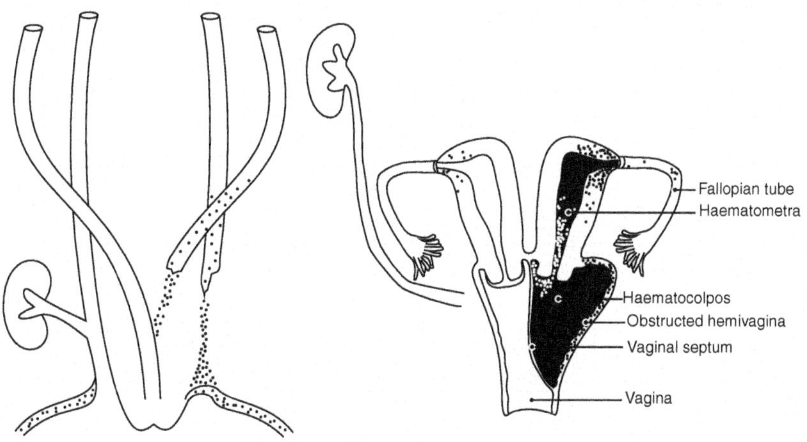

Fig. 3.6 Rokitansky sequence. Ipsilateral failure of caudal growth of the Wolffian duct leads to absence of the ureteric bud and agenesis or dysgenesis of the ipsilateral kidney. In addition, the Müllerian duct cannot migrate caudally in the absence of the Wolffian duct as a guide, which leads to an obstructed hemi-uterus and hemi-vagina with haematocolpos at the onset of menstruation

3.2.2 Anti-Müllerian Hormone (AMH or MIS)

Anti-Müllerian hormone (AMH) was first synthesised in the 1980s and is a glycoprotein dimer (~MW 140,000 Da) produced by Sertoli cells. It is also secreted like testosterone into the Wolffian duct and then diffuses laterally into the adjacent Müllerian duct to trigger its cranio-caudal regression in the male. It may also have some secondary role in the development of the gubernaculum and has postnatal functions in the ovarian cycle (Seifer and Maclaughlin 2007; Hutson and Lopez-Marambio 2017).

3.2.3 Insulin-Like Hormone (INSL3)

Insulin-like hormone 3 (INSL3) was discovered in the 1990s and is a protein with homology to insulin that is produced by Leydig cells. It stimulates the growth of the genito-inguinal ligament, or gubernaculum, which is important for the first phase of testicular descent (Zimmerman et al. 1999).

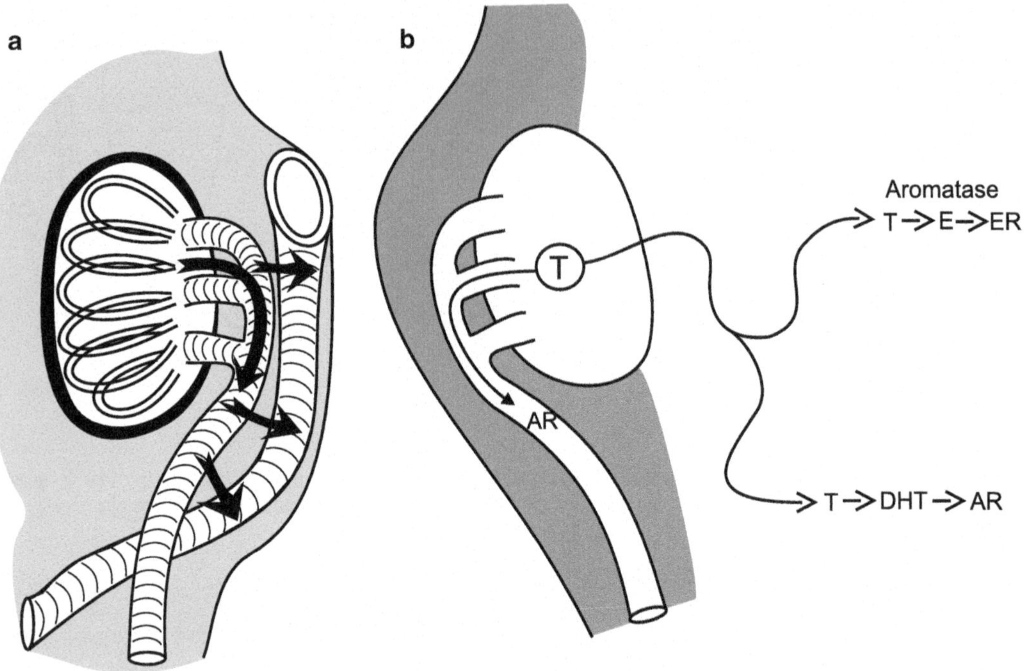

Fig. 3.7 (**a**) Schema of urogenital ridge at 8–10 weeks showing developing testis and ducts. Testosterone and anti-Müllerian hormone (AMH) (or MIS) produced in the testis by Leydig cells and Sertoli cells diffuse into the duct system and pass in an exocrine manner down the mesonephric (Wolffian) duct. The testosterone is present in a very high concentration, which causes preservation of the Wolffian duct and differentiation into epididymis, vas deferens and seminal vesicle caudally. Where there is gonadal dysgenesis or a block in androgen synthesis, only the cranial segment of the Wolffian duct is preserved. AMH also passes down the Wolffian duct and diffuses into the adjacent Müllerian duct to trigger regression. As with testosterone, the degree of regression is proportional to the amount of exocrine hormone reaching the duct system. (**b**) Testosterone acts by both exocrine and endocrine pathways in early development. Endocrine levels of the hormone are low, presumably because the developing testis is initially very tiny, so adaptations have arisen to augment endocrine function at this stage. In some parts of the brain (in some animals), testosterone is converted to oestrogen, which then acts through the oestrogen receptor. Circulating oestrogens in females are bound to α-fetoprotein, which prevents crossing the blood–brain barrier, while testosterone can enter the brain freely. In the external genitalia and prostate, the testosterone is converted by 5-alpha-reductase type-2 to dihydrotestosterone (DHT), which binds five to ten times more tightly to androgen receptors than the testosterone itself. Without this effective concentrating factor, the external genitalia cannot be masculinised by the testis, as its testosterone production is insufficient. However, at puberty, the testis is now so much larger that testosterone is capable of virilising remote tissues as the blood levels are more than 10–100 times higher than that in the early foetus

3.3 External Genitalia

The external genitalia remain undifferentiated until 8 weeks of development (Fig. 3.8a). Initially, they contain a central genital tubercle surrounded by inner and outer genital folds. Between the inner genital folds lies the endodermal urethral plate and the urogenital sinus opening. Masculine development is triggered by DHT, which causes the growth of the genital tubercle into a penis, as well as growth of the perineal body to cover the urogenital sinus, canalisation of the endodermal urethral plate to form the urethra and fusion of the outer genital folds to form the scrotum (Fig. 3.8b–d). In the female, the genital tubercle enlarges only a small amount to form the clitoris. In addition, in the absence of androgens, there is apoptosis of the ventrally placed endoderm of the urethral plate, which leads to bending of the clitoral shaft. The inner genital folds remain sepa-

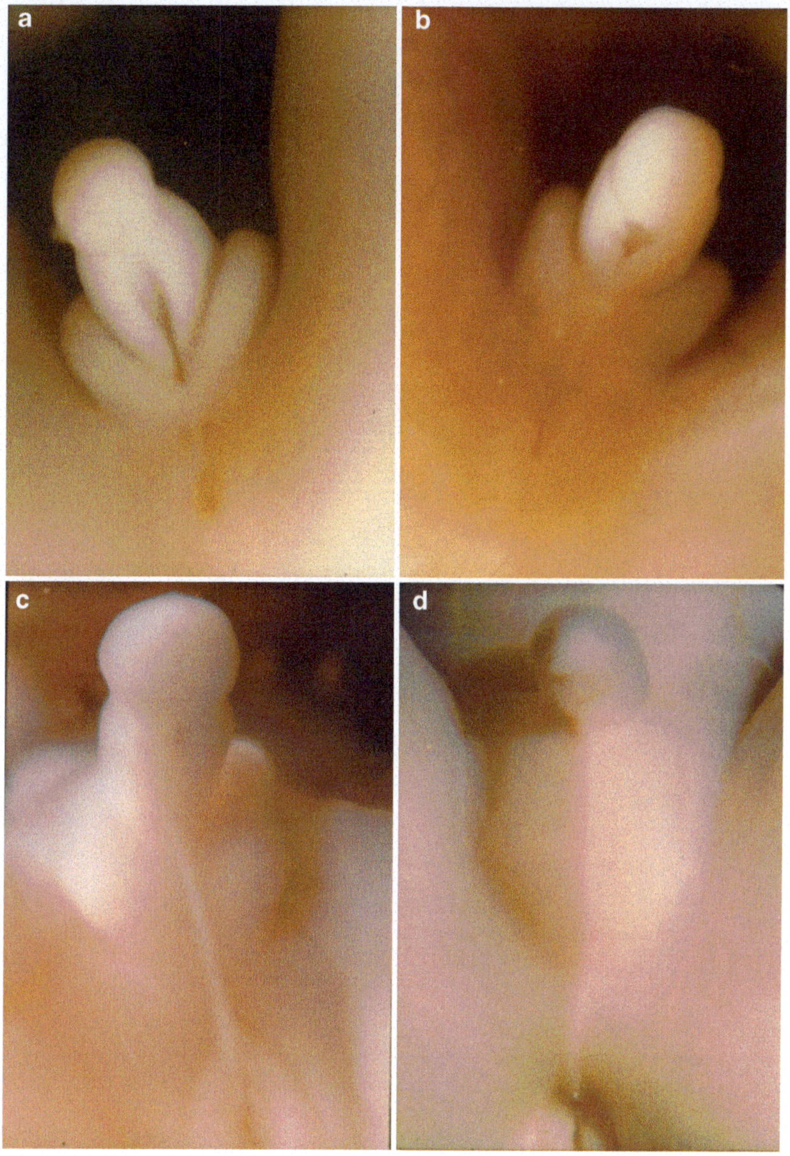

Fig. 3.8 Transformation of the undifferentiated genitalia into that of a male over 8–12 weeks of gestation. (**a**) The external genitalia of an 8- to 9-week human embryo showing the undifferentiated stage, just before the onset of sexual differentiation. (**b**) Week 9: partially fused urogenital folds. (**c**) Week 10: urogenital fusion progressing. (**d**) Week 12: fused urogenital folds (Clarnette et al. 1997; Miller et al. 2004) (Reproduced with permission from England 1983 (England 1983; Clarnette et al. 1997))

rate to become the labia minora, while the outer genital folds remain separate and develop into the labia majora. The urogenital sinus remains open to form the vestibule of the introitus (Fig. 3.9a–d).

3.4 Gonadal Descent

The ovary descends relatively passively in the abdomen, as the Müllerian ducts and their mesentery, the broad ligament, do not grow as quickly as the lower part of the abdominal cavity (Fig. 3.10). By contrast, the position of the testis is changed radically by exposure to testicular hormones. Between 8 and 15 weeks, INSL3 stimulates the gubernaculum to enlarge, known as the swelling reaction, which actively holds the testis close to the future inguinal canal as the abdomen enlarges. This anchoring of the testis close to the inguinal canal means that the testis remains in relatively the same position as enlargement of the abdominal cavity results in everything else moving further away. The passive nature of this process is probably the reason that this mechanism is rarely

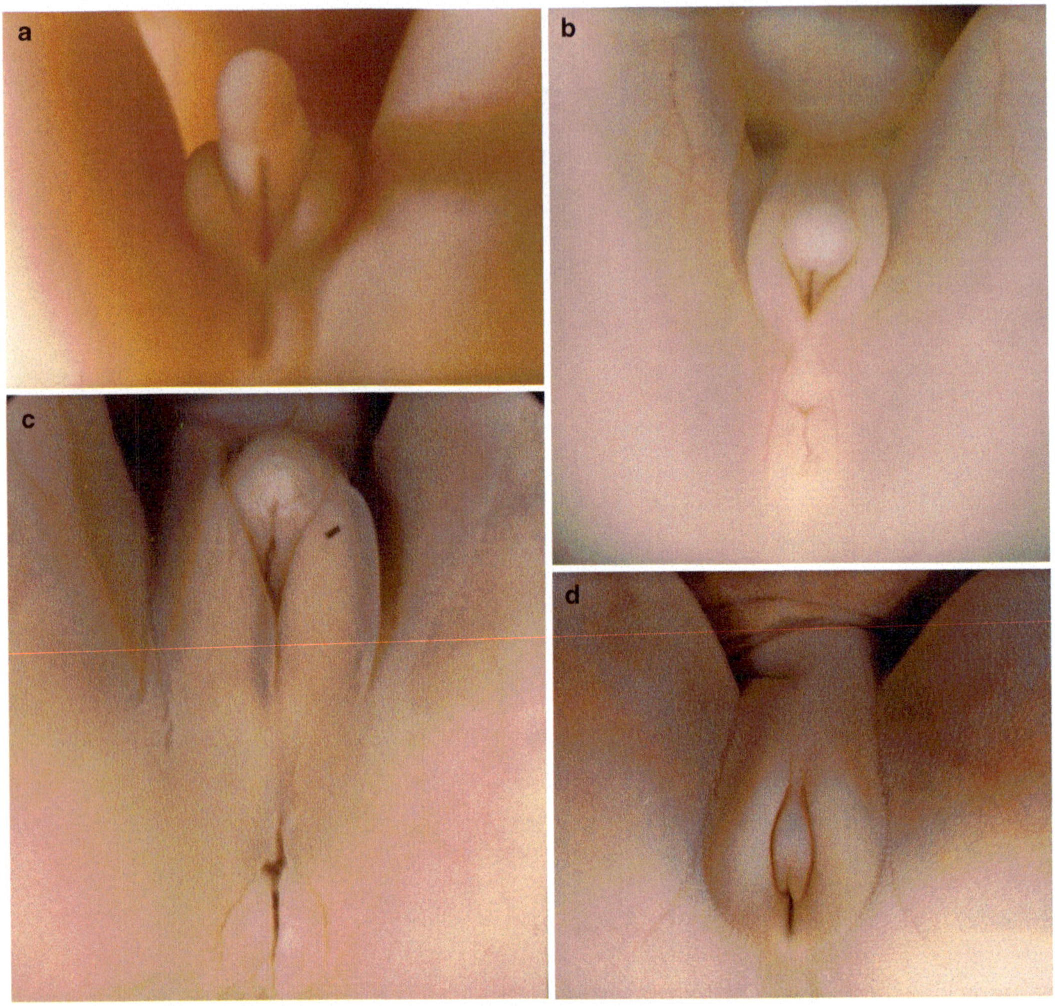

Fig. 3.9 Development of the external genitalia in female foetuses between 8 and 20 weeks. (**a**) Week 9: The clitoris is growing, but at a much slower rate than the rest of the foetus, making it look progressively smaller. (**b**) Week 13: The folding of the clitoris, caused by apoptosis of the endoderm forming the urethral plate, is visible. (**c**) Week 17. (**d**) Week 20 (Reproduced with permission from England (1983))

abnormal, and hence, undescended testes inside the peritoneal cavity are rare. Around the same time, testosterone causes regression of the cranial suspensory ligament, which is the residual cranial mesentery of the urogenital ridge. In many mammals, the gonadal position is the vector sum of traction of the cranial and caudal ligaments (Fig. 3.11).

Between 25 and 35 weeks of gestation, testosterone stimulates the gubernaculum to grow out of the abdominal wall guided by the genitofemoral nerve, which releases a neurotransmitter (calcitonin gene-related peptide, CGRP) from its sensory nerve endings, which is thought to provide a chemotactic gradient for the gubernaculum to follow (Hutson and Hasthorpe 2005). The processus vaginalis grows inside the elongating gubernaculum, as does the cremaster muscle. Formation of the processus vaginalis inside the gubernaculum enables the intra-abdominal testis on its mesentery, the mesogenitale, to reach the scrotum while still inside an extension of the peri-

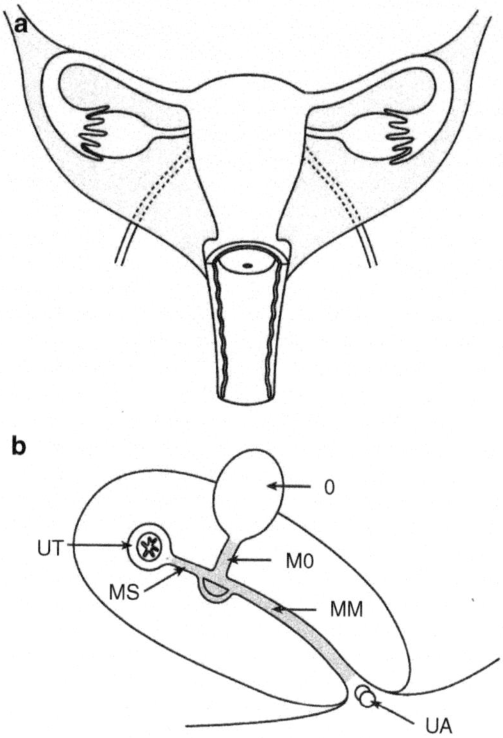

Fig. 3.10 Drawing of broad ligament (shaded) in an adult female human shown from the back (**a**) and from the side (**b**). *UT* uterine tube, *O* ovary, *MO* mesovarium, *MS* mesosalpinx, *MM* mesometrium, *UA* uterine artery (Redrawn from Gray's Anatomy (Williams et al. 1995), and reproduced with permission from Miller et al. (2004))

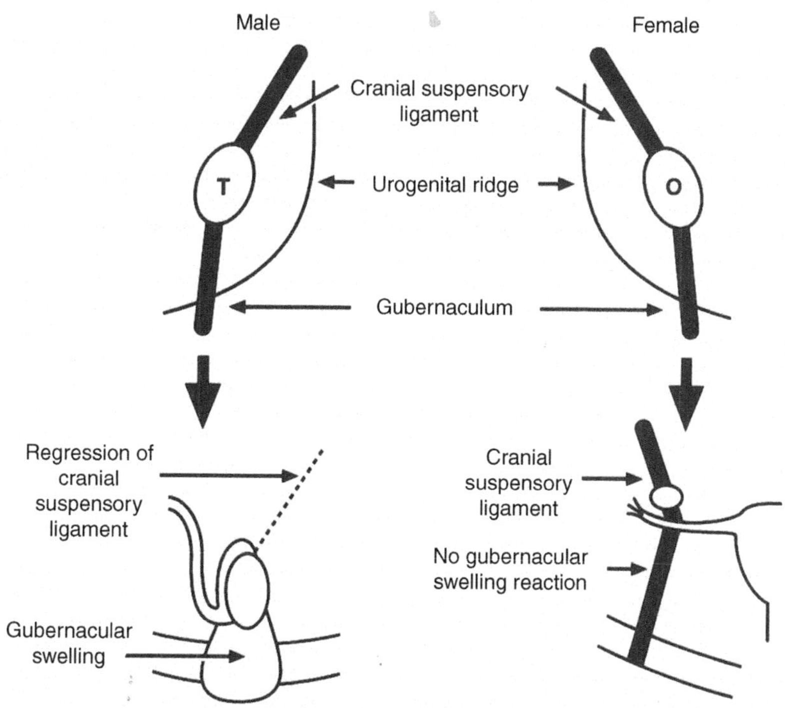

Fig. 3.11 Schematic diagram illustrating the role of the gubernaculum and cranial suspensory ligaments in the final position of the gonad. In the male, a combination of gubernacular swelling and regression of the cranial suspensory ligament allows the testis to remain close to the internal inguinal ring. In females, the gubernaculum remains long and thin, allowing the ovary to move away from the inguinal region with growth of the embryo. The cranial suspensory ligament helps to maintain the position of the ovary on the posterior abdominal wall (Reproduced with permission from Clarnette et al. (1997))

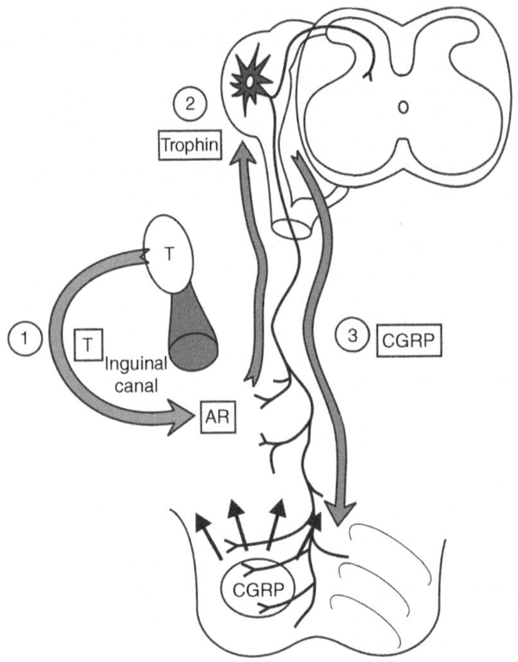

Fig. 3.12 The inguino-scrotal phase of testicular descent occurs between 25 and 35 weeks of gestation, under the control of androgen. However, the mechanism is very complex and indirect, with androgen acting mostly indirectly through the androgen receptors in the inguinal region to trigger masculinisation (through an unknown trophin) of the genitofemoral nerve, which releases a neurotransmitter through its sensory nerve endings in the groin and scrotum (calcitonin gene-related peptide; CGRP). CGRP provides a chemotactic gradient for the migrating gubernaculum to the scrotum

toneal cavity (Hutson and Beasley 1992). During migration of the gubernaculum, it is thought to release enzymes to dissolve the surrounding extracellular matrix so that it can migrate through the tissues like an icebreaker (Churchill et al. 2011). This second phase of testicular descent, requiring migration of the gubernaculum in the correct direction, is very complex mechanically (Hutson et al. 2010), and hence, failure of this process, leading to undescended testis, is common (Fig. 3.12).

References

Churchill JA, Buraundi S, Farmer PJ, et al. Gubernaculum as icebreaker: do matrix metalloproteinases in rodent gubernaculum and inguinal fat pad permit testicular descent? J Pediatr Surg. 2011;46(12):2353–7.

Clarnette T, Sugita Y, Hutson JM. Genital anomalies in the human and animal models reveal the mechanisms and hormones governing testicular descent. Br J Urol. 1997;79:99–112.

Di Spiezio Sardo A, Campo R, Gordts S, et al. The comprehensiveness of the ESHRE/ESGE classification of female genital tract congenital anomalies: a systematic review of cases not classified by the AFS system. Hum Reprod. 2015;30(5):1046–58.

England M. A colour atlas of life before birth. Normal fetal development. Weert: Wolfe Medical Publishers; 1983.

Handelsman DJ. Testosterone: use, misuse and abuse. Med J Aust. 2006;185(8):436–9.

Hutson J. Development of the urogenital system. Gray's anatomy. 4th ed. London, Chapter 78: S. Standring; 2008. p. 1305–25.

Hutson J, Beasley S. Descent of the testis. London: Edward Arnold; 1992.

Hutson JM, Hasthorpe S. Testicular descent and cryptorchidism: the state of the art in 2004. J Pediatr Surg. 2005;40(2):297–302.

Hutson JM, Lopez-Marambio FA. The possible role of AMH in shortening the gubernacular cord in testicular descent: A reappraisal of the evidence. J Pediatr Surg. 2017;52(10):1656–60.

Hutson JM, Balic A, Nation T, et al. Cryptorchidism. Semin Pediatr Surg. 2010;19(3):215–24.

Miller A, Hong MK, Hutson J. The broad ligament: a review of its anatomy and development in different species and hormonal environments. Clin Anat. 2004;17:244–51.

Nef S, Parada LF. Cryptorchidism in mice mutant for Insl3. Nat Genet. 1999;22(3):295–9.

Seifer DB, Maclaughlin DT. Mullerian inhibiting substance is an ovarian growth factor of emerging clinical significance. Fertil Steril. 2007;88(3):539–46.

Stephens FD, Smith ED, Hutson JM. Congenital anomalies of the kidney, urinary and genital tracts. London: Martin Dunitz; 2002.

Tong SYC, Hutson JM, Watts LM. Does testosterone diffuse down the Wolffian duct during sexual differentiation? J Urol. 1996;155:2057–9.

Williams P, Bannister LH, Berry MM, Collins P, Dyson M, Dussek JE, Ferguson MWJ, editors. Gray's anatomy. 38th ed. New York: Churchill Livingstone; 1995. p. 198–217.

Zimmerman S, Steding G, Emmen J, et al. Targeted disruption of the INSL3 gene causes bilateral cryprotchidism. Mol Endocrinol. 1999;13:681–91.

Hormones Regulating Sex Development

4

John M. Hutson

4.1 Introduction

The hormones regulating sex development are produced by the placenta, adrenal glands and developing gonads, with some signal processing also occurring in the target organs. Androgens synthesised by the Leydig cells from 8 to 9 weeks of gestation are one of the key regulators controlling Wolffian duct and external genital development. Anti-Müllerian hormone (AMH) is produced by the Sertoli cells and is one of the first hormones made, controlling regression of the Müllerian ducts. Insulin-like hormone 3 (INSL3) is made by Leydig cells and stimulates the swelling reaction in the gubernaculum as part of the first phase of testicular descent. Oestrogens from the foetal (or maternal) ovary have a role in the differentiation of the female genital tract, but their precise role is hard to identify, as oestrogens are essential for maintaining placental (and therefore foetal) viability.

J. M. Hutson (✉)
Department of Urology, The Royal Children's Hospital, Melbourne, VIC, Australia

Murdoch Children's Research Institute, Melbourne, VIC, Australia

Department of Paediatrics, University of Melbourne, Melbourne, VIC, Australia
e-mail: john.hutson@rch.org.au

4.2 Testicular Hormones

4.2.1 Testosterone Synthesis

In the adrenal gland, the raw material for testosterone and other steroid synthesis is cholesterol. Cholesterol enters the developing Leydig cells where it must reach the mitochondria (Warne and Kanumakala 2002). In the placenta, cholesterol can reach the mitochondria directly, but in the adrenal cortex and developing testis, cholesterol needs to be actively transported across the mitochondrial membrane by steroid acute regulatory protein (StAR). The gene for this key protein is on chromosome 8p11.2, and mutations cause a rare anomaly known as lipoid adrenal hyperplasia. In this condition, steroid production is defective in both the testis and adrenal gland, and accumulation of large droplets of lipid in the adrenal cortical cells leads to hyperplasia. As steroid production in the placenta is unaffected, steroid deficiency does not present until shortly after birth (with adrenal crisis in phenotypic females, regardless of XX or XY chromosomes).

At about the sixth week of gestation, Leydig cells begin to synthesise testosterone from cholesterol. As outlined below, this process is dependent on a multi-step pathway of a number of specific enzymes. Genetic variants resulting in reduced activity of any enzyme in this pathway can therefore lead to differences in genital appearance.

J. M. Hutson et al. (eds.), *Disorders|Differences of Sex Development*,
https://doi.org/10.1007/978-981-13-7864-5_4

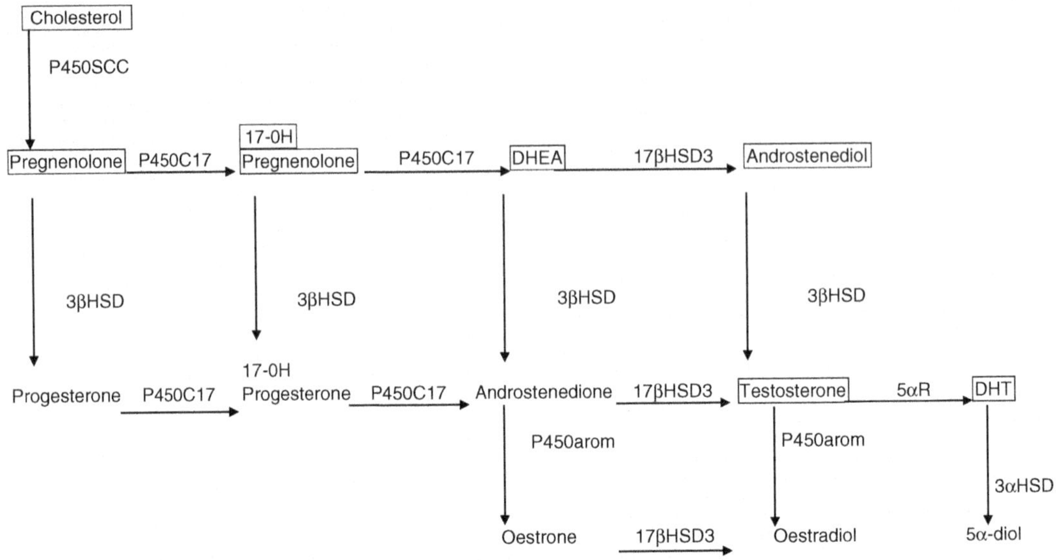

Fig. 4.1 The pathways for steroid hormone synthesis in the adrenal glands and gonads

Once cholesterol enters the mitochondria, its conversion to Δ^5-pregnenolone is catalysed by cholesterol side-chain cleavage enzyme ($P450_{scc}$), which is also known as CYPIIA (Fig. 4.1). The gene for this enzyme, which also catalyses two other steroid conversions (20-hydroxylation and 22-hydroxylation), is on chromosome 15q23-24. Mutations in $P450_{scc}$ are lethal, as steroid synthesis is disrupted in the placenta as well as in the foetus.

Pregnenolone can be converted into 17-OH-pregnenolone and then dehydroepiandrosterone (DHEA) by the enzyme P450C17 (the gene is on chromosome 10q24.3) or progesterone by 3β-hydroxysteroid dehydrogenase (3β-HSD). $P450_{C17}$ also converts progesterone into 17-hydroxyprogesterone and then androstenedione at a lower level. Incomplete virilisation can occur in 46,XY foetuses due to a block in testosterone synthesis when 3β-HSD function is altered; however, salt losing is the most prominent presenting feature in neonates. In 46,XX foetuses, genital appearance is most commonly typically female, although some mild virilisation may occur.

DHEA is converted to androstenediol by the enzyme 17β-hydroxysteroid dehydrogenase-3 (17β-HSD3), which can also convert androstenedione to testosterone and oestrone to oestradiol. Androstenediol is converted to testosterone (T) by 3β-hydroxysteroid dehydrogenase/$\Delta^5\Delta^4$ isomerase. Testosterone activity occurs in both a paracrine and an endocrine manner. P450 aromatase ($P450_{arom}$) can convert testosterone into oestradiol (E_2), but a more important pathway in virilisation is the intracellular conversion of testosterone to 5α-dihydrotestosterone (DHT) in androgen-target tissues by the enzyme 5 alpha reductase. DHT binds five to ten times more tightly to androgen receptors than testosterone itself. DHT is essential for androgen-induced phallic growth and masculinisation of the external genitalia in early foetal life, at a time (8–12 weeks) when circulating testosterone levels are otherwise probably too low to stimulate genital virilisation.

This is likely to be because the developing testis is still too small to produce enough hormones for normal endocrine function. By stimulating the differentiation of the urogenital swelling, the genital tubercle and the urethral folds into penis and scrotum, DHT also induces the formation of the prostate. Alterations in 5-alpha reductase-2 enzymatic activity result in lower levels of DHT production and hence may lead to DSD with atypical genital appearance at birth. However, because testosterone is secreted directly into the Wolffian duct, this is still virilised normally. In addition, once puberty is reached, 5α-reductase-2 is no longer as crucial, as the circulating testosterone levels are now higher (because of increased Leydig cell volume in the larger pubertal testes), and further virilisation at this stage is common (Figs. 4.2 and 4.3).

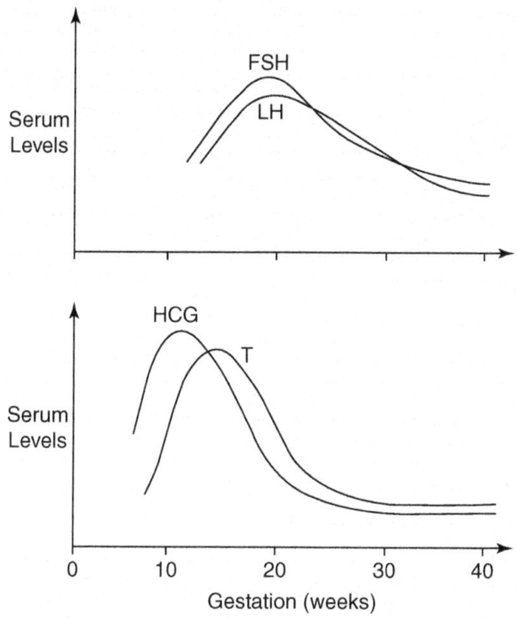

Fig. 4.2 Serum levels of follicle-stimulating hormone (FSH), luteinising hormone (LH) (upper panel), human chorionic gonadotrophin (hCG) and testosterone (T) (the lower panel) during gestation in a male foetus (Redrawn from Grumbach et al. (2003))

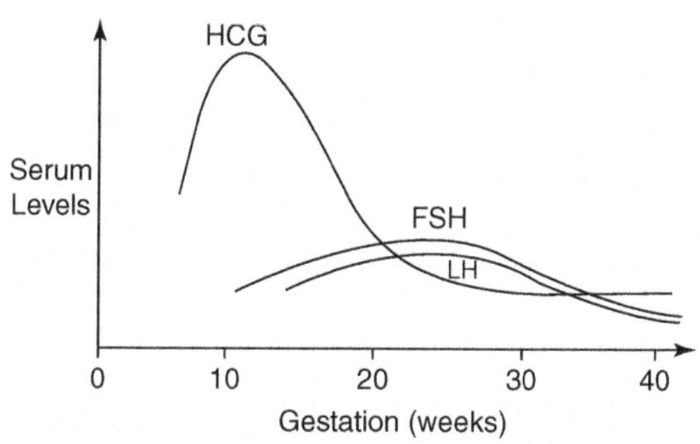

Fig. 4.3 Serum levels of human chorionic gonadotrophin (hCG), follicle-stimulating hormone (FSH) and luteinising hormone (LH) in a developing female foetus (Redrawn from Grumbach et al. (2003))

DHT is converted by 3α-hydroxysteroid dehydrogenase (3α-HSD) to 5α-androstanediol, which in marsupials is the key androgen regulating development of the prostate and may be the key androgen circulating in the blood (Shaw et al. 2000; Wilson et al. 2003). It is still unknown whether this is relevant for humans but is a theoretical cause of under-virilisation in some 46,XY DSD patients with no obvious problem in androgen synthesis.

While 5α-reduction of T is the classical biosynthetic pathway to DHT production, an alternative 'backdoor' pathway has also been demonstrated. Initial studies of testes of tammar wallaby pouch young (Shaw et al. 2000; Wilson et al. 2003) showed that 17-hydroxyprogesterone (17-OHP) can be converted to 5α-reduced 21-carbon (C21) precursor 5α-pregnane-3α,17α-diol-20-one (pdiol) and subsequently to DHT through this alternative pathway. Subsequent human studies have shown that this alternative pathway is active in individuals with 21-hydroxylase deficiency congenital adrenal hyperplasia (21-OHD CAH) and may contribute to virilisation in this cohort (Kamrath et al. 2012).

Variants in 17β-HSD3 are a relatively uncommon cause of 46,XY DSD overall but may result in such a reduction in androgen production in foetal life that minimal androgen-induced virilisation of the external genitalia (hence female phenotype) occurs in a 46,XY baby. Thereafter, affected individuals may present in infancy if virilisation occurs due to additional androgen exposure during the 'mini-puberty' of the early months of life or at any age with palpable swellings (testes) in the groin, or alternatively on investigation of virilisation or primary amenorrhoea in a teenage girl (Boehmer et al. 1999).

Both androstenedione and testosterone can be substrates for P450 aromatase ($P450_{arom}$), which is present in some peripheral tissues (brain, hair follicles, fat, muscle and liver) but is most active in the developing ovary and the placenta. The role of placental P450 aromatase is crucial during pregnancy, as it prevents foetal androgens in a male foetus from reaching the maternal circulation and virilising their mother. In addition, it metabolises any intermediate androgenic metabolites in a female foetus to oestrogens. Variants in the gene for $P450_{arom}$ cause virilisation of the mother as well as minor virilisation of the female foetus.

4.2.2 Androgen Receptor

The androgen receptor (AR) is a key component of the androgenic signalling pathway that is encoded by a gene with eight exons on the X chromosome. It is a member of the nuclear receptor family, which includes the steroid receptors as well as receptors for retinoic acid, vitamin D and thyroid hormone. The first exon contains a variable sequence of trinucleotide repeats associated with an adult-onset neurological disorder of spinal and bulbar muscular atrophy known as Kennedy's disease (Chamberlain et al. 1994). The second and third exons encode the DNA-binding region, which is similar in all nuclear receptors. The fourth to eight exons encode the androgen-binding region. The AR has several heat shock proteins (HSP56, 70 + 90), as well as a large number of other co-activators and co-repressors that may be linked to it, and dissociate on steroid binding. DHT has significantly higher affinity for the AR than testosterone, which is probably the reason why 5α-reductase-2 has evolved in peripheral tissues such as the external genitalia, effectively increasing the concentration of androgens fivefold to tenfold. This concentrating effect is not needed in the Wolffian duct, as it is exposed to much higher levels of testosterone that are secreted in an exocrine manner down the duct (Tong et al. 1996).

Variants in the AR causing androgen insensitivity in the foetus with 46,XY karyotype are common (Eggers et al. 2016). As the AR is on the X chromosome and only a single allele is present in 46,XY individual (Lobaccaro et al. 1994), this variation does not impact significantly on 46,XX individuals, although women who carry this variation on one of their X chromosomes (usually identified in the setting of having an affected offspring), may have sparse pubic and axillary hair. In 46,XY-affected individuals, variants in the gene coding for the AR that completely eliminate receptor binding or function cause complete androgen insensitivity syndrome (CAIS), while some others diminish androgen function only to a variable degree, causing partial androgen insensitivity syndrome (PAIS). Individuals with CAIS have a typically female external genital phenotype, while signs of reduced androgen effect on the external genitalia at birth are a common presenting feature in PAIS (see Chap. 7).

4.2.3 Control of Testosterone Levels

Testosterone is first produced by the developing testes at about 8–9 weeks of development (Siiteri and Wilson 1974). However, receptors for human chorionic gonadotrophin/luteinising hormone (hCG/LH) are not found until 10–12 weeks of gestation, suggesting that, initially, androgen production is autonomous (Grumbach et al. 2003). Peak levels of testosterone are reached by 15–16 weeks of gestation, by which time external genital masculinisation is complete. Interestingly, this is before the foetal hypothalamic–pituitary axis is fully functional, which occurs at about 15 weeks of development. After the peak of testosterone levels at 16 weeks, the serum level falls to about half (3.5 nmol/L) until about 24 weeks, after which it is lower but still measurable.

The serum levels of foetal testosterone mirror that of hCG, suggesting that the placenta has an important role in the early events of male sexual development (Kaplan et al. 1976). The key masculinising effects during the second half of gestation (i.e. growth of the penis and scrotum and testicular descent) are probably regulated by the foetal hypothalamus, as babies with congenital hypopituitarism and anencephaly have normal early masculinisation, but micropenis and hypoplastic scrotum with cryptorchidism (Grumbach et al. 2003). In infants born prematurely with severe intrauterine growth restriction (IUGR) due to placental insufficiency, incomplete virilisation of the external genitalia is a recognised association. This is consistent with inadequate placental hCG to stimulate testosterone production from the foetal Leydig cells during a critical phase of sex development.

4.2.4 Anti-Müllerian Hormone (AMH)

This large glycoprotein (140 KDa) secreted by the developing Sertoli cells is one of the first substances produced by the differentiating testis. AMH is secreted into the Wolffian duct and diffuses into the adjacent Müllerian duct to trigger its regression. Identification and purification of AMH took nearly 40 years after Alfred Jost first proposed that there must be another testicular hormone apart from testosterone involved in male sexual differentiation.

AMH is secreted by the testis from 8 to 9 weeks of gestation, and postnatally, there is an increase in secretion coincident with 'minipuberty', after which the blood levels decline but remain measurable until the onset of puberty (Yamanaka et al. 1991). After puberty, AMH is very low in the bloodstream in males but still measurable in the semen (where its function remains unknown). Recent evidence suggests that AMH has a role in brain and lung functions (McLennan and Chong 2017).

In females, the granulosa cells of the ovary produce AMH, but secretion does not begin until well after sexual differentiation is complete, around the time of birth (Seifer and Maclaughlin 2007). During the ovarian cycle, AMH has an important role in follicular physiology and is now used as a marker of ovarian function and reserve (Pankhurst et al. 2016).

The *AMH* gene contains five exons and is located on chromosome 19. The signals controlling activation of the gene at the onset of sexual differentiation are under active analysis, with *SOX9*, *SF1*, *WT1* and *GATA4* known to be involved. There is keen interest in this area because AMH is one of the first secreted factors to be produced after activation of the SRY gene in developing males (see Chap. 2 for details).

AMH acts through two receptors, AMHR-1 and AMHR-2. The ligand binds to AMHR-2, which is a transmembrane serine/threonine kinase, which then phosphorylates the type-1 receptor. The active unit is a tetramer of two molecules each of the type-1 and -2 receptor, which on AMH binding initiates an intracellular signalling cascade leading to gene activation. Regression of the Müllerian duct occurs in a cranial-to-caudal wave of apoptosis as AMH diffuses down the Wolffian ducts and into the adjacent Müllerian duct, at the same time as the distal Müllerian duct is still migrating to the cloaca.

Anomalies in the *AMH* gene or its receptors cause persistence of the Fallopian tubes, uterus and upper vagina in males (Josso et al. 1983). In mice with homozygous deletion of *amh*, the Wolffian ducts become obstructed by persistence of the Müllerian ducts, leading to infertility. In addition, the Leydig cells show hyperplasia (Josso et al. 2001). Over-expression of human *AMH* in mice causes loss of the Müllerian ducts in females and inadequate virilisation in males, secondary to suppression of steroidogenesis in the Leydig cells (Behringer et al. 1990).

Humans with variants in *AMH* or *AMHR-2* show a similar, but not identical phenotype. In addition to persistence of internal Müllerian structures, boys with this rare difference, known as the **p**ersistent **M**üllerian **d**uct **s**yndrome (PMDS), have typical virilisation of the external genitalia but testicular descent is commonly incomplete. By contrast, in the rodent, testicular descent is normal. The cord of the gubernaculum in humans with PMDS is elongated, so much so that it resembles an elongated round ligament in a female. This suggests that AMH has an important role in gubernacular development and testicular descent, at least in humans. The absence of obvious morphological effects of *amh* mutation in the mouse gubernaculum, despite the presence of amhr-2, suggests that AMH has only a minor role in gubernacular development in the rodent. Cryptorchidism in humans with PMDS has been postulated to be secondary to mechanical effects of the retained uterus (Josso et al. 1983), although the unusually long gubernacular cords and mobility of the internal genitalia do not support this (Hutson and Baker 1994). Indeed, the excessively mobile testes appear to be at a higher risk of prenatal torsion, causing the vanishing testis (Imbeaud et al. 1995).

4.2.5 Insulin-Like Hormone 3 (INSL3)

It was known for many years that the swelling reaction in the rodent gubernaculum was caused by a low-molecular-weight factor, but it remained unidentified until 1999. The missing hormone was called 'descendin' (Fentener van Vlissingen et al. 1988). The mystery was eventually solved from another part of biology, when transgenic mice were generated with variants in a gene related in structure to insulin and relaxin. The male mice with these genes had intra-abdominal testes with absence of the swelling reaction in the gubernaculum, supporting the proposal that so-called 'descendin' was actually insulin-like hormone 3 (INSL3), also known as relaxin-like factor (RLF) (Nef and Parada 1999; Zimmerman et al. 1999).

INSL3 is partly homologous with relaxin, consistent with both hormones evolving from a common precursor gene. Duplication of this ancestral gene occurred about the time of early mammalian evolution, with relaxin becoming involved in breast development and INSL3 acting on the gubernaculum (Park et al. 2008). INSL3 and relaxin have separate receptors (LGR8 and LGR7, respectively), but with some overlap in binding between alternate ligands and receptors.

A mutant mouse with a partial chromosomal deletion (GREAT) was identified with a similar phenotype to that of *insl3* mutant mice and was subsequently found to have a deleted LGR8 receptor (Gorlov et al. 2002). The *insl3* receptor (LGR8) has been localised to the foetal gubernaculum (Park et al. 2008), and addition of synthesised human INSL3 to rat gubernaculum in organ culture caused the expected swelling reaction (Kubota et al. 2002). Auxiliary roles were found for dihydrotestosterone (DHT) and AMH, and the AMHR-2 receptor was also present in the gubernaculum, along with LGR8, but not LGR7 (Kubota et al. 2002).

Release of INSL3 from the foetal Leydig cells occurs at the time of the swelling reaction during the first phase of descent (10–15 weeks in humans), but the regulation of its secretion is not yet known. AMH may play a role, as there are AMHR-2 receptors on Leydig cells, and transgenic mice with over-expression of *Amh* have interference with Leydig cell function. AMH is quite likely to have a more significant role in humans than in rodents, as evidenced by the unusually long gubernacular cord in boys with PMDS (Hutson et al. 1987, 1994).

4.3 Ovarian Hormones

Oestrogen synthesis is possible in the developing ovary, even as early as 8–9 weeks of gestation (George and Wilson 1979). However, the cell within the early ovary that can synthesise oestrogen may well be an interstitial cell, rather than the granulosa cells, which are not yet fully formed (Gondos and Hobel 1973). There are no gonadotrophin receptors in the early ovary between 8 and 16 weeks of development, so that the foetal ovary becomes sensitive to gonadotrophins between 16 and 20 weeks of development, which is probably important for the later development and maintenance of the ovarian follicles (Grumbach et al. 2003).

The role of oestrogens in development of the female genital tract remains difficult to determine, as models of oestrogen deficiency are not compatible with pregnancy. It is quite likely that both maternal oestrogens, along with foetal ovarian oestrogens in the second and third trimesters have key (as yet unidentified roles) in uterine and vaginal differentiation.

4.4 The Placenta

The placenta has several key roles in sex development. Human chorionic gonadotrophin (hCG) secreted by the placenta is structurally similar to luteinising hormone (LH) and has similar biological effects. It is therefore the likely main regulator of testosterone production during the crucial phase of sexual differentiation between 8 and 12 to 15 weeks, when the internal and external phenotypes are modified. Later, in gestation, this regulatory function is mostly taken over by the foetal hypothalamic–pituitary axis, which oversees gonadal hormone production to allow penile and scrotal growth, as well as testicular descent in males, and uterine and vaginal development in females. However, it is possible that hCG later in gestation may have other functions in sex development, and some authors have suggested a role in testicular descent (Hadziselimovic et al. 2016)

Another key placental function is to aromatise any gonadal or adrenal androgens in the foetal bloodstream, thereby preventing masculinisation of both the mother and a female foetus (Grumbach and Auchus 1999).

4.5 The Foetal Hypothalamic–Pituitary Axis

Development of the male genitalia requires a functional hypothalamic–pituitary–gonadal axis but only in the second half of pregnancy, after sexual differentiation of the external genitalia is complete at about 12–15 weeks of gestation. Initially, androgen production is autonomous but is probably quickly brought under the control of placental hCG. Baby boys with hypothalamic or pituitary disorders show typical male external genitalia but show limited phallic growth with micropenis and scrotal hypoplasia and cryptorchidism. Since the first phase of testicular descent is controlled by INSL3, stimulating the swelling reaction in the gubernaculum, the testes are nearly always descended to the inguinal region where they are palpable just outside the external inguinal rings.

4.6 Postnatal Hormone Levels and Implications (Fig. 4.4)

Shortly after birth, levels of both LH and FSH are low in both sexes. As a result, serum levels of androgens and AMH fall to basal levels, so that in the first week, they may be low or barely detectable. However, following clearance of placental hormones in the early days of life, gonadotrophin levels start to rise and ultimately peak between 1 week and 3 months of life. This surge of gonadotrophins triggers a corresponding rise in testosterone production, with levels usually seen to rise

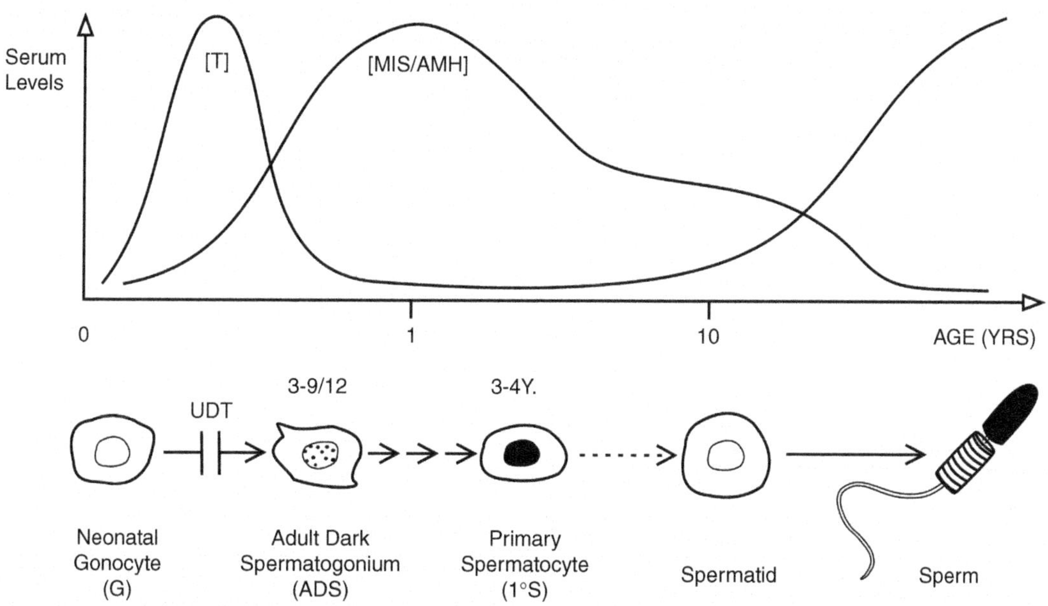

Fig. 4.4 Schema of serum levels of testosterone (T) and Anti-Müllerian Hormone (AMH) from birth to puberty, along with the testicular germ cell development. Note the hormone peaks in the first year and the block in germ cell maturation from gonocytes to adult dark spermatogonia caused by undescended testes (UDT)

from the second week of life. This transient postnatal peak in androgen levels is known as 'mini-puberty' (Kuiri-Hanninen et al. 2014). Circulating testosterone levels typically peak between 1 and 3 months of age, when they may be similar to those in adolescent boys. There is speculation that 'mini-puberty' is important for early postnatal germ cell development (Hadziselimovic et al. 2007; Li et al. 2017). We have also suggested that it may be required for ensuring complete obliteration of the processus vaginalis to prevent inguinal hernia development (Clarnette et al. 1997). In other mammals and birds, there is good evidence that this short burst of androgens after birth/hatching not only is present and similar to humans but has also been shown to be crucial for subsequent masculine behaviour in the adult animal (Hrabovszky and Hutson 2002). Like testosterone, there is also a postnatal rise in AMH, but this occurs slightly later at about 6 months, and it then reaches a peak at 12 months and remains high throughout childhood, not falling again until the onset of puberty (Fig. 4.4) (Baker et al. 1990; Baker and Hutson 1993; Thorup et al. 2015). Compared to testosterone, much less is known about the possible functions of AMH, but there is speculation that it may also have a role in germ cell development (Zhou et al. 1993). More research is needed to understand the place of postnatal hormones in sex development, as it is quite likely to have important clinical implications.

References

Baker ML, Hutson JM. Serum levels of Müllerian inhibiting substance in boys throughout puberty and in the first two years of life. J Clin Endocrinol Metab. 1993;76(1):245–7.

Baker ML, Metcalfe SA, Hutson JM. Serum levels of mullerian inhibiting substance in boys from birth to 18 years, as determined by enzyme immunoassay. J Clin Endocrinol Metab. 1990;70(1):11–5.

Behringer RR, Cate RL, Froelick GJ, et al. Abnormal sexual development in transgenic mice chronically expressing Müllerian inhibiting substance. Nature. 1990;345(6271):167–70.

Boehmer AL, Brinkmann AO, Sandkuijl LA, et al. 17Beta-hydroxysteroid dehydrogenase-3 deficiency: diagnosis, phenotypic variability, population genetics, and worldwide distribution of ancient and de novo mutations. J Clin Endocrinol Metab. 1999;84(12):4713–21.

Chamberlain NL, Driver ED, Miesfeld RL. The length and location of CAG trinucleotide repeats in the androgen receptor N-terminal domain affect transactivation function. Nucleic Acids Res. 1994;22(15):3181–6.

Clarnette T, Sugita Y, JM H. Genital anomalies in the human and animal models reveal the mechanisms and hormones governing testicular descent. Br J Urol. 1997;79:99–112.

Eggers S, Sadedin S, van den Bergen JA, Robevska G, Ohnesorg T, Hewitt J, Lambeth L, Bouty A, Knarston IM, Tan TY, Cameron F, Werther G, Hutson J, O'Connell M, Grover SR, Heloury Y, Zacharin M, Bergman P, Kimber C, Brown J, Webb N, Hunter MF, Srinivasan S, Titmuss A, Verge CF, Mowat D, Smith G, Smith J, Ewans L, Shalhoub C, Crock P, Cowell C, Leong GM, Ono M, Lafferty AR, Huynh T, Visser U, Choong CS, McKenzie F, Pachter N, Thompson EM, Couper J, Baxendale A, Gecz J, Wheeler BJ, Jefferies C, MacKenzie K, Hofman P, Carter P, King RI, Krausz C, van Ravenswaaij-Arts CM, Looijenga L, Drop S, Riedl S, Cools M, Dawson A, Juniarto AZ, Khadilkar V, Khadilkar A, Bhatia V, Dũng VC, Atta I, Raza J, Thi Diem Chi N, Hao TK, Harley V, Koopman P, Warne G, Faradz S, Oshlack A, Ayers KL, Sinclair AH. Disorders of sex development: insights from targeted gene sequencing of a large international patient cohort. Genome Biol. 2016;17(1):243.

Fentener van Vlissingen MF, van Zoelen EJJ, Ursem PJF, et al. In vitro model of the first phase of testicular descent: identification of a low molecular weight factor from fetal testis involved in proliferation of gubernaculum testis cells and distinct from specified polypeptide growth factors and fetal gonadal hormones. Endocrinology. 1988;123:2868–77.

George F, Wilson J. The regulation of androgen and estrogen formation in fetal gonads. Ann Biol Anim Biochim Biophys. 1979;19(4B):1297–306.

Gondos B, Hobel C. Interstitial cells in the human fetal ovary. Endocrinology. 1973;93:736–9.

Gorlov IP, Kamat A, Bogatcheva NV, et al. Mutations of the GREAT gene cause cryptorchidism. Hum Mol Genet. 2002;11(19):2309–18.

Grumbach MM, Auchus RJ. Estrogen: consequences and implications of human mutations in synthesis and action. J Clin Endocrinol Metab. 1999;84(12):4677–94.

Grumbach M, Hughes I, Conte F. Disorders of sex differentiation. In: Larsen KH, PR MS, Polonsky KS, editors. Williams Textbook of Endocrinology. Philadelphia: WB Saunders; 2003. p. 842–968.

Hadziselimovic F, Hocht B, Herzog B, et al. Infertility in cryptorchidism is linked to the stage of germ cell development at orchidopexy. Horm Res. 2007;68(1):46–52.

Hadziselimovic F, Gegenschatz-Schmid K, Verkauskas G, et al. Gene expression changes underlying idiopathic central hypogonadism in cryptorchidism with defective mini-puberty. Sex Dev. 2016;10(3):136–46.

Hrabovszky Z, Hutson JM. Surgical treatment of intersex abnormalities: a review. Surgery. 2002;131(1):92–104.
Hutson JM, Baker M. A hypothesis to explain abnormal gonadal descent in persistent Müllerian duct syndrome. Pediatr Surg Int. 1994;9:542–3.
Hutson J, Chow C, Ng W. Persistent Müllerian duct syndrome with transverse testicular ectopia. an experiment of nature with clues for understanding testicular descent. Pediatr Surg Int. 1987;2:191–4.
Hutson JM, Davidson P, Reece L, et al. Failure of gubernacular development in the persistent Müllerian duct syndrome allows herniation of the testes. Pediatr Surg Int. 1994;9:544–6.
Imbeaud S, Rey R, Berta P, et al. Testicular degeneration in three patients with the persistent Müllerian duct syndrome. Eur J Pediatr. 1995;154(3):187–90.
Josso N, Fekete C, Cachin O, et al. Persistence of Müllerian ducts in male pseudohermaphroditism, and its relationship to cryptorchidism. Clin Endocrinol. 1983;19(2):247–58.
Josso N, di Clemente N, Gouedard L. Anti-Müllerian hormone and its receptors. Mol Cell Endocrinol. 2001;179(1–2):25–32.
Kamrath C, Hochberg Z, Hartmann MF, et al. Increased activation of the alternative "backdoor" pathway in patients with 21-hydroxylase deficiency: evidence from urinary steroid hormone analysis. J Clin Endocrinol Metab. 2012;97(3):E367–75.
Kaplan SL, Grumbach MM, Aubert ML. The ontogenesis of pituitary hormones and hypothalamic factors in the human fetus: maturation of central nervous system regulation of anterior pituitary function. Recent Prog Horm Res. 1976;32:161–243.
Kubota Y, Temelcos C, Bathgate RA, et al. The role of insulin 3, testosterone, Müllerian inhibiting substance and relaxin in rat gubernacular growth. Mol Hum Reprod. 2002;8(10):900–5.
Kuiri-Hanninen T, Sankilampi U, Dunkel L. Activation of the hypothalamic-pituitary-gonadal axis in infancy: minipuberty. Horm Res Paediatr. 2014;82(2):73–80.
Li R, Vannitamby A, Yue SSK, et al. Mouse minipuberty coincides with gonocyte transformation into spermatogonial stem cells: a model for human minipuberty. Reprod Fertil Dev. 2017;29(12):2430–6.
Lobaccaro JM, Lumbroso S, Poujol N, et al. Molecular genetics of androgen insensitivity syndromes. Cell Mol Biol (Noisy-le-Grand). 1994;40(3):301–8.
McLennan IS, Chong YH. Does testicular anti-Müllerian hormone extend life? Endocrine. 2017;55(1):1–2.
Nef S, Parada LF. Cryptorchidism in mice mutant for Insl3. Nat Genet. 1999;22(3):295–9.
Pankhurst MW, Chong YH, McLennan IS. Relative levels of the proprotein and cleavage-activated form of circulating human anti-Müllerian hormone are sexually dimorphic and variable during the life cycle. Physiol Rep. 2016;4(9).
Park JI, Semyonov J, Chang CL, et al. Origin of INSL3-mediated testicular descent in therian mammals. Genome Res. 2008;18(6):974–85.
Seifer DB, Maclaughlin DT. Müllerian inhibiting substance is an ovarian growth factor of emerging clinical significance. Fertil Steril. 2007;88(3):539–46.
Shaw G, Renfree MB, Leihy MW, et al. Prostate formation in a marsupial is mediated by the testicular androgen 5 alpha-androstane-3 alpha,17 beta-diol. Proc Natl Acad Sci U S A. 2000;97(22):12256–9.
Siiteri P, Wilson J. Testosterone formation and metabolism during male sexual differentiation in the human embryo. J Clin Endocrinol Metab. 1974;38:113–25.
Thorup J, Clasen-Linde E, Thorup SC, et al. Pre- and postoperative status of gonadotropins (FSH and LH) and inhibin-B in relation to testicular histopathology at orchiopexy in infant boys with unilateral undescended testes. J Pediatr Urol. 2015;11(1):25 e21–5.
Tong SY, Hutson JM, Watts LM. Does testosterone diffuse down the Wolffian duct during sexual differentiation? J Urol. 1996;155(6):2057–9.
Warne GL, Kanumakala S. Molecular endocrinology of sex differentiation. Semin Reprod Med. 2002;20(3):169–80.
Wilson JD, Auchus RJ, Leihy MW, et al. 5alpha-androstane-3alpha,17beta-diol is formed in tammar wallaby pouch young testes by a pathway involving 5alpha-pregnane-3alpha,17alpha-diol-20-one as a key intermediate. Endocrinology. 2003;144(2):575–80.
Yamanaka J, Baker M, Metcalfe S, et al. Serum levels of Müllerian inhibiting substance in boys with cryptorchidism. J Pediatr Surg. 1991;26(5):621–3.
Zhou B, Watts LM, Hutson JM. Germ cell development in neonatal mouse testes in vitro requires Müllerian inhibiting substance. J Urol. 1993;150(2 Pt 2):613–6.
Zimmerman S, Steding G, Emmen J, et al. Targeted disruption of the INSL3 gene causes bilateral cryprotchidism. Mol Endocrinol. 1999;13:681–91.

Embryology in DSD

5

John M. Hutson and Aurore Bouty

5.1 Sex Determination

The first step in sexual differentiation is the activation of the *SRY* gene to trigger testicular development at 7–8 weeks of development. When there is a variation or deletion of *SRY*, or one of the early downstream genes in gonadal differentiation, such as *SOX9*, then the gonads do not mature into either ovary or testis and become non-functional streak gonads. The streak gonad is unable to support the germ cells, which are lost. Failure of testicular development leads to absent male hormones required for masculinisation of both the internal and external genitalia. This leads to regression of the mesonephric (Wolffian) duct and preservation of the paramesonephric (Müllerian) duct. The external genitalia continue on the female developmental pathway, leading to a complete external female phenotype at birth. The fallopian tubes, uterus and vagina form normally in the absence of AMH, while absent INSL3 leads to an absence of the swelling reaction in the gubernaculum, so the streak gonads occupy the position of ovaries, in an intra-abdominal position.

A similar developmental pathway occurs in individuals with non-disjunction of the sex chromosomes, leading to the 45,X genotype (Turner syndrome). In this circumstance, the primitive germ cells migrate from the caudal yolk-sac into the bi-potential gonad, but absence of the second X chromosome leads to the follicles undergoing premature senescence usually either in early childhood or in puberty. Although there is a substantial loss in germ cells in all 46,XX individuals from a peak of 20×10^6 at 20 weeks of gestation to 1×10^6 at birth, this loss of germ cells is faster in those with 45,X. Biopsy of the gonad at birth or shortly after may show some primary follicles, but they regress leaving the non-functional streak ovary that is the hallmark of Turner Syndrome (Fig. 5.1) (Ngan and Mitchell 1997). The vast majority of pregnancies with 45,X (98–99%) end as a first trimester pregnancy loss. Occasionally, ovarian function persists until later in life, particularly in those patients with 45,X/46,XX mosaicism (known as Turner-Ullrich syndrome). In some individuals who have 45,X/46,XY mosaicism, with a small percentage of 46,XY cells, the presence of the Y material predisposes to malignant change in the streak gonads. Removal of the

J. M. Hutson (✉)
Department of Urology, The Royal Children's Hospital, Melbourne, VIC, Australia

Murdoch Children's Research Institute, Melbourne, VIC, Australia

Department of Paediatrics, University of Melbourne, Melbourne, VIC, Australia
e-mail: john.hutson@rch.org.au

A. Bouty
Department of Urology, The Royal Children's Hospital, Melbourne, VIC, Australia

Murdoch Children's Research Institute, Melbourne, VIC, Australia
e-mail: aurore.bouty@rch.org.au

J. M. Hutson et al. (eds.), *Disorders|Differences of Sex Development*,
https://doi.org/10.1007/978-981-13-7864-5_5

streak, non-functioning gonads is indicated in this circumstance, as there is no fertility potential and no hormonal production.

In some rare forms of atypical sex determination, there is complete sex reversal, with XY females or XX males. In the latter case, the common cause is translocation of a small segment of the Y chromosome that includes the *SRY* gene, onto the X chromosome, usually at Yp11.3 (Table 5.1). This is now recognised by fluorescent *in situ* hybridisation (FISH) with a marker for the *SRY* gene.

5.2 46,XY Complete Gonadal Dysgenesis

In this condition, there is a variation of the Y chromosome affecting the region of the *SRY* gene. In 15–30% of patients, a variation in this region can be identified (see Chap. 21).

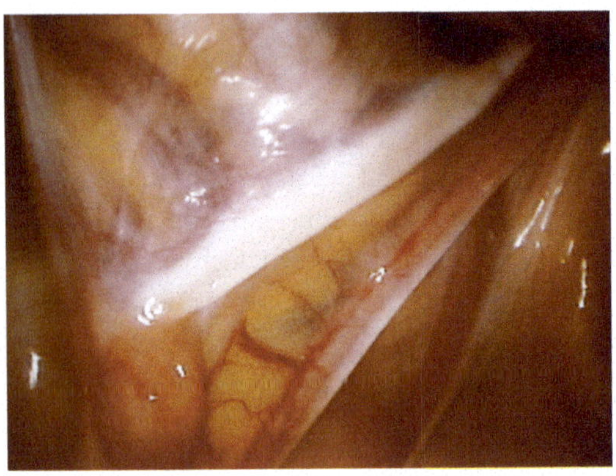

Fig. 5.1 A streak gonad seen at laparoscopy

Because *SRY* signalling is disrupted, the bipotential gonads do not differentiate into testes and remain as non-functional streak gonads. Absence of testosterone and AMH allows female external development, and internally, there is persistence of the Müllerian ducts into a female genital tract.

Individuals usually present at puberty with primary amenorrhoea and/or delayed development of secondary sex characteristics. Their stature is normal or tall, rather than short, in contrast to those with Turner syndrome. More recently, some of these individuals are recognised at birth, when there is discordance between antenatal testing, which identified a 46,XY complement and the baby with completely female external genitalia.

There is a high risk of development of a gonadal tumour by late adolescence, and in one series of eight patients presenting between 13 and 18 years of age, six had tumours (gonadoblastoma and/or dysgerminoma) at the time of diagnosis (Zielinska et al. 2007). Overall, the risk for tumours in individuals with 46,XY complete GD has been reported to be as high as 54% (Wolffenbuttel et al. 2016) and to occur in individuals <10 years old (Frasier et al. 1964)

5.3 Incomplete Testicular Differentiation (and Mixed Gonadal Dysgenesis)

The genetic pathway regulating testicular development after *SRY* activation remains largely unknown. Although the downstream genes themselves remain obscure, it is possible to predict

Table 5.1 Sex reversal syndromes

Syndrome	OMIM no.	Genetics	Clinical features
Autosomal sex reversal syndrome	154230	DMTI gene deleted on 9p24	Females with 46,XY and pure gonadal dysgenesis
Campomelic dysplasia	114290	SOX9 haplo-insufficiency at 17q24.3-q25.1	Females with 46,XY gonadal dysgenesis and bowed long bones
Dosage-sensitive sex reversal	300018	DAX1 duplication at Xp21.2-21.3	Females with 46,XY gonadal dysgenesis
Rutledge lethal multiple anomaly syndrome	268670	7-Dehydrocholesterol reductase gene variant at 11q12-13	Females with 46,XY and polydactyly Congenital heart defects Renal + pulmonary hypoplasia
46,XY complete gonadal dysgenesis	306100	SRY variant/deletion at Xp21.2-22	Females with 46,XY gonadal dysgenesis
XX male syndrome	278850	SRY translocation to X chromosome (Yp11.3)	Males with 46,XX

that variants in these genes may produce various forms of gonadal dysgenesis (Fig. 5.2). This may include decrease in overall testicular size (testicular hypoplasia), so that the total volume of hormone production is significantly decreased. This will lead to impaired virilisation of both the internal and external genitalia (Fig. 5.3). Also, delayed onset of testicular differentiation may produce a testis with apparently normal function postnatally, but the delay will result in impaired sexual differentiation, which is required to occur in a narrow window of time between 8 and 12 weeks of development.

A more common cause of testicular maldevelopment occurs in mixed chromosomal DSD, also known as mixed gonadal dysgenesis (45,X/46,XY)

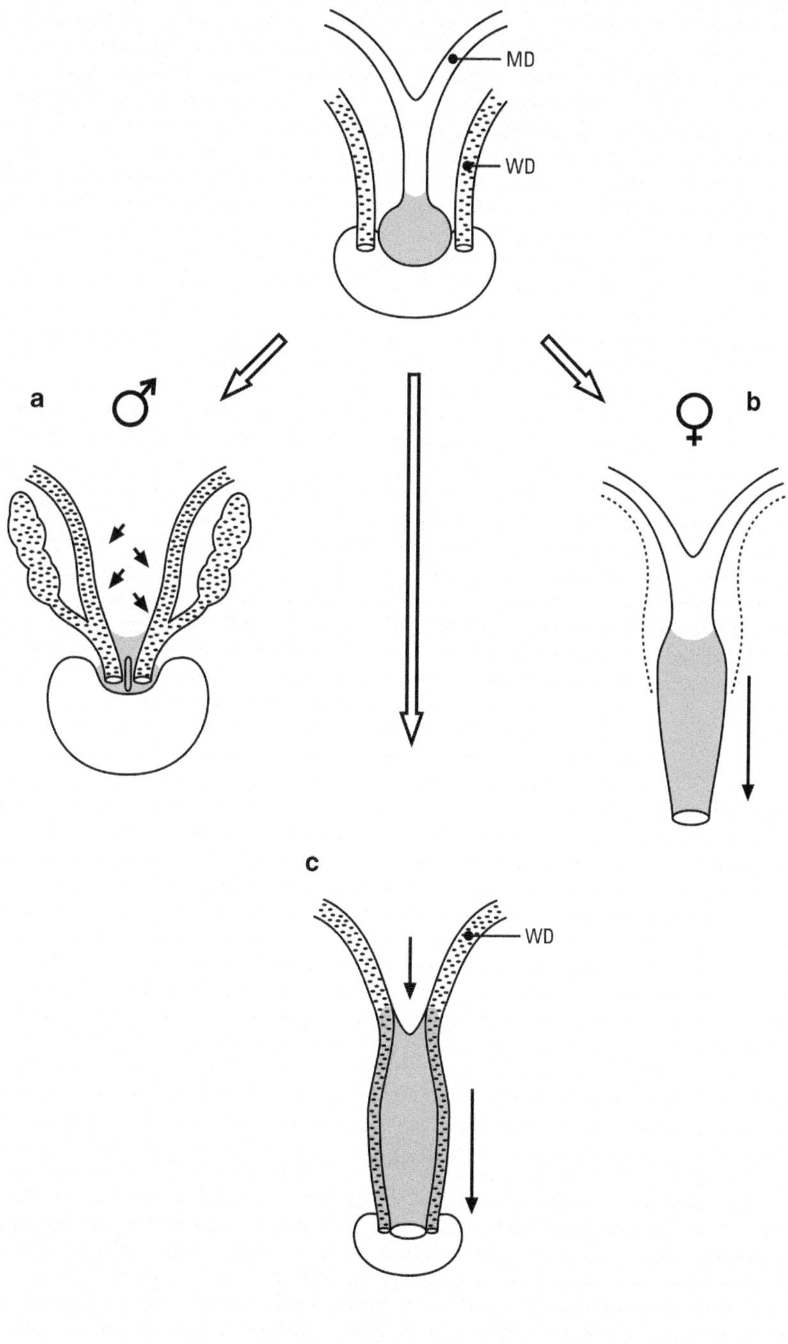

Fig. 5.2 (**a**) Müllerian duct (MD) regressed with normal AMH levels in a male. (**b**) Normal downward growth of vaginal plate to vestibule and regression of Wolffian ducts in a female. (**c**) Wolffian ducts (WD) incorporated into the side of vaginal plate secondary to moderate testosterone levels in 5α-reductase deficiency. Partially inhibited downward growth of conjoined urogenital sinus opening secondary to inadequate DHT levels (Reproduced with permission from Ben-Meir and Hutson (2005))

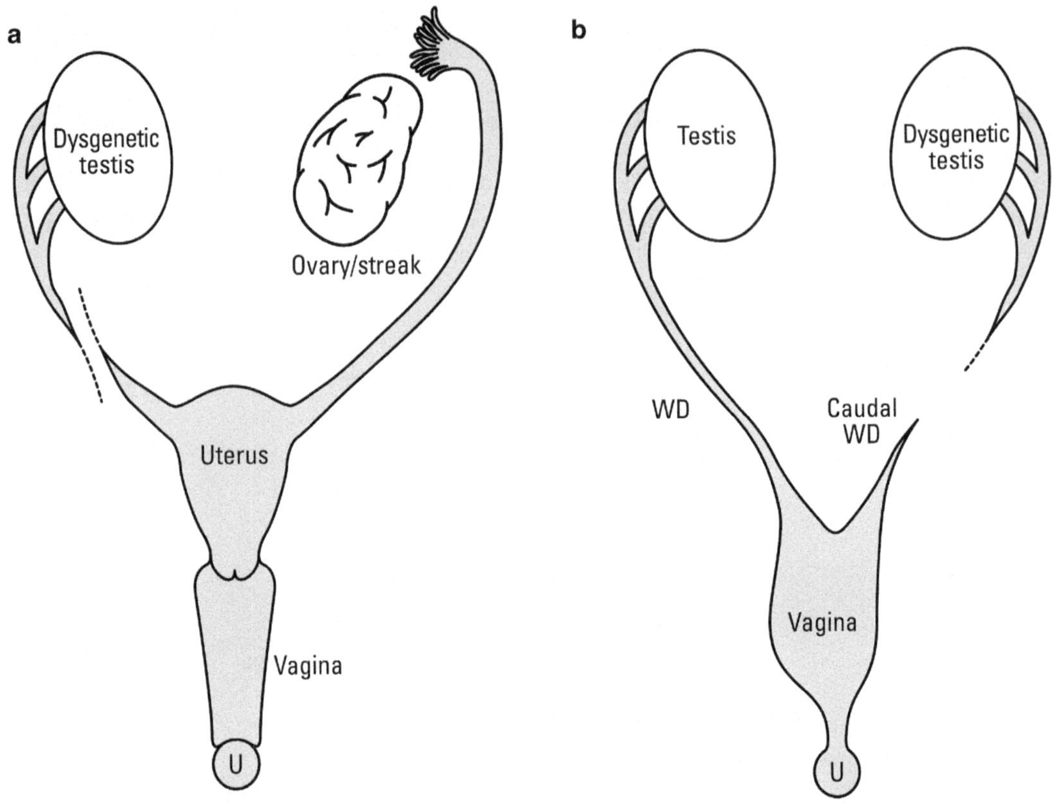

Fig. 5.3 (**a**) Variant of gonadal dysgenesis (as in MGD or ovo-testicular DSD): unilateral, poorly developed testis leads to local epididymal preservation only, with persistence of contralateral as well as distal ipsilateral Müllerian duct, secondary to inadequate exocrine function. Vagina is also preserved because of inadequate endocrine function. (**b**) Variant of gonadal dysgenesis (MGD): unilateral well-developed testis leads to complete ipsilateral Wolffian duct as well as the caudal end of contralateral duct. Contralateral dysgenetic gonad produces only enough androgen to preserve the epididymis. Inadequate AMH secretion leads to incomplete Müllerian regression. *U* urethra, *WD* Wolffian duct (Reproduced with permission from Ben-Meir and Hutson (2005))

related to mosaicism of the sex chromosomes. This may result in two dysplastic testes, but commonly, the mosaicism is segregated so that one gonad develops into a testis (with or without variable dysplasia), while the other gonad becomes a non-functional streak. This form of DSD produces a variable degree of virilisation on each side of the internal genitalia, as the male hormones are present only on one side, leading to the preservation of part or all of the Wolffian duct on the testicular side, while the Müllerian duct is preserved on the side of the streak gonad (Fig. 5.3) (Nonaka et al. 1998; Marszalek et al. 1999; Takeda et al. 1999; Ben-Meir and Hutson 2005) (Box 5.1).

Box 5.1: Asymmetry of the Urogenital Ridges in Normal Birds and Humans with DSD

The overriding asymmetry of the body of vertebrates is mostly concealed in the urogenital tract, although it is not only obvious but also completely normal in birds (Hutson et al. 1983). In the chick embryo, the urogenital ridges are symmetrical in males, but in the female embryo, there is distinctive asymmetry. Initial ambisexual stages of development are symmetrical, but once the gonads begin to develop, the left gonad forms a normal ovary, but the right gonadal development is partly testicular, forming an ovo-testis. Indeed, the right gonad produces sufficient AMH to cause regression of the right Müllerian duct, so that the female ends up with a uterus forming from only the left Müllerian duct (Hutson et al. 1983). Although the AMH circulates through the blood, the left Müllerian duct is relatively resistant to regression, related to different expression of oestrogen receptors, which protect it from regression. The right ovo-testis is vestigial in a young hen but may degenerate later in life with development of gonadal tumours with full-blown development of testicular hormones, which may masculinise the aging hen (Hutson et al. 1983).

The asymmetrical urogential ridge in birds shows that the two sides can differentiate differently, with the right side being more 'masculine'. It is fascinating to observe similar sidedness in humans with asymmetrical gonadal development, where, as in birds, the right side of the body is more likely to be the masculine side. In babies with mixed gonadal dysgenesis and ovo-testicular DSD, it is the right gonad that is more likely to be a testis, while the left gonad is more frequently an ovo-testis, streak gonad or ovary (Forest 2006).

5.4 Anatomy of Caudal Internal Ducts in DSD

The Wolffian duct persists as epididymis and vas deferens in most patients with 45,X/46,XY MGD ipsilateral to the gonad that has formed into a testis (albeit dysgenetic) (Zah et al. 1975). In a series of 15 patients with MGD, Alvarez-Nava and co-authors found only one child with Wolffian duct structures on the same side as the streak gonad (Alvarez-Nava et al. 1999). In another series of 14 patients with MGD, seven had a vas deferens on the same side as the dysgenetic testis (Donahoe et al. 1979). These cases suggest that there had been some exocrine function arising from the gonad/testes, although at the time of assessment, the gonad was now considered a streak and non-functional. At the caudal end of the internal ducts, the vas deferens has been reported to enter into a persisting Müllerian duct or vaginal remnant (Hrabovszky and Hutson 2002; Ben-Meir and Hutson 2005). This has also been reported in ovo-testicular DSD (Nihoul-Fekete et al. 1984).

The association of internal genital ducts with ipsilateral gonadal development was likely to be caused by the male hormones (testosterone and AMH) being secreted down the Wolffian duct in an exocrine fashion (Tong et al. 1996). In an *in vitro* study of the urogenital ridge, fluorescent androgen injected into the testis did not diffuse radially from the site of injection within the testis but was immediately transported into and along the Wolffian duct, so that within a few hours of culture, nearly all the fluorescence was found within the distal Wolffian duct, consistent with active transport along the duct system. This putative exocrine secretion of hormones into the Wolffian duct is not surprising, when one appreciates that it was functioning just before sexual development as the mesonephric, excretory duct of the 'middle kidney', or mesonephros, and that some small amounts of 'urine' pass down the duct to the cloaca.

The anatomy of the caudal ends of the Wolffian and Müllerian ducts is predictable when it is assumed that testosterone and AMH pass down the Wolffian duct from the ipsilateral gonad. When a dysgenetic testis is produced, the amount of ipsilateral Wolffian duct that persists would then be predicted to be directly proportional to the amount of testosterone that is manufactured. If the testis is well formed, the entire Wolffian duct will be preserved. By contrast, however, when the gonad forms a dysplastic testis, only the most proximal part of the Wolffian duct will persist to form epididymis and some proximal vas deferens. Regression of the Müllerian duct is the mirror-image of this, so that where only the proximal Wolffian duct is preserved, the distal Müllerian duct may persist as a blind-ending fallopian tube or uterine horn. By contrast, inhibition of development of the vaginal plate to form the vagina requires circulating androgens and conversion of testosterone to DHT. This can lead to unusual variants where the Wolffian duct has been preserved by exocrine action of androgen secreted down the duct, but there is inadequate endocrine function of androgens so that there is a vaginal remnant and deficient seminal vesicles (Fig. 5.3).

5.5 Placental Failure

In the developing embryo, the initial production of testicular hormones was thought to be autonomous, as the foetal hypothalamus and pituitary are not functional until around 15 weeks of development (Forest 2006). Recent evidence, however, suggests that the early testis is probably responding to stimulation by the placenta, which produces chorionic gonadotrophin (hCG). This trophic effect of placental hormones may be more important than once thought, as demonstrated in some babies with severe intra-uterine growth restriction (IUGR) and extreme prematurity. We now see some extremely premature male infants with severe IUGR with under-virilisation of the external genitalia, suggesting insufficient androgen production between 8 and 12 weeks, secondary to placental failure. By the time the foetal hypothalamic–pituitary axis is functional, the incomplete genital development is permanent. Subsequent investigations postnatally have revealed no endocrinopathy, although the placentas were reported to be very hypoplastic (Mouriquand et al. 2016).

5.6 Failure of the Hypothalamic–Pituitary–Gonadal Axis

The foetal nervous system develops at a different rate from the urogenital tract, and variations of hypothalamic or pituitary function have a characteristic appearance in males. As mentioned above, the pituitary begins producing trophic hormones (follicle-stimulating hormone (FSH) and luteinising hormone (LH)) to regulate testicular function at about 15 weeks of development. Where there is a structural anomaly (e.g. septo-optic dysplasia) or a molecular defect in hormone-signalling pathways (LH mutation, LH receptor mutations), the internal and external genitalia will have masculinised normally in a male by 15 weeks. However, development thereafter will be inhibited by lack of testicular hormone secretion, leading to cessation of phallic growth. Male babies with hypothalamic or pituitary disorders have completely formed male external genitalia (indicating normal hormone levels between 8 and 12 weeks) but inadequate subsequent penile growth, leading to micropenis. In addition, because testicular descent occurs later in development, and the second step, the inguino-scrotal phase, requires androgens, this is likely to be disrupted, leaving undescended testes palpable in the inguinal regions (Fig. 5.4).

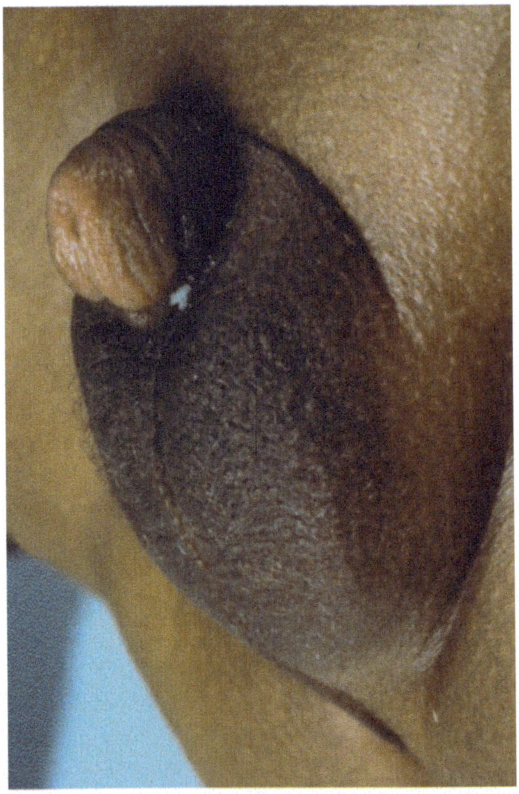

Fig. 5.4 External genitalia of a boy with micropenis, secondary to inadequate androgenic stimulation in the second half of pregnancy, when the foetal hypothalamic–pituitary–gonadal axis should be functioning

5.7 Failure of Hormone Action

5.7.1 INSL3

INSL3 is produced by the Leydig cells and is known to cause the swelling reaction in the gubernaculum, enabling its distal end to enlarge in males. The enlarged gubernaculum remains short with progressive foetal growth, while in the female, the gubernaculum elongates into the round ligament and ligament of the ovary. The result is that the testes descend from their initial embryonic position high in the abdominal cavity to the internal inguinal ring. The swelling reaction occurs at about 10–15 weeks of development in the human. Failure of INSL3 production, or variants in its gene or receptor (LGR8), would produce failure of the transabdominal phase of testicular descent. A number of authors have screened boys with cryptorchidism for anomalies in the *INSL3* or *LGR8* genes, but to date, only a small number of cases have been reported (Adham and Agoulnik 2004; Chavez-Saldana et al. 2018; Lu et al. 2018).

5.7.2 AMH

Sertoli cells produce AMH, which diffuses down the Wolffian duct to reach the adjacent ipsilateral Müllerian duct. Mutations in the *AMH* gene or its receptor produce a unique genital anomaly known as the persistent Müllerian duct syndrome (PMDS) (Hutson et al. 1987; Hutson et al. 1994; Hutson and Baker 1994; Hutson and Lopez-Marambio 2017). In this rare anomaly, the Müllerian ducts persist as a female genital tract in an otherwise completely virilised male, whose only other anomaly is cryptorchidism. Although INSL3 is known to be the primary hormone regulating the swelling reaction in rodents, AMH has been shown to have a subsidiary role in gubernacular enlargement in organ culture and the gubernaculum contains AMH receptors (Kubota et al. 2002; Fu et al. 2004).

It is quite likely that the role of AMH on gubernacular development is more significant in humans than in rodents, as in boys, there is a very tight link between Müllerian duct regression and ipsilateral descent of the testis (Scott 1987; Abe and Hutson 1994; Hutson and Lopez-Marambio 2017).

In boys with PMDS, there are three main clinical presentations, depending on the location of the testes (Fig. 5.5). Because androgenic function is normal, the cranial suspensory ligament has regressed, and despite the persistence of the Müllerian ducts, the broad ligament is hypoplastic (because of the absence of oestrogens). Abnormality of the swelling reaction, with failure of the gubernacular cord to remain short, leads to the gubernaculum being unusually long, even longer than a normal round ligament in a girl. As androgen production and action is unimpeded, the second phase of testicular descent, migration of the caudal end of the gubernaculum to the scrotum, appears to be relatively normal, despite abnormality of the transabdominal phase of descent. This leaves the inguinal canals open with a patent *processus vaginalis* extending into the hemiscrotum. The testis, however, rather than being within the scrotum and attached by a very short gubernacular cord to the inside of the *processus vaginalis*, is usually located within the abdomen attached to a greatly elongated gubernacular cord (Fig. 5.6).

In the commonest clinical variant described in the literature (60–70%), both testes are in an 'ovarian' position within the abdomen and the inguinal hernial sacs remain empty. There is a smaller group, comprising 20%–30% of all cases described, where one testis is located within an inguinal hernia, along with its attached Fallopian tube and infantile uterus. This variety is known as '*hernia uteri inguinalis*'. In the remaining 10% of patients, both testes are found within the same patent *processus vaginalis*, producing transverse testicular ectopia. At operation, the testes are not anchored to the inside of the *processus vaginalis* in the normal way, as the gubernaculum is so long that it can permit herniation of one testis out into a contralateral hernial sac! In one of these cases witnessed by JMH, delivery of the contents of a right inguinal hernia in a phenotypic boy with a left cryptorchid testis (palpable in the groin), led to the left testis disappearing into the

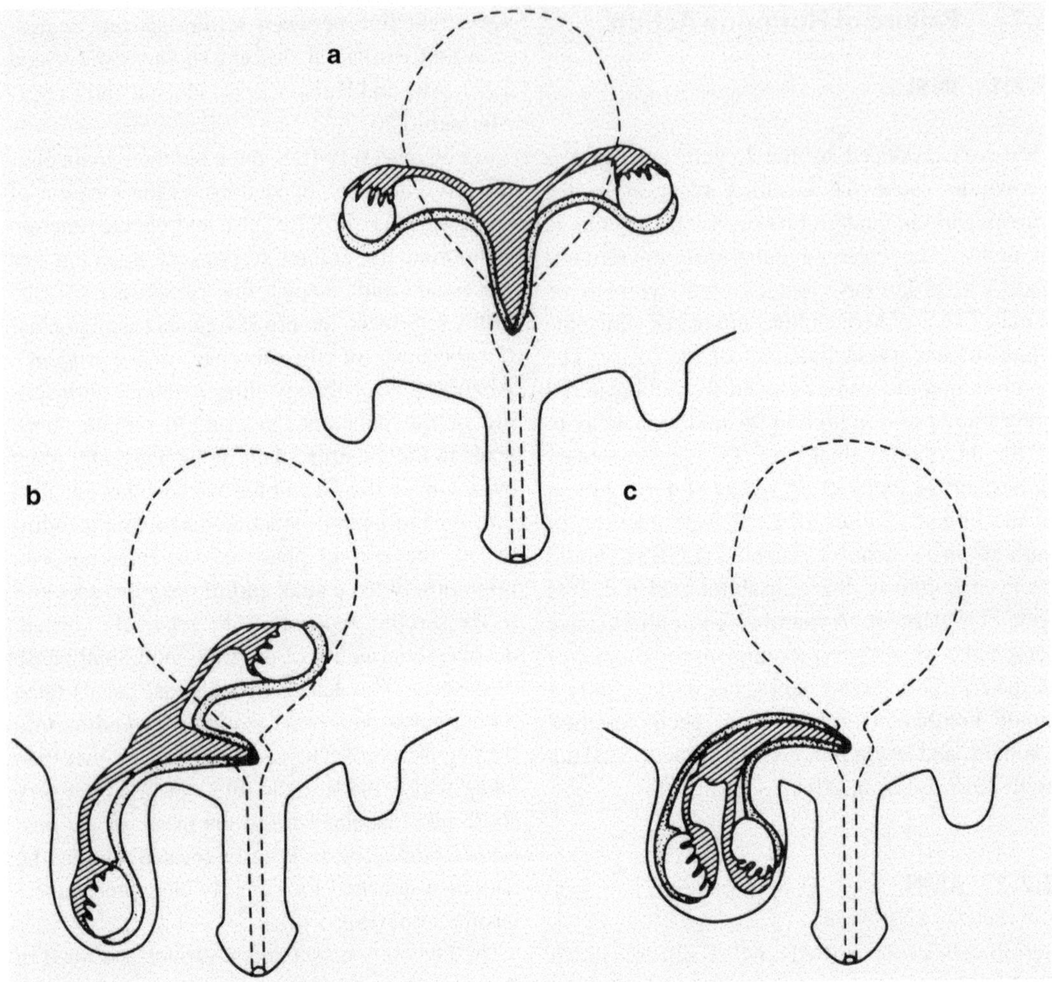

Fig. 5.5 The three clinical presentations of persistent Müllerian duct syndrome (PMDS). The testis is highly mobile due to regression of the cranial suspensory ligament and the presence of a long and thin gubernacular cord. (**a**) Most (60%–70%) patients have testes in the normal position of ovaries and the inguinal sacs remain patent but empty. (**b**) A smaller group (20%–30%) have one testis in an inguinal hernia along with its attached tube and uterus. This is known as '*hernia uteri inguinalis*'. (**c**) About 10% of patients have both testes herniated into one processus vaginalis (transverse testicular ectopia) (Reproduced with permission from Hutson and Lopez-Marambio (2017))

abdominal cavity and reappearing in the right inguinal hernia! These findings suggest that 'descent' of the testis into the groin or scrotum in PMDS is actually prolapse of a highly mobile genital tract, rather than normal testicular migration (Hutson and Lopez-Marambio 2017).

Many authors have come to a contrary explanation for cryptorchidism in PMDS, concluding that testicular descent was passively impeded by the attachments of the broad ligaments and Fallopian tubes (Josso et al. 1993). The highly mobile genital tract in PMDS, however, is such that the entire internal genital tract can be delivered out of a laparotomy wound for photography, in a way which is not usually possible in either males or females (Fig. 5.7). By contrast, if the cause of cryptorchidism was merely passive prevention of gonadal descent by the persistent Müllerian ducts, one would expect the testes to be closely bound to each internal inguinal ring by a normal gubernacular cord. Clearly, this is not the case in PMDS.

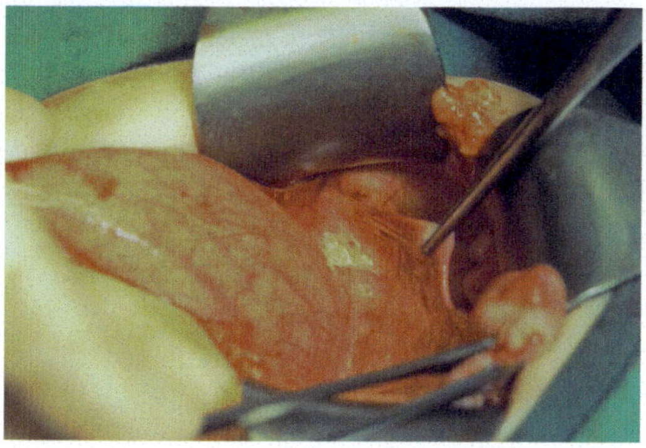

Fig. 5.6 Intra-operative photograph of a boy with PMDS showing the elongated gubernacular cord more than 10 cm long extending from the right internal inguinal ring to the right testis out of focus in the foreground

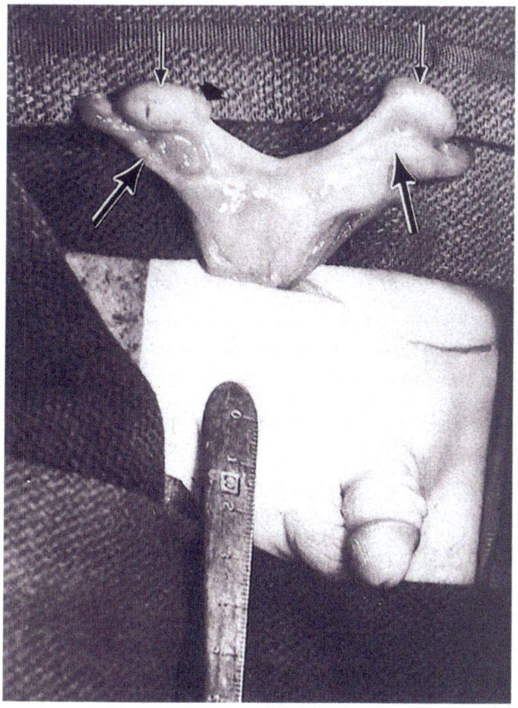

Fig. 5.7 Photograph of the genital tract being delivered from the wound during a laparotomy for a boy with PMDS (Miller et al. 2004) (reproduced with permission of the publisher)

The most useful deduction from understanding the anatomy of PMDS is the tight link between Müllerian duct regression and testicular descent in babies with DSD. Where the testis is palpable in the groin in a baby with atypical genitalia, we can predict that the ipsilateral Müllerian duct has undergone regression, and hence, there will be no Fallopian tube and uterine horn on that side.

5.7.3 Androgen

Failure of androgen production is most commonly caused by a variant in the enzyme 17β-hydroxysteroid dehydrogenase-3 (17β-HSD3). Androgen synthesis is frequently substantially reduced, such that the external genitalia are completely or nearly completely female at birth, where the foetal testis is unable to synthesise enough androgen for virilisation of the external genitalia. The first clue to this variation may be primary amenorrhoea at puberty and signs of virilisation caused by the larger adolescent testis now being able to produce sufficient androgen despite the reduced functioning of the enzyme. Despite 46,XY chromosomes and undescended testes in the inguinal canals or groins, these individuals usually have a female gender orientation, suggesting that significant androgens are necessary during foetal development or in the postnatal 'minipuberty' for gender development (Hrabovszky and Hutson 2002). Minor virilisation at puberty is probably related to excessive hypothalamic drive (because negative feedback is lacking), which causes testicular enlargement and allows testosterone production to increase even when the variant has deactivated the enzyme by 95%.

Variations of the androgen receptor gene lead to complete or partial androgen insensitivity syndrome (CAIS or PAIS) depending on the remaining function of the receptor. The external genitalia are completely feminine in CAIS, confirming that androgens are essential for masculinisation. As the testis has normal Sertoli and Leydig cell function, AMH production is normal and the Müllerian ducts regress. Absence of negative feedback leads to testicular hypertrophy from pituitary stimulation. The testes are in the inguinal canals or groins, as the first phase of testicular descent is normal (Fig. 5.8). Gender orientation is female in CAIS, and either male or female in

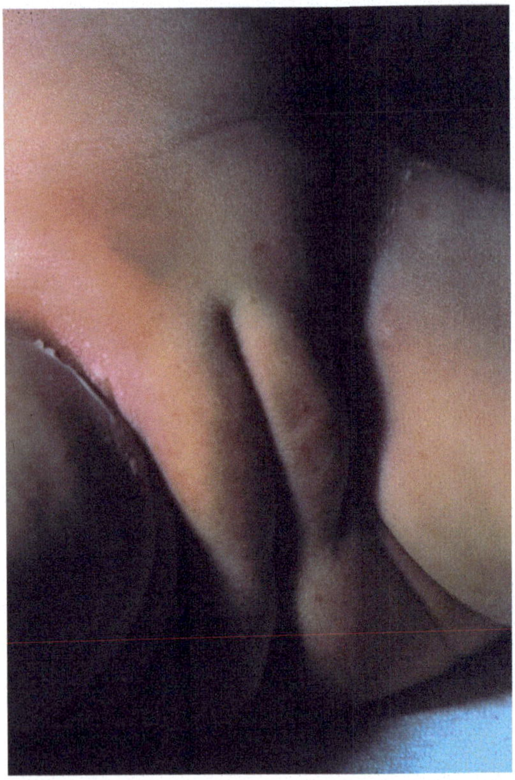

Fig. 5.8 A 1-week-old girl (46,XY) with complete androgen insensitivity syndrome and female phenotype. The trans-abdominal migration of the testes is normal, but inguinoscrotal migration is absent, leaving the testes in the groin (Clarnette et al. 1997), reproduced with permission

PAIS, depending on the level of androgen receptor function and the amount of exposure, although the exact predictors for brain sex remain to be determined (Hrabovszky and Hutson 2002).

Aromatase variations lead to virilisation of both foetus and mother, as not only the foetus but also the placenta is unable to neutralise any foetal androgens by conversion to oestrogens in females.

Mixed effects on the 46,XY foetus are seen where there is a 5α-reductase-2 gene variant, leaving the external genitalia under-virilised. Masculinisation of the brain, however, seems less affected, as patients are reported to develop male gender identity at puberty, when testicular growth occurs. This suggests that 5α-reductase-2 is less important in the brain than the genitalia, perhaps because sexual dimorphism of the brain is occurring later in gestation when circulating androgen levels may be higher than that at 8–12 weeks when the testis first develops (Hrabovszky and Hutson 2002; Veale et al. 2010)

5.8 Morphogenesis of the Genitalia (See Also Chap. 9)

Failure of ingrowth of mesenchyme from the periumbilical region and from the primitive streak to migrate around the cloacal membrane may prevent typical development of the lower anterior abdominal wall and genital tubercle, which may lead to bladder exstrophy. Recent evidence suggests that genes involving differentiation of abdominal wall muscle and the anterior bladder muscle may be involved (Ngan and Mitchell 1997; Lund and Hendren 2001; Reiner and Gearhart 2004; Cheng et al. 2006), and P63 has been identified as a possible candidate, as knockout mice develop bladder exstrophy (Ngan and Mitchell 1997; Lund and Hendren 2001; Reiner and Gearhart 2004; Cheng et al. 2006).

The genitalia are affected because of failure of fusion of the pubic bones and loss of formation of the anterior abdominal wall in the hypogastrium, along with absence of the anterior wall of the bladder. This leaves the bladder and urethral mucosa exposed as a flat plate. In females, the glans of the clitoris is as two separate halves, and the vagina is oriented almost directly forwards, rather than downwards. In males, the urethral plate is on the dorsal surface of the corpora cavernosa, which are short and curved upwards, producing reversed chordee. In both sexes, the anterior abdominal wall is deficient, with not only exposure of the bladder mucosa but also foreshortening of the distance between the umbilicus and the perineum (Fig. 5.9a).

An even more severe anomaly of the urogenital tract may occur that includes failure of separation of the hindgut from the urogenital sinus in the primitive cloaca. This leads to the rare defect of cloacal exstrophy, where the external

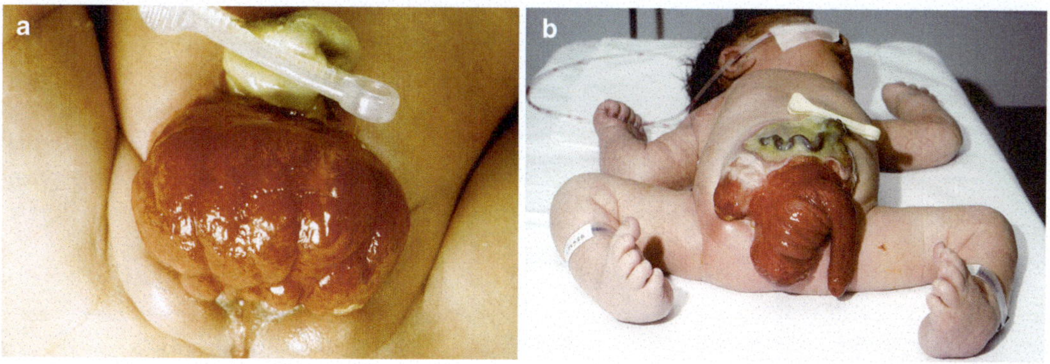

Fig. 5.9 (**a**) Genital variation secondary to bladder exstrophy, where the primary anomaly lies in failure of development of the mesoderm, forming the anterior lower abdominal wall. (**b**) The rare defect of cloacal exstrophy, where not only the anterior abdominal wall is deficient, but also subdivision of the primitive cloaca into the urogenital tract anteriorly and hindgut posteriorly does not occur

genitalia are disrupted by the presence of not only the open bladder plate (in 2 halves) laterally but also the dysplastic hindgut and midgut, represented by the open caecum (Fig. 5.9b). The internal genital tracts are widely separated and often obstructed, leading to haematometra and/or haematocolpos in adolescent girls. Unlike other conditions, the associated renal tract anomalies are not necessarily on the same side as the Müllerian anomaly. The cause of this complex variant remains unknown, but it is recognised to be associated with numerous other malformations, including neural tube defects and hindgut anomalies. It has also been suggested to be caused by *forme fruste* conjoined twinning.

Formation of the genital tubercle may be altered in the rare cases of penile agenesis. In this condition, the genital tubercle is entirely absent in an otherwise completely phenotypic male with testes descended into the scrotum (Fig. 5.10). When the median scrotal raphe is absent, then there is a very high incidence of severe urinary tract anomalies, including absent kidneys (Srinivasan et al. 2003). The urethra is usually connected to the anterior rim of the anal canal, consistent with aberrant separation of the urinary and gastrointestinal tracts. Urine is seen to dribble from the anus through this ectopic urethra,

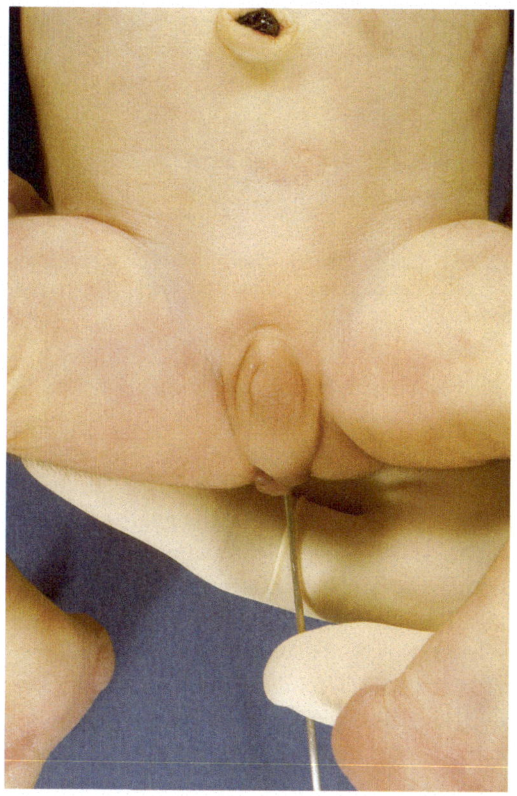

Fig. 5.10 Agenesis of the phallus in a baby with an empty scrotum with no midline septum (Srinivasan et al. 2003) (reproduced with permission of the publisher). (Probe in perineal fistula, as anus is absent)

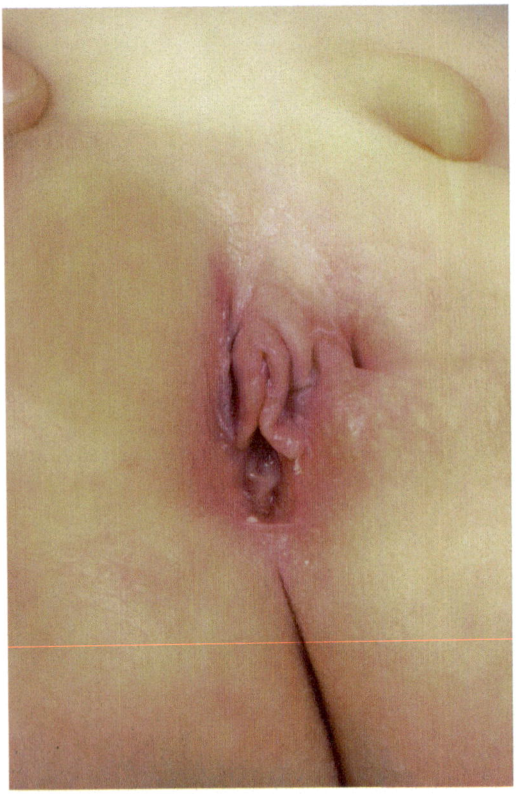

Fig. 5.11 Ectopic labium, which is likely to be caused by external compression deformity from the heel of one of the feet

which is similar in anatomy to an H-fistula in some rare variants of anorectal malformations (Holschneider and Hutson 2006) The ectopic urethra usually has some erectile tissue around it analogous to aberrant *corpus spongiosum*.

The genital folds may sometimes be aberrant and may fail to be present or be located ectopically. The latter anomaly leads to ectopic scrotum or labia (Fig. 5.11). When the hemi-scrotum is ectopic, it is usual for the testis to descend into it, suggesting that its innervation by the genitofemoral nerve is intact, and the gubernaculum has migrated into the ectopic scrotum under correct chemotactic guidance by the genitofemoral nerve (as described in Chap. 3). An ectopic location of the genital fold on one side, especially if found to be in two separate locations, is well described as a secondary anomaly caused by external compression of the foetus. The usual problem is one foot of the foetus becoming trapped in the perineum, leading to displacement or atrophy of the genital fold (Stephens et al. 1996). External compression of the genitalia by the heel of the foot is also reported to cause 'exstrophy' of the testis and primary urethral fistulae in the presence of a normal distal urethra (Heyns 1990) by development of a pressure sore.

5.9 Internal Genital Tract

5.9.1 Wolffian Ducts

5.9.1.1 In the Female

Gartner duct cysts are embryonic remnants of the mesonephric duct in females (Hoogendam and Smink 2017).

5.9.1.2 In the Male

Epididymis

Epididymal disjunction (ED) is the failure of the efferent ducts to reach the testis and might reflect the failure of the ducts to elongate or coil during their development. It has been reported that 30%–79% of boys with undescended testis have Wolffian duct anomalies, of which 25% display ED. It is important that epididymal anomalies be detected at orchidopexy to better classify those cases of infertility that would otherwise remain idiopathic (Murashima et al. 2015).

Vas Deferens

Congenital bilateral absence of vas deferens (CBAVD) affects 1%–2% of males with infertility and 60%–90% of men of European descent harbour at least one associated cystic fibrosis transmembrane conductance regulator (CFTR) gene variant. This is presumably secondary to late foetal involution and atresia of the Wolffian duct due to various gene variants. *PAX2*, *WT1* and *FGF* genes could be some of the candidate genes (Murashima et al. 2015).

Although rare, unilateral agenesis of a *vas deferens* has also been reported in Klinefelter syndrome (Akinsal et al. 2017).

Seminal Vesicles (SV)

Cysts

Congenital seminal vesicle cysts usually develop and become symptomatic during adulthood, although some pre-pubertal boys examined for epididymitis and recurrent urinary tract infections were found with cysts, which are thought to arise from the seminal vesicle. A cyst is the result of accumulation of secretions from the gland owing to insufficient drainage or atresia (Slaoui et al. 2016).

Due to their common embryologic origin, associated anomalies of the Wolffian ducts and ipsilateral kidney are common, as part of the Rokitansky sequence. However, ectopic ureters entering seminal vesicle cysts associated with ipsilateral renal agenesis are rare (Sheih et al. 1990).

Zinner syndrome is a rare congenital malformation that includes a triad of obstruction of the ejaculatory ducts, ipsilateral seminal vesicle cyst and ipsilateral renal agenesis (Casey et al. 2008).

Agenesis and Hypoplasia

Seminal vesicle agenesis is the most common congenital pathology. The vast majority are bilateral and associated with atresia of the *vas deferens* in the context of cystic fibrosis.

Seminal vesicle hypoplasia is also mainly bilateral.

5.9.2 Müllerian Ducts

5.9.2.1 In the Female

Müllerian duct anomalies (MDAs) in females can arise during early development, including variations in fusion or septal reabsorption (Behr et al. 2012; Luvero et al. 2017) (Table 5.2).

Anomalies of Development

A new European Society of Human Reproduction and Embryology/European Society for Gynaecological Endoscopy classification system for Müllerian tract anomalies allows the

Table 5.2 ESHRE/ESGE classification of Müllerian anomalies (Grimbizis et al. 2013)

ESHRE/ESGE classification
Female genital tract anomalies

	Uterine anomaly	
	Main class	***Sub-class***
U0	Normal uterus	
U1	Dysmorphic uterus	**a.** T-shaped **b.** Infantilis **c.** Others
U2	Septate uterus	**a.** Partial **b.** Complete
U3	Bicorporeal uterus	**a.** Partial **b.** Complete **c.** Bicorporeal septate
U4	Hemi-uterus	**a.** With rudimentary cavity (communicating or not horn) **b.** Without rudimentary cavity (horn without cavity / no horn)
U5	Aplastic	**a.** With rudimentary cavity (bi- or unilateral horn) **b.** Without rudimentary cavity (bi- or unilateral uterine remnants / Aplasia)
U6	Unclassified Malformations	
U		

Cervical / Vaginal anomaly	
Co-existent class	
C0	*Normal cervix*
C1	*Septate cervix*
C2	*Double "normal" cervix*
C3	*Unilateral cervical aplasia*
C4	*Cervical Aplasia*
V0	*Normal vagina*
V1	*Longitudinal non-obstructing vaginal septum*
V2	*Longitudinal obstructing vaginal septum*
V3	*Transverse vaginal septum and/or imperforate hymen*
V4	*Vaginal aplasia*
C	***V***

description of the fusion and cavitation anomalies of the uterus, cervix and vagina separately (Grimbizis et al. 2013), which allows a better classification than previous systems.

Aplasia and Hypoplasia

Aplasia or hypoplasia of the upper third of vagina, cervix and/or uterus results from the interruption of Müllerian duct development. The most severe form of MDAs with aplasia of all three structures occurs as uterovaginal agenesis or the Mayer-Rokitansky-Küster-Hauser syndrome (MRKH) (see Chap. 18). Interestingly, renal anomalies, due to concomitant abnormal development of the Wolffian ducts, are seen in approximately 40% of patients (Strubbe et al. 1993).

Aplasia can occur unilaterally or bilaterally; hence, it is possible to have unilateral aplasia of the uterus and/or unilateral aplasia of the cervix.

Unicornuate Uterus

Unicornate uterus results from the absence or near-complete absence or failure of canalisation of one of the Müllerian ducts, while the contralateral duct develops completely. The unicornuate horn will usually function without problems from a pregnancy perspective. On the contralateral side, there is a range of possible variations including cavitated and non-cavitated horns that are separate or communicating. If tubal fimbriae are present, they do pose a risk for ectopic pregnancy, and if the incompletely formed contralateral horn is cavitated, it has the potential to cause pain when menstruation commences.

Ipsilateral renal anomalies are present in approximately 40% of cases of unicornuate uterus. Renal agenesis is the most common (67%) (Behr et al. 2012).

Anomalies of Fusion

Uterus Didelphys

Uterus didelphys results from complete failure of fusion of otherwise two fully developed Müllerian ducts. Therefore, the patient presents two uterine horns, two cervices and normal upper third of the vagina. Unless a duplicated proximal vagina with transverse hemi-vaginal septum is associated, uterus didelphys is usually asymptomatic.

Bicornuate Uterus

Bicornuate uterus results from incomplete fusion of the Müllerian ducts. The duplicated endometrial cavity may be associated with a duplicated cervix (bicornuate bicollis) or not (bicornuate unicollis). A longitudinal vaginal septum is also present in 25% of cases (Behr et al. 2012).

Anomalies of Septal Reabsorption

Septate Uterus

This is the most common form of Müllerian duct anomalies (55%) and results from the complete or partial failure of reabsorption of the utero-vaginal septum. The septum originates from the midline and is composed of various proportions of fibrous tissue and myometrium. Recognition is important, as it is associated with repeated miscarriage and is amenable to surgical correction (Behr et al. 2012).

Arcuate Uterus

Arcuate uterus occurs when reabsorption of the utero-vaginal septum is nearly complete. This is the mildest form of Müllerian duct anomaly and is generally asymptomatic, with argument as to whether it should even be classified as a variant or anomaly.

5.9.2.2 In the male

See Sect. 5.7.2.

5.10 External Genitalia

5.10.1 Gonads

Testicular descent occurs in two morphologically distinct phases (Hutson et al. 2015):

The intra-abdominal phase, between 8 and 15 weeks of gestation, where Leydig cells produce insulin-like hormone 3 (INSL3), which causes the gubernaculum to swell and anchor the testis to the future inguinal canal. Concomitantly, testosterone leads to regression of the cranial suspensory ligament, increasing the effect of this first phase.

Between 25 and 35 gestational weeks, under the control of testosterone, the gubernaculum migrates into the scrotum, attracting the testis down. This is known as the inguino-scrotal phase. Disruption of any of these steps can lead to an undescended testis, in isolation or in the context of a DSD.

5.10.2 Genital Folds

Androgen secretion will cause the genital folds to fuse in the midline, commencing posteriorly, to create the penile shaft and the scrotum in males. Failure to do so will result in a bifid scrotum.

In females, the absence of androgens leads the inner genital folds to remain separate and differentiate into the labia minora and the outer folds into the labia majora. When androgens are produced in a XX foetus, they will lead to variable fusion of the genital folds and masculinisation of the external genitalia (rugosity and pigmentation).

5.10.3 Genital Tubercle and Urogenital Sinus

Masculine development of the genital tubercle into a penis is triggered by dihydrotestosterone (DHT). This happens in two phases (Cimador et al. 2015):

- Before 13 gestational weeks, the urogenital folds fuse along the midline to become the penile urethra. When this process is incomplete it leads to hypospadias.
- After 13 gestational weeks, the penis is formed and will enlarge under the influence of DHT. When this influence is absent, a typically formed but micropenis occurs.

In the female, the urogenital sinus remains open to form the vestibule of the introitus. Therefore, virilisation of an XX foetus with exposure to elevated androgens, such as in congenital adrenal hyperplasia (CAH), leads to various degrees of closure of the urethral plate and persistence of a urogenital sinus depending on the amount of adrenal androgens produced and their timing of production.

References

Abe T, Hutson JM. Gonadal migration in ambiguous genitalia. Pediatr Surg Int. 1994;9:547–50.

Adham IM, Agoulnik AI. Insulin-like 3 signalling in testicular descent. Int J Androl. 2004;27(5):257–65.

Akinsal EC, Baydilli N, Imamoglu H, et al. Three cases of Klinefelter's syndrome with unilateral absence of vas deferens. Andrologia 2017;49(9).

Alvarez-Nava F, Gonzalez S, Soto S, et al. Mixed gonadal dysgenesis: a syndrome of broad clinical, cytogenetic and histopathologic spectrum. Genet Couns. 1999;10(3):233–43.

Behr SC, Courtier JL, Qayyum A. Imaging of Müllerian duct anomalies. Radiographics. 2012;32(6):E233–50.

Ben-Meir DB, Hutson JM. The anatomy of the caudal vas deferens in patients with a genital anomaly. J Pediatr Urol. 2005;1(5):349–54.

Casey RG, Stunell H, Buckley O, et al. A unique radiological pentad of mesonephric duct abnormalities in a young man presenting with testicular swelling. Br J Radiol. 2008;81(963):e93–6.

Chavez-Saldana M, Vigueras-Villasenor RM, Yokoyama-Rebollar E, et al. Single nucleotide polymorphisms associated with nonsyndromic cryptorchidism in Mexican patients. Andrologia. 2018;50(1).

Cheng W, Jacobs WB, Zhang JJ, et al. DeltaNp63 plays an anti-apoptotic role in ventral bladder development. Development. 2006;133(23):4783–92.

Cimador M, Catalano P, Ortolano R, et al. The inconspicuous penis in children. Nat Rev Urol. 2015;12(4):205–15.

Clarnette T, Sugita Y, Hutson JM. Genital anomalies in the human and animal models reveal the mechanisms and hormones governing testicular descent. Br J Urol. 1997;79:99–112.

Donahoe PK, Crawford JD, Hendren WH. Mixed gonadal dysgenesis, pathogensis, and management. J Pediatr Surg. 1979;14(3):287–300.

Forest MG. Diagnosis and treatment of disorders of sexual development. In: DeGroot LJ, Jameson JL, editors. Endocrinology. Philadelphia, PA: Elsevier Saunders. . III; 2006. p. 2779–829.

Frasier SD, Bashore RA, Mosier HD. Gonadoblastoma associated with pure gonadal dysgenesis in monozygous twins. J Pediatr. 1964;64:740–5.

Fu P, Layfield S, Ferraro T, et al. Synthesis, conformation, receptor binding and biological activities of monobiotinylated human insulin-like peptide 3. J Pept Res. 2004;63(2):91–8.

Grimbizis GF, Gordts S, Di Spiezio Sardo A, et al. The ESHRE-ESGE consensus on the classification of female genital tract congenital anomalies. Gynecol Surg. 2013;10(3):199–212.

Heyns CF. Exstrophy of the testis. J Urol. 1990;144:724–5.

Holschneider A, Hutson JM. (editors). Anorectal malformations in children. Berlin: Springer; 2006.

Hoogendam JP, Smink M. Gartner's duct cyst. N Engl J Med. 2017;376(14):e27.

Hrabovszky Z, Hutson JM. Surgical treatment of intersex abnormalities: a review. Surgery. 2002;131(1):92–104.
Hutson J, Chow CW, Ng W. Persistent mullerian duct syndrome with transverse testicular ectopia. An experiment of nature with clues for understanding testicular descent. Pediatr Surg Int. 1987;2:191–4.
Hutson J, Davidson P, Reece L, et al. Failure of gubernacular development in the persistent mullerian duct syndrome allows herniation of the testes. Pediatr Surg Int. 1994;9:544–6.
Hutson JM, Baker M. A hypothesis to explain abnormal gonadal descent in persistent Müllerian duct syndrome. Pediatr Surg Int. 1994;9:542–3.
Hutson JM, Li R, Southwell BR, et al. Regulation of testicular descent. Pediatr Surg Int. 2015;31(4):317–25.
Hutson JM, Lopez-Marambio FA. The possible role of AMH in shortening the gubernacular cord in testicular descent: a reappraisal of the evidence. J Pediatr Surg. 2017;52(10):1656–60.
Hutson JM, MacLaughlin DT, Ikawa H, et al. Regression of the Müllerian ducts during sexual differentiation in the chick embryo: a reappraisal. In: Greep RO, editor. Vol. IV, Chapt. 5 Reproductive physiology; 1983. p. 177–224.
Josso N, Cate RL, Picard JY, et al. Anti-mullerian hormone: the Jost factor. Recent Prog Horm Res. 1993;48:1–59.
Kubota Y, Temelcos C, Bathgate RA, et al. The role of insulin 3, testosterone, Müllerian inhibiting substance and relaxin in rat gubernacular growth. Mol Hum Reprod. 2002;8(10):900–5.
Lu P, Wang Y, Wang F, et al. Genetic analysis of HOXA11 gene in Chinese patients with cryptorchidism. Andrologia. 2018;50(1).
Lund DP, Hendren WH. Cloacal exstrophy: a 25-year experience with 50 cases. J Pediatr Surg. 2001;36(1):68–75.
Luvero D, Plotti F, Capriglione S, et al. Undescended or absent ovary without uterine anomalies: systematic review and a single center's experience. Minerva Ginecol. 2017;69(1):35–40.
Marszalek JR, Ruiz-Lozano P, Roberts E, et al. Situs inversus and embryonic ciliary morphogenesis defects in mouse mutants lacking the KIF3A subunit of kinesin-II. Proc Natl Acad Sci U S A. 1999;96(9):5043–8.
Miller A, Hong MK, Hutson J. The broad ligament: a review of its anatomy and development in different species and hormonal environments. Clin Anat. 2004;17:244–51.
Mouriquand PD, Gorduza DB, Gay CL, et al. Surgery in disorders of sex development (DSD) with a gender issue: if (why), when, and how? J Pediatr Urol. 2016;12(3):139–49.
Murashima A, Xu B, Hinton BT. Understanding normal and abnormal development of the Wolffian/epididymal duct by using transgenic mice. Asian J Androl. 2015;17(5):749–55.
Ngan JH, Mitchell ME. Exstrophic anomalies: recent advances and long-term outlook. Indian J Pediatr. 1997;64(3):327–38.
Nihoul-Fekete C, Lortat-Jacob S, Cachin O, et al. Preservation of gonadal function in true hermaphroditism. J Pediatr Surg. 1984;19(1):50–5.
Nonaka S, Tanaka Y, Okada Y, et al. Randomization of left-right asymmetry due to loss of nodal cilia generating leftward flow of extraembryonic fluid in mice lacking KIF3B motor protein. Cell. 1998;95(6):829–37.
Reiner WG, Gearhart JP. Discordant sexual identity in some genetic males with cloacal exstrophy assigned to female sex at birth. N Engl J Med. 2004;350(4):333–41.
Scott JE. The Hutson hypothesis. A clinical study. Br J Urol. 1987;60(1):74–6.
Sheih CP, Hung CS, Wei CF, et al. Cystic dilatations within the pelvis in patients with ipsilateral renal agenesis or dysplasia. J Urol. 1990;144(2 Pt 1):324–7.
Slaoui A, Regragui S, Lasri A, et al. Zinner's syndrome: report of two cases and review of the literature. Basic Clin Androl. 2016;26:10.
Srinivasan J, McDougall P, Hutson JM. When is 'intersex' not intersex? A case of penile agenesis demonstrates how to distinguish non-endocrine disorders in neonates with genital anomaly. J Paediatr Child Health. 2003;39(8):629–31.
Stephens FD, Smith ED, Hutson JM. Congenital anomalies of the urinary and genital tracts. Oxford: I. M. Medica; 1996. p. 80–90.
Strubbe EH, Willemsen WN, Lemmens JA, et al. Mayer-Rokitansky-Kuster-Hauser syndrome: distinction between two forms based on excretory urographic, sonographic, and laparoscopic findings. Am J Roentgenol. 1993;160(2):331–4.
Takeda S, Yonekawa Y, Tanaka Y, et al. Left-right asymmetry and kinesin superfamily protein KIF3A: new insights in determination of laterality and mesoderm induction by kif3A−/− mice analysis. J Cell Biol. 1999;145(4):825–36.
Tong SY, Hutson JM, Watts LM. Does testosterone diffuse down the Wolffian duct during sexual differentiation? J Urol. 1996;155(6):2057–9.
Veale JF, Clarke DE, Lomax TC. Biological and psycholsocial correlates of adult gender-variant identities: a review. Personal Individ Differ. 2010;48(4):357–66.
Wolffenbuttel KP, Hersmus R, Stoop H, et al. Gonadal dysgenesis in disorders of sex development: diagnosis and surgical management. J Pediatr Urol. 2016;12(6):411–6.
Zah W, Kalderon AE, Tucci JR. Mixed gonadal dysgenesis. Acta Endocrinol Suppl (Copenh). 1975;197:1–39.
Zielinska D, Zajaczek S, Rzepka-Gorska I. Tumors of dysgenetic gonads in Swyer syndrome. J Pediatr Surg. 2007;42(10):1721–4.

46,XX DSD

6

Michele A. O'Connell, Sonia R. Grover, and Aurore Bouty

6.1 Clinical Presentations of Individuals with 46,XX DSD

An infant or child with one of the 46,XX DSD may present with the following:

- *Atypical genitalia*. More than half of all infants born with atypical (sometimes referred to as ambiguous) genitalia are 46,XX. Their atypical genital appearance, which is due to varying degrees of phallic enlargement and labial fusion, results from *in utero* exposure to excess androgen. The source of the excess androgen may be *adrenal* (as in congenital adrenal hyperplasia (CAH)) or *testicular* (with 46,XX being the most common karyotype associated with ovo-testicular DSD (Krob et al. 1994) see Chap. 8 for a full description). Sometimes the source of androgens is maternal ingestion or maternal androgen-secreting tumours.
- *A complex congenital malformation*, such as cloaca, bladder exstrophy or cloacal exstrophy (these are described in Chap. 9).
- *Gradual enlargement of the clitoris during childhood, with or without other signs of virilisation*. This may be seen in girls with non-classic CAH (see Chap. 13).
- *Atypical development at puberty* (see Table 6.1, Chap. 14). The girl may have primary amenorrhoea and either *no* breast and pubic hair development (46,XX gonadal dysgenesis, steroid biosynthetic defects); *or normal breast and pubic/axillary hair development* (Müllerian duct agenesis); or normal breast, pubic and axillary hair ± onset of menses with excessive virilisation due to an androgen-producing tumour.

M. A. O'Connell (✉)
Department of Endocrinology and Diabetes, The Royal Children's Hospital, Melbourne, VIC, Australia

Murdoch Children's Research Institute, Melbourne, VIC, Australia
e-mail: Michele.Oconnell@rch.org.au

S. R. Grover
Department of Gynaecology, The Royal Children's Hospital, Melbourne, VIC, Australia

Murdoch Children's Research Institute, Melbourne, VIC, Australia

Department of Paediatrics, University of Melbourne, Melbourne, VIC, Australia
e-mail: Sonia.grover@rch.org.au

A. Bouty
Department of Urology, The Royal Children's Hospital, Melbourne, VIC, Australia

Murdoch Children's Research Institute, Melbourne, VIC, Australia
e-mail: aurore.bouty@rch.org.au

J. M. Hutson et al. (eds.), *Disorders|Differences of Sex Development*,
https://doi.org/10.1007/978-981-13-7864-5_6

Table 6.1 46 XX conditions that may present with atypical development at puberty

Condition	Breast/pubic hair development	Menstruation	Distinguishing feature
46,XX gonadal dysgenesis	–	–	Increased FSH and LH, decreased E2. FSH receptor gene mutation
17α-Hydroxylase deficiency	–	–	Hypertension, hypokalaemia. Increased mineralocorticoids, decreased cortisol and sex steroids. Mutation in *CYP17*
Steroidogenic factor-1 deficiency	±	Primary amenorrhoea or premature ovarian in sufficiency	Mutation in *NR5A1*
Müllerian duct agenesis	+	–	Normal hormone levels, anatomical anomaly seen on imaging. *WNT4* mutations in some cases

6.2 Congenital Adrenal Hyperplasia (CAH)

CAH is a *family* of genetically determined conditions caused by deficiencies of steroidogenic enzymes in the adrenal cortex (Hughes 1990a, b). In some forms of CAH, such as lipoid CAH, ovarian steroidogenesis is also impaired (Table 6.2). In relation to each type of CAH, the terms *classic* and *non-classic* are used to distinguish grades of severity. In the *classic* form, prenatal development of the genitalia is affected, whereas in the non-classic form, the first effects on sex development occur after birth. The classic form is usually further divided into salt wasting (SW) and simple virilising (SV)

6.2.1 21-Hydroxylase Deficiency

The classic form of 21-hydroxylase deficiency is the single most common cause of atypical genitalia. It is potentially lethal, in that 75% of cases have the *salt-wasting* (SW) form, and from the end of the first week of life, they are at risk of an adrenal crisis or sudden death. Many countries have established newborn screening programs for CAH, aimed at preventing these deaths (White and Medscape 2009). Infants with salt-wasting CAH will inevitably die unless the correct diagnosis is made and appropriate treatment promptly started. The other 25% of cases have the *simple virilising* (SV), or non-salt-wasting form; they have milder adrenal insufficiency, are able to maintain normal electrolyte homeostasis and have a lower risk of adrenal crisis.

Deficiency of 21-hydroxylase impairs the conversion of 17-hydroxyprogesterone to 11-deoxycortisol in the zona fasciculata of the adrenal cortex, resulting in cortisol deficiency. This stimulates an increase in pituitary ACTH secretion, which increases the production of adrenal androgens (DHEA and androstenedione); these androgens are in turn converted to testosterone and DHT, inducing virilisation of the genitalia in a female foetus. The enzyme deficiency also impairs the conversion of progesterone to 11-deoxycorticosterone in the mineralocorticoid pathway, lowering aldosterone production. While only the SW form of CAH is associated with severe aldosterone deficiency and serum electrolyte imbalance, aldosterone production is also impaired in the SV form; in most cases, plasma renin activity and plasma angiotensin II are increased (Rosler et al. 1977), indicating salt depletion. Angiotensin II stimulates ACTH secretion, so when there is salt depletion and levels of angiotensin II are elevated, the pituitary is relatively resistant to the negative feedback from cortisol and higher glucocorticoid doses will be needed to treat the patient (Rosler et al. 1977).

Table 6.2 Summary of the different types of CAH causing 46,XX DSD

Type of CAH	OMIM #	Expressed in adrenal	Expressed in ovary	Virilisation	Hypertension	Salt wasting
21-Hydroxylase deficiency	201910	+	–	+	–	+
11β-Hydroxylase deficiency	202010	+	–	+	+	Transient neonatal (before treatment)
3β-HSD[a] deficiency	201810	+	+	+	–	+
P450-oxidoreductase deficiency	124015	+	+	+	–	±
17α-Hydroxylase deficiency	202110	+	+	–	+	–
Lipoid adrenal hyperplasia	201710	+	+	–	–	+

[a]3β-Hydroxysteroid dehydrogenase

6.2.1.1 Clinical Features

A typical 46,XX infant with classic 21-hydroxylase deficiency will have the following:

- Atypical genitalia with evidence of androgen exposure, but no palpable gonads (Fig. 6.1).
- Hyperpigmentation of the genital skin due to excess ACTH.
- Female internal genital tract: normal uterus, cervix, Fallopian tubes and ovaries. The lower third of the vagina may be narrow or shared with the lower urinary tract depending on the extent of virilisation.
- Evidence of a possible metabolic disturbance if steroid treatment has been delayed—hypoglycaemia, hyponatraemia and hyperkalaemia (classic SW form, after the first week).
- Absence of any dysmorphic features that might suggest aneuploidy.
- A normally placed anus that rules out a cloaca.

6.2.1.2 Diagnosis

- Elevated serum 17-hydroxyprogesterone (>700 nmol/L in the classic form; 70–500 nmol/L in the non-classic form) (Levine et al. 1981).
- Urine steroid analysis by gas chromatography–mass spectrometry (Wudy et al. 2000). Characteristic peaks of pregnanetriol and pregnanetriolone confirm the diagnosis of 21-hydroxylase deficiency and differentiate it from other virilising forms of CAH, such as 11β-hydroxylase deficiency.
- Serum electrolytes—after the first week in an untreated infant with the SW form, serum sodium falls and potassium rises.
- Blood glucose—may be low due to cortisol deficiency.
- Imaging studies (see Chap. 12).
  - Pelvic ultrasound confirms presence of uterus and ovaries and typically demonstrates enlarged adrenal glands.
  - Urogenital sinugram (which is not necessarily undertaken) defines length of the urogenital sinus and site of junction between urethra and vagina.

6.2.1.3 Genetics

Deficiency of 21-hydroxylase is inherited as an autosomal recessive trait. The gene frequency in the general community is 1:55 (Baumgartner-Parzer et al. 2005). The gene that encodes this enzyme is *cytochrome P450c21* (also known as *CYP21A2*; OMIM 201910), which is located on chromosome 6p21.3, contiguous with genes for complement and the major HLA loci (Levine et al. 1978). Close by is a pseudogene called *CYP21A1*, which, compared to the *CYP21A2* gene, has missing eight base pairs from exon 2, making it inactive. The presence of the pseudogene complicates mutational analysis (Koppens et al. 2002). To date, more than 174 *CYP21A2* deletions and missense variants have been reported (Concolino et al. 2010; Finkielstain et al. 2010). These may be exonic or intronic (in fact, the commonest mutation is an intron two frameshift mutation) (Speiser and White 2003).

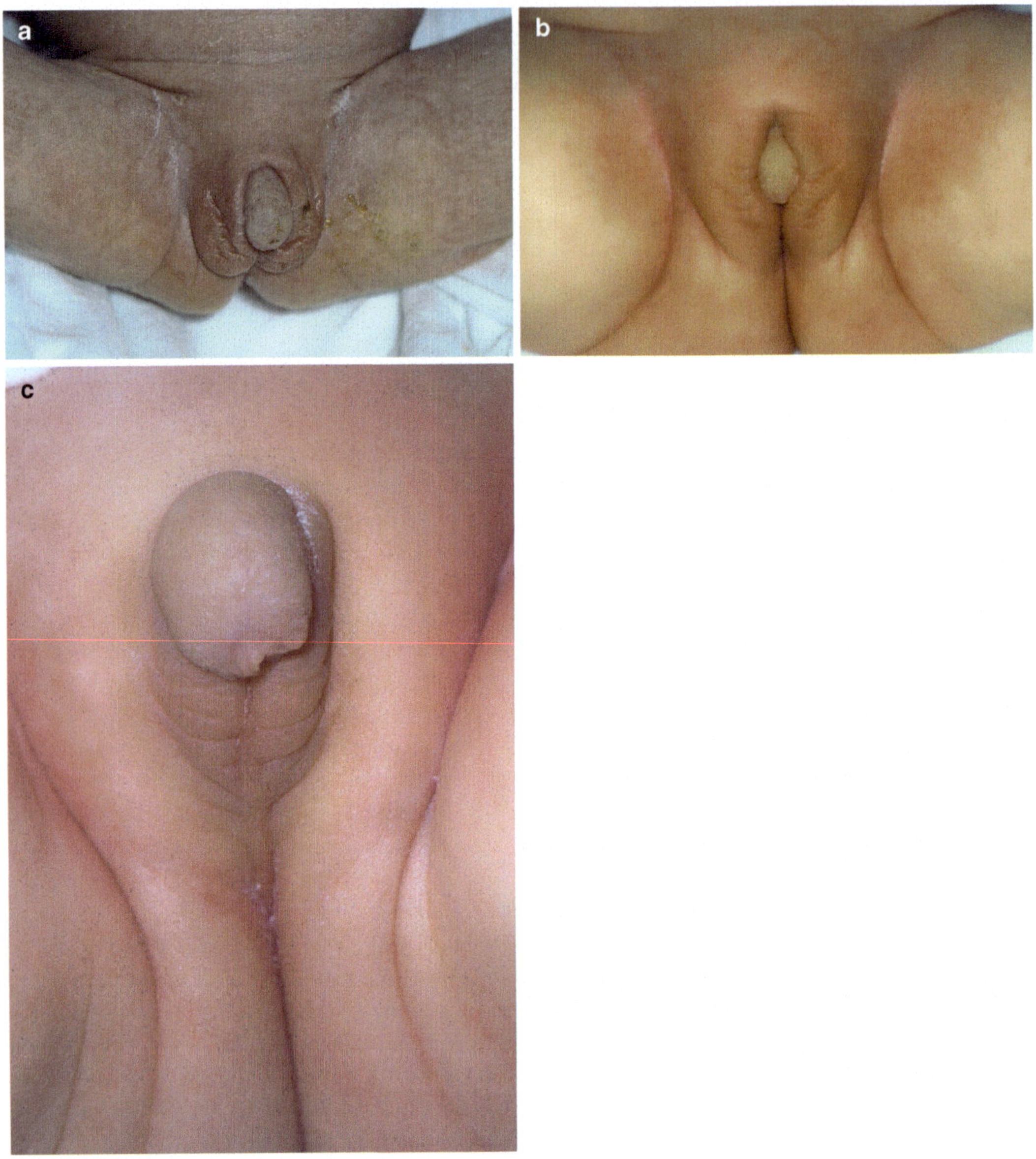

Fig. 6.1 (**a**) External evidence of exposure to androgens in this 46,XX female with CAH and Prader 3 virilisation at birth. Note pigmentation and wrinkling of fused labio-scrotal folds but no visible gonads. (**b**) The same baby at 8 weeks of age, showing some regression of the virilisation after commencing steroid treatment. (**c**) Another baby girl with 46,XX DSD with CAH caused by a more severe defect in 21-hydroxylase, leading to more marked virilisation (Prader 4–5)

Many of the point variants are examples of *gene conversion*, that is, the structure of the active gene has reverted to that of the pseudogene (Higashi et al. 1986). Structure–function correlations have been studied for the most common allele variants (Chung et al. 1995; Robins et al. 2006). In one large series, 79% of individuals with CAH were compound heterozygotes. Genotype accurately predicted phenotype in 90.5%, 85.1% and 97.8% of patients with salt-wasting, simple virilising and non-classic forms, respectively (Finkielstain et al. 2010).

6.2.1.4 Monitoring of Treatment

In children with CAH, growth velocity, weight gain, blood pressure, development and general well-being are followed at three to four monthly intervals (Halper et al. 2017). The aim of treatment is to allow appropriate growth and weight gain, for blood pressure to be normal and for general health to be good, without episodes of adrenal crisis. Parents need education in how to prevent adrenal crises and are given several rules to follow. These are as follows:

- That they should never stop the child's steroid medications unless instructed to do so by their treating endocrinologist/team.
- That inter-current illnesses, especially those associated with fever, should be covered by trebling the child's usual glucocorticoid dose (to give ~35–50 mg/m2/day minimum) for 2–3 days, then doubling for 2 days before resuming usual glucocorticoid doses.
- That if the child is vomiting or has diarrhoea, hydrocortisone should be given by injection until the medication can be tolerated by mouth.

Monitoring for adequacy of steroid dosing also includes exploring for features of over- and under-dosing of steroids on the basis of history, clinical examination and biochemical tests.

Details on history include seeking information regarding energy levels, sport and physical activity tolerance and adrenal crises.

Clinical examination involves checking weight, monitoring for postural blood pressure drop and looking for evidence of increasing pigmentation. In the past, it was common practice to monitor the genital appearance of 46,XX children with CAH to identify if there was progressive or increasing virilisation occurring. The genital examination does not contribute to decision-making regarding steroid dose and repeated genital examination has a negative impact on self-esteem and body image with girls with CAH (Tonkin-Hill, 2018). Advocacy groups have rightly challenged this practice (Feder and Dreger 2016; Darlington Statement 2017), which should no longer be routine.

Studies exploring body image and self-esteem in individuals with 46,XX CAH have demonstrated that obesity, skin pigmentation, acne and height are sources of major concern (Zainuddin et al. 2020).

Biochemical monitoring is important in CAH, although different clinics monitor this in different ways. As serum 17OHP is subject to diurnal variation, some clinics ask patients to collect a series of dried blood spots on a filter paper across 24 h and to mail them to the laboratory. Others compromise and measure only an early morning 17OHP and also measure plasma renin activity. Decisions about changing doses of hydrocortisone and fludrocortisone are then made using the collated clinical and biochemical information. It is undesirable to completely suppress serum 17OHP, even to the normal range, because adrenal androgens are more readily suppressed than 17OHP and because over-treatment will suppress or slow linear growth and cause excessive weight gain. It has been recommended (Hughes 1990a, b) that early morning 17OHP levels should be maintained in the range of 30–70 nmol/L and that the dose of hydrocortisone should be 12–15 mg/m^2/day in divided doses. The dose of fludrocortisone is generally in the range of 0.1–0.15 mg/day and is adjusted to maintain plasma renin activity within the normal range.

6.2.1.5 Gender Identity and Sexuality in 46,XX Individuals with CAH

All girls with the classic form of 21-hydroxylase deficiency have had prenatal exposure to levels of adrenal androgens that are higher than for unaffected girls; some have had additional postnatal exposure to excess androgens, and some have experienced severe dehydration and salt depletion after birth. Some neuropsychological effects have been reported in a number of studies (Kelso et al. 2000; Berenbaum 2001; Hines et al. 2004; Hamed et al. 2018). Prepubertal girls with CAH exhibit tomboyish behaviour more commonly (Hall et al. 2004; Berenbaum et al. 2018). Some girls with CAH experience gender dysphoria; however this is uncommon (Razzaghy-Azar et al. 2017). Higher rates of same sex attraction are also reported (Wisniewski et al. 2000; Dessens et al. 2005; Meyer-Bahlburg et al. 2008). Historically, many women CAH reported they abstain from sexual relations (Mulaikal et al. 1987). Fertility rates for the classic forms of CAH are low, being lower for the salt-losing form than for the simple virilising form (Meyer-Bahlburg 1999; Jaaskelainen et al. 2001), although some of this reduction relates to not seeking fertility rather than infertility itself.

6.2.1.6 Bilateral Adrenalectomy in the Treatment of CAH

Management of some patients with CAH can be very difficult with conventional management. For example, it may be impossible to achieve suppression of hyper-androgenism without causing obesity or other symptoms of hyper-cortisolism. In 1996, bilateral adrenalectomy was proposed (Van Wyk et al. 1996) as a treatment to consider in such situations, especially when the patient has a null mutation in the *CYP21A2* gene. Subsequent experience in 18 patients followed up for an average post-operative duration of 59 months supports the view that these selected patients generally benefited by the procedure (Van Wyk and Ritzen 2003; MacKay et al. 2018) although the potential risks and benefits must be weighed and discussed carefully in each individual case.

6.2.2 11β Hydroxylase Deficiency

This is the second most common type of CAH after 21-hydroxylase deficiency, accounting for 5%–8% of cases of CAH (except in the Middle East, where it is more prevalent (Rosler et al. 1992)), and like that condition, it causes virilisation of a female foetus. The nature of the biochemical defect was first discovered in 1956 (Bongiovanni and Eberlein 1956). It is inherited as an autosomal recessive condition. The 11β-hydroxylase enzyme is needed for the conversion of 11-deoxycortisol to cortisol and of 11-deoxycorticosterone to corticosterone. The accumulation of 11-deoxycorticosterone results in arterial hypertension and sometimes clinically significant hypokalaemia, but paradoxically, infants with this condition may show transient salt-wasting before the commencement of treatment (al-Jurayyan 1995), and an incorrect diagnosis of 21-hydroxylase deficiency can be made. The hypertension can develop soon after birth and be severe enough to cause seizures (Rosler et al. 1988). The *CYP11B1* (OMIM # 610613) gene is located on chromosome 8q21. Prenatal virilisation occurs in the classic form, and expression studies have shown that there is little or no enzyme activity present in these individuals. There is, in addition, a non-classic form of 11β-hydroxylase deficiency, in which enzyme activity may be 25%–40% of wild-type (Parajes et al. 2010). The diagnosis of 11β-hydroxylase deficiency is established by marked elevations of both 11-deoxycortisol and 11-deoxycorticosterone in blood and through the detection of excessive amounts of tetrahydro-11-deoxycortisol in the urine by GC-MS analysis. Treatment with hydrocortisone suppresses ACTH, and as the levels of deoxycorticosterone fall, blood pressure returns to normal. Treatment is monitored by tracking serial measurements of 11-deoxycortisol and 11-deoxycorticosterone in the blood, along with linear growth and blood pressure measurements. Occasionally, the hypertension can be very resistant to conventional treatment with steroids and anti-hypertensive drugs; bilateral adrenalectomy has been successfully used in several cases (John et al. 2009; Kacem et al. 2009).

6.2.3 3β-Hydroxysteroid Dehydrogenase Deficiency

This is a rare type of CAH, which can cause atypical genitalia in both 46,XX and 46,XY foetuses. Mutations are found in the 3β-HSD Type 2 gene (*HSD3B2*, OMIM #201810; chromosome 1p13.1). The enzyme is required for the conversion of pregnenolone to progesterone, 17-hydroxypregnenolone to 17-hydroxyprogesterone and dehydroepiandrosterone to androstenedione in the adrenal glands and gonads. In 46,XX individuals, the overproduction of dehydroepiandrosterone by the adrenals causes clitoral enlargement and labial fusion. Not all patients have atypical genitalia; some present with salt-losing in the neonatal period without evidence of excess androgen exposure. Most patients with the classic form of the condition have both atypical genitalia and are salt-losing (Simard et al. 2002). Biochemically, 3β-HSD deficiency is characterized by elevated levels of serum 17-hydroxypregnenolone and DHEA (Lutfallah et al. 2002). Because 17OHP and androstenedione levels are also increased, misdiagnosis of 21-hydroxylase deficiency can occur (Nordenstrom et al. 2007).

6.2.4 P450 Oxidoreductase Deficiency

In this rare form of CAH, 46,XX infants are born with atypical genitalia, and some infants have craniosynostosis and other skeletal features of Antley-Bixler syndrome (OMIM #201750). The biochemical profile suggests a combination of 21-hydroxylase deficiency and 17α-hydroxylase deficiency (Fujieda and Tajima 2005), with impaired cortisol biosynthesis, increased ACTH and 17-hydroxyprogesterone and altered androgen biosynthesis. Paradoxically, androgens are produced by an alternative pathway, and in some cases, both the mother and her female foetus were simultaneously virilised (Fluck et al. 2008) (as also occurs in placental aromatase deficiency). Mutations are found in the *POR* gene (OMIM # 124015; chromosome 7q11.12).

6.2.5 17α-Hydroxylase Deficiency

In common with 11β-hydroxylase deficiency, 17α-hydroxylase deficiency causes the accumulation of mineralocorticoid precursors (in this case, corticosterone and deoxycorticosterone) and arterial hypertension; it also causes a reduction in cortisol biosynthesis and an increase in ACTH secretion. Unlike 11β-hydroxylase deficiency, however, 17α-hydroxylase deficiency is associated with reduction in androgen synthesis, so that both 46,XX and 46,XY affected individuals may be born with phenotypically female external genitalia. The ovaries are unable to make oestrogen because the pathway is through the aromatization of testosterone. In either sex, the diagnosis may be delayed until the second decade, when puberty fails to occur; the discovery of the hypertension, associated with hypokalaemia, is the vital clue. The enzyme that is deficient is actually steroid 17-mono-oxygenase, which has both 17α-hydroxylase and 17,20-lyase activities. Treatment of a 46,XX individual would be with a glucocorticoid (which will usually correct the hypertension) and a combination of oestrogen and a progestogen. Mutations have been found in the *CYP17A1* gene (OMIM #609300) (Tian et al. 2009; Rosa et al. 2010). A high prevalence of the condition is found in Mennonite populations in Brazil, Canada and The Netherlands (Imai et al. 1992; Costa-Santos et al. 2004; Miller 2004), but it is rare elsewhere.

6.2.6 Lipoid Congenital Adrenal Hyperplasia

This condition gets its name from the appearance of the adrenal glands, which are convoluted, lipid-laden and bright yellow. The gonads in both males and females are also affected. The underlying cause is a mutation in the gene encoding the steroid acute regulatory protein (*STAR*, OMIM #201710), which is needed for the transport of cholesterol, the substrate for all steroid biosynthesis, to the inner mitochondrial membrane (Bose et al. 1996; Arakane et al. 1998). Cholesterol accumulates in the cytoplasm and has a toxic effect on the cell. In classic lipoid CAH, a 46,XX infant will have a hyperpigmented appearance and develop hypoglycaemia soon after birth; salt wasting becomes evident towards the end of the first week. The urine steroid profile on GC-MS analysis is flat. Milder phenotypes have been reported, with some presenting only as familial glucocorticoid deficiency (Baker et al. 2006). A Japanese report (Fujieda et al. 1997) describes a 46,XX patient with lipoid CAH who entered puberty spontaneously, and women who have had pregnancies have been reported (Khoury et al. 2009). If correctly diagnosed and treated with glucocorticoid, mineralocorticoid and later sex hormone replacement, the condition has a good prognosis.

6.3 Steroidogenic Factor-1 Deficiency

In its most severe form, deficiency of a nuclear receptor, steroidogenic factor-1 (SF-1; also known as NR5A1), results in failure of development in both the adrenals and the gonads (Achermann et al. 1999). There are, however, milder and varied phenotypes. In 46,XX individuals, it can manifest as primary ovarian insufficiency (with either primary or secondary amenorrhoea) without evidence of glucocorticoid deficiency (Lourenco et al. 2009). The reverse is also possible: a girl with functioning ovaries may have or develop glucocorticoid deficiency (Biason-Lauber and Schoenle 2000).

6.4 46,XX Gonadal Dysgenesis

A familial form of 46,XX gonadal dysgenesis due to a mutation in the FSH receptor gene was reported from Finland (Aittomaki et al. 1996; Tapanainen et al. 1998). Ovarian dysgenesis and premature ovarian insufficiency may also occur in *NR5A1* deficiency, as described above. The possibility of sex chromosome aneuploidy needs to be borne in mind; absence of low-level aneuploidy in peripheral blood does not exclude the possibility of mosaicism in the ovary. Sex chromosome micro-array analysis facilitates the detection of X-chromosomal deletions and rearrangements.

6.5 46,XX Premature Ovarian Insufficiency (POI)

This may present in a variety of ways, ranging from delayed puberty, to primary amenorrhoea (with normal breast, pubic and axillary hair development) or as secondary amenorrhoea, often with associated climacteric symptoms. By definition, POI is ovarian insufficiency in 46,XX individuals <40 years of age and occurs in 1 in 100 women, including 1 in 1000 before the age of 30 years (Tucker et al. 2016). A number of the underlying causes for POI have now been identified due to the increasing capacity to undertake detailed genetic testing (see Chaps. 2 and 21).

6.6 Müllerian Duct Agenesis

Vaginal agenesis, usually associated with absent uterus and proximal Fallopian tubes, but with normal ovarian development, is found in approximately 1 in 4000–5000 female births. This is also known as the Mayer-Rokitansky-Kuster-Hauser (MRKH) syndrome. There is an increased risk for associated renal (43%), skeletal (mostly vertebral 30%) and cardiac anomalies (15%), and a number of individuals will have their Müllerian agenesis as part of other syndromes (Klippel-Feil—7%, and MURCS association—7%). There may be a vaginal opening present with a hymen, although in one-fourth of these, there may be a hymenal variation present in the form of a cribriform, septate or arcuate hymen. The hymen will be absent in about one-third, and in these individuals, there is likely to be an associated absent kidney (Kimberley et al. 2012). Some degree of Müllerian variation is reported to occur in 7% of the female population (Vallerie and Breech 2010), although many of these will be very minor variations. Familial clusters have been reported, and although a great deal of attention has been focused on the *WNT4* gene, mutations in that gene appear rarely to be involved, except perhaps in a small subset of cases with hyperandrogenism (Biason-Lauber et al. 2007) (see Chap. 21).

6.7 46,XX Testicular DSD

Approximately one in every 20,000 individuals with male genitalia and testes has a 46,XX karyotype. In the majority, a translocation of *SRY* to the tip of one of the X-chromosomes has occurred. In SRY-negative cases (Kolon et al.

1998), there is intense research activity to try and identify mutations in other genes capable of regulating testicular development. Some evidence points to *SOX3* (Sutton et al. 2011). Recently, duplications in upstream enhancers of SOX9 have been shown to be associated with 46XX sex reversal (Croft et al. 2018). There are some phenotypic similarities between 46,XX men and those with Klinefelter syndrome (KS), but 46,XX men tend to be shorter than men with KS (Vorona et al. 2007). Both syndromes are associated with low semen volume and oligospermia (Aksglaede et al. 2009).

6.8 46,XX Ovo-Testicular DSD

Ovo-testicular DSD is a specific type of gonadal dysgenesis characterised by the presence of ovarian follicles and seminiferous tubules in the gonads of one individual. In all populations studied, the 46,XX karyotype is the one most frequently found. A more complete discussion is found in Chap. 8.

6.9 Cloacal Exstrophy and Bladder Exstrophy

These complex anomalies affect the lower abdominal wall and perineum, leading to abnormal external genital development. A detailed description is found in Chap. 9.

Acknowledgements With acknowledgements and thanks to the original writers of this chapter: Professor Garry L. Warne, Dr. Jacqueline Hewitt.

References

Achermann JC, Ito M, Hindmarsh PC, et al. A mutation in the gene encoding steroidogenic factor-1 causes XY sex reversal and adrenal failure in humans. Nat Genet. 1999;22(2):125–6.

Aittomaki K, Herva R, Stenman UH, et al. Clinical features of primary ovarian failure caused by a point mutation in the follicle-stimulating hormone receptor gene. J Clin Endocrinol Metab. 1996;81(10):3722–6.

Aksglaede L, Jorgensen N, Skakkebaek NE, et al. Low semen volume in 47 adolescents and adults with 47,XXY Klinefelter or 46,XX male syndrome. Int J Androl. 2009;32(4):376–84.

al-Jurayyan NA. Congenital adrenal hyperplasia due to 11 beta-hydroxylase deficiency in Saudi Arabia: clinical and biochemical characteristics. Acta Paediatr. 1995;84(6):651–4.

Arakane F, Kallen CB, Watari H, et al. Steroidogenic acute regulatory protein (StAR) acts on the outside of mitochondria to stimulate steroidogenesis. Endocr Res. 1998;24(3–4):463–8.

Baker BY, Lin L, Kim CJ, et al. Nonclassic congenital lipoid adrenal hyperplasia: a new disorder of the steroidogenic acute regulatory protein with very late presentation and normal male genitalia. J Clin Endocrinol Metab. 2006;91(12):4781–5.

Baumgartner-Parzer SM, Nowotny P, Heinze G, et al. Carrier frequency of congenital adrenal hyperplasia (21-hydroxylase deficiency) in a middle European population. J Clin Endocrinol Metab. 2005;90(2):775–8.

Berenbaum SA. Cognitive function in congenital adrenal hyperplasia. Endocrinol Metab Clin N Am. 2001;30(1):173–92.

Berenbaum SA, Beltz AM, Bryk K, et al. Gendered peer involvement in girls with congenital adrenal hyperplasia: effects of prenatal androgens, gendered activities, and gender cognitions. Arch Sex Behav. 2018;47(4):915–29.

Biason-Lauber A, De Filippo G, Konrad D, et al. WNT4 deficiency–a clinical phenotype distinct from the classic Mayer-Rokitansky-Kuster-Hauser syndrome: a case report. Hum Reprod. 2007;22(1):224–9.

Biason-Lauber A, Schoenle EJ. Apparently normal ovarian differentiation in a prepubertal girl with transcriptionally inactive steroidogenic factor 1 (NR5A1/SF-1) and adrenocortical insufficiency. Am J Hum Genet. 2000;67(6):15z.

Bongiovanni AM, Eberlein WR. Plasma and urinary corticosteroids in the hypertensive form of congenital adrenal hyperplasia. J Biol Chem. 1956;223(1):85–94.

Bose HS, Sugawara T, Strauss JF 3rd, et al. The pathophysiology and genetics of congenital lipoid adrenal hyperplasia. International congenital lipoid adrenal hyperplasia consortium. N Engl J Med. 1996;335(25):1870–8.

Chung BC, Hu MC, Guzov VM, et al. Structure and expression of the CYP21 (P450c21, steroid 21-hydroxylase) gene with respect to its deficiency. Endocr Res. 1995;21(1–2):343–52.

Concolino P, Mello E, Zuppi C, et al. Molecular diagnosis of congenital adrenal hyperplasia due to 21-hydroxylase deficiency: an update of new CYP21A2 mutations. Clin Chem Lab Med. 2010;48(8):1057–62.

Costa-Santos M, Kater CE, Auchus RJ. Two prevalent CYP17 mutations and genotype-phenotype correlations in 24 Brazilian patients with 17-hydroxylase deficiency. J Clin Endocrinol Metab. 2004;89(1):49–60.

Croft B, Ohnesorg T, Hewitt J, et al. Human sex reversal is caused by duplication or deletion of core enhancers upstream of SOX9. Nat Commun. 2018;9(1):5319.

Darlington Statement. 2017. https://darlington.org.au.

Dessens AB, Slijper FME, Drop SLS. Gender dysphoria and gender change in chromosomal females with congenital adrenal hyperplasia. Arch Sex Behav. 2005;34(4):389–97.

Feder EK, Dreger A. Still ignoring human rights in intersex care. J Pediatr Urol. 2016;12(6):436–7.

Finkielstain GP, Chen W, Mehta SP, et al. Comprehensive genetic analysis of 182 unrelated families with congenital adrenal hyperplasia due to 21-hydroxylase deficiency. J Clin Endocrinol Metab. 2010;96(1):E161–72.

Fluck CE, Pandey AV, Huang N, et al. P450 oxidoreductase deficiency–a new form of congenital adrenal hyperplasia. Endocr Dev. 2008;13:67–81.

Fujieda K, Tajima T. Molecular basis of adrenal insufficiency. Pediatr Res. 2005;57(5 Pt 2):62R–9R.

Fujieda K, Tajima T, Nakae J, et al. Spontaneous puberty in 46,XX subjects with congenital lipoid adrenal hyperplasia. Ovarian steroidogenesis is spared to some extent despite inactivating mutations in the steroidogenic acute regulatory protein (StAR) gene. J Clin Invest. 1997;99(6):1265–71.

Hall CM, Jones JA, Meyer-Bahlburg HFL, et al. Behavioral and physical masculinization are related to genotype in girls with congenital adrenal hyperplasia. J Clin Endocrinol Metab. 2004;89(1):419–24.

Halper A, Hooke MC, Gonzalez-Bolanos MT, et al. Health-related quality of life in children with congenital adrenal hyperplasia. Health Qual Life Outcomes. 2017;15(1):194.

Hamed SA, Metwalley KA, Farghaly HS. Cognitive function in children with classic congenital adrenal hyperplasia. Eur J Pediatr. 2018;177(11):1633–40.

Higashi Y, Yoshioka H, Yamane M, et al. Complete nucleotide sequence of two steroid 21-hydroxylase genes tandemly arranged in human chromosome: a pseudogene and a genuine gene. Proc Natl Acad Sci U S A. 1986;83(9):2841–5.

Hines M, Brook C, Conway GS. Androgen and psychosexual development: core gender identity, sexual orientation and recalled childhood gender role behavior in women and men with congenital adrenal hyperplasia (CAH). J Sex Res. 2004;41(1):75–81.

Hughes IA. Congenital adrenal hyperplasia. Trends Endocrinol Metab. 1990a;1(3):123–8.

Hughes IA. Monitoring treatment in congenital adrenal hyperplasia. Arch Dis Child. 1990b;65(3):333.

Imai T, Yanase T, Waterman MR, et al. Canadian mennonites and individuals residing in the Friesland region of The Netherlands share the same molecular basis of 17 alpha-hydroxylase deficiency. Hum Genet. 1992;89(1):95–6.

Jaaskelainen J, Tiitinen A, Voutilainen R. Sexual function and fertility in adult females and males with congenital adrenal hyperplasia. Horm Res. 2001;56(3–4):73–80.

John M, Menon SK, Shah NS, et al. Congenital adrenal hyperplasia 11beta-hydroxylase deficiency: two cases managed with bilateral adrenalectomy. Singap Med J. 2009;50(2):e68–70.

Kacem M, Moussa A, Khochtali I, et al. Bilateral adrenalectomy for severe hypertension in congenital adrenal hyperplasia due to 11beta-hydroxylase deficiency: long term follow-up. Ann Endocrinol. 2009;70(2):113–8.

Kelso WM, Nicholls ME, Warne GL, et al. Cerebral lateralization and cognitive functioning in patients with congenital adrenal hyperplasia. Neuropsychology. 2000;14(3):370–8.

Khoury K, Barbar E, Ainmelk Y, et al. Gonadal function, first cases of pregnancy, and child delivery in a woman with lipoid congenital adrenal hyperplasia. J Clin Endocrinol Metab. 2009;94(4):1333–7.

Kimberley N, Hutson JM, Southwell BR, et al. Vaginal agenesis, the hymen, and associated anomalies. J Pediatr Adolesc Gynecol. 2012;25(1):54–8.

Kolon TF, Ferrer FA, McKenna PH. Clinical and molecular analysis of XX sex reversed patients. J Urol. 1998;160(3 Pt 2):1169–72. discussion 1178.

Koppens PF, Hoogenboezem T, Degenhart HJ. Duplication of the CYP21A2 gene complicates mutation analysis of steroid 21-hydroxylase deficiency: characteristics of three unusual haplotypes. Hum Genet. 2002;111(4–5):405–10.

Krob G, Braun A, Kuhnle U. True hermaphroditism: geographical distribution, clinical findings, chromosomes and gonadal histology. Eur J Pediatr. 1994;153(1):2–10.

Levine LS, Dupont B, Lorenzen F, et al. Genetic and hormonal characterization of cryptic 21-hydroxylase deficiency. J Clin Endocrinol Metab. 1981;53(6):1193–8.

Levine LS, Zachmann M, New MI, et al. Genetic mapping of the 21-hydroxylase-deficiency gene within the HLA linkage group. N Engl J Med. 1978;299(17):911–5.

Lourenco D, Brauner R, Lin L, et al. Mutations in NR5A1 associated with ovarian insufficiency. N Engl J Med. 2009;360(12):1200–10.

Lutfallah C, Wang W, Mason JI, et al. Newly proposed hormonal criteria via genotypic proof for type II 3beta-hydroxysteroid dehydrogenase deficiency. J Clin Endocrinol Metab. 2002;87(6):2611–22.

MacKay D, Nordenstrom A, Falhammar H.Bilateral adrenalectomy in congenital adrenal hyperplasia: a systematic review and meta-analysis. J Clin Endocrinol Metab. 2018. https://doi.org/10.1210/jc.2018-00217.

Meyer-Bahlburg HF. What causes low rates of childbearing in congenital adrenal hyperplasia? J Clin Endocrinol Metab. 1999;84(6):1844–7.

Meyer-Bahlburg HF, Dolezal C, Baker SW, et al. Sexual orientation in women with classical or non-classical congenital adrenal hyperplasia as a function of degree of prenatal androgen excess. Arch Sex Behav. 2008;37(1):85–99.

Meyer-Bahlburg HF, Gruen RS, New MI, et al. Gender change from female to male in classical congenital adrenal hyperplasia. Horm Behav. 1996;30(4):319–32.

Miller WL. Steroid 17alpha-hydroxylase deficiency–not rare everywhere. J Clin Endocrinol Metab. 2004;89(1):40–2.
Mulaikal RM, Migeon CJ, Rock JA. Fertility rates in female patients with congenital adrenal hyperplasia due to 21-hydroxylase deficiency. N Engl J Med. 1987;316(4):178–82.
Nordenstrom A, Forest MG, Wedell A. A case of 3beta-hydroxysteroid dehydrogenase type II (HSD3B2) deficiency picked up by neonatal screening for 21-hydroxylase deficiency: difficulties and delay in etiologic diagnosis. Horm Res. 2007;68(4):204–8.
Parajes S, Loidi L, Reisch N, et al. Functional consequences of seven novel mutations in the CYP11B1 gene: four mutations associated with nonclassic and three mutations causing classic 11{beta}-hydroxylase deficiency. J Clin Endocrinol Metab. 2010;95(2):779–88.
Razzaghy-Azar M, Karimi S, Shirazi E. Gender identity in patients with congenital adrenal hyperplasia. Int J Endocrinol Metab. 2017;15(3):e12537.
Robins T, Carlsson J, Sunnerhagen M, et al. Molecular model of human CYP21 based on mammalian CYP2C5: structural features correlate with clinical severity of mutations causing congenital adrenal hyperplasia. Mol Endocrinol. 2006;20(11):2946–64.
Rosa S, Steigert M, Lang-Muritano M, et al. Clinical, genetic and functional characteristics of three novel CYP17A1 mutations causing combined 17alpha-hydroxylase/17,20-lyase deficiency. Horm Res Paediatr. 2010;73(3):198–204.
Rosler A, Leiberman E, Cohen T. High frequency of congenital adrenal hyperplasia (classic 11 beta-hydroxylase deficiency) among Jews from Morocco. Am J Med Genet. 1992;42(6):827–34.
Rosler A, Levine LS, Schneider B, et al. The interrelationship of sodium balance, plasma renin activity and ACTH in congenital adrenal hyperplasia. J Clin Endocrinol Metab. 1977;45(3):500–12.
Rosler A, Weshler N, Leiberman E, et al. 11 Beta-hydroxylase deficiency congenital adrenal hyperplasia: update of prenatal diagnosis. J Clin Endocrinol Metab. 1988;66(4):830–8.
Simard J, Moisan AM, Morel Y. Congenital adrenal hyperplasia due to 3beta-hydroxysteroid dehydrogenase/Delta(5)-Delta(4) isomerase deficiency. Semin Reprod Med. 2002;20(3):255–76.
Speiser PW, White PC. Congenital adrenal hyperplasia. N Engl J Med. 2003;349(8):776–88.
Sutton E, Hughes J, White S, et al. Identification of SOX3 as an XX male sex reversal gene in mice and humans. J Clin Investig. 2011;121(1):328–41.
Tapanainen JS, Vaskivuo T, Aittomaki K, et al. Inactivating FSH receptor mutations and gonadal dysfunction. Mol Cell Endocrinol. 1998;145(1–2):129–35.
Tian Q, Yao F, Sha G, et al. Genotyping of a Chinese family with 46,XX and 46,XY 17-hydroxylase deficiency. Gynecol Endocrinol. 2009;25(8):485–90.
Tonkin-Hill G. Identifying the resource needs of adolescents with Differences of Sex Development. Faculty of Medicine, University of Melbourne, Melbourne; 2018.
Tucker EJ, Grover SR, Bachelot A, et al. Premature ovarian insufficiency: new perspectives on genetic cause and phenotypic spectrum. Endocr Rev. 2016;37(6):609–35.
Vallerie AM, Breech LL. Update in Müllerian anomalies: diagnosis, management, and outcomes. Curr Opin Obstet Gynecol. 2010;22(5):381–7.
Van Wyk JJ, Gunther DF, Ritzen EM, et al. The use of adrenalectomy as a treatment for congenital adrenal hyperplasia. J Clin Endocrinol Metab. 1996;81(9):3180–90.
Van Wyk JJ, Ritzen EM. The role of bilateral adrenalectomy in the treatment of congenital adrenal hyperplasia. J Clin Endocrinol Metab. 2003;88(7):2993–8.
Vorona E, Zitzmann M, Gromoll J, et al. Clinical, endocrinological, and epigenetic features of the 46,XX male syndrome, compared with 47,XXY Klinefelter patients. J Clin Endocrinol Metab. 2007;92(9):3458–65.
White PC, Medscape. Neonatal screening for congenital adrenal hyperplasia. Nat Rev Endocrinol. 2009;5(9):490–8.
Wisniewski AB, Migeon CJ, Meyer-Bahlburg HF, et al. Complete androgen insensitivity syndrome: long-term medical, surgical, and psychosexual outcome. J Clin Endocrinol Metab. 2000;85(8):2664–9.
Wudy SA, Hartmann M, Homoki J. Hormonal diagnosis of 21-hydroxylase deficiency in plasma and urine of neonates using benchtop gas chromatography-mass spectrometry. J Endocrinol. 2000;165(3):679–83.
Zainuddin AA, Grover SR, Soon CH, et al. A Multi-center cross-sectional study of Malaysian females with congenital adrenal hyperplasia: Their body image and their persepctives on feminizing surgery. J Pediatr Adolesc Gynecol. 2020 (epub ahead of print 3 May 2020).

46,XY DSD

7

Michele A. O'Connell, Aurore Bouty, and Sonia R. Grover

Atypical sex development can occur through interruption of testicular development, the hormonal hypothalamic–pituitary–gonadal axis or morphogenesis of the urogenital region. These three broad groups of DSD aetiology are termed gonadal dysgenesis, hormonal dysfunction (in either production or response) and atypical morphogenesis, respectively (Table 7.1).

Thus, there is a wide spectrum of presentations of these individuals.

Table 7.1 Causes of 46,XY DSD

Causes of 46,XY DSD	
Gonadal dysgenesis	Partial gonadal dysgenesis Mixed gonadal dysgenesis Complete gonadal dysgenesis Testicular regression syndrome Ovo-testicular DSD
Hormone dysfunction	
Gonadotrophin dysfunction	Isolated gonadotrophin deficiency Multiple pituitary hormone deficiency LH receptor defect
Steroidogenesis dysfunction	Steroidogenic acute regulatory protein Cholesterol side chain cleavage enzyme 17α-Hydroxylase deficiency 17,20-Lyase deficiency 3β-Hydroxysteroid dehydrogenase-2 deficiency P450 oxidoreductase deficiency Cytochrome b5 deficiency 17β-Hydroxysteroid dehydrogenase-3 deficiency 5α-Reductase-2 deficiency
Androgen insensitivity	Partial androgen insensitivity syndrome (mild, moderate and severe) Complete androgen insensitivity syndrome
AMH dysfunction	Persistent Müllerian duct syndrome
Atypical morphogenesis	Bladder and cloacal exstrophy

M. A. O'Connell (✉)
Department of Endocrinology and Diabetes, The Royal Children's Hospital, Melbourne, VIC, Australia

Murdoch Children's Research Institute, Melbourne, VIC, Australia
e-mail: michele.oconnell@rch.org.au

A. Bouty
Department of Urology, The Royal Children's Hospital, Melbourne, VIC, Australia

Murdoch Children's Research Institute, Melbourne, VIC, Australia
e-mail: aurore.bouty@rch.org.au

S. R. Grover
Department of Gynaecology, The Royal Children's Hospital, Melbourne, VIC, Australia

Murdoch Children's Research Institute, Melbourne, VIC, Australia

Department of Paediatrics, University of Melbourne, Melbourne, VIC, Australia
e-mail: Sonia.grover@rch.org.au

J. M. Hutson et al. (eds.), *Disorders|Differences of Sex Development*,
https://doi.org/10.1007/978-981-13-7864-5_7

7.1 Clinical Presentation

DSD in a 46,XY individual can present within a wide clinical spectrum. This includes discordant (female) phenotype at birth when antenatal testing has indicated 46,XY individual, atypical genital appearance at birth, absence of development of secondary sex characteristics in an adolescent boy or primary amenorrhoea in an adolescent with a female phenotype (with or without some secondary sexual characteristics). The variation in clinical presentation is due to two factors: the degree of disturbance of androgen production or action and the temporal point at which this disturbance occurred during sex development.

The anatomic variations may be divided into those describing the external genitalia and those describing the presence or absence of Müllerian structures. Evaluation of the infant should include assessment of the presence of gonads in the labioscrotal folds, the fusion of the labioscrotal folds (e.g., fused/bifid), the size of the phallus and the site of the urinary meatus on the phallus. An atypical site of the urethral opening is described as being a hypospadias when the urethral opening is on the ventral aspect of the penis at the glans, midshaft, penoscrotal or perineal level. These external features can be individually scored to provide an aggregate score, the external masculinisation score (EMS) (Ahmed et al. 2000) (Fig. 7.1).

Variations may therefore include the following features:

- Complete absence of androgen action, due to any cause, from the time of early foetal development, results in a child with a typical female external phenotype. This child will most commonly present either at birth with discordant phenotype from that predicted by antenatal testing or as an adolescent with primary amenorrhoea.
- Partial action of androgen during foetal development may cause hypospadias, with position of the urethral opening further down penile shaft reflecting more significant androgen dysfunction between 8 and 12 weeks of gestation.
- Smaller than typical stretched penile length (previously termed 'micropenis', where the

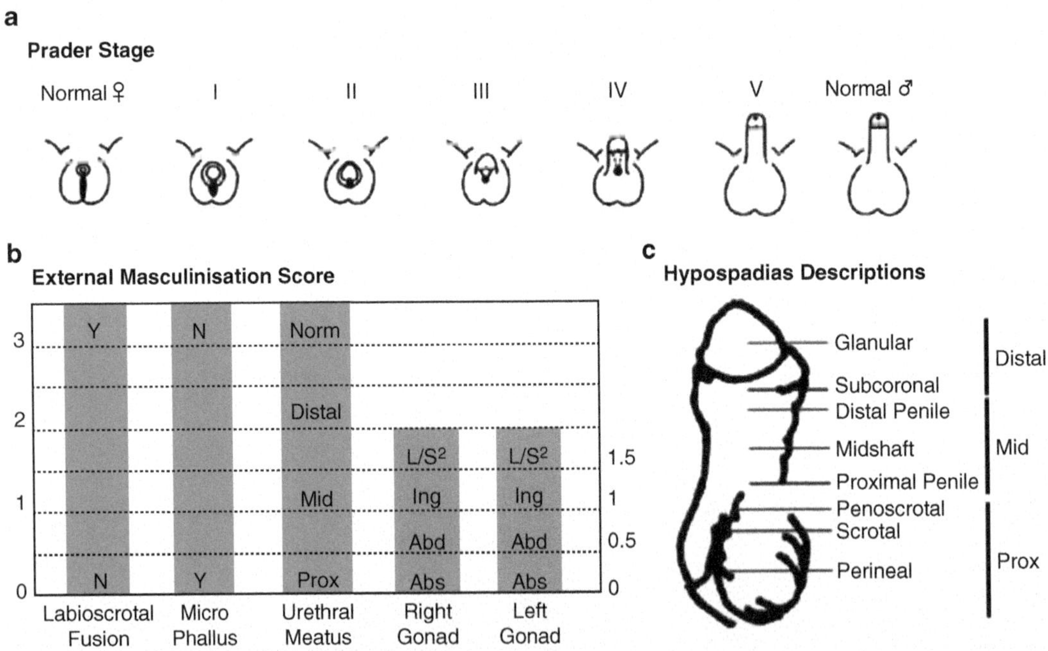

Fig. 7.1 Assessment of external genitalia. (**a**) Prader Stage. (**b**) External masculinisation score. (**c**) Classification of hypospadias (Reproduced with permission from Ahmed and Rodie (2010))

stretched penile length at birth is less than 2 cm), can also occur with limited androgen action later in gestation (Lee et al. 1980).
- Cryptorchidism, or undescended testes, can result from developmental androgen deficiency, and small or absent testes suggest testicular dysgenesis (Kearsey and Hutson 2017).
- Absence of androgen action with onset at later time points can cause disruption of puberty in an adolescent boy.

In 46,XY DSD, Müllerian structures may be present or absent. In 46,XY individuals with functioning Sertoli cells and anti-Müllerian hormone (AMH) receptors, the Müllerian structures regress in a typical manner. In contrast, where embryonic testes do not develop functioning Sertoli cells, AMH is not released and Müllerian structures will remain as the female genital tract. It is important to determine if Müllerian structures are present in an individual with features suggestive of 46,XY DSD, as this may have a bearing on potential future fertility options. The morphology of Müllerian structures is now best described or classified with a system that allows a separate description of vaginal, cervical and uterine anomalies (Grimbizis et al. 2013).

Cryptorchidism occurs where the multimodal mechanisms controlling testicular descent are altered. These mechanisms include roles of androgen, molecular factors such as INSL3 and LGR8 and mechanical factors associated with the abdominal wall (Foresta et al. 2008; Hutson et al. 2010).

When the clinical presentation of 46,XY DSD is with atypical genital appearance, such that sex is not obvious (based on genital appearance) at birth, the question regarding optimal sex of rearing is important. The decision-making around this has changed substantially over the last few decades and is further discussed in Chaps. 12 and 16.

46,XY ovo-testicular DSD are discussed in Chap. 8.

7.2 Incidence

Due to the varied clinical presentation of 46,XY DSD, a comprehensive incidence for this group of conditions is not known. The most common presentation, hypospadias, is understood to occur in 1 in 125 to 1 in 300 male births. The more common, isolated distal hypospadias, where the scrotum is fused and both testes are descended, is not typically classified as a 'DSD'. The inclusion of mild isolated hypospadias in some literature regarding DSD is the source of the significantly higher rate of reported incidence of DSD/Intersex. More significant degrees of hypospadias carry a greater likelihood of an underlying genetic cause and are less common.

In addition to the wide spectrum of clinical presentation, 46,XY DSD are further complicated by difficulty in ascertaining a clear underlying diagnosis/cause. Recent data from 122 boys with genital variations and a median EMS of 9 (range 1–11) reported detection of an underlying endocrine problem in 28 (23%). Median EMS was statistically higher in those with normal endocrine testing results (median 9 cf. 8.3), but as there was a lot of overlap between groups, EMS scores were not discriminatory. Of 21 boys with a genetic variant identified on either array-comparative genomic hybridisation or a limited seven-gene panel, 11 (52%) had normal endocrine investigations (Nixon et al. 2017).

Despite thorough hormonal and molecular-genetic investigations therefore, a definitive diagnosis is difficult to achieve in the majority of 46,XY DSD cases (Hughes 2008; Bhullar et al. 2011; Nixon et al. 2017). The recent availability of targeted next-generation sequencing gene panels for genetic variants associated with DSD has been shown to improve diagnostic rates with a likely genetic diagnosis reported in 43% of all 46,XY DSD in a recent large study (n = 278 46,XY DSD individuals included) (Eggers et al. 2016). The genetic diagnosis rate rose to 60% in the cohort with 46, XY DSD relating to differences of androgen synthesis and action. Overall, given the lack of a clear association between clinical assessment/EMS and presence of identifiable endocrine and genetic variations, both endocrine and genetic investigations are warranted in many cases of suspected XY DSD. Much research effort continues to be directed to understanding the aetiology of 46,XY DSD so that diagnostic accuracy can be improved.

7.3 Undefined 46,XY DSD (Hypospadias and Cryptorchidism)

DSD due to milder forms of hypospadias represent a large patient group (incidence of 1 in 125 live male births) with wide geographical differences and varying reports of a rising incidence. Hypospadias is thought to relate to a combination of genetic and environmental factors (Bouty et al. 2015). Altered hormonal exposure *in utero* may be an underlying cause; this may be due to an inherent DSD or to placental insufficiency, resulting in lower hCG and hence lower testosterone stimulation in the early weeks of gestation. The potential role of environmental endocrine disruptors is the subject of much scrutiny (Fisch et al. 2010; Kalfa et al. 2015). For example, chemicals such as phthalates and bisphenol A, which are used in manufacturing, are thought to act by reducing testosterone production antenatally in the developing male foetus (Morales-Suarez-Varela et al. 2011).

In boys with genital differences, a chromosomal variation has previously been described in approximately 3% of those with isolated cryptorchidism, 7% of those with hypospadias and 13% of those with a combination of cryptorchidism and hypospadias (Moreno-Garcia and Miranda 2002).

The apparent rising incidence of hypospadias has been associated with a rising incidence of cryptorchidism and testicular germ cell cancer in population-based studies, and the concept of a 'testicular dysgenesis syndrome' due to environmental exposures has been proposed to explain these increases (Olesen et al. 2007). Some authors doubt this hypothesis and have argued that the rising hypospadias incidence may not be real but may relate to improved ascertainment (Fisch et al. 2010). A large study in Denmark found evidence that hypospadias or cryptorchidism increased the relative risk for testicular germ cell cancer by twofold to fourfold (Schnack et al. 2010). This risk was increased only in affected individuals and not if there was a family history for disease, supporting the 'testicular dysgenesis syndrome" association.

In children with more severe degrees of hypospadias and cryptorchidism, the likelihood of a germ-line genetic mutation is more likely, and investigations to determine aetiology are warranted (Ollivier et al. 2018).

7.3.1 Management

Cryptorchidism resolves spontaneously over the first 3 months of life in up to 70% of children (Berkowitz et al. 1993). If this does not occur in the early postnatal months, intervention to bring the testes to the scrotum is recommended. The use of hCG to assist testicular descent is no longer routine due to limited evidence and unclear distinctions of cryptorchidism aetiology and severity. The effectiveness of hCG is reported to range from 0% to 55% (Henna et al. 2004). In addition, concerns have been raised regarding mild inflammatory infiltrate noted at testicular biopsy after hCG administration in older children; however, this may be a normal physiological process associated with the usual FSH and LH surge during early infancy (Hjertkvist et al. 1993). The vast majority of cryptorchidism, however, is managed with a reported 95% success rate by surgical orchidopexy (Ritzen et al. 2007). Orchidopexy should be timed to occur at 6–12 months to minimise the risk of infertility and germ cell cancer (Hutson et al. 2010; Thorup and Cortes 2016).

In the setting of associations with increased risk of testicular germ cell cancer and infertility, it is prudent to arrange follow-up of these boys at the time of puberty to counsel them on testicular self-examination, give advice on management of future infertility or testicular failure and to ensure normal pubertal development.

7.4 46,XY Gonadal Dysgenesis

Gonadal dysgenesis results when the process of gonadal development is disrupted, leading to variable degrees of gonadal function. This developmental pathway involves activation of a complex gene cascade (see Chap. 2). Perhaps in part due to our incomplete understanding of the entire process of human testicular development, causative genetic variants cannot be determined for all affected individuals (Hughes 2008; Bhullar et al. 2011), although detection rates are improving with newer gene panels and exome sequencing (Baxter et al. 2015; Eggers et al. 2016).

The diagnosis of gonadal dysgenesis is therefore often based on clinical features and evidence of less than typical gonadal function. In those with 46,XY karyotype, gonadal dysgenesis is easier to discern in individuals with minimal (severe partial) or no (complete dysgenesis) evidence of genital virilisation than for those with a milder partial change in function, where the phenotypic spectrum can overlap with differences in androgenic synthesis or action. Gonadal dysgenesis of significant severity will lead to small, underdeveloped, poorly differentiated gonads (testes) with markedly reduced androgen production capacity, presence of Müllerian structures due to absence of sufficient AMH to cause regression *in utero* and elevated gonadotrophin levels from the time of puberty, due to primary gonadal insufficiency.

Given the spectrum of 46,XY gonadal dysgenesis, these variations are classified into partial gonadal dysgenesis (PGD), mixed gonadal dysgenesis (MGD) and complete gonadal dysgenesis (CGD).

In 46,XY partial and mixed gonadal dysgenesis, there is some element of testicular development, evidenced by virilisation of the external genitalia at birth, albeit with some variation from typical development (Fig. 7.2). Mixed gonadal dysgenesis refers to marked asymmetry in gonadal development, with a dysgenetic testis on one side and a streak gonad on the other (Donahoe et al. 1979). It is more often associated with mixed sex chromosome (aneuploidy) DSD but can occur in 46,XY DSD. External genital appearance relates to the degree of androgen production and effect and can vary widely; similarly, Müllerian structures may or may not be present, depending on amount of Sertoli cell function. As AMH acts in an ipsilateral manner by local exocrine secretion, there can also be asymmetric Müllerian findings such as a hemi-uterus in mixed gonadal dysgenesis. This is discussed in more detail in Chap. 8.

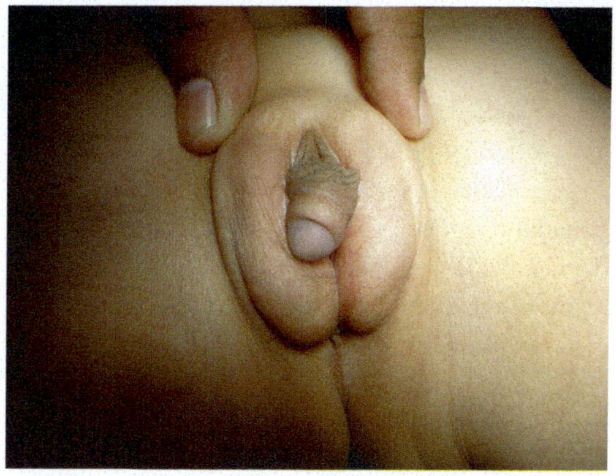

Fig. 7.2 46,XY gonadal dysgenesis with low amounts of early androgen production (leading to bifid scrotum and severe chordee of phallus) but greater androgen production later in gestation, leading to growth of the hypospadiac phallus

An individual with 46,XY complete gonadal dysgenesis has bilateral streak gonad development and therefore typical female phenotype with developed Müllerian structures (due to complete absence of testicular/gonadal androgen and AMH production *in utero*). This may be diagnosed at birth when an antenatal karyotype performed as part of antenatal screening is discordant with the phenotype, or when a karyotype is requested in a girl with delayed or absent puberty. The advent of non-invasive prenatal testing (NIPT) and its relative frequency of uptake in developed countries is causing a shift in the age of detection of some DSD from adolescence to the neonatal period.

The causes of partial or mixed gonadal dysgenesis are loss-of-function mutations in the genes associated with testicular sex determination, or gain-of-function of genes associated with ovarian sex determination. These genes include those at the level of the bipotential gonad, such as *CBX2*, *NR5A1*, *WT1* and *GATA4*, those at the level of early testis determination such as *SRY* and *DMRT1/DMRT2* and those that act in the testis determination cascade such as *SOX9*, *NR0B1*, *DHH*, *ATRX*, *MAMLD1*, *TSPYL1* and *WNT4*.

There are specific phenotypic associations with variants in some of these genes, while others have a diverse presentation. NR5A1 is expressed in the urogenital ridge and acts at an early stage of gonadal development; its gene product, SF-1, activates the expression of SRY (de Santa Barbara et al. 2001). Functional mutations in *NR5A1* (also called *SF1*) have been reported to lead to a spectrum of phenotypes. These range from adrenal and gonadal dysgenesis through to isolated gonadal dysgenesis and penoscrotal hypospadias (Lin et al. 2007; Kohler et al. 2009). In contrast to many of the other genes involved in gonadal dysgenesis where the aetiology explains only infrequent cases, *NR5A1* contributes to a relatively large proportion of DSD. It is thought to be associated with approximately 15% of 46,XY partial gonadal dysgenesis and can also cause complete gonadal dysgenesis (Kohler and Achermann 2010; Philibert et al. 2010).

WT1 is a zinc-finger transcription factor expressed in the genital ridge, foetal gonads and developing kidneys. *WT1* has a tumour suppressor function in addition to its role in organogenesis, and variants are associated with high risk of germ cell cancer. There are many isoforms of the WT1 protein, with variants leading to the (−) KTS isoform resulting in Frasier syndrome, characterised by gonadal dysgenesis, progressive glomerulopathy and renal failure but not Wilms tumour. Mutations in WT1 with the (+)KTS isoform lead to Denys-Drash syndrome, with gonadal dysgenesis, diffuse mesangial sclerosis and frequent development of germ cell cancer and Wilms tumour of the kidney (Wagner et al. 2003). The association of Wilms tumour, aniridia, genitourinary anomalies/gonadoblastoma and intellectual disability occurs with larger 11p13 deletions, which include the *WT1* gene, and is termed WAGR syndrome. Mutations in *GATA4* are associated with atrial septal congenital heart defects and gonadal dysgenesis due to the role of this gene in cardiac and testis development (Lourenco et al. 2011).

The key testis-determining factor on the Y chromosome is *SRY* and variants in this gene lead to complete gonadal dysgenesis. Such variants were previously estimated at explaining 10–15% of 46,XY CGD cases (Cameron and Sinclair 1997; Harley et al. 2003), although they were reported in a much smaller proportion of 46,XY DSD in a recent study of massively parallel sequencing-targeted DSD gene panel (four variants in 276 46,XY DSD cases) (Eggers et al. 2016). Variants in *SOX9* lead to gonadal dysgenesis and campomelic dysplasia due to its role in both gonadal and cartilage development. Seventy-five per cent of 46,XY individuals with a *SOX9* variant are either phenotypically female or have atypical genital appearance (Foster et al. 1994). Variants in regulatory elements surrounding the coding region for *SOX9* now indicate that there could be gonad-specific loss of *SOX9* function with normal skeletal development in some 46,XY DSD patients (Cox et al. 2011). These findings for *SOX9* regulation are significant, as variants in regulatory elements of other genes are also likely to lead to gene dysfunction.

NR0B1 is considered an 'anti-testis' gene because, in humans, duplication of the chromosomal region Xp21 which includes *NR0B1*, leads to 46,XY gonadal dysgenesis. *NR0B1* (also known as *DAX1*) leads to 46,XY DSD by an unusual mechanism—so-called dosage-sensitive sex reversal. That is, duplications of *NR0B1* in a 46,XY individual leads to complete gonadal dysgenesis (Bardoni et al. 1994). In contrast, loss-of-function mutations in *NR0B1* result in congenital adrenal hypoplasia and hypogonadotrophic hypogonadism, but not DSD.

DMRT1 and *DMRT2* are associated with gonadal dysgenesis when they are deleted in contiguous distal 9p monosomy disorders, however, dysfunction in a single gene has not yet been reported to cause 46,XY DSD. This suggests that there may be some redundancy between the genes in the region, with a larger deletion required to cause loss of function (Ottolenghi et al. 2000).

DHH variants are associated with 46,XY partial gonadal dysgenesis and mini-fascicular polyneuropathy, consistent with the phenotype of the mouse model (Umehara et al. 2000). *ATRX* mutations are associated with the rare disorder X-linked alpha thalassaemia, intellectual disability and 46,XY DSD (Tang et al. 2011). *MAMLD1* is thought to be associated with a less marked virilisation deficit form of 46,XY DSD phenotype and penoscrotal hypospadias (Ogata et al. 2008). *TSPYL1* mutations have been associated with sudden infant death and dysgenesis of the testis (Puffenberger et al. 2004).

MAP3K1 encodes a signal transduction regulator in the sex determination pathway and is emerging as one of the more common genes responsible for 46,XY DSD presenting as complete or partial gonadal dysgenesis (Eggers et al. 2014; Granados et al. 2017). It is postulated that *Cbx2* is required for the expression of *sry* in gonadal development. Compound heterozygous variants in *CBX2* have been reported in one 46,XY female with histologically normal ovaries, an uncommon phenotype (Biason-Lauber et al. 2009).

In addition to loss-of-function of genes involved in testis development, gain of function in genes involved in ovarian development can also cause 46,XY DSD. This has been reported for *WNT4* duplications (Jordan et al. 2003). More detailed information on the genetics of DSD can be found in Chapter 2.

7.4.1 Management

The initial concern for many families of individuals with 46,XY gonadal dysgenesis recognised at birth is the optimal sex of rearing for a child. While future gender identity can never be predicted with 100% accuracy in any child, some DSD are known to have a more common gender identity. It is important that parents are fully informed about what is known and as yet unknown in this regard; the possibility of future gender diversity and acceptance of divergence from sex of rearing should also be discussed and promoted from early interactions with the family and throughout childhood.

In individuals with 46,XY severe partial or complete gonadal dysgenesis, female gender identity has been most frequently reported for those with a female phenotype with presence of Müllerian structures (McCarty et al. 2006). Where there is evidence of functional testicular tissue (i.e., evidence of some, but less than typical, external genital virilisation at birth), male sex of rearing is increasingly considered. This is because the peripheral tissues' response to androgen is not altered in gonadal dysgenesis, allowing the potential for further virilisation in response to future endogenous testosterone at puberty (albeit that this may be in lower-than-typical amounts in PGD). In the case of 46, XY gonadal dysgenesis with female sex of rearing, feminising genitoplasty should not be routinely undertaken in early childhood, as this procedure may irreversibly remove tissues which may be desired later should the individual identify as male. Due consideration of the ethical principles involved (Gillam et al. 2010) would therefore recommend no intervention until such time as the individual is older and can be involved in the decision as to whether this is desired.

Previously, gonadectomy in early childhood was undertaken in some individuals with 46,XY partial gonadal dysenesis, where female sex assignment had been determined. This was performed both to prevent any further virilisation (thought to be unwanted if female sex of rearing had been assigned) and due to the higher risk of malignancy in those with 46,XY PGD (Pleskacova et al. 2010; Pyle and Nathanson 2017). In light of increased awareness of dissatisfaction and regret at such procedures in those who subsequently identified as male, such surgeries are no longer be considered appropriate in infancy. Deferral until the individual is old enough to be involved in decisions relating to removal or preservation of their gonads is now a preferred approach. Discussions around these decisions should be broached in late first decade / peri-pubertally as the risk of malignancy increases thereafter. In addition, assessment of the young person's gender identity in the context of anticipated and experienced pubertal hormone exposure is also important. Pre-natal androgen is also thought to have specific effects on the developing brain, which may influence subsequent gender identity (Latronico and Arnhold 2012; Peper and Koolschijn 2012); however this potential effect cannot be quantified/extrapolated from assessment of the level of genital virilisation. In all situations regarding difficult choice of the sex of rearing, ethical considerations should be balanced and weighed (Gillam et al. 2010) (see Chap. 15).

In individuals with 46,XY gonadal dysgenesis with persisting Müllerian duct structures who are raised male, the Müllerian tissue in the past was removed, but currently, the preference at our institution and many other centres is for these structures to be ligated and left *in situ* for decisions regarding removal or otherwise to be made at a later date by the affected individual. Surgical intervention may be re-appraised if these structures should be associated with intrusive symptoms (e.g., recurrent UTIs).

Gonadectomy may be recommended for patients with 46,XY DSD and intra-abdominal testes, which cannot be brought to the scrotum for cancer surveillance or adequately monitored with imaging. Biopsy should be performed in patients at risk of germ cell cancer with testes *in situ*. Regular, intermittent cancer surveillance and monitoring for hormonal testicular failure should occur on a lifelong basis, with fertility assistance as required. Affected individuals and their families should also be informed of the limitations of available monitoring tools. For those in whom there is no spontaneous endogenous gonadal function, or where gonads have been removed, discussions regarding appropriate hormone replacement therapy should be undertaken. Prior to commencing such therapy, it should be ensured that the choice of hormone replacement aligns with an individual's gender identity; this should not be assumed based on either sex chromosomal make-up or sex of rearing but rather based on open discussions with the individual themelves. This is particularly important when puberty, and hence the development of secondary sex characteristics, is to be induced with exogenous hormone therapy. Conversely, for those with endogenous hormone function, if gender identity diverges from sex of rearing and is causing distress, pubertal progression may be 'blocked' temporarily using gonadotrophin-releasing hormone analogue (GnRHa) therapy to allow time for further decision-making.

7.4.2 46,XY Testicular Regression Syndrome

Testicular regression syndrome is also variously termed anorchia or vanishing testes syndrome. The common phenotype is the absence of structural testicular tissue in a 46,XY individual with clinical evidence in external genital phenotype of previously normal testicular function, hence, testicular regression. Testicular regression can occur antenatally or postnatally, with the eventual clinical finding of absence of palpable testes, confirmed biologically and/or at surgical exploration. There may be a residual nodule on exploration for testicular tissue, containing haemosiderin-laden macrophages or dystrophic calcification (Spires et al. 2000). The aetiology is unknown; however, the histological findings in residual nodules are consistent with antenatal testicular torsion and ischaemic damage as a cause. This aetiology would, however, seem more likely for unilateral rather than bilateral cases. Analysis of candidate gene mutations to explain the aetiology in bilateral cases has revealed an association with *NR5A1* variants in a small proportion of patients (Philibert et al. 2007). Management involves long-term sex hormone replacement and fertility assistance; testicular prostheses can also be offered if desired.

7.5 Hormonal causes of 46,XY DSD

7.5.1 Gonadotrophin deficiency or resistance

Atypical pituitary gland production of gonadotrophins and alterations of LH receptor function result in hypogonadotrophic hypogonadism, which is associated with 46,XY DSD if primary sex development is affected (Fig. 7.3). Gonadotrophin deficiency due to LH or LHRH deficiency in the developing 46,XY foetus typically results in an infant born with smaller than typical penis and cryptorchidism. There are a series of genes that can cause hypothalamo-pituitary gondadotrophin deficiency, including the *KAL* genes, GnRH receptor, *FGFR*-1 and *GPR54* (Iovane et al. 2004). *KAL-1* gene mutations are additionally associated with congenital anosmia. Conditions associated with multiple pituitary hormone deficiency may also be associated with gonadotrophin deficiency; these

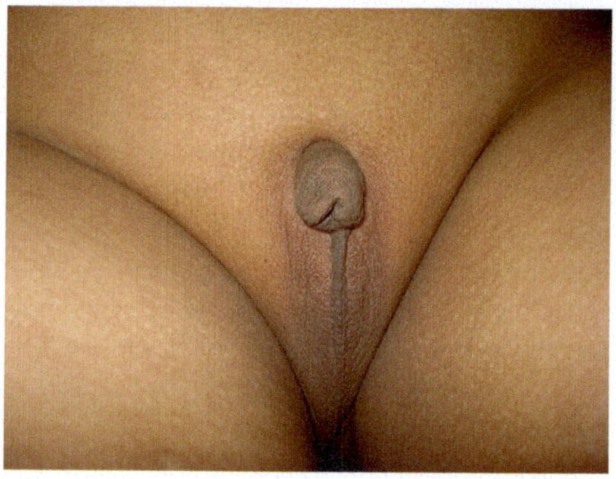

Fig. 7.3 Gonadotrophin deficiency causes failure of growth of the phallus to produce smaller than typical penile size, but early male sexual differentiation is complete, as this is controlled by placental hCG

include isolated pituitary disorders associated with gene variants such as in *PIT-1*, *PROP-1* and *HESX-1*, and syndromic DSD associations such as Bardet-Biedl, Prader-Willi or CHARGE syndrome (the latter representing **c**oloboma, **h**eart defects, **a**tresia of the nasal choanae, growth **r**estriction and developmental delay, **g**enital anomalies and **e**ar anomalies) (Aminzadeh et al. 2010). Loss of function at the LH receptor arises due to variants in the luteinising hormone/chorionic gonadotrophin receptor (*LHCGR)* gene. Clinically, affected individuals may present with varying phenotype, from typical female appearance and absence of secondary sex differentiation at puberty in those with more severe LH receptor resistance to milder genital, variation in those with more LH receptor function (Themmen and Verhoef-Post 2002; Latronico 2012, #1003; Latronico and Arnhold 2012).

Measurement of FSH and LH in the newborn period will often reveal absence of the normal early infantile gonadotrophin surge (known as 'minipuberty') where dysfunction in gonadotrophin synthesis exists. In the case of LH receptor defects, a typical level of FSH is found in association with elevated LH levels; basal as well as hCG-stimulated testosterone levels are low without evidence of higher testosterone biosynthesis precursors. The testes have only slightly reduced size but a cardinal feature is Leydig cell hypoplasia (absent or scarce Leydig cells) on testicular histology. Müllerian structures are absent.

7.5.2 Management

Testosterone administration to supplement the absent sex steroid hormone that would otherwise be typical in the infantile period may provide some supplemental penile growth, but is not universally clinically indicated. In this particular group, if hormonal replacement is thought appropriate treatment with hCG to assist testicular descent and increase in testicular volume would be a reasonable consideration. Treatment with pulsatile LHRH, or FSH and hCG, at induction of puberty may assist with testicular development and spermatogenesis (Christiansen and Skakkebaek 2002; Rohayem et al. 2017). Pubertal induction and lifelong exogenous sex hormone replacement (congruent with gender) will be required from adolescence.

Sex of rearing and subsequent gender identity in 46,XY individuals with central hypothalamo-pituitary causes is most commonly male; however, in the severe form of LH receptor variant with marked Leydig cell hypoplasia and female phenotype with absence of virilisation, female sex of rearing may be considered.

7.5.3 Altered Androgen Biosynthesis

Androgen production occurs according to the same synthesis pathway in the adrenal glands and testes, although some enzymes are testis-specific. Dysfunction of an enzyme will lead to accumulation of metabolites prior to the enzyme block and deficiency of subsequent metabolites.

The extent of virilisation of external genitalia is dependent on the degree of the enzyme block and can therefore vary widely. As Sertoli cell function is typically preserved, Müllerian structures will be absent, except for severe Smith-Lemli-Opitz syndrome, where there is poor basic cholesterol synthesis with an effect on testis development (Kelley and Hennekam 2000).

Unfortunately, there have been many terms and gene symbols used to refer to the same protein or enzyme and its coding gene, although there has been a move towards general use of the approved OMIM nomenclature. These proteins include steroidogenic acute regulatory protein (StAR), cholesterol side chain cleavage enzyme or 11α-hydroxylase (CYP11A1/P450scc), 17α-hydroxylase and 17,20-lyase (CYP17/P450c17), p450 oxidoreductase (POR), 3β-hydroxysteroid dehydrogenase-2 (HSD3B2), 17β-hydoxysteroid dehydrogenase-3 (HSD17B3) and 5α-reductase-2 (SRD5A2).

Most of these gene products influence the production of hormones within both the adrenal gland and testis, so there may be cortisol or aldosterone insufficiency requiring replacement therapy in addition to the under-virilisation. Glucocorticoid synthesis reserve should be assessed by an ACTH-stimulation test, and insufficiency treated with maintenance and stress steroid replacement, or stress steroid administration alone in those with adequate basal cortisol but insufficient ACTH response (typically defined as <550 nmol/L 60 min post administration of 250 mcg of synthetic ACTH ['Synacthen']). Mineralocorticoid insufficiency results in low sodium and high potassium, with elevated plasma renin activity, and can be treated with fludrocortisone replacement; sodium supplementation is often required in infancy. Sex steroid replacement, if required, should occur in the standard fashion in accordance with the individual's gender identity.

Elevated levels of some metabolites due to the enzyme deficiency can result in specific phenotypic effects in 46,XY individuals; the most notable are hypertension in 17α-hydroxylase deficiency due to increased deoxycorticosterone levels and partial virilisation in 3β-hydroxysteroid dehydrogenase-2 deficiency due to DHEA excess.

The two enzymes that act at the level of the testes only and which are therefore not associated with glucocorticoid deficiency, are 17β-hydroxysteroid dehydrogenase-3 and 5α-reductase-2. 46,XY infants born with these enzyme deficiencies can have partially virilised or typically female-appearing external genitalia due to lower testosterone production and exposure *in utero*. Higher levels of androgen production that will result in virilising effects are, however, expected at puberty and beyond; hence, if identified early in life, greater consideration of male sex of rearing is appropriate. Spontaneous virilisation at puberty has been reported to be associated with male gender identification in ~60% (Cohen-Kettenis 2005). For some children, signs of androgen effects on the external genitalia may only become evident during the early months of life ('mini-puberty') in a child where female assignment has already occurred. In individuals raised female, there can be a transition to identification with the male gender at puberty (Mieszczak et al. 2009). Consideration of genital/gonadal surgical interventions is therefore best deferred until adolescence, when the young person can be involved in the decision making process. Open discussions with the young person in relation to their gender identity may help to both normalise gender diversity and establish their true identity. For those raised female, blockade of pubertal progression with GnRHa therapy from the early pubertal period may be appropriate until the individual feels able to make a decision regarding their identity and desired sex hormone exposure. Possible advantages of such an approach are to defer potentially unwanted irreversible masculinising effects (if female gender identity), to allow further maturity in relation to decision-making and to ensure the young person has had time to be fully informed about and involved in decisions relating to their desired development; however, studies of outcomes of such an approach are lacking.

7.5.4 Androgen Insensitivity Syndrome

Reduced function of the androgen receptor leads to varying degrees of androgen insensitivity and incomplete virilisation of a 46,XY individual.

The clinical spectrum ranges from completely phenotypic females with absent or minimal pubic hair to phenotypical males with sub- or infertility or reduced body hair (Fig. 7.4).

Classification has typically been to divide the degree of insensitivity into complete androgen insensitivity syndrome (CAIS) and partial androgen insensitivity syndrome (PAIS). A large num-

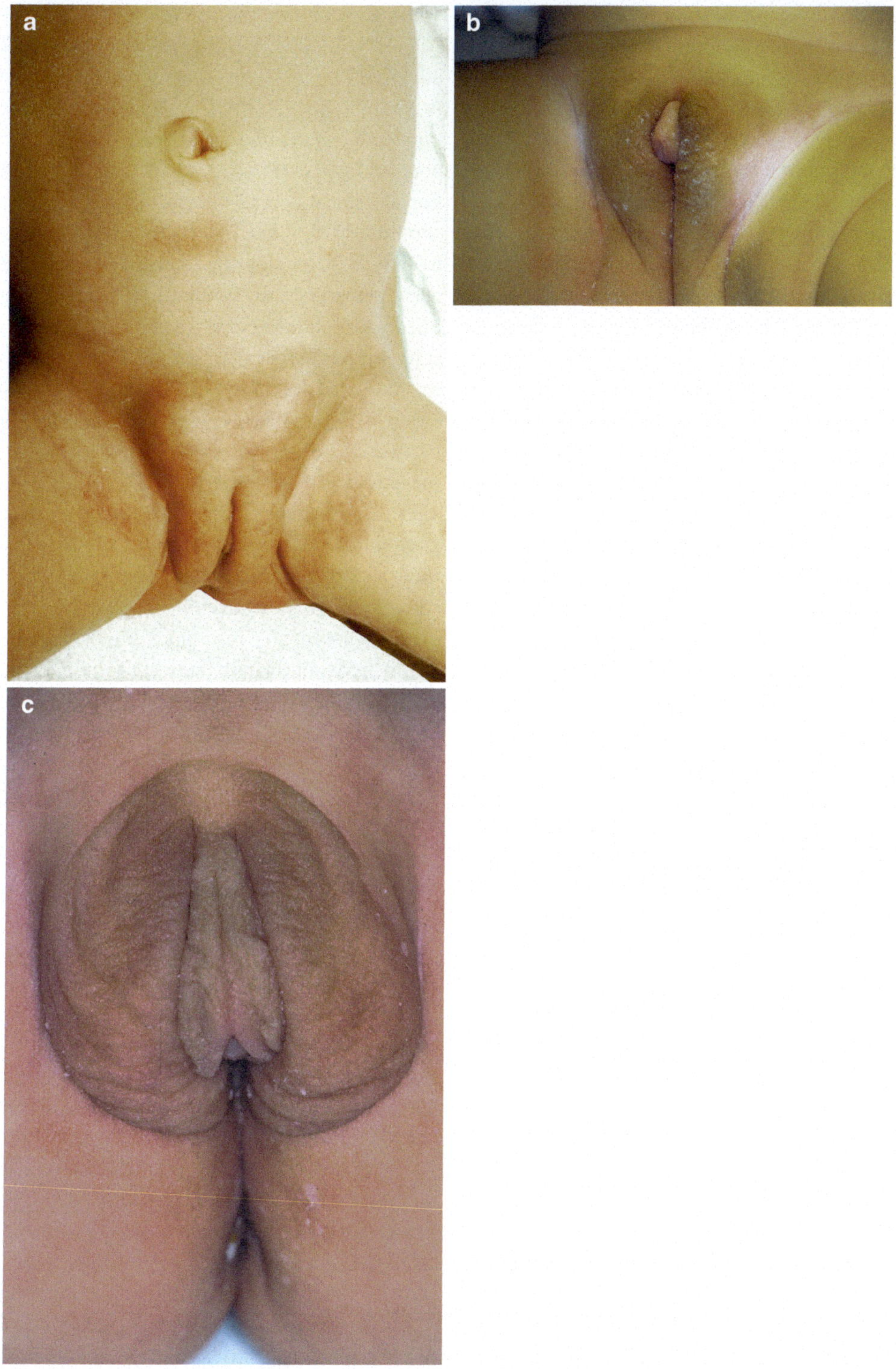

Fig. 7.4 (**a**) Complete androgen insensitivity syndrome (CAIS) showing female external genitalia, but visible gonads in the groin, just outside the inguinal canals. The testes have enlarged secondary to loss of negative feedback in gonadotrophin secretion. (**b**) Partial androgen insensitivity syndrome (PAIS), showing minimal virilisation of phallus and genital folds. (**c**) PAIS, where the genitalia show unfused labio-scrotal folds, but pigmentation and wrinkling are more noticeable and the phallus is much larger than that in Fig. 7.4b

ber of variations in the androgen receptor gene (AR) have been reported. Earlier studies reported coding region variants in nearly all CAIS patients but only 20% of PAIS patients (Deeb et al. 2005), although rates of detection of causative genes are higher with newer forms of genetic testing such as massively parallel sequencing targeted DSD gene panels (Eggers et al. 2016). Lower rates of detection in earlier studies may also relate to clinical misclassification of other conditions associated with lower than typical levels of virilisation as presumptive 'PAIS'.

Complete androgen insensitivity syndrome is defined as significant impairment of androgen receptor function, leading to an unvirilised or typically female phenotype and absence of pubic hair. Testes produce usual or elevated levels of testosterone in utero and from puberty; however the altered androgen receptor function does not allow typical virilisation. Luteinising hormone and sex hormone-binding globulin levels are often elevated. At puberty, circulating testosterone is aromatised to oestrogen with spontaneous development of female secondary sex characteristics. As AMH production in testes of individuals with CAIS is in the typical male range, Müllerian structures are absent. The epididymis and vas deferens are usually absent. The testes are usually situated very near the inguinal canal.

Individuals with CAIS may be diagnosed as an incidental finding due to incongruence between the female phenotype and 46,XY sex chromosome complement found on a karyotype performed for other reasons (increasingly as antenatal NIPT in developed countries), upon presentation with 'inguinal hernia' in infancy, or with primary amenorrhoea despite progression of breast development in puberty. Gender identity is nearly exclusively female (Hines 2004). Germ cell cancer risk in CAIS in early life is now estimated at no more than ~2% (Looijenga et al. 2007; Cools and Looijenga 2017). As a result, many people with CAIS retain their testes to allow endogenous hormone exposure, at least in puberty. At present, the associated risk, if any, of this approach is unknown. This must be balanced with the potential for malignant transformation, which, although thought to be low pre-puberty (estimated at 0.8%–2.0%) (Cools et al. 2006a, b), appears to increase with age such that the risk for adult women may be ~14% (0%–22%) (Deans et al. 2012; Cools et al. 2017). The factors that influence progression to malignancy are not well defined, although knowledge is evolving (see Sect. 7.6.1.1). Careful counselling in this regard is important, where gonadectomy is both considered and declined. It should also be noted that there is no consensus as to how best to monitor retained testes to detect early signs of malignancy in AIS. The utility of ultrasound and magnetic resonance imaging as a screening tool prior to gonadectomy has been explored and found to perform poorly for assessment of gonadoblastoma or malignancy (Alaniz et al. 2016). Intermittent biopsy is considered by many to be the best way to monitor for pre-malignant or malignant change, but this is an invasive procedure with higher complexity if testes are intra-abdominal. Cure rates are relatively high should malignancy develop.

A phenotype that resembles complete androgen insensitivity, but where there are minimal signs of virilisation in an otherwise phenotypically female individual, occurs in the form of partial androgen insensitivity syndrome where there is some, but very limited, response to androgens. This has been known as 'severe' partial androgen insensitivity, but alternative terminology may be warranted for this group in order to assist phenotypic classification in a clinically meaningful manner.

In individuals with CAIS or near-complete AIS, the vaginal dimensions may be less than that in a 46,XX individual due to some loss in length as a result of effects of AMH from the functioning testes. In our experience, this rarely requires surgical management and responds to functional use and dilators if required.

The genes for AIS are on the X chromosome, and this condition thus occurs either as a spontaneous variation or may be inherited from the maternal side. Mothers carrying this gene may have markedly reduced pubic and axillary hair.

A third group of clinical presentations of androgen insensitivity syndrome involves males with evidence of varying degrees of reduced virilisation of the external genitalia including hypospadias, cryptorchidism, incomplete labio-scrotal fusion, Wolffian duct development or Müllerian remnant presence and, later in life, sparse chest or facial hair (Grino et al. 1988) with or without infertility. Testosterone aromatisation commonly leads to gynaecomastia in this group from puberty. Germ cell cancer risk is as yet undefined in scrotal gonads; however, it is thought to be less than that for non-scrotal gonads. Sexual dysfunction is higher in men in this group than in unaffected men (Bouvattier et al. 2006).

Individuals with PAIS raised male or female identify with their sex of rearing in the majority; however, presence of gender dysphoria exists in up to 30% individuals, regardless of sex assigned at birth (Migeon et al. 2002; Veale et al. 2010; T'Sjoen et al. 2011).

7.5.4.1 Management

Assessment of possible androgen insensitivity syndrome involves measurement of hormone profile, sequencing of the AR gene, imaging to locate the testes and for cancer surveillance, and if desired by the individual, possible trial of testosterone ester administration to assess effect.

If testes are not palpable where there is biological evidence that testes are present (PAIS), a laparoscopy is indicated. In contrast, in 'simple' cryptorchidism, an ultrasound scan is usually requested to look for a Müllerian remnant.

If stretched penile length is less than typical (e.g., <2 cm), clinical response to a trial of testosterone administration in infancy, using 25 mg testosterone esters monthly for 3 months, can provide an indication of the potential for androgen responsiveness and ultimately further genital virilisation potential at puberty (when consistently higher levels of testosterone will be expected to be produced due to greater Leydig cell volume). The absence of clinical response (e.g. increase in phallic size) to exogenous androgen makes a more significant functional change in androgen receptor activity more likely, and discussions and counselling around the potential for low virilisation potential at puberty and in adulthood should occur with the family; however definitive predictions in this regard cannot be made on this basis alone. Encouraging and supporting the family's openness to future gender diversity (including the potential for non-binary identities) and normalising these concepts with the young person over time is important. Avoiding interventions in infancy/early childhood with a view to re-appraising their desirability peri-pubertally, may therefore be considered preferable.

In puberty, gynaecomastia is not infrequently associated with testosterone aromatisation; this may be problematic for some. While physiological gynaecomastia is very common in pubertal males in the general population, this typically resolves spontaneously after 2–3 years, whereas gynaecomastia associated with PAIS is more likely to persist. Mastectomy may be considered, but typically only if expressly desired and requested by the adolescent or young adult (e.g., to align with their affirmed gender identity) in a situation where gynaecomastia is persistent beyond 2–3 years. Sub- or infertility can be treated with assisted reproduction technology, using the individual's own gametes if viable, or donor gametes. Germ cell cancer should be managed according to the risk stratification by regular examination and annual imaging and tumour marker analysis from puberty. Testicular biopsy is recommended in the peri-pubertal period to assess testicular histology for evidence of premalignant changes and histological risk factors (e.g., OCT 3/4 or c-kit ligand positivity - see Sect. 7.6.1 below); if the latter are positive, risk-reducing gonadectomy (Cools et al. 2017) may be considered and discussed with the adolescent and their family.

Sex of rearing decisions are relatively straightforward for individuals with complete or near-complete androgen insensitivity or mild partial androgen insensitivity. However, in more significant grades of partial androgen insensitivity, where external masculinisation scores (EMS) are lower, decisions regarding sex of rearing can be difficult. There is evidence that the EMS in infancy may be a reasonable predictor of virilisation at puberty (Hughes et al. 2012). In recent years, there has been an increasing trend towards male sex of rearing for those with XY karyotype and genital variations recognised in infancy (Kolesinska et al. 2014). Regardless of sex of rearing, frank discussions with parents in relation to both the possibility of future gender diversity and also unknown degree of future additional androgen effect (hence, virilisation) are important. Optimal management, regardless of sex of rearing, would allow preservation of future options for anatomically congruent gender identity; for example, not removing erectile tissue from the phallus and not removing gonads that have hormonal or fertility production potential (albeit with significantly reduced androgen receptor activity). In this group, rigorous consideration of ethical principles should accompany decision-making.

7.5.5 Persistent Müllerian Duct Syndrome

Variants in the gene encoding anti-Müllerian hormone (AMH) or its receptor will lead to persistence of Müllerian duct organs in a 46,XY individual (Fig. 7.5). These are inherited in an autosomal recessive manner. The usual presentation is of a phenotypic male with cryptorchidism, although the Müllerian remnant may become apparent with thorough investigation in the newborn period or later with inguinal herniation of Müllerian tissue or incidentally at laparoscopy for other reasons (Hutson et al. 1987; Hutson et al. 1994; Colacurci et al. 1997).

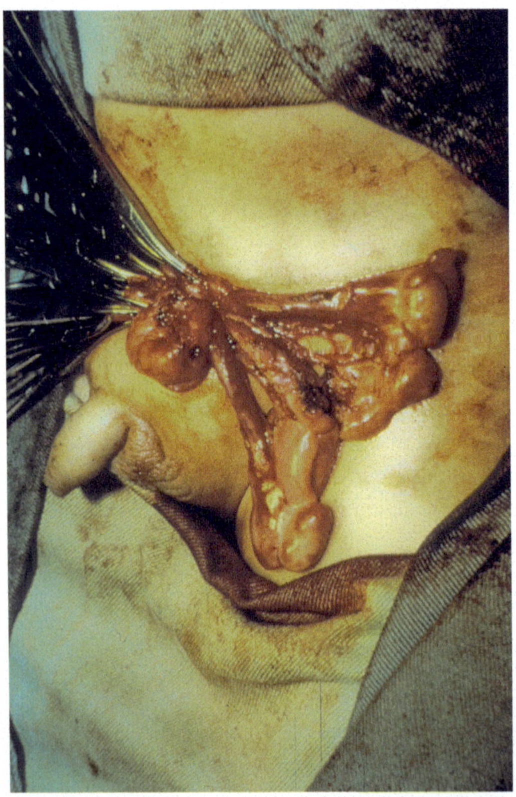

Fig. 7.5 Boy presenting with undescended testes and inguinal hernia found at operation to have persistent M llerian duct syndrome (PMDS). The hernia sac contains a loop of bowel as well as two testes and spermatic cords, as well as oedematous Fallopian tubes and a small uterus

Today, management involves conservation of the Müllerian structures and orchidopexy for cryptorchidism with usual follow-up for those with a history of undescended testes. Removal of Müllerian structures is not considered routine unless there are associated troublesome symptoms (e.g., recurrent UTIs); otherwise decisions in relation to such surgery are best delayed until the individual is old enough to decide for themselves how to proceed in this regard.

7.6 Additional Management Considerations

Accurate diagnosis allows for improved clinical management of 46,XY DSD and its potential associations, including gonadal germ cell tumour risk, as well as variations in fertility potential, sexual function and psychosocial concerns. The likelihood of different associations varies according to both the underlying diagnosis and its impact.

7.6.1 Germ Cell Tumours

The risk of gonadal germ cell tumour is of primary importance in 46,XY DSD management. Malignant tumours include seminoma of the testis or dysgerminoma of the ovary or dysgenetic gonad and the various nonseminomatous tumours. Their non-invasive counterparts are Germ cell Neoplasia *in situ* (GCNIS) (in a testicular environment) and gonadoblastoma (in the dysgenetic gonad) (Oosterhuis and Looijenga 2005). The precursor lesion within the testicular environment, previously known as carcinoma *in situ*, is now referred to as GCNIS according to the newest WHO classification (Moch et al. 2016). Broadly, germ cell tumours occur with increased frequency in gonads that arise in the presence of Y-chromosomal material but which are underdeveloped. The search for associated oncogenes on the Y chromosome has revealed candidate genes such as GBY and TSPY (Cools et al. 2006a, b). Germ cell tumours are the result of Y chromosome-mediated up-regulation of genes associated with pluri-potentiality, such as *PLAP*, *OCT3/4*, *c-KIT* and its ligand, Stem Cell Factor, in the poorly matured germ cells of DSD gonads. Germ cells with arrested development and in the presence of the Y chromosome undergo transformation into one of two pre-malignant states: GCNIS in a testis and gonadoblastoma in a dysplastic gonad or an ovary. Malignant transformation can occur towards any of the various germ cell cancers due to the pluri-potential capacity; these cancers include seminoma, non-seminomatous teratoma, yolk sac tumour or choriocarcinoma.

GCNIS and gonadoblastoma are early forms of neoplasia, in which there is no invasion of surrounding tissue by the pre-malignant cells. GCNIS cells, as germ cell cancer precursors, are situated within the spermatic tubules and appear gonocyte-like, with abundant cytoplasm. Gonadoblastoma cells comprise a proliferative admixture of immature germ cells and sex cord-stromal cells within the spermatic tubules. In general terms, gonads that are less advanced along the pathway of typical testicular development are effectively less differentiated and at higher risk for germ cell neoplasia. Another postulated contributing factor is the persistence of pluripotent germ cells, called gonocytes, in AIS testes.

Differentiation of GCNIS or gonadoblastoma from the appearance of simple maturational delay in a DSD gonad can be difficult, and histological staining for markers of pluri-potentiality such as AP-2γ or (more commonly) OCT3/4 is suggested (Fig. 7.6). Delayed maturation of germ cells is a common finding in all conditions characterised by altered hormonal and/or cellular environment and can be recognised by the presence of OCT3/4-positive luminal germ cells well beyond birth (Hannema et al. 2006). This is not a premalignant condition *per se*, therefore, differentiating between maturational delay and pre-malignancy to avoid overdiagnosis of GCNIS is very important. As OCT3/4 is physiologically expressed in the early months after birth, interpretation of aberrant findings is much easier after the first year of life (noting, however, that OCT3/4-positive germ cells can be found in AIS gonads of young children). Importantly, (pre-) GCNIS areas, but not germ cells with simple maturational delay, display aberrant c-kit ligand expression. Thus, the finding of c-kit ligand positivity in a suspected lesion substantially corroborates the diagnosis of (pre-) GCNIS (Stoop et al. 2008).

In individuals at high risk for germ cell tumour, testicular biopsy should be analysed for pre-malignant lesions after the onset of puberty. While this is currently recommended practice, the inherent limitations of a biopsy as a diagnostic tool must also be recognised. It is currently thought that only a small number of GCNIS cells and 50% of gonadoblastoma cells will eventually undergo malignant transformation (Cools et al. 2017; Looijenga et al. 2007).

The germ cell tumour risk in 46,XY DSD has been defined in a diagnosis-specific manner according to currently available follow-up data. It is reported to be up to 60% for some diagnoses, such as those associated with *WT1* mutations (Looijenga et al. 2007). It is, however, recognised that the accuracy of these estimations is limited by a number of factors, including the absence of an accurate underlying genetic diagnosis in a significant proportion of individuals with 46,XY DSD included in reported case series, as well as small numbers and the retrospective nature of many reported cohorts. It is important that such datasets are regularly re-appraised to ensure optimal accuracy. This can be challenging, as interventions such as early prophylactic gonadectomy will alter assessment of natural history. As malignancy in a pre-pubertal gonad that is not completely dysgenetic or 'streak' (and hence non functioning) is rare, removal of gonads that are predicted to have some endogenous function (with potential for hormone production or fertility) is now rarely indicated in childhood. Deferring decisions on such procedures until adolescence when the individual themselves can be involved are largely preferable where practical.

Malignant testicular germ cell tumours are classified into seminomatous and non-seminomatous tumours. The former arises purely

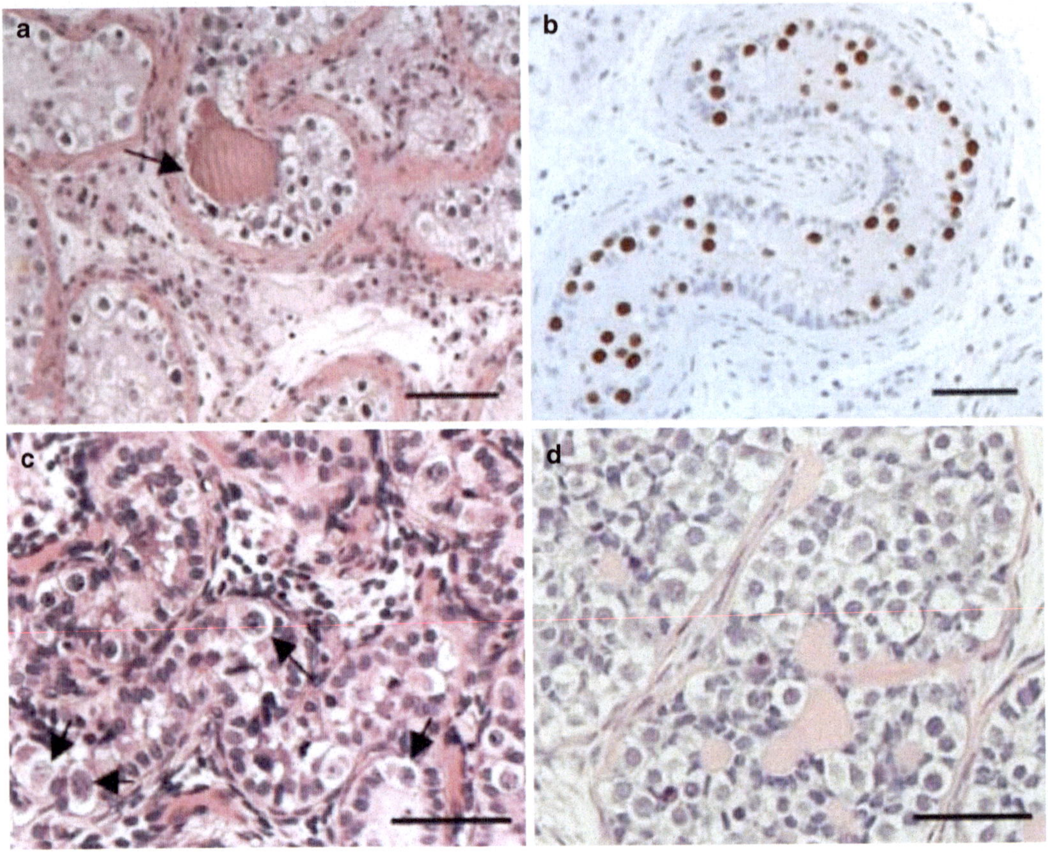

Fig. 7.6 Histological appearance of pre-invasive changes. (**a**) Germ Cell Neoplasia *in situ* (GCNIS) in the contralateral testis of an adult man with a testicular germ cell cancer. Arrow indicates a microlith. (**b**) GCNIS cells in a tubule with undifferentiated Sertoli cells; GCNIS cells stained for AP-2γ (a marker of pluripotency). (**c**) Arrow indicates GCNIS in the testis of a pre-pubertal girl with mixed gonadal dysgenesis 46,XY/45,X. (**d**) Gonadoblastoma in an adolescent boy with mosaicism for sex chromosome aneuploidy. (Scale bar = 50 micron) (Reproduced with permission from Rajpert-de Meyts and Hoei-Hansen (2007))

from the primordial germ cell lineage and the latter represents pluri-potential differentiation along various lineages, including teratoma, choriocarcinoma, yolk sac carcinoma and embryonal carcinoma. The overall 5-year survival rate is now over 95%; however, late tumour recurrence is reported (Oldenburg et al. 2006). Seminomas are sensitive to adjuvant radiotherapy after resection, and non-seminomatous tumours are sensitive to chemotherapy. Tumour staging allows stratification of good- and poor-risk patients. Poor risk occurs in 10%–25% and is associated with high serum tumour markers, metastases and mediastinal, non-seminomatous tumours (Bosl and Motzer 1997).

Testicular germ cell tumours typically present with a mass or a painless swelling of one testis, although pain can be a presenting feature in a minority. Ultrasonography is the initial investigation tool and can distinguish, and under ideal conditions, it can localise testicular lesions as small as 1–2 mm in diameter, especially if calcified. Serum tumour markers produced by non-seminomatous tumour types include α-fetoprotein and human chorionic gonadotrophin β-subunit. Further anatomical imaging by MRI or CT scan along with chest X-ray may help to define the anatomy of the tumour and any regional lymphadenopathy or distant metastases.

Mitigation of the germ cell tumour risk can occur through various means, dependent on the risk associated with the underlying DSD aetiology. In the situation of simple hypospadias and cryptorchidism, there is a twofold to fourfold increased risk of testicular germ cell tumour in early adulthood, and regular, thorough testicular self-examination is recommended (Schnack et al. 2010). In partial androgen insensitivity syndrome (PAIS) or mild gonadal dysgenesis, where the child is raised male and the testes are secured in a scrotal position, the testes may be left *in situ* with strict cancer surveillance. Biopsy and analysis for premalignant lesions at commencement of puberty, subsequent regular testicular self-examination (palpation) and annual tumour marker analysis with intermittent ultrasound are suggested for follow-up of patients at long-term risk of testicular germ cell cancer (Looijenga et al. 2007; Schmoll et al. 2010). The limitations of imaging (ultrasound and MRI) for detection of pre-malignant change such as GCNIS are, however, well recognised (Cools and Looijenga 2017).

In individuals with perceived high risk of germ cell tumour such as 46,XY complete gonadal dysgenesis (where cancer risk approximates 30%), or PAIS with intra-abdominal gonads (where cancer risk was formerly estimated to approximately 50%), risk-reducing prophylactic gonadectomy has been recommended (Looijenga et al. 2007. As outlined above, however, it is noted that this advice rests on retrospective studies of overall small numbers (Table 7.2)

Table 7.2 Previous estimates of germ cell cancer risk in various DSD. Newer data are available for some diagnostic groups, notably PAIS, which **no longer falls in a high-risk group** (ref Cools and Looijenga 2017; see text), hence recommended actions have evolved in the years since this publication (Wolfenbuttel et al 2016). The table remains to highlight the very low cohort numbers on which some previous estimates were based, hence caution is urged when extrapolating risk to a given individual.

Risk of type-II germinal cell tumors (GCTs) in the various categories of disorders of sex development (DSD) patients, classified into high-, intermediate-, low- and no-risk groups.

Risk group	Disorder	Malignancy risk (%)	Recommended action	Studies (n)	Patients (n)
High	GD[a] (+Y)[b] intra-abdominal	15–35	Gonadectomy[c]	12	>350
	PAIS non-scrotal	50	Gonadectomy[c]	2	24
	Frasier	60	Gonadectomy[c]	1	15
	Denys–Drash (+Y)	40	Gonadectomy[c]	1	5
Intermediate	Turner (+Y)	12	Gonadectomy[c]	11	43
	17β-HSD	28	Monitor	2	7
	GD (+Y)[c]	Unknown	Biopsy[d] and irradiation?	0	0
	PAIS scrotal gonad	Unknown	Biopsy[d] and irradiation?	0	0
Low	CAIS	2	Biopsy[d] and ???	2	55
	Ovotestis DSD	3	Testis tissue removal?	3	426
	Turner (– Y)	1	None	11	557
No (?)	5α-reductase	0	Unresolved	1	3
	Leydig cell hypoplasia	0	Unresolved	2	

CAIS, complete androgen insensitivity syndrome; 17β-HSD, 17β-hydroxysteroid dehyrdrogenase deficiency; PAIS, partial androgen insensitivity syndrome.

[a] Gonadal dysgenesis (including not further specified, 46XY, 46X/46XY, mixed, partial, complete).

[b] GBY region positive, including the *TSPY* gene.

[c] At time of diagnosis.

[d] At puberty, allowing investigation of at least 30 seminiferous tubules, with diagnosis preferably based on OCT3/4 immunohistochemistry.

Reproduced with permission from Looijenga et al. (2007)

and prospective natural history studies are lacking. Newer studies that call these data and recommendations into question are outlined below.

The functional impact of a given DSD will also affect the decision-making process, particularly if irreversible surgery such as gonadectomy is being considered. In CGD, gonads are completely dysgenetic or 'streak' and therefore have no inherent testicular function. In tandem with this, their state of maturational arrest has been shown to be associated with much higher risk of progression to germ cell tumour (Cools et al. 2006a, b). CGD gonads are classically intra-abdominal and difficult to identify on standard imaging. As estimated risk of malignancy is high, can occur in infancy or toddler years and gonadal tissue has no potential for endogenous hormonal or fertility potential, the recommendation for early gonadectomy (soon after diagnosis) will minimise risk from gonadal tumour while having no impact on function (which, by definition, is absent in CGD). In contrast in PAIS, where gonads have some inherent endocrine function and possibly some fertility potential (albeit low if not scrotal in position), the optimal pathway is less straightforward. If gonads can be brought to the scrotum to increase ease of monitoring (annual exam and imaging), then this is reasonable; however, the best approach for those with intra-abdominal gonads with some (albeit likely less) potential for function, but higher malignancy risk is unknown. As malignancy in PAIS is rare pre-pubertally, gonadal biopsy and decisions in relation to need for gonadectomy have increasingly been deferred until puberty (Lee et al. 2016) with clinical monitoring by palpation also in place.

It is also important to acknowledge that 'group' risk can not be directly extrapolated to everyone with a particular DSD; refinement of this risk can be achieved with gonadal biopsy and immunohistochemical staining. Decisions in each person should therefore be made based on assessment of the level of gonadal function (in terms of hormonal production and potential fertility), estimated malignancy risk profile (individual's age, gonadal location, biopsy findings and the availability of appropriate monitoring tools) and the individual's preferences in relation to surgery or surveillance pathways once this information is ascertained (Wolffenbuttel KP et al. 2016). As absolute germ cell tumour risk is central to defining the strategy for risk reduction, including decision on gonadectomy, further prospective and longitudinal work to clarify both diagnostic grouping and diagnosis-specific cancer risks and natural history of individual conditions without intervention will be important.

7.6.1.1 Germ Cell Tumour Risk in AIS

Although an increasing proportion of 46,XY women with CAIS now elect to retain their gonads, there are no prospective studies aimed at ascertaining the gonadal malignancy risk in this group. A literature review in 2012 found four studies reporting outcomes in adult women (>18 years) with CAIS. Taking into account the limitations of combining historical retrospective data, this study estimated the risk of gonadal malignancy in adulthood at 14% (range 0%–22%) (Deans et al. 2012). This is markedly higher than the 0.08%–2% (Cools et al. 2006a, b) quoted in childhood; hence, it is important that age-appropriate estimates are used in conversations with affected individuals, as these data suggested an apparent potential for risk to change (increase) with age.

Studies that include only those with genetically proven AIS also offer additional condition-specific insights. Notwithstanding the limitations of combining retrospective/cross-sectional data, a recent report of four such studies found GCNIS risk of 11/117 adolescent or adult AIS individuals (9.4%), of which 10/102 (9.8%) had CAIS and 1/15 (6.6%) had PAIS (Cools and Looijenga 2017). In contrast to what has previously been thought from historical studies (where the clinical diagnosis of PAIS may have included some with other forms of 46,XY DSD and hence different malignancy risk) (Cools et al. 2006a, b), these data indicate that PAIS individuals do *not* seem to be at a higher risk of gonadal tumour than women who have CAIS. Interestingly, no individual in these studies had developed an invasive testicular germ cell tumour (TGCT) at the time of gonadectomy, suggesting either that progression of GCNIS to invasiveness is a rare event in AIS, or that this takes place at older ages than covered in the mentioned studies.

A further recent cross-sectional study reported the prevalence of malignant TGCT and its precursors, (pre-) GCNIS, in 97 gonadal samples prophylactically removed from 52 late teenagers and adults (median age 17.5 years; range 14–54 years) with AIS; the impact of an individual's genetic susceptibility to development of TGCT was also examined (Cools et al. 2017). In this cohort, pre-GCNIS was present in 14% of individuals with complete and 10% of those with partial AIS at a median age of 16 years. Importantly, no GCNIS or invasive TGCT was found. Among the 14 TGCT-associated SNPs studied, important roles for risk alleles G at KITLG (rs995030) and C at ATFZIP (rs2900333) were suggested. These data indicate that genetic susceptibility likely contributes to pre-GCNIS development in AIS, but factors related to malignant progression remain unclear. Although data in older adults with AIS remain scarce (due to the previous more widespread practice of earlier gonadectomy), results of this study indicate that the prevalence of *in situ* germ cell tumours in those with PAIS in particular, is lower than that previously estimated and that overall, malignant progression appears to be rare in AIS. The natural history of the premalignant lesion remains unknown, however. The authors' conclusion therefore, was that the practice of routine prophylactic gonadectomy in adults with AIS now appears questionable and the individual's preference, once fully informed in relation to their own individual circumstance (including biopsy findings and possibly genetic susceptibility in future), should be decisive in this matter.

It is possible that progression from premalignant to invasive malignant tumour differs in AIS gonads as compared with dysgenetic gonads. In addition to the relatively normal testicular architecture (unlike dysgenetic gonads where the arrested development is associated with higher malignancy risk), this may relate to the fact that germ cells in AIS undergo apoptosis during childhood, hence offering the testis some protection from malignant degeneration. Germ cell numbers also decrease with age in AIS. The lack of paracrine androgen effect within the testis may also be important (Cools and Looijenga 2017).

These emerging data appear to re-frame historical estimates of tumour risk in AIS in particular, and prospective studies are needed to more accurately define risk over time.

7.6.2 Fertility

Reduced fertility to varying degrees is not infrequently encountered in 46,XY DSD. For individuals with mild hypospadias or cryptorchidism, fertility may be possible without the need for assisted reproductive technology. Successful attempts for paternity occur in 93% of men with fully descended testes, 90% of those with unilateral cryptorchidism and 65% of those with bilateral cryptorchidism (Lee and Coughlin 2001; Thorup and Cortes 2016). For other forms of 46,XY DSD, fertility may be more significantly reduced. Advances in assisted reproduction continue and now allow for successful use of germ cells developed to the level of round spermatids in intra-cytoplasmic sperm injection (Tesarik et al. 1995). Unfortunately, in many individuals with DSD, the developing germ cells do not even reach this minimal stage of development, and therefore, the sperm cannot be used.

Testicular biopsy tissue can be analysed for germ cell and sperm development in addition to cancer risk. Should there be viable sperm in a gonad which is to be removed prophylactically or therapeutically for germ cell tumour, sperm salvage and storage by cryopreservation should be offered (Sanders et al. 2018). Adolescents and young adults should be afforded the opportunity to have open and frank discussions in relation to their parenting desires (with recognition that this can change over time), likelihood of fertility as well as the potential impact of gonadal surgery (if proposed) on these factors (Sanders et al. 2018). Other options for parenting such as gamete donation or adoption/fostering should also be discussed.

In the case of female individuals with 46,XY complete gonadal dysgenesis, the presence of Müllerian structures allows consideration of donor-egg embryo implantation and carriage of pregnancy to term.

7.6.3 Hormonal and Sexual Function

Testicular failure in male 46,XY DSD individuals can occur before or after puberty, or may be induced by prophylactic gonadectomy. Regular hormonal assessment is therefore important and affected individuals should be counselled on the symptoms of androgen deficiency.

In those with a male/masculine gender identity with evidence of testicular insufficiency, male puberty can be induced with oral (testosterone undecanoate 40 mg daily), intramuscular (testosterone esters 50–100 mg monthly) or transdermal testosterone (2.5 g daily), using a gradually increasing dose to adult replacement over 6–12 months (Ambler 2009). Adolescents and young adults should be counselled on the importance of continuous sex hormone replacement for the purposes of metabolic and bone health in addition to subjective wellbeing. Metabolic parameters and bone densitometry should be monitored periodically for individuals who are taking exogenous hormone replacement.

Long-term follow-up studies of men with smaller than typical penile size indicate that genital and sexual function can be satisfactory; however, there may be dissatisfaction with body image (Wisniewski et al. 2001).

In female 46,XY DSD individuals, risk-reducing gonadectomy is recommended to be indicated pre-puberty in those with CGD, as malignant transformation (including, albeit uncommonly, invasive or metastatic disease) is well described in early childhood. Additionally, by virtue of their arrested development (complete gonadal dysgenesis), there is no inherent gonadal fertility or hormonal function to preserve, hence leaving the gonads *in situ* offers no functional benefit (but rather poses a risk) to the individual. In conditions such as CGD, as gonads are non-functioning even if left *in situ*, there will be a requirement for hormone replacement therapy; if recognised in childhood, this may begin with induction of puberty from the age of 10–12 years. Female gender identity is most common in CGD, but nonetheless, it should not be assumed. As hormone replacement therapy will stimulate development of secondary sex characteristics, gender identity and the desire for associated bodily changes should be established in discussions with peri-pubertal youth with CGD prior to starting treatment. For those with a female gender identity, oestrogen can be commenced in low-dose oral (oestradiol valerate 250 mcg daily or 500 mcg alternate daily) or trans-dermal (oestradiol 6.25 mcg per day) forms, increasing the dose gradually to adult replacement over ~2 years. If a uterus is present (as is typical in CGD), addition of progestogen is then also indicated (de Muinck Keizer-Schrama 2007; Hewitt and Warne 2009), and this may be used either in a cyclic (allowing intermittent menses) or a continuous (suppressing menses) manner. Induction of secondary sex characteristics should occur slowly in females to follow the natural development and progression.

As outlined previously, females with 46,XY CAIS may choose to defer prophylactic gonadectomy as malignancy risk pre-pubertally is low. Aromatisation of her own endogenous testosterone production will allow development of secondary female sex characteristics and usually, adequate bone density development without the need for hormonal replacement therapy (Bertelloni et al. 2017), although this may be required later in life.

Women with absence of Müllerian structures will usually have the lower third of the vagina; serial vaginal dilatation prior to penetrative sexual intercourse may therefore be offered if desired by the young woman. Graduated solid dilators are applied with pressure against the vaginal dimple daily for a minimum of 30 min after a warm bath. Functional success is reported in approximately 90% of women with vaginal agenesis after 18 months (Sanders et al. 2018; Gargollo et al. 2009). In individuals in whom non-surgical treatment is not successful, creation of a neovagina can occur through a variety of different techniques (Perera et al. 2012; McQuillan and Grover 2014).

7.6.4 Urinary Function

Depending on the clinical significance and impact of a variation, multiple surgical procedures may be undertaken to construct the penile urethra. Long-term follow-up of males who had surgery for a DSD demonstrated a high prevalence of persisting urological difficulties, including wetting (25%), spraying of urine (31%) and recurrent infections (25%) (Moriya et al. 2007; Rynja et al. 2009; Gonzalez and Ludwikowski 2011; Perera et al. 2012; Andersson et al. 2015; Ortqvist et al. 2015). Urological function and management are discussed further in Chap. 17.

7.6.5 Psychosocial Considerations

A 46,XY DSD diagnosis may be a significant stressor for both the affected individual and their family and partners. Long-term psychosocial support is recognised as an essential part of medical care; however, it remains the realm in which care providers are thought to perform most poorly as reported by patients (Crawford et al. 2009; Jones et al. 2009). In long-term follow-up, most patients report a good quality-of-life outcome (Fagerholm et al. 2012; Jurgensen et al. 2014; Amaral et al. 2015; Rapp et al. 2018; Thyen et al. 2018; Warne et al. 2005; Warne 2008); however, in some individuals, distress can lead to significant functional impairment, with risk of self-harm (Schutzmann et al. 2009).

As outlined above, with limited evidence to guide decisions in relation to optimal sex assignment at birth, some individuals will have a gender identity that is discordant from sex of rearing, and some may develop gender dysphoria (Raveenthiran 2017). Long-term outcome studies from small cohorts indicate that gender diversity and dysphoria can exist regardless of sex of rearing for many DSD (Migeon et al. 2002; Veale et al. 2010; Berenbaum and Meyer-Bahlburg 2015; Kreukels et al. 2018; Rapp et al. 2018). Identification with a gender other than male or female is also increasingly reported (Kreukels et al. 2018), and it is important that clinicians are aware and supportive of non-binary gender identities and avoid assumptions that relate to a gender binary (Kreukels et al. 2018). It is of course also the case that gender diversity and dysphoria occur in individuals without DSD. As the prevalence of gender non-conformity with sex assigned at birth in the general population is unknown, comparisons to rates in those with a DSD are difficult to quantify. Gender diversity and dysphoria can be significant issues for individual self-understanding, and access to psychological support while exploring one's gender identity is considered essential.

Female assignment at birth is more commonly the case for individuals with 46,XY DSD associated with a typical female appearance to the external genitalia (e.g., CAIS or CGD) as evidence supports female gender identity in the majority; this may relate to the relative absence of androgen exposure and hence effect on the brain. For babies with 46,XY karyotype and some, but less obvious degrees of virilisation, decisions in relation to optimal sex of rearing can be difficult. Whilst historically, significantly under-virilised 46,XY DSD infants were relatively frequently assigned a female sex of rearing, this approach is now less common. Those with 46,XY DSD who have evidence of inherent endogenous testicular function are increasingly raised male in recent times, (Diamond and Beh 2008), albeit with an understanding that future gender identity, degree of virilisation and fertility cannot be reliably predicted or guaranteed. Reasons for the change in preferred sex of rearing are multiple, and include the understanding that while most individuals as adults identify with their original sex of rearing, this is not something that can be predicted by genital appearance alone. Families must be fully informed of the basis for a given decision/recommendation in their child and also made aware of possibility of future gender non-conformity with their sex of rearing. Normalising, and where appropriate, affirming this concept with both the young person themselves and their extended family is important.

With these considerations in mind, raising a 46,XY child with some virilisation of their external genitalia as male, with an open attitude to gender diversity and future decision making by the individual is increasingly thought appropriate. Men with micropenis (as previously described) are known to have potential for satisfactory sexual outcomes. It is also the case that historically, decisions in relation to interventions previously undertaken to 'align' with sex of rearing, were potentially biased towards cis- / heterosexual 'norms'; awareness of this is important to consider and discuss openly. For example, feminising genitoplasty may involve the irreversible removal of erectile tissue, which may be regretted in an individual raised female later identifying as male. Furthermore, there is some evidence that individuals with a 46,XY karyotype and some level of prenatal virilisation, in addition to potential for spontaneous or induced pubertal virilisation, can have difficulty accepting a female sex of rearing and have significant gender dysphoria (Reiner and Gearhart 2004).

Male sex is now more routinely considered for children with 46,XY karyotype who have 17β-hydroxysteroid dehydrogenase (17β-HSD3) deficiency, 5α-reductase-2 deficiency, bladder exstrophy or diagnoses consistent with androgen responsiveness (Mieszczak et al. 2009; Hughes et al. 2006). For similar reasons to those outlined above, if a female sex is decided for a 46,XY child with any of these DSD, deferring irreversible interventions until an age where the child is old enough to contribute to decision making and consent to such procedures if desired, is preferable. At puberty, termporary blockade of pubertal hormones if incongruent with the young person's gender identity, is a reversible therapeutic option that may be beneficial in such an instance, while decisions regarding future management are made.

7.6.6 Genetic Counselling and Disclosure

Many causes of 46,XY DSD arise de novo and lead to significantly reduced fertility or infertility in the affected individual, so for many variations, there is a low risk of recurrence in a family. Others can be inherited in an X-linked, autosomal recessive or even autosomal dominant fashion. Genetic counselling should be offered regarding testing of extended family members, risk of recurrence in future offspring of the parents and in time to the affected individual themselves (most commonly, first offered in adolescence with further offers later in young adulthood if initially declined).

Discussions in relation to an individual's own circumstances and their specific diagnosis should occur in a staged and developmentally appropriate manner, with the aim for open and complete dialogue including explanation of known associations by the completion of puberty (see Chap. 19).

7.7 Conclusion

46,XY DSD comprise a heterogeneous group of conditions with varying natural history and complication risk stratifications. Although rates of accurate genetic diagnoses have increased significantly in recent years, an underlying causative genetic variant or aetiology is still not identified in many affected individuals. Where possible, there is a clinical responsibility to provide an accurate genetic/genomic diagnosis, to optimise provision of appropriate medical care. Our understanding and management of these conditions, in particular in relation to prophylactic gonadectomy due to risk of cancer, has changed in recent years and continues to evolve. Input from affected individuals and advocacy groups has been and remains central to informing newer approaches. In concert with this is an obligation to pursue research which will seek to improve diagnostic rates and further illuminate genotype-phenotype associations, as well as long-term diagnosis-specific outcomes and optimal medical management and counselling.

Acknowledgements With thanks and acknowledgement to the authors of the original chapter: Dr. Jacqueline Hewitt, Professor Garry L. Warne AM.

References

Ahmed SF, Khwaja O, Hughes IA. The role of a clinical score in the assessment of ambiguous genitalia. BJU Int. 2000;85(1):120–4.

Ahmed SF, Rodie M. Investigation and initial management of ambiguous genitalia. Best Pract Res Clin Endocrinol Metab. 2010;24(2):197–218. https://doi.org/10.1016/j.beem.2009.12.001.

Alaniz VI, Kobernik EK, Dillman J, et al. Utility of ultrasound and magnetic resonance imaging in patients with disorders of sex development who undergo prophylactic gonadectomy. J Pediatr Adolesc Gynecol. 2016;29(6):577–81.

Amaral RC, Inacio M, Brito VN, et al. Quality of life of patients with 46,XX and 46,XY disorders of sex development. Clin Endocrinol. 2015;82(2):159–64.

Ambler GR. Androgen therapy for delayed male puberty. Curr Opin Endocrinol Diabetes Obes. 2009;16(3):232–9.

Aminzadeh M, Kim HG, Layman LC, et al. Rarer syndromes characterized by hypogonadotropic hypogonadism. Front Horm Res. 2010;39:154–67.

Andersson M, Doroszkiewicz M, Arfwidsson C, et al. Normalized urinary flow at puberty after tubularized incised plate urethroplasty for hypospadias in childhood. J Urol. 2015;194(5):1407–13.

Bardoni B, Zanaria E, Guioli S, et al. A dosage sensitive locus at chromosome Xp21 is involved in male to female sex reversal. Nat Genet. 1994;7(4):497–501.

Baxter RM, Arboleda VA, Lee H, et al. Exome sequencing for the diagnosis of 46,XY disorders of sex development. J Clin Endocrinol Metab. 2015;100(2):E333–44.

Berenbaum SA, Meyer-Bahlburg HF. Gender development and sexuality in disorders of sex development. Horm Metab Res. 2015;47(5):361–6.

Berkowitz GS, Lapinski RH, Dolgin SE, et al. Prevalence and natural history of cryptorchidism. Pediatrics. 1993;92(1):44–9.

Bertelloni S, Meriggiola MC, Dati E, et al. Bone mineral density in women living with complete androgen insensitivity syndrome and intact testes or removed gonads. Sex Dev. 2017;11(4):182–9.

Bhullar K, Grover S, Hutson JM, et al. Spectrum of disorders of sex development in children aged 0-10 years. J Pediatr Adolesc Gynecol. 2011;24(2):50.

Biason-Lauber A, Konrad D, Meyer M, et al. Ovaries and female phenotype in a girl with 46,XY karyotype and mutations in the CBX2 gene. Am J Hum Genet. 2009;84(5):658–63.

Bosl GJ, Motzer RJ. Testicular germ-cell cancer. N Engl J Med. 1997;337(4):242–53.

Bouty A, Ayers KL, Pask A, et al. The genetic and environmental factors underlying hypospadias. Sex Dev. 2015;9(5):239–59.

Bouvattier C, Mignot B, Lefevre H, et al. Impaired sexual activity in male adults with partial androgen insensitivity. J Clin Endocrinol Metab. 2006;91(9):3310–5.

Cameron FJ, Sinclair AH. Mutations in SRY and SOX9: testis-determining genes. Hum Mutat. 1997;9(5):388–95.

Christiansen P, Skakkebaek NE. Pulsatile gonadotropin-releasing hormone treatment of men with idiopathic hypogonadotropic hypogonadism. Horm Res. 2002;57(1–2):32–6.

Cohen-Kettenis PT. Gender change in 46,XY persons with 5alpha-reductase-2 deficiency and 17beta-hydroxysteroid dehydrogenase-3 deficiency. Arch Sex Behav. 2005;34(4):399–410.

Colacurci N, Cardone A, De Franciscis P, et al. Laparoscopic hysterectomy in a case of male pseudohermaphroditism with persistent Mullerian duct derivatives. Hum Reprod. 1997;12(2):272–4.

Cools M, Drop SL, Wolffenbuttel KP, et al. Germ cell tumors in the intersex gonad: old paths, new directions, moving frontiers. Endocr Rev. 2006a;27(5):468–84.

Cools M, Looijenga L. Update on the pathophysiology and risk factors for the development of malignant testicular germ cell tumors in complete androgen insensitivity syndrome. Sex Dev. 2017;11(4):175–81.

Cools M, Stoop H, Kersemaekers AM, et al. Gonadoblastoma arising in undifferentiated gonadal tissue within dysgenetic gonads. J Clin Endocrinol Metab. 2006b;91(6):2404–13.

Cools M, Wolffenbuttel KP, Hersmus R, et al. Malignant testicular germ cell tumors in postpubertal individuals with androgen insensitivity: prevalence, pathology and relevance of single nucleotide polymorphism-based susceptibility profiling. Hum Reprod. 2017;32(12):2561–73.

Cox JJ, Willatt L, Homfray T, et al. A SOX9 duplication and familial 46,XX developmental testicular disorder. N Engl J Med. 2011;364(1):91–3.

Crawford JM, Warne G, Grover S, et al. Results from a pediatric surgical centre justify early intervention in disorders of sex development. J Pediatr Surg. 2009;44(2):413–6.

de Muinck Keizer-Schrama SM. Introduction and management of puberty in girls. Horm Res. 2007;68(Suppl 5):80–3.

de Santa Barbara P, Mejean C, Moniot B, et al. Steroidogenic factor-1 contributes to the cyclic-adenosine monophosphate down-regulation of human SRY gene expression. Biol Reprod. 2001;64(3):775–83.

Deans R, Creighton SM, Liao LM, et al. Timing of gonadectomy in adult women with complete androgen insensitivity syndrome (CAIS): patient preferences and clinical evidence. Clin Endocrinol. 2012;76(6):894–8.

Deeb A, Mason C, Lee YS, et al. Correlation between genotype, phenotype and sex of rearing in 111 patients with partial androgen insensitivity syndrome. Clin Endocrinol. 2005;63(1):56–62.

Diamond M, Beh HG. Changes in the management of children with intersex conditions. Nat Clin Pract Endocrinol Metab. 2008;4(1):4–5.

Donahoe PK, Crawford JD, Hendren WH. Mixed gonadal dysgenesis, pathogensis, and management. J Pediatr Surg. 1979;14(3):287–300.

Eggers S, Ohnesorg T, Sinclair A. Genetic regulation of mammalian gonad development. Nat Rev Endocrinol. 2014;10(11):673–83.

Eggers S, Sadedin S, van den Bergen JA, et al. Disorders of sex development: insights from targeted gene sequencing of a large international patient cohort. Genome Biol. 2016;17(1):243.

Fagerholm R, Mattila AK, Roine RP, et al. Mental health and quality of life after feminizing genitoplasty. J Pediatr Surg. 2012;47(4):747–51.

Fisch H, Hyun G, Hensle TW. Rising hypospadias rates: disproving a myth. J Pediatr Urol. 2010;6(1):37–9.

Foresta C, Zuccarello D, Garolla A, et al. Role of hormones, genes, and environment in human cryptorchidism. Endocr Rev. 2008;29(5):560–80.

Foster JW, Dominguez-Steglich MA, Guioli S, et al. Campomelic dysplasia and autosomal sex reversal caused by mutations in an SRY-related gene. Nature. 1994;372(6506):525–30.

Gargollo PC, Cannon GM Jr, Diamond DA, et al. Should progressive perineal dilation be considered first line therapy for vaginal agenesis? J Urol. 2009;182(4 Suppl):1882–9.

Gillam LH, Hewitt JK, Warne GL. Ethical principles for the management of infants with disorders of sex development. Horm Res Paediatr. 2010;74:412–8.

Gonzalez R, Ludwikowski BM. Importance of urinary flow studies after hypospadias repair: a systematic review. Int J Urol. 2011;18(11):757–61.

Granados A, Alaniz VI, Mohnach L, et al. MAP3K1-related gonadal dysgenesis: six new cases and review of the literature. Am J Med Genet C Semin Med Genet. 2017;175(2):253–9.

Grimbizis GF, Gordts S, Di Spiezio Sardo A, et al. The ESHRE-ESGE consensus on the classification of female genital tract congenital anomalies. Gynecol Surg. 2013;10(3):199–212.

Grino PB, Griffin JE, Cushard WG Jr, et al. A mutation of the androgen receptor associated with partial androgen resistance, familial gynecomastia, and fertility. J Clin Endocrinol Metab. 1988;66(4):754–61.

Hannema SE, Scott IS, Rajpert-De Meyts E, et al. Testicular development in the complete androgen insensitivity syndrome. J Pathol. 2006;208(4): 518–27.

Harley VR, Clarkson MJ, Argentaro A. The molecular action and regulation of the testis-determining factors, SRY (sex-determining region on the Y chromosome) and SOX9 [SRY-related high-mobility group (HMG) box 9]. Endocr Rev. 2003;24(4):466–87.

Henna MR, Del Nero RG, Sampaio CZ, et al. Hormonal cryptorchidism therapy: systematic review with metanalysis of randomized clinical trials. Pediatr Surg Int. 2004;20(5):357–9.

Hewitt JK, Warne GL. Management of disorders of sex development. Pediatr Health. 2009;3(1):51–65.

Hines M. Psychosexual development in individuals who have female pseudohermaphroditism. Child Adolesc Psychiatr Clin N Am. 2004;13(3):641–656, ix.

Hjertkvist M, Lackgren G, Ploen L, et al. Does HCG treatment induce inflammation-like changes in undescended testes in boys? J Pediatr Surg. 1993;28(2):254–8.

Hoei-Hansen CE, Olesen IA, Jorgensen N, Carlsen E, Holm M, Almstrup K, Leffers H, Rajpert-De Meyts E. Current approaches for detection of carcinoma in situ testis. Int J Androl. 2007;30(4):398–404; discussion 404-5.

Hughes IA. Disorders of sex development: a new definition and classification. Best Pract Res Clin Endocrinol Metab. 2008;22(1):119–34.

Hughes IA, Davies JD, Bunch TI, et al. Androgen insensitivity syndrome. Lancet. 2012;380(9851):1419–28.

Hughes IA, Houk C, Ahmed SF, et al. Consensus statement on management of intersex disorders. Arch Dis Child. 2006;91(7):554–63.

Hutson J, Chow CW, Ng WD. Persistent Müllerian duct syndrome with transverse testicular ectopia. An experiment of nature with clues for understanding testicular descent. Pediatr Surg Int. 1987;2:191–4.

Hutson JM, Balic A, Nation T, et al. Cryptorchidism. Semin Pediatr Surg. 2010;19(3):215–24.

Hutson JM, Davidson P, Reece L, et al. Failure of gubernacular development in the persistent Müllerian duct syndrome allows herniation of the testes. Pediatr Surg Int. 1994;9:544–6.

Iovane A, Aumas C, de Roux N. New insights in the genetics of isolated hypogonadotropic hypogonadism. Eur J Endocrinol. 2004;151(Suppl 3):U83–8.

Jones BC, O'Brien M, Chase J, et al. Early hypospadias surgery may lead to a better long-term psychosexual outcome. J Urol. 2009;182(4 Suppl):1744–9.

Jordan BK, Shen JH, Olaso R, et al. Wnt4 overexpression disrupts normal testicular vasculature and inhibits testosterone synthesis by repressing steroidogenic factor 1/beta-catenin synergy. Proc Natl Acad Sci U S A. 2003;100(19):10866–71.

Jurgensen M, Lux A, Wien SB, et al. Health-related quality of life in children with disorders of sex development (DSD). Eur J Pediatr. 2014;173(7):893–903.

Kalfa N, Paris F, Philibert P, et al. Is hypospadias associated with prenatal exposure to endocrine disruptors? A French collaborative controlled study of a cohort of 300 consecutive children without genetic defect. Eur Urol. 2015;68(6):1023–30.

Kearsey I, Hutson JM. Disorders of sex development (DSD): not only babies with ambiguous genitalia. A practical guide for surgeons. Pediatr Surg Int. 2017;33(3):355–61.

Kelley RI, Hennekam RC. The Smith-Lemli-Opitz syndrome. J Med Genet. 2000;37(5):321–35.

Kohler B, Achermann JC. Update-steroidogenic factor 1 (SF-1, NR5A1). Minerva Endocrinol. 2010;35(2):73–86.

Kohler B, Lin L, Mazen I, et al. The spectrum of phenotypes associated with mutations in steroidogenic factor 1 (SF-1, NR5A1, ad4BP) includes severe penoscrotal hypospadias in 46,XY males without adrenal insufficiency. Eur J Endocrinol. 2009;161(2):237–42.

Kolesinska Z, Ahmed SF, Niedziela M, et al. Changes over time in sex assignment for disorders of sex development. Pediatrics. 2014;134(3):e710–5.

Kreukels BPC, Kohler B, Nordenstrom A, et al. Gender dysphoria and gender change in disorders of sex development/intersex conditions: results from the dsd-life study. J Sex Med. 2018;15(5):777–85.

Latronico AC, Arnhold IJ. Inactivating mutations of the human luteinizing hormone receptor in both sexes. Semin Reprod Med. 2012;30(5):382–6.

Latronico AC, Arnhold IJ. Inactivating mutations of the human luteinizing hormone receptor in both sexes. Semin Reprod Med. 2012;30(5):382–6. https://doi.org/10.1055/s-0032-1324721. Epub 2012 Oct 8.

Lee PA, Coughlin MT. Fertility after bilateral cryptorchidism. Evaluation by paternity, hormone, and semen data. Horm Res. 2001;55(1):28–32.

Lee PA, Mazur T, Danish R, et al. Micropenis. I. Criteria, etiologies and classification. Johns Hopkins Med J. 1980;146(4):156–63.

Lee PA, Nordenstrom A, Houk CP, et al. Global disorders of sex development update since 2006: perceptions, approach and care. Horm Res Paediatr. 2016;85(3):158–80.

Lin L, Philibert P, Ferraz-de-Souza B, Kelberman D, Homfray T, Albanese A, Molini V, Sebire NJ, Einaudi S, Conway GS, Hughes IA, Jameson JL, Sultan C, Dattani MT, Achermann JC. Heterozygous missense mutations in steroidogenic factor 1 (SF1/Ad4BP, NR5A1) are associated with 46,XY disorders of sex development with normal adrenal function. J Clin Endocrinol Metab. 2007;92(3):991–9.

Looijenga LH, Hersmus R, Oosterhuis JW, et al. Tumor risk in disorders of sex development (DSD). Best Pract Res Clin Endocrinol Metab. 2007;21(3):480–95.

Lourenco D, Brauner R, Rybczynska M, et al. Loss-of-function mutation in GATA4 causes anomalies of human testicular development. Proc Natl Acad Sci U S A. 2011;108(4):1597–602.

Moch H, Cubilla AL, Humphrey PA, Reuter VE, Ulbright TM. The 2016 WHO Classification of Tumours of the Urinary System and Male Genital Organs-Part A: Renal, Penile, and Testicular Tumours. Eur Urol. 2016;70(1):93–105. https://doi.org/10.1016/j.eururo.2016.02.029. Epub 2016 Feb 28.

McCarty BM, Migeon CJ, Meyer-Bahlburg HF, et al. Medical and psychosexual outcome in women affected by complete gonadal dysgenesis. J Pediatr Endocrinol Metab. 2006;19(7):873–7.

McQuillan SK, Grover SR. Systematic review of sexual function and satisfaction following the management of vaginal agenesis. Int Urogynecol J. 2014;25(10):1313–20.

Mieszczak J, Houk CP, Lee PA. Assignment of the sex of rearing in the neonate with a disorder of sex development. Curr Opin Pediatr. 2009;21(4):541–7.

Migeon CJ, Wisniewski AB, Gearhart JP, et al. Ambiguous genitalia with perineoscrotal hypospadias in 46,XY individuals: long-term medical, surgical, and psychosexual outcome. Pediatrics. 2002;110(3):e31.

Morales-Suarez-Varela MM, Toft GV, Jensen MS, et al. Parental occupational exposure to endocrine disrupting chemicals and male genital malformations: a study in the Danish National Birth Cohort study. Environ Health. 2011;10(1):3.

Moreno-Garcia M, Miranda EB. Chromosomal anomalies in cryptorchidism and hypospadias. J Urol. 2002;168(5):2170–2.

Moriya K, Kakizaki H, Tanaka H, et al. Long-term patient reported outcome of urinary symptoms after hypospadias surgery: norm related study in adolescents. J Urol. 2007;178(4 Pt 2):1659–62. discussion 1662.

Nixon R, Cerqueira V, Kyriakou A, et al. Prevalence of endocrine and genetic abnormalities in boys evaluated systematically for a disorder of sex development. Hum Reprod. 2017;32(10):2130–7.

Ogata T, Fukami M, Wada Y. MAMLD1 (CXorf6) is a new gene for hypospadias. Clin Pediatr Endocrinol. 2008;17(4):87–93.

Oldenburg J, Martin JM, Fossa SD. Late relapses of germ cell malignancies: incidence, management, and prognosis. J Clin Oncol. 2006;24(35):5503–11.

Olesen IA, Sonne SB, Hoei-Hansen CE, et al. Environment, testicular dysgenesis and carcinoma in situ testis. Best Pract Res Clin Endocrinol Metab. 2007;21(3):462–78.

Ollivier M, Paris F, Philibert P, et al. Family history is underestimated in children with isolated hypospadias: a French multicenter report of 88 families. J Urol. 2018;200(4):890–4.

Ono M, Harley VR. Disorders of sex development: new genes, new concepts. Nat Rev Endocrinol. 2013;9(2):79–91.

Oosterhuis JW, Looijenga LH. Testicular germ-cell tumours in a broader perspective. Nat Rev Cancer. 2005;5(3):210–22.

Ortqvist L, Fossum M, Andersson M, et al. Long-term followup of men born with hypospadias: urological and cosmetic results. J Urol. 2015;193(3):975–81.

Ottolenghi C, Veitia R, Quintana-Murci L, et al. The region on 9p associated with 46,XY sex reversal contains several transcripts expressed in the urogenital system and a novel doublesex-related domain. Genomics. 2000;64(2):170–8.

Peper JS, Koolschijn PC. Sex steroids and the organization of the human brain. J Neurosci. 2012;32(20):6745–6.

Perera M, Jones B, O'Brien M, et al. Long-term urethral function measured by uroflowmetry after hypospadias surgery: comparison with an age matched control. J Urol. 2012;188(4 Suppl):1457–62.

Philibert P, Leprieur E, Zenaty D, et al. Steroidogenic factor-1 (SF-1) gene mutation as a frequent cause of primary amenorrhea in 46,XY female adolescents with low testosterone concentration. Reprod Biol Endocrinol. 2010;8:28.

Philibert P, Zenaty D, Lin L, et al. Mutational analysis of steroidogenic factor 1 (NR5a1) in 24 boys with bilateral anorchia: a French collaborative study. Hum Reprod. 2007;22(12):3255–61.

Pleskacova J, Hersmus R, Oosterhuis JW, et al. Tumor risk in disorders of sex development. Sex Dev. 2010;4(4–5):259–69.

Puffenberger EG, Hu-Lince D, Parod JM, et al. Mapping of sudden infant death with dysgenesis of the testes syndrome (SIDDT) by a SNP genome scan and identification of TSPYL loss of function. Proc Natl Acad Sci U S A. 2004;101(32):11689–94.

Pyle LC, Nathanson KL. A practical guide for evaluating gonadal germ cell tumor predisposition in differences of sex development. Am J Med Genet C Semin Med Genet. 2017;175(2):304–14.

Rapp M, Mueller-Godeffroy E, Lee P, et al. Multicentre cross-sectional clinical evaluation study about quality of life in adults with disorders/differences of sex development (DSD) compared to country specific reference populations (dsd-LIFE). Health Qual Life Outcomes. 2018;16(1):54.

Raveenthiran V. Neonatal sex assignment in disorders of sex development: a philosophical introspection. J Neonatal Surg. 2017;6(3):58.

Reiner WG, Gearhart JP. Discordant sexual identity in some genetic males with cloacal exstrophy assigned to female sex at birth. N Engl J Med. 2004;350(4):333–41.

Ritzen EM, Bergh A, Bjerknes R, et al. Nordic consensus on treatment of undescended testes. Acta Paediatr. 2007;96(5):638–43.

Rohayem J, Hauffa BP, Zacharin M, et al. Testicular growth and spermatogenesis: new goals for pubertal hormone replacement in boys with hypogonadotropic hypogonadism? -a multicentre prospective study of hCG/rFSH treatment outcomes during adolescence. Clin Endocrinol. 2017;86(1):75–87.

Rynja SP, Wouters GA, Van Schaijk M, et al. Long-term followup of hypospadias: functional and cosmetic results. J Urol. 2009;182(4 Suppl):1736–43.

Sanders C, Hall J, Sanders C, et al. Involving individuals with disorders of sex development and their parents in exploring new models of shared learning: proceedings from a DSDnet COST action workshop. Sex Dev. 2018.

Schmoll HJ, Jordan K, Huddart R, et al. Testicular seminoma: ESMO clinical practice guidelines for diagnosis, treatment and follow-up. Ann Oncol. 2010;21(Suppl 5):v140–6.

Schnack TH, Poulsen G, Myrup C, et al. Familial coaggregation of cryptorchidism, hypospadias, and testicular germ cell cancer: a nationwide cohort study. J Natl Cancer Inst. 2010;102(3):187–92.

Schutzmann K, Brinkmann L, Schacht M, et al. Psychological distress, self-harming behavior, and suicidal tendencies in adults with disorders of sex development. Arch Sex Behav. 2009;38(1):16–33.

Spires SE, Woolums CS, Pulito AR, et al. Testicular regression syndrome: a clinical and pathologic study of 11 cases. Arch Pathol Lab Med. 2000;124(5):694–8.

Stoop H, Honecker F, van de Geijn GJ, Gillis AJ, Cools MC, de Boer M, Bokemeyer C, Wolffenbuttel KP, Drop SL, de Krijger RR, Dennis N, Summersgill B, McIntyre A, Shipley J, Oosterhuis JW, Looijenga LH. Stem cell factor as a novel diagnostic marker for early malignant germ cells. J Pathol. 2008;216(1):43–54. https://doi.org/10.1002/path.2378.

T'Sjoen G, De Cuypere G, Monstrey S, et al. Male gender identity in complete androgen insensitivity syndrome. Arch Sex Behav. 2011;40(3):635–8.

Tang P, Frankenberg S, Argentaro A, et al. Comparative analysis of the ATRX promoter and 5′ regulatory region reveals conserved regulatory elements which are linked to roles in neurodevelopment, alpha-globin regulation and testicular function. BMC Res Notes. 2011;4:200.

Tesarik J, Mendoza C, Testart J. Viable embryos from injection of round spermatids into oocytes. N Engl J Med. 1995;333(8):525.

Themmen AP, Verhoef-Post M. LH receptor defects. Semin Reprod Med. 2002;20(3):199–204.

Thorup J, Cortes D. Long-term follow-up after treatment of cryptorchidism. Eur J Pediatr Surg. 2016;26(5):427–31.

Thyen U, Ittermann T, Flessa S, et al. Quality of health care in adolescents and adults with disorders/differences of sex development (DSD) in six European countries (dsd-LIFE). BMC Health Serv Res. 2018;18(1):527.

Umehara F, Tate G, Itoh K, et al. A novel mutation of desert hedgehog in a patient with 46,XY partial gonadal dysgenesis accompanied by minifascicular neuropathy. Am J Hum Genet. 2000;67(5):1302–5.

Veale JF, Clarke DE, Lomax TC. Biological and psychol-social correlates of adult gender-variant identities: a review. Personal Individ Differ. 2010;48(4):357–66.

Wagner KD, Wagner N, Schedl A. The complex life of WT1. J Cell Sci. 2003;116(Pt 9):1653–8.

Warne G, Grover S, Hutson J, et al. A long-term outcome study of intersex conditions. J Pediatr Endocrinol Metab. 2005;18(6):555–67.

Warne GL. Long-term outcome of disorders of sex development. Sex Dev. 2008;2(4–5):268–77.

Wisniewski AB, Migeon CJ, Gearhart JP, et al. Congenital micropenis: long-term medical, surgical and psychosexual follow-up of individuals raised male or female. Horm Res. 2001;56(1–2):3–11.

Wolffenbuttel KP, Hersmus R, Stoop H, Biermann K, Hoebeke P, Cools M, Looijenga LHJ. Gonadal dysgenesis in disorders of sex development: Diagnosis and surgical management. Journal of Pediatric Urology. 2016;12:e411–6.

8 Sex Chromosome DSD

Michele A. O'Connell

8.1 Introduction

Sex chromosome aneuploidy is a variation in the number of X or Y chromosomes, with the addition or loss of one or more sex chromosomes. It is extremely common, with an incidence of ~1:400 births. In some individuals, it may affect all cells. The most common aneuploid karyotypes found are 47,XXY (1:576 boys), 47,XYY (1:851 boys), 47,XXX (1:897 girls), and 45,X (1:2130 girls). Alternatively, the aneuploidy may form part of a mosaic karyotype. The most common of these are 45,X/46,XX, 45,X/46,XY, 46,XX/47,XXX and 46,XY/47,XXY. Sex chromosome aneuploidy and sex chromosome mosaicism are included in the DSD classification system established in 2005. In many conditions associated with sex chromosome aneuploidy or mosaicism, the development of the gonad is affected, and therefore puberty, fertility and even primary sex differentiation, may be atypical.

In the past, some unwarranted assumptions were made about the phenotype of individuals with sex chromosome aneuploidy and mosaicism. A very different picture emerged from long-term follow-up of individuals detected through cytogenetic surveys of the newborn that were begun in collaboration between a number of centres in North America and Europe in the 1960s. Out of 199,898 consecutive newborn live births screened by examination of amniotic membranes, buccal smear or cord blood, 307 individuals were identified and invited to participate in follow-up studies, along with age- and sex-matched controls. The results showed that "most of these individuals with sex chromosome aneuploidy fall within the normal range in development and that marked abnormality is not usually seen" (Linden et al. 1996). Further, unbiased information emerged from follow-up studies of infants born following intra-uterine diagnosis. A very surprising finding at the time was that 95% of infants with prenatally diagnosed 45,X/46,XY mosaicism had a male phenotype rather than the more typical presentations of, for example, mosaic Turner syndrome (TS) that clinicians were more used to seeing in patients diagnosed after birth (Chang et al. 1990). This is important information to share with parents where non-invasive prenatal testing (NIPT) with cell-free DNA (cfDNA) or other antenatal genetic testing reveals such a chromosomal complement, although importantly at the time of writing, cfDNA should still not be considered a diagnostic test (Shaffer and Norton 2018). Nonetheless, as described in Sect. 8.2.2 later, intermittent follow-up of such infants through to adulthood is recommended.

M. A. O'Connell (✉)
Department of Endocrinology and Diabetes, The Royal Children's Hospital, Melbourne, VIC, Australia

Murdoch Children's Research Institute, Melbourne, VIC, Australia
e-mail: michele.oconnell@rch.org.au

J. M. Hutson et al. (eds.), *Disorders|Differences of Sex Development*,
https://doi.org/10.1007/978-981-13-7864-5_8

8.2 45,X/46,XY Mosaicism

This is the most common chromosomal variant associated with atypical genitalia and, together with congenital adrenal hyperplasia (CAH) and androgen insensitivity syndrome (AIS), one of the three most common causes of atypical genitalia overall. The atypical anatomy in 45,X/46,XY mosaicism results from gonadal dysgenesis and the phenotype (degree of virilisation) will depend on the proportion of each cell line. When one gonad is a streak (consisting of fibrous tissue without any germ cells) and the other is an underdeveloped or dysgenetic testis, the individual is said to have *mixed* gonadal dysgenesis. When both gonads are dysgenetic, the term used is *partial* gonadal dysgenesis. The histological characteristic of testicular dysgenesis is a cortical network of anastomosing seminiferous cords that penetrate a thin tunica albuginea. In streak gonads, the 45,X cell line predominates over the 46,XY line, while, in dysgenetic testes, the two cell lines are more equally balanced (Chemes et al. 2003).

8.2.1 Phenotype of 45,X/46,XY DSD

A wide range of phenotypes is possible with this karyotype. At one end of the spectrum, representing 95% of the total number of affected individuals, are those with an apparently complete male phenotype. Follow-up of these boys has shown that many have short stature and dysgenetic testes (Telvi et al. 1999). The risk of gonadal cancer in this group is unknown but is likely to exceed that of the background male population.

Recent data from a retrospective longitudinal study of outcomes of 40 boys with 45,X/46,XY mosaicism considered to have typical male phenotype at birth have reported that longer-term follow-up of such boys into adulthood is indeed warranted (Dumeige et al. 2018). Features in their cohort ($n = 20$ of whom were diagnosed antenatally and $n = 20$ diagnosed postnatally) included short stature (mean adult height of 158 ±7.6 cm [−2.3 SD of expected MPH]), minor external genital variations (22/40), structural cardiac (6/23 investigated) and renal variations (3/19 investigated) and, in one boy, testicular embryonic carcinoma suggesting partial gonadal dysgenesis. Spontaneous puberty occurred in 93%, but 71% ($n = 5$) of those evaluated at the end of puberty showed low inhibin B levels and increased follicle-stimulating hormone (FSH) levels, suggesting lower than typical Sertoli cell function. As azoospermia diagnosed in adulthood is recognised in this cohort, follow-up through puberty with early fertility preservation if warranted may be beneficial.

At the other end of the spectrum are those with a female phenotype and features of Turner syndrome. Estimates of the number of girls with Turner syndrome whose karyotype contains Y chromosome material vary, depending on the detection technique used (Hanson et al. 2001; Yorifuji et al. 2001; Nishi et al. 2002), and the ideal method of screening for this has not been clearly defined. The incidence of GB in women with 45,X Turner syndrome is low, but it is significantly higher in those with all or part of a Y chromosome. GB was found in resected gonads of 4/14 (28%) 45X/46XY children in one recent retrospective study; however, no dysgerminoma cases were found in that series (Coyle et al. 2016). The presence of *TSPY* has been postulated to be the best indicator of cancer risk (Hersmus et al. 2008). A high frequency (47%) of Y chromosome deletions has been identified in patients with sex chromosome mosaicism, and these are believed to contribute to Y chromosome instability (Patsalis et al. 2005).

Infants with mixed gonadal dysgenesis often have atypical genitalia that have an asymmetrical appearance, due to the presence of a descended testis on one side and an impalpable, intra-abdominal streak gonad on the other (Fig. 8.1). The size of the better-differentiated testis is usually smaller than typical testicular size. Around 75% have a Müllerian remnant, usually on the side of the streak gonad, due to insufficient foetal gonadal secretion of AMH. Endometrial cancer has also been reported in women with mixed gonadal dysgenesis (MGD) with a retained uterus treated with oestrogen (Robboy et al. 1982; Wallace and Levin 1990). Either a large prostatic utricle or a Müllerian remnant may be present, and this may predispose to recurrent urinary tract infections and epididymo-orchitis if there is backfilling with urine. Short stature is common, with no apparent benefit of growth hormone on adult height. A study of 20 men with 45X/46XY MGD to adulthood reported mean

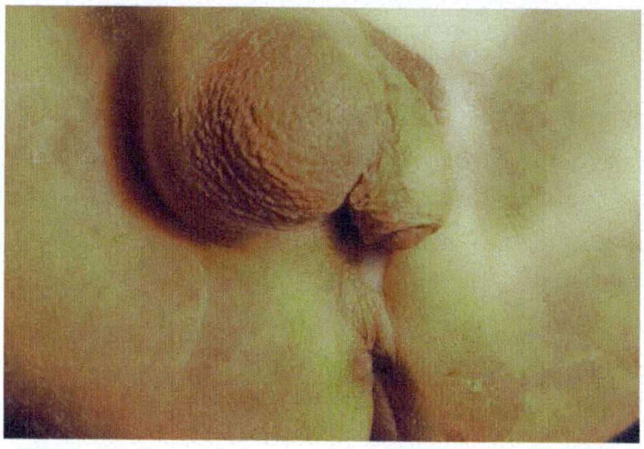

Fig. 8.1 In 45,X/46,XY mixed gonadal dysgenesis, the gonadal mosaicism leads to asymmetrical external genital development. In this patient, the right gonad was a testis that had descended into the hemi-scrotum, while on the left side the gonad was an intra-abdominal streak gonad, producing striking genital asymmetry. A vaginal cavity was present inside the common urogenital opening, as can be predicted from the presence of vaginal mucus below the phallus (stimulated by maternal hormones). He was raised as a boy, with the gonads left *in situ*. He re-presented in adolescence with a malignant tumour arising from the streak gonad

adult height of 156.9 ± 2 cm, regardless of GH treatment (Martinerie et al. 2012). In this same cohort, 17/20 boys had spontaneous onset of puberty, although 6/17 ultimately needed supplemental exogenous testosterone therapy to complete puberty, and a majority (67%) of the remaining cohort also showed signs of declining testicular function at the end of puberty (high FSH and low inhibin). Variations in Y chromosome structure known to be associated with reduced fertility were also found in 10/16 studied. Abnormalities of the urinary tract (axial rotation of the kidney, ureteric duplication, horseshoe kidney, renal dysplasia) and cardiovascular system (arterial hypertension, coarctation of the aorta, bicuspid aortic valve) may be present (Telvi et al. 1999). Some affected individuals have learning difficulties; an increased risk of deafness due to recurrent otitis media and dysmorphic features resembling those of Turner syndrome are also reported.

8.2.2 Malignancy Risk and Risk Management

Histological features of dysgenetic testes may also include two pre-malignant types of germ cell: gonadoblastoma (GB), the precursor to dysgerminoma and germ cell neoplasia *in situ (GCNIS)*, the precursor for germ cell tumours (*GCT*; previously referred to as carcinoma *in situ*) (Looijenga et al. 2007; Berney et al. 2016). The features of a gonadoblastoma are germ cell proliferation and sex cord derivatives frequently surrounding small round deposits containing amorphous hyaline material (Gorosito et al. 2010).

Presence of GB, possibly in combination with GCNIS, in a scrotal testis, is indicative of an underlying DSD (Hersmus et al. 2012). GB may be bilateral and may be present from birth, or they may develop later. All are thought to have the potential to transform into malignant germ cell tumours, known as dysgerminomas, over time. GCNIS cells are found lining seminiferous tubules in dysgenetic testes. They resemble immature germ cells and cannot therefore be diagnosed early in life, when such cells are normally present, but if found in the testes of an older infant or child, they are pathological and are capable of transforming into GCT. Expression of two genetic markers—OCT3/4 and *TSPY*—can be found in either germ cells presenting delayed maturation or GCNIS (Looijenga et al. 2010). Additional staining with c-KIT ligand (KITLG, also known as Stem Cell Factor) differentiates between these, as KITLG is regarded as pathognomonic of GCNIS (Wolffenbuttel et al. 2016). The risk of gonadal cancer in an individual with severe gonadal dysgenesis and 45,X/46,XY mosaicism is considered mildly to moderately elevated, especially if the gonad is intra-abdominal (Hughes et al. 2006). The risk in a more differentiated, scrotal testis is somewhat lower but still too high to be ignored. Risk management strategies need to take these factors into account.

It is widely recommended that intra-abdominal dysgenetic testes and streak gonads be removed as soon as possible after diagnosis; reports of very early evidence of both pre-malignant and malignant changes in gonads removed from children aged <1 year appear to support this practice. Earlier advice would have also been to remove the better-differentiated scrotal or inguinal testis, given the high likelihood of infertility, hormonal insufficiency needing replacement therapy and the risk of malignancy. However, the removal of gonadal tissue that is at higher risk for malignant potential but which has the potential for inherent function is a less straightforward decision.

The external masculinisation score (EMS) reflects gonadal differentiation and appears inversely related to tumour risk in individuals with 45,X/46,XY (Cools et al. 2011). In boys, testosterone production may be sufficient, at least in early puberty/adolescence, hence leaving inguinal or scrotal gonads *in situ* to allow endogenous hormone production is appropriate; however strict follow-up is warranted to mitigate the malignancy risk. In phenotypic 45,Y/46,XY girls (indicating severe gonadal dysgenesis), as gonads are intra-abdominal (higher malignancy risk) and too dysgenetic to offer hormonal production or fertility potential, gonadectomy to remove malignancy risk from a non functioning gonad that is small and very difficult to monitor radiologically is widely considered to be a reasonable option. Optimal timing of gonadectomy in 45,X/46,XY girls has not yet been established and rates of pre-malignany/ malignant change vary widely (2.2% to 50%). If a dysgenetic testis is to be retained, a risk management strategy is mandatory (Wolffenbuttel et al. 2016). This would include bringing an inguinal testis down to the scrotum for examination purposes, regular clinical follow-up and biopsy after the onset of puberty, with specialised pathological examination (including staining for OCT3/4, TSPY and KITLG—see Chap. 7 for further discussion), to exclude GCNIS. If evidence of GCNIS is found, the testis can be either removed or irradiated (Skakkebaek 1994). The reason for waiting until after the onset of puberty to biopsy is that by that time, GCNIS cells may have spread to involve more/all of the seminiferous tubules, and sampling error is thought to be lower. As previously stated, it would be less helpful to perform the biopsy in a very young child, when it may be very difficult to differentiate GCNIS cells from immature germ cells. If this is undertaken (e.g. if gonadal biopsy is performed when a young child is having a general anaesthetic/surgical procedure for another indication) staining for presence of KITLG may be helpful in identifying GCNIS.

8.2.3 Management

A risk management strategy to prevent undiagnosed invasive malignancy is most important in all patients with sex chromosome mosaicism including a Y chromosome or a marker derived from the Y chromosome. Completely dysgenetic or 'streak' gonads, which by their nature have no potential for endogenous hormonal production or fertility but a high malignancy risk, can be removed laparoscopically. The decision as to the removal or retention of a partially dysgenetic testis will depend upon several factors: the EMS, the perceived malignancy risk (based on available evidence at the time and acknowledging the inherent limitations of currently available data), the likelihood that the testis will secrete enough testosterone for pubertal development, the possibility of fertility and the position of the testis that would make it amenable to easy clinical follow-up and self-examination. Ethically, an important aim should be to minimise physical harm to the child (Gillam et al. 2010), and the elimination of malignancy risk could justify removing a dysgenetic gonad. Maximising the potential for fertility would mitigate against removing it, but if a biopsy showed a complete absence of germ cells, there would be no chance of fertility (unless in the future, germ cell transplantation or stem cell therapy offered a solution), and therefore gonadectomy may be reasonable if hormonal function is absent. Hormonal function is usually inadequate to initiate and sustain puberty in intra-abdominal/severely dysgenetic testes, making hormone replacement therapy necessary in most cases.

The absolute risk of development of germ cell malignancy over a lifespan is difficult to quantify, in part due to the relatively low number of affected adults with preserved dysgenetic gonads. A retrospective review of 94 individuals with DSD comprising dysgenetic gonads and Y chromosome aged 1.2–32 years (47 pre-pubertal and 47 post-pubertal) reported germ cell neoplasia in 53.2% of patients (51.1% in children, 55.3% in pubertal/adults). Invasive GCT was identified in 11.7% of cases, of which 90.9% were in pubertal/adult patients. Other neoplastic lesions included gonadoblastoma (16% prevalence) and testicular carcinoma *in situ* (25.5%). Raised FSH was found in 81% of the younger cohort, and the majority of pubertal/adult-aged individuals had hypergonadotrophic hypogonadism (Slowikowska-Hilczer et al. 2015). These data confirm the high risk of both GCT and primary gonadal insufficiency in a relatively large cohort of individuals with dysgenetic gonads and Y material and can inform discussions with families in relation to decisions around consideration of gonadectomy.

The decision about the sex of rearing was 'traditionally' closely related to the degree of virilisation in the external genitalia (Cameron et al. 1997). While the individual nuances of every case must be respected, current recommendations suggest the principle factors to be considered in relation to male or female sex of rearing include likely future gender identity, fertility potential, evidence of potential foetal central nervous system (CNS) exposure to androgens, gonadal malignancy risk, surgical options/indications, future sexual function and psychosocial factors (familial, social and cultural) (Lee et al. 2016). While the likelihood of future gender identity is a central consideration, it is well recognised that gender identity cannot reliably be predicted from the genital anatomy (Hughes et al. 2006; Warne 2008) and may differ from sex of rearing. While in the majority of cases, the affirmed gender identity will match the sex assigned at birth, some will experience severe gender dysphoria. In one study of 19 adults with mixed or partial gonadal dysgenesis, all 10 who were raised as male had a male gender identity, while 2 of 9 raised as females reported gender incongruence and dysphoria (Szarras-Czapnik et al. 2007). Therefore, where sex of rearing is female, the key ethical considerations include keeping future options open. Thus, today, early feminising genitoplasty should be avoided. The wishes and beliefs of the parents will also come in to the decision-making process. Where strong preferences are expressed for cultural reasons (Warne and Raza 2008), a male sex of rearing is often favoured.

Long-term management will include hormone replacement therapy (Warne et al. 2005a, b), with oestrogen for those with streak (non-hormonally active) gonads which were removed and who have a female/feminine gender identity (combined with a progestogen when a uterus is present), and testosterone for those who idenitfy as male/masculine. If gonads are retained, hormone replacement therapy is required to ensure adequate sex steroid exposure in the majority of adolescents and adults with MGD due to primary gonadal insufficiency (Slowikowska-Hilczer et al. 2015). Referral of girls to a paediatric and adolescent gynaecologist at around age 10–12 years allows counselling about physical development, sexual and reproductive health, gender identity and fertility options (see Chap. 18). The involvement of an experienced mental health professional is also strongly recommended.

Those who have had hypospadias surgery and who have been raised as males are often in the care of a paediatric urologist and an endocrinologist (for monitoring of growth and pubertal development). Long-term follow-up studies have revealed a high incidence (44%) of persisting urinary difficulties (Warne et al. 2005a, b). Boys may also have poor self-esteem because of their perceived small penis, even when it is in the typical range (Aulagne et al. 2010; Xu et al. 2016) for age. Long-term outcome studies of adolescents who were born with either atypical genital appearance or smaller than typical penile length show that they experience a range of challenges (Brinkmann et al. 2007; de Vries et al. 2007), yet services caring for these boys and men frequently include little provision in terms of professional mental health support, which is suboptimal.

8.3 Ovo-Testicular DSD

In ovo-testicular DSD, ovarian follicles and seminiferous tubules are present in the gonads of the one individual. Their distribution in the gonads varies. One pole of a gonad may consist of ovarian tissue, while the other pole consists of testicular tissue. Another variation is that one gonad is an ovary, while the other is a dysgenetic testis. In 89% of ovo-testes, however, the ovarian and tes-

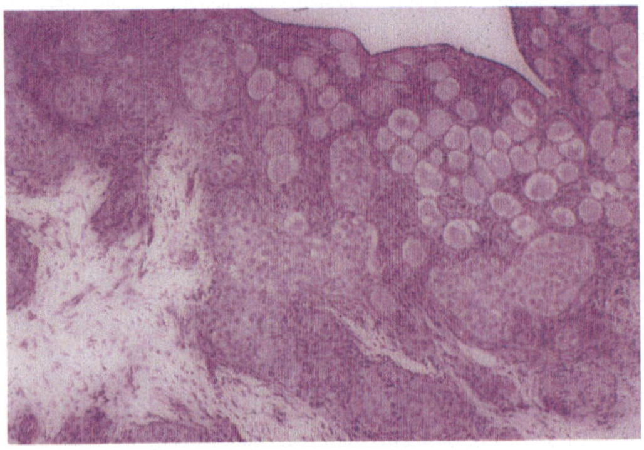

Fig. 8.2 Gonadal histology in a baby with ovo-testicular DSD. The section shows relatively normal seminiferous tubules adjacent to ovarian stroma with follicles

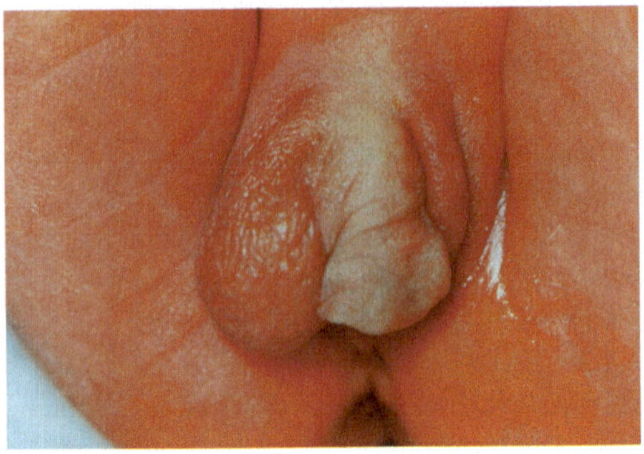

Fig. 8.3 Ovo-testicular DSD in a baby with external asymmetry. On the right, the descended gonad was a testis, while the undescended left gonad was an ovo-testis

ticular elements are evenly distributed throughout, making it impossible to distinguish one from the other at the macroscopic level (Fig. 8.2) (Wiersma and Ramdial 2009).

The testicular tissue in ovo-testicular DSD undergoes atresia at a faster rate than the ovarian tissue. Pregnancy has been reported in a small number of women with ovo-testicular DSD (n = 14 women with 26 pregnancies and 20 live-born babies reported 1975–2017); however, male fertility leading to paternity has not been reported to date (Bayraktar 2018).

The karyotype in ovo-testicular DSD is most commonly 46,XX, but 45,X/46,XY and 46,XY ovo testicular DSD are seen (Krob et al. 1994). Occasional 46,XX/46,XY chimeras are also seen. The cancer risk in ovo-testicular DSD with a 46,XX karyotype has not been determined (Looijenga et al. 2010; Wolffenbuttel et al. 2016), but the risk in patients with a Y chromosome is assumed to be higher.

The phenotype varies, depending on the gonadal status, but one easily recognisable pattern is when there is a testis on one side (often the right), and an ovo-testis or ovary on the other side (Fig. 8.3).

In a recent retrospective analysis of 64 ovotesticular DSD cases in South Africa, the most common karyotype was 46,XX (88%), followed by 46,XY (8%), 46,XY/45,X (3%) and 46,XX/46,XY. Predominant sex of rearing was male in two-thirds of individuals, with gender dysphoria noted in n = 8 (11%) at a median of 6.4 years; long-term follow-up revealed dysphoria in two cases and neuropsychiatric diagnoses in four cases (Ganie et al. 2017).

8.3.1 Management of Ovo-Testicular DSD

The gonad most likely to function in an individual with ovo-testicular DSD is the ovary. The uterus may be normal, hypoplastic or absent (Yordam et al. 2001). Of 36 Brazilian patients with ovo-testicular DSD, female sex of rearing was assigned in 56% (Damiani et al. 2005). Given that the gonadal cancer risk in 46,XX ovo-testicular DSD is difficult to determine, but likely not on the higher side, and that fertile oocytes may be present in the ovarian tissue, but spermatogenesis is likely to be absent it has been recommended that the testicular component be excised if it can be identified (Wiersma 2001). In recent years, in keeping with a broader preference to preserve gonadal tissue with the potential for function, early surgical excision is less frequently considered. Rather, a preferred option for many is to leave the ovo-testis *in situ*, review the hormonal status at puberty and potentially then remove tissue that is producing unwanted hormones (which may involve excision of the whole gonad). GnRHa therapy can be used to temporarily block pubertal hormone production while the young person has time to consider their options in the context of their gender identity.

8.4 Klinefelter Syndrome: 47,XXY and Variants

The most common karyotype in patients with Klinefelter syndrome (KS) is 47,XXY, but other variants are also reported (Fruhmesser and Kotzot 2011). Genital variations at birth are rare in males with a 47,XXY karyotype (Lee et al. 2007), although progressive deterioration of testicular function is a feature in the majority of patients (Wikstrom and Dunkel 2008) and testosterone replacement therapy to sustain typical adult male range testosterone levels is prescribed for many men (Forti et al. 2010). One of the potential benefits of sex hormone replacement therapy is the prevention of osteoporosis, which is present in 40% of men with Klinefelter syndrome (KS) (Ferlin et al. 2010); however, the long-term effects of testosterone have not been rigorously evaluated in men with KS, and these studies are required (Gravholt et al. 2017). Although relatively uncommon overall, gender dysphoria and female gender identity are reported in KS cohorts, hence assessment of gender identity should be undertaken if sex hormone replacement therapy is being considered.

Classically described characteristics of KS include small testes, infertility, hypergonadotrophic hypogonadism and learning/cognitive difficulties. Most men with KS are oligospermic or azoospermic, with high levels of FSH and LH. A significant proportion of those with KS are diagnosed in the context of investigation for subfertility (potentially indicating the absence of troublesome clinical symptoms until early adulthood). Until the turn of the millennium, infertility was thought to be almost universal in KS; however, this is no longer the case. Significantly improved rates of sperm retrieval have been reported with assisted reproductive technologies, particularly intra-cytoplasmic sperm injection (ICSI) (Paduch et al. 2009) and more recently with testicular sperm extraction—ICSI (TESE-ICSI) (Plotton et al. 2014). A recent systematic review and meta-analysis has reported that performing TESE/micro-TESE in men with KS results in sperm retrieval rates, pregnancy rates and live birth rates that are all close to 50%, with results being independent of any clinical or biochemical parameters (Corona et al. 2017).

Spermatozoa have occasionally been identified in ejaculate of adult KS men but very exceptionally in KS adolescents. Spermatozoa can, however, be retrieved in testicular tissue of KS adolescents. The testis may also harbour spermatogonia and incompletely differentiated germ cells. Optimal age at sperm extraction is unknown, although rates of positive sperm extraction are reported as higher at an earlier age. In a recent retrospective cohort study of 111 azoospermic KS men undergoing TESE, successful sperm recovery was reported in $n = 38$ (34.2%). Age at TESE, anthropometric measures, testis volume, sex hormone levels and semen parameters were not predictive parameters of sperm retrieval rate (SRR). In those treated with testosterone, gonadotrophin levels were, however, significantly lower in those with failure in sperm retrieval (Garolla et al. 2018).

Males with KS tend to be taller than average. In comparison with siblings, a deficit of 10–15 IQ points has been reported, although intelligence falls within the normal range (Linden et al. 1996). Verbal IQ is affected more than performance IQ. Social cognitive functioning (e.g. interpretation of facial expression/cues) may also be affected (van Rijn et al. 2018). At puberty, gynaecomastia occurs in one-third of boys. There is an increased lifetime risk of breast cancer. Men with KS are also at increased risk of non-testicular germ cell cancers, especially in the mediastinum, although absolute incidence is low (Hiramatsu et al. 2008). The spectrum in which KS may affect someone is important to consider when counselling a couple who have a pregnancy with antenatal KS diagnosis (increasingly common, given the relatively high uptake of NIPT in developed countries).

8.5 Turner Syndrome: Monosomy X and Variants

Loss of one of the two X chromosomes results in a wide range of changes in foetal development. All except 1% of 45,X foetuses are estimated to be spontaneously aborted (Linden et al. 1996).

The phenotypes of live-born girls with TS vary markedly, but may include short stature and reduced linear growth velocity (average untreated adult height is 144 cm), atypical gonadal/ovarian differentiation causing premature ovarian insufficiency and sub- or infertility, as well as variations in development of the cardiovascular, lymphatic and renal systems, the eyes and ears and other organs. Infants may be born with webbing of the neck, which is a consequence of intra-uterine cystic hygroma resulting from obstruction to the thoracic duct. Other lymphatic abnormalities are responsible for lymphoedema of the hands and feet, which can be troublesome. Typical cardiovascular variations are bicuspid aortic valve and coarctation of the aorta. Hypertension is a risk during adolescence and adulthood. Girls with TS are prone to obstruction of their Eustachian tubes and are therefore prone to otitis media, conductive deafness and cholesteatoma. In addition, sensorineural deafness, which is independent of the conductive deafness, tends to develop towards the end of the second decade, and by middle age, more than a quarter of women with TS require a hearing aid (Hultcrantz et al. 1994; Beckman et al. 2004; Morimoto et al. 2006; Bergamaschi et al. 2008). Other head and neck features include high-arched palate, downturned angles of the mouth, strabismus and epicanthic folds. There is often an increased number of pigmented cutaneous naevi, and wound healing is often with keloid scarring. Horseshoe or ectopic, pelvic kidney occurs frequently. As with all sex chromosome aneuploidies detected on antenatal testing, the spectrum in which TS may affect someone is important to consider when consulting a couple who have a pregnancy with likely TS diagnosis.

There are some psychological characteristics that may affect learning, even though mean IQ is within the normal range for the general community. Individual IQ in comparison to that of siblings is reduced by an average of 9 points, while a number of Wechsler scores (particularly Arithmetic, Block Design, Object Assembly and Picture Arrangement) are lower in TS females as a group (Loesch et al. 2005).

Over a life course, the main issues that may affect quality of life for girls and women with TS include short stature, infertility and deafness, in addition to increased risk for the metabolic syndrome, autoimmune diseases (most commonly hypothyroidism and coeliac disease) and osteoporosis due to relative oestrogen deficiency. A particular long-term concern that needs lifelong monitoring is the risk of dilatation of the aortic root as, if unrecognised and progressive, this may result in catastrophic aortic dissection. This occurs most commonly in women with bicuspid aortic valve but can also occur in those without previously detectable cardiac anomalies. Sudden death may occur in early adult life due to dissecting aneurysm, and strategies aimed at preventing it have been proposed (Conway 2009). Spontaneous pregnancies have been reported in 4.8–7.6% of women with TS but foetal outcomes are affected with higher rates of spontaneous abortion and chromosomal anomalies in the infant (Georgopoulos et al. 2009; Mortensen et al. 2010). Women with TS who have premature ovarian insufficiency have high rates of parenting desire and are very interested in assisted reproductive technologies (Huang et al. 2008; Cabanes et al. 2010). The maternal risks are however considerable, including 100-fold increase in pregnancy-related complications, including the risk of aortic dissection. Recent international consensus guidelines for the management of TS recommend counselling females with TS that their ability to spontaneously conceive decreases rapidly with age, hence consideration should be given to offering fertility treatment at a young age (Gravholt et al. 2017). Young women with mosaic TS who have persistent ovarian function should be counselled that oocyte cryopreservation after controlled ovarian hyperstimulation is a possible fertility preservation option. Oocyte retrieval for fertility preservation of young TS girls before the age of 12 years is not recommended. All women with TS should be counselled about the increased cardiovascular risk of pregnancy, and oocyte donation for fertility should only be offered after thorough screening and appropriate counselling.

8.5.1 Detecting Mosaicism in Turner Syndrome

Around 30% of individuals with TS have sex chromosome mosaicism. Those with 45,X/46,XX mosaicism have a better chance of fertility than those with 45,X, and it has been proposed that cryopreservation of ovarian tissue before all of the oocytes have undergone atresia may improve reproductive chances (Huang et al. 2008).

Some women with TS have 45,X/46,XY mosaicism and because of the Y chromosome, as outlined earlier, are at increased risk for germ cell cancer (Looijenga et al. 2010). The rate of gonadoblastoma among TS patients with Y chromosome sequences that were detected by PCR or FISH varies from 4% to 60% in 14 studies, and data on the long-term outcome of this cohort are incomplete. Putting all data together, approximately 10% may develop a gonadoblastoma, although there is considerable variation in risk estimates, possibly related to methodology, sample size and potential selection bias. It is therefore currently recommended that in TS women with Y chromosome material, the streak gonads should be removed (Cools et al. 2006; Gravholt et al. 2017). The difficulty lies in detecting low levels of mosaicism. Ideally, 100 cells need to be counted to exclude low-level mosaicism in those who appear to have a 45,X karyotype (Wolff et al. 2010). Standard karyotype is recommended by recent guidelines as although chromosomal microarray is increasingly utilised in a clinical setting, its prognostic utility remains to be ascertained in TS. Quantitative PCR is also able to detect very small amounts of Y-derived DNA. FISH with X and Y centromere probes are recommended to determine the origin of ring or small marker chromosomes; however, it is thought no longer clinically indicated to use FISH with SRY probes to exclude cryptic Y material. This latter recommendation relates to the fact that the gonadoblastoma locus is mapped adjacent to the centromere to a region that does not include the SRY gene; therefore, SRY probes are not required (Gravholt et al. 2017).

Issues relating to hormonal management of Turner syndrome are discussed in more detail in Chap. 16.

Acknowledgements With thanks and acknowledgement to the original authors of this chapter Dr. Jacqueline Hewitt, Professor Garry L. Warne AM.

References

Aulagne MB, Harper L, de Napoli-Cocci S, et al. Long-term outcome of severe hypospadias. J Pediatr Urol. 2010;6(5):469–72.

Bayraktar Z. Potential autofertility in true hermaphrodites. J Matern Fetal Neonatal Med. 2018;31(4):542–7.

Beckman A, Conway GS, Cadge B. Audiological features of Turner's syndrome in adults. Int J Audiol. 2004;43(9):533–44.

Bergamaschi R, Bergonzoni C, Mazzanti L, et al. Hearing loss in Turner syndrome: results of a multicentric study. J Endocrinol Investig. 2008;31(9):779–83.

Berney DM, Looijenga LH, Idrees M, et al. Germ cell neoplasia in situ (GCNIS): evolution of the current nomenclature for testicular pre-invasive germ cell malignancy. Histopathology. 2016;69(1):7–10.

Brinkmann L, Schuetzmann K, Richter-Appelt H. Gender assignment and medical history of individuals with different forms of intersexuality: evaluation of medical records and the patients' perspective. J Sex Med. 2007;4(4 Pt 1):964–80.

Cabanes L, Chalas C, Christin-Maitre S, et al. Turner syndrome and pregnancy: clinical practice. Recommendations for the management of patients with Turner syndrome before and during pregnancy. Eur J Obstet Gynecol Reprod Biol. 2010;152(1):18–24.

Cameron FJ, Montalto J, Byrt EA, et al. Gonadal dysgenesis: associations between clinical features and sex of rearing. Endocr J. 1997;44(1):95–104.

Chang HJ, Clark RD, Bachman H. The phenotype of 45,X/46,XY mosaicism: an analysis of 92 prenatally diagnosed cases. Am J Hum Genet. 1990;46(1):156–67.

Chemes HE, Muzulin PM, Venara MC, et al. Early manifestations of testicular dysgenesis in children: Pathological phenotypes, karyotype correlations and precursor stages of tumour development. APMIS. 2003;111(1):12–24.

Conway GS. Adult care of pediatric conditions: lessons from Turner's syndrome. J Clin Endocrinol Metab. 2009;94(9):3185–7.

Cools M, Stoop H, Kersemaekers AM, et al. Gonadoblastoma arising in undifferentiated gonadal tissue within dysgenetic gonads. J Clin Endocrinol Metab. 2006;91(6):2404–13.

Cools M, Pleskacova J, Stoop H, Hoebeke P, Van Laecke E, Drop SL, Lebl J, Oosterhuis JW, Looijenga LH, Wolffenbuttel KP, Mosaicism Collaborative Group. Gonadal pathology and tumor risk in relation to clinical characteristics in patients with 45,X/46,XY mosaicism. J Clin Endocrinol Metab. 2011;96(7): E1171–80.

Corona G, Pizzocaro A, Lanfranco F, et al. Sperm recovery and ICSI outcomes in Klinefelter syndrome: a systematic review and meta-analysis. Hum Reprod Update. 2017;23(3):265–75.

Coyle D, Kutasy B, Han Suyin K, et al. Gonadoblastoma in patients with 45,X/46,XY mosaicism: a 16-year experience. J Pediatr Urol. 2016;12(5):283 e281–7.

Damiani D, Guedes DR, Damiani D, et al. True hermaphroditism: experience with 36 patients. Arq Bras Endocrinol Metabol. 2005;49(1):71–8.

Dumeige L, Chatelais L, Bouvattier C, et al. Should 45,X/46,XY boys with no or mild anomaly of external genitalia be investigated and followed up? Eur J Endocrinol. 2018;179(3):181–90.

Ferlin A, Schipilliti M, Di Mambro A, et al. Osteoporosis in Klinefelter's syndrome. Mol Hum Reprod. 2010;16(6):402–10.

Forti G, Corona G, Vignozzi L, et al. Klinefelter's syndrome: a clinical and therapeutical update. Sex Dev. 2010;4(4–5):249–58.

Fruhmesser A, Kotzot D. Chromosomal variants in Klinefelter syndrome. Sex Dev. 2011;5(3):109–23.

Ganie Y, Aldous C, Balakrishna Y, et al. The spectrum of ovotesticular disorders of sex development in South Africa: a single-centre experience. Horm Res Paediatr. 2017;87(5):307–14.

Garolla A, Selice R, Menegazzo M, et al. Novel insights on testicular volume and testosterone replacement therapy in Klinefelter patients undergoing testicular sperm extraction. A retrospective clinical study. Clin Endocrinol. 2018;88(5):711–8.

Georgopoulos NA, Adonakis G, Papadopoulos V, et al. Feto-maternal risks associated with pregnancy achieved through oocyte donation in a woman with Turner syndrome. Gynecol Endocrinol. 2009;25(6):383–6.

Gillam LH, Hewitt JK, Warne GL. Ethical principles for the management of infants with disorders of sex development. Horm Res Paediatr. 2010;74:412–8.

Gorosito M, Pancera B, Sarancone S, et al. Gonadoblastoma: an unusual ovarian tumor. Ann Diagn Pathol. 2010;14(4):247–50.

Gravholt CH, Andersen NH, Conway GS, et al. Clinical practice guidelines for the care of girls and women with Turner syndrome: proceedings from the 2016 Cincinnati International Turner Syndrome Meeting. Eur J Endocrinol. 2017;177(3):G1–G70.

Hanson L, Bryman I, Barrenas ML, et al. Genetic analysis of mosaicism in 53 women with Turner syndrome. Hereditas. 2001;134(2):153–9.

Hersmus R, de Leeuw BH, Wolffenbuttel KP, et al. New insights into type II germ cell tumor pathogenesis based on studies of patients with various forms of disorders of sex development (DSD). Mol Cell Endocrinol. 2008;291(1–2):1–10.

Hersmus R, Stoop H, White SJ, et al. Delayed recognition of disorders of sex development (DSD): a missed opportunity for early diagnosis of malignant germ cell tumors. Int J Endocrinol. 2012;2012:671209.

Hiramatsu H, Morishima T, Nakanishi H, et al. Successful treatment of a patient with Klinefelter's syndrome complicated by mediastinal germ cell tumor and AML(M7). Bone Marrow Transplant. 2008;41(10):907–8.

Huang JY, Tulandi T, Holzer H, et al. Cryopreservation of ovarian tissue and in vitro matured oocytes in a female with mosaic Turner syndrome: Case Report. Hum Reprod. 2008;23(2):336–9.

Hughes IA, Houk C, Ahmed SF, et al. Consensus statement on management of intersex disorders. Arch Dis Child. 2006;91(7):554–63.

Hultcrantz M, Sylven L, Borg E. Ear and hearing problems in 44 middle-aged women with Turner's syndrome. Hear Res. 1994;76(1–2):127–32.

Krob G, Braun A, Kuhnle U. True hermaphroditism: geographical distribution, clinical findings, chromosomes and gonadal histology. Eur J Pediatr. 1994;153(1):2–10.

Lee YS, Cheng AW, Ahmed SF, et al. Genital anomalies in Klinefelter's syndrome. Horm Res. 2007;68(3):150–5.

Lee PA, Nordenstrom A, Houk CP, et al. Global disorders of sex development update since 2006: perceptions, approach and care. Horm Res Paediatr. 2016;85(3):158–80.

Linden MG, Bender BG, Robinson A. Intrauterine diagnosis of sex chromosome aneuploidy. Obstet Gynecol. 1996;87(3):468–75.

Loesch DZ, Bui QM, Kelso W, et al. Effect of Turner's syndrome and X-linked imprinting on cognitive status: analysis based on pedigree data.[Erratum appears in Brain Dev. 2006 Mar;28(2):134 Note: Bergman, Paul [corrected to Bergman, Philip B]]. Brain and Development. 2005;27(7):494–503.

Looijenga LH, Hersmus R, Oosterhuis JW, et al. Tumor risk in disorders of sex development (DSD). Best Pract Res Clin Endocrinol Metab. 2007;21(3):480–95.

Looijenga LH, Hersmus R, de Leeuw BH, et al. Gonadal tumours and DSD. Best Pract Res Clin Endocrinol Metab. 2010;24(2):291–310.

Martinerie L, Morel Y, Gay CL, et al. Impaired puberty, fertility, and final stature in 45,X/46,XY mixed gonadal dysgenetic patients raised as boys. Eur J Endocrinol. 2012;166(4):687–94.

Morimoto N, Tanaka T, Taiji H, et al. Hearing loss in Turner syndrome. J Pediatr. 2006;149(5):697–701.

Mortensen KH, Rohde MD, Uldbjerg N, et al. Repeated spontaneous pregnancies in 45,X Turner syndrome. Obstet Gynecol. 2010;115(2 Pt 2):446–9.

Nishi MY, Domenice S, Medeiros MA, et al. Detection of Y-specific sequences in 122 patients with Turner syndrome: nested PCR is not a reliable method.[Erratum appears in Am J Med Genet. 2002 Nov 15;113(1):116-7]. Am J Med Genet. 2002;107(4):299–305.

Paduch DA, Bolyakov A, Cohen P, et al. Reproduction in men with Klinefelter syndrome: the past, the present, and the future. Semin Reprod Med. 2009;27(2):137–48.

Patsalis PC, Skordis N, Sismani C, et al. Identification of high frequency of Y chromosome deletions in patients with sex chromosome mosaicism and correlation with the clinical phenotype and Y-chromosome instability. Am J Med Genet A. 2005;135(2):145–9.

Plotton I, Brosse A, Cuzin B, et al. Klinefelter syndrome and TESE-ICSI. Ann Endocrinol (Paris). 2014;75(2):118–25.

van Rijn S, de Sonneville L, Swaab H. The nature of social cognitive deficits in children and adults with Klinefelter syndrome (47,XXY). Genes Brain Behav. 2018;17(6):e12465.

Robboy SJ, Miller T, Donahoe PK, et al. Dysgenesis of testicular and streak gonads in the syndrome of mixed gonadal dysgenesis: perspective derived from a clinicopathologic analysis of twenty-one cases. Hum Pathol. 1982;13(8):700–16.

Shaffer BL, Norton ME. Cell-Free DNA screening for aneuploidy and microdeletion syndromes. Obstet Gynecol Clin N Am. 2018;45(1):13–26.

Skakkebaek NE. Management and biology of carcinoma in situ and cancer of the testis. Histopathology. 1994;25(1):97–8.

Slowikowska-Hilczer J, Szarras-Czapnik M, Wolski JK, et al. The risk of neoplasm associated with dysgenetic testes in prepubertal and pubertal/adult patients. Folia Histochem Cytobiol. 2015;53(3):218–26.

Szarras-Czapnik M, Lew-Starowicz Z, Zucker KJ. A psychosexual follow-up study of patients with mixed or partial gonadal dysgenesis. J Pediatr Adolesc Gynecol. 2007;20(6):333–8.

Telvi L, Lebbar A, Del Pino O, et al. 45,X/46,XY mosaicism: report of 27 cases. Pediatrics. 1999;104(2 Pt 1):304–8.

de Vries ALC, Doreleijers TAH, Cohen-Kettenis PT. Disorders of sex development and gender identity outcome in adolescence and adulthood: understanding gender identity development and its clinical implications. Pediatr Endocrinol Rev. 2007;4(4):343–51.

Wallace TM, Levin HS. Mixed gonadal dysgenesis. A review of 15 patients reporting single cases of malignant intratubular germ cell neoplasia of the testis, endometrial adenocarcinoma, and a complex vascular anomaly. Arch Pathol Lab Med. 1990;114(7):679–88.

Warne GL. Long-term outcome of disorders of sex development. Sex Dev. 2008;2(4–5):268–77.

Warne GL, Raza J. Disorders of sex development (DSDs), their presentation and management in different cultures. Rev Endocr Metab Disord. 2008;9(3):227–36.

Warne G, Grover S, Hutson J, et al. A long-term outcome study of intersex conditions. J Pediatr Endocrinol. 2005a;18(6):555–67.

Warne GL, Grover S, Zajac JD. Hormonal therapies for individuals with intersex conditions: protocol for use. Treat Endocrinol. 2005b;4(1):19–29.

Wiersma R. Management of the African child with true hermaphroditism. J Pediatr Surg. 2001;36(2):397–9.

Wiersma R, Ramdial PK. The gonads of 111 South African patients with ovotesticular disorder of sex differentiation. J Pediatr Surg. 2009;44(3):556–60.

Wikstrom AM, Dunkel L. Testicular function in Klinefelter syndrome. Horm Res. 2008;69(6):317–26.

Wolff DJ, Van Dyke DL, Powell CM, et al. Laboratory guideline for Turner syndrome. Genet Med. 2010;12(1):52–5.

Wolffenbuttel KP, Hersmus R, Stoop H, et al. Gonadal dysgenesis in disorders of sex development: Diagnosis and surgical management. J Pediatr Urol. 2016;12(6):411–6.

Xu L, Zhao M, Yang Z, et al. Modified penile augmentation by dermal-fat graft in post-hypospadias adults. Aesthet Plast Surg. 2016;40(1):120–9.

Yordam N, Alikasifoglu A, Kandemir N, et al. True hermaphroditism: Clinical features, genetic variants and gonadal histology. J Pediatr Endocrinol Metab. 2001;14(4):421–7.

Yorifuji T, Muroi J, Mamada M, et al. Analysis of the SRY gene in Turner syndrome patients with Y chromosomal material. J Med Genet. 2001;38(11):E41.

Non-hormonal DSD

9

John M. Hutson and Aurore Bouty

9.1 Introduction

Variations of genital development that lead to DSD are usually secondary to altered gonadal or hormonal function, but there is also a large group of congenital malformations affecting the abdominal wall and perineum that may lead to genital variants. Two groups are distinguished here: those with a defect in the morphogenesis of the genital tract alone and those with a more widespread abdominal or perineal defect, affecting the genitalia as well (Table 9.1) (Stephens et al. 2002).

The key to recognition of these variants is that the external anatomy is outside the range between male and female. In particular, there is an anatomical defect that is beyond the effects of androgens acting on the genital tubercle and genital folds. By contrast, in hormonal causes of DSD, the morphological development is otherwise normal, and the dysmorphology is merely a consequence of abnormal androgenic or anti-Müllerian hormone (AMH) function.

Table 9.1 Classification of non-hormonal DSD

Site of dysmorphogenesis	Disorder
Internal genital ducts	Urogenital ridge or gonadal duplication/agenesis Müllerian duct malunion Vaginal duplication/agenesis Rokitansky sequence
External genitalia	Penile agenesis Ectopic labium/scrotum Urogenital sinus
Lower abdominal wall	Bladder exstrophy Epispadias
Perineum	Anorectal malformations – Cutaneous fistula – Recto-bulbar fistula Acquired anomalies secondary to embryonic/foetal compression
Cloacal development	Partial twinning Cloacal anomaly Cloacal exstrophy Caudal regression

9.2 Internal Genitalia

The commonest anomaly of the internal genital development is failure of normal fusion of the Müllerian ducts, leading to various degrees of uterine and vaginal separation. There may be a completely duplicated genital tract through to a partial

J. M. Hutson (✉)
Department of Urology, The Royal Children's Hospital, Melbourne, VIC, Australia

Murdoch Children's Research Institute, Melbourne, VIC, Australia

Department of Paediatrics, University of Melbourne, Melbourne, VIC, Australia
e-mail: john.hutson@rch.org.au

A. Bouty
Department of Urology, The Royal Children's Hospital, Melbourne, VIC, Australia

Murdoch Children's Research Institute, Melbourne, VIC, Australia
e-mail: aurore.bouty@rch.org.au

J. M. Hutson et al. (eds.), *Disorders|Differences of Sex Development*,
https://doi.org/10.1007/978-981-13-7864-5_9

bicornuate uterus or arcuate uterus. Whilst simple inspection of the introitus may occasionally identify an apparent duplication of the vagina, this does not necessarily represent complete Müllerian duplication. Thus, most variations in development of the female genitalia are only documented at endoscopy or laparoscopy, or on imaging studies (Fig. 9.1). A new classification system for

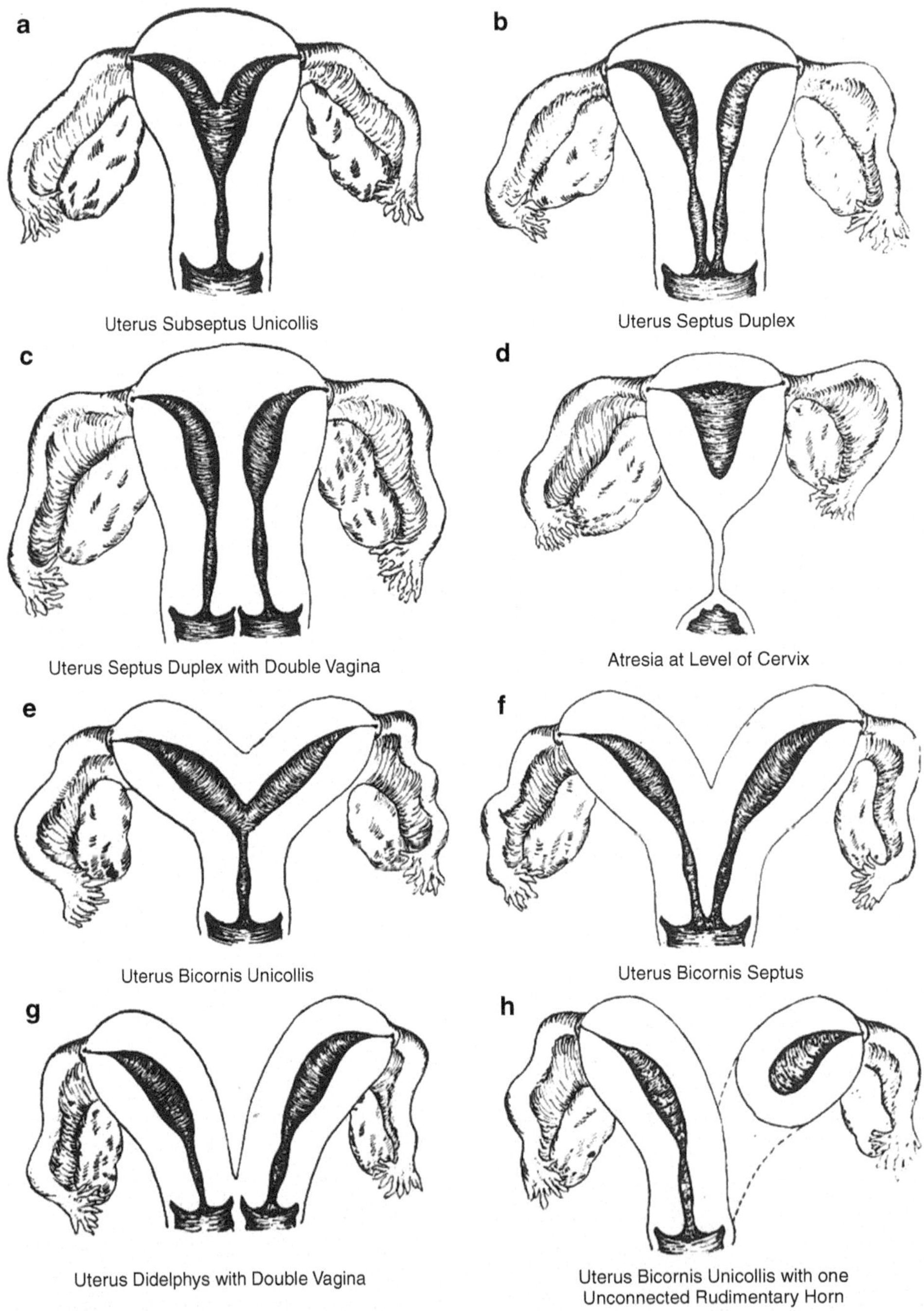

Fig. 9.1 Schematic diagrams of variations in fusion of the paired Müllerian ducts and types of atresia (Reproduced with permission from Stephens et al. (2002))

Müllerian anomalies has been developed that enables careful complete classification of these anomalies (Grimbizis et al. 2013).

Complete or partial duplication in the urogenital ridge is well described, and this may present clinically as an extra testis.

Agenesis of the female genital tract has important implications for the woman in both function and psychological development (Box 9.1). One of the key causes for Müllerian duct agenesis is a primary anomaly in the mesonephros and its duct, the mesonephric or Wolffian duct. The latter is an intrinsic organiser of Müllerian development, as the Müllerian ducts use the Wolffian ducts to guide their migration to the cloaca between 6 and 8 weeks of gestation. The elongating solid tips of the Müllerian ducts grow along the basement membrane of the adjacent Wolffian ducts. Failure of the Wolffian duct to reach the cloaca by 4 weeks of gestation may prevent the ureter budding from the lower Wolffian duct (leading to ipsilateral renal agenesis) as well as distal agenesis of the Müllerian duct (Rokitansky sequence). This is the classic Mayer-Rokitansky-Küster-Hauser (MRKH) syndrome type II (Stephens et al. 2002). When such a change occurs later, for example, between 8 and 12 weeks of development, the vagina may fail to canalise, leading to atresia, but the urinary tract is not affected, thereby leading to MRKH syndrome type 1 (Table 9.2).

Box 9.1 Mayer-Rokitansky-Küster-Hauser (MRKH) Syndrome

MRKH syndrome (OMIM 277000) with agenesis of part or whole of the female genital tract is present in about 1/4500 females. It can be classified into two subgroups: with or without associated anomalies.

MRKHS Type I (OMIM 277000): Isolated Müllerian duct agenesis with absent uterus and vagina.

MRKHS Type II (OMIM 601076): Müllerian duct agenesis with associated anomalies of the urogenital ridge (Wolffian duct development, ureteric bud development, renal dysplasia) and cervical somites (also called MURCS association. *Mü*llerian duct agenesis, *R*enal anomalies, *C*ervical *S*omite anomalies). This may also be called Genital Renal Ear Syndrome (GRES; OMIM 267400) when there are anomalies of the middle ear, with associated deafness (Morcel et al. 2007; Bernardini et al. 2009).

Table 9.2 Timing of events in urogenital tract

Weeks	Crown-rump length (mm)	Urinary tract	Genital tract
4	5	Wolffian duct (WD) reaches cloaca Ureteric bud forms	
5	8	Ureter + pelvis form Kidney "ascending"	
6	12	Ureter separates from WD	Müllerian duct forms
7	17	Urogenital membrane ruptures	
8			Müllerian ducts reach cloaca and sexual differentiation begins
10	40	Kidneys make urine	Wolffian duct regressing in female
12	55–65	Ureteric orifice in bladder	Uterus canalising Vaginal plate migrating
20	150		Vaginal lumen forms Hymen ruptures

From Stephens, Smith & Hutson, Congenital Anomalies of the Kidney, Urinary and Genital Tracts (second Edn, 2002)

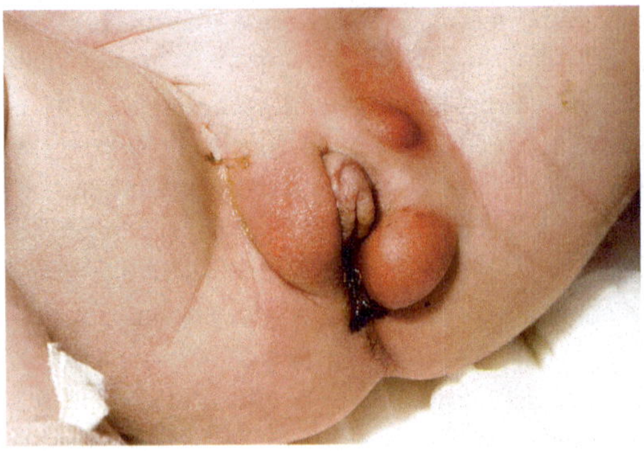

Fig. 9.2 Ectopic labium majorum, secondary to failure of the outer genital fold to develop around the cloacal membrane, in a baby with a recto-vestibular fistula

9.3 External Genitalia

Isolated variations of the external genitalia may be readily confused with hormonal causes of DSD, but the overriding feature is that the altered anatomy cannot be explained by atypical hormonal effects. Failure of the genital folds to form around the cloacal membrane is a sign of an early anomaly of fundamental embryogenesis and hence is relatively uncommon in surviving babies. Such anomalies include ectopia of the outer genital fold, leading to ectopic hemi-scrotum or labium majorum (Fig. 9.2), although these differences may be caused by pressure from the heel of the foetus. More fundamental nonhormonal DSD may include complete absence of the genital tubercle, which causes penile agenesis in boys. In this rare anomaly, the urethra usually opens via a meatus located within the anterior tip of the anal canal, if present. An important clue to the prognosis is the presence of a median raphe in the scrotum: when this is absent, there is a very high likelihood of renal dysplasia or agenesis (Fig. 9.3) (Srinivasan et al. 2003).

During the formation of the vaginal plate, if there is insufficient caudal elongation and migration to the vestibule, then the baby girl is born with a common opening for the urinary and genital tracts, known as a urogenital sinus. This is not related to androgenic suppression of vaginal plate development, as the vagina is otherwise well formed; the variation lies in the genetic regulation of migration of Müllerian tubercle and vaginal plate to the vestibule. Acquired adhesion of the labia minora is occasionally misdiagnosed as a congenital anomaly; however, this is not present at birth and develops as a result of mild inflammation of the atrophic labial surfaces and secondary labial adherence during healing. Labial adhesions are rarely noticed below 6 months of age and frequently present from 6 months up to 2–3 years (Leung et al. 1993), and evidence suggests they spontaneously resolve as they are almost never found in post-menarchal girls (Norris et al. 2018).

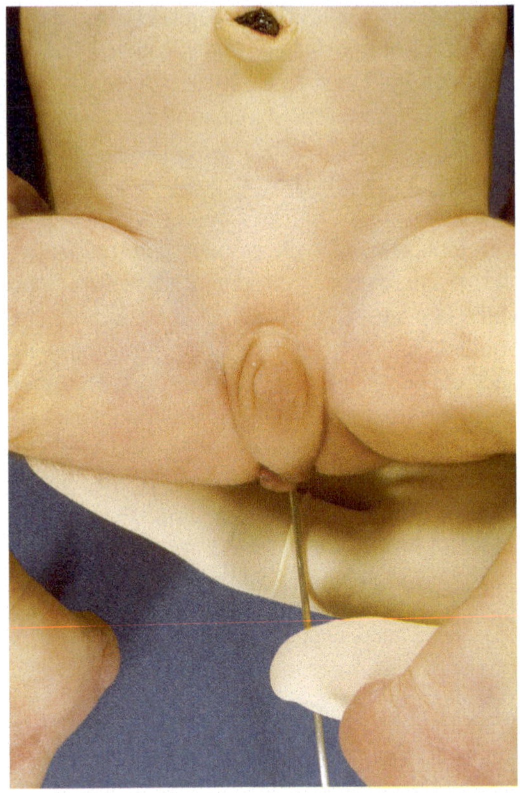

Fig. 9.3 Penile agenesis, showing empty scrotum, which has no median raphe. The baby had cystic dysplasia of ectopic pelvic kidneys (Reproduced from Srinivasan et al. (2003); with permission of the publisher)

9.4 Lower Abdominal Wall Defects

The lower anterior abdominal wall is formed by the ectoderm during embryonic folding, as well as by migration of the lateral plate mesoderm around the developing trunk to form the muscles of the abdominal wall. Migration of mesodermal cells between the umbilical stalk and the immediately adjacent cloacal membrane leads to proliferation of muscle precursors that will form the abdominal wall musculature as well as contribute to the development of the anterior bladder wall. Failure of this mesenchymal expansion may lead to various defects in the lower anterior abdominal wall, from classic bladder exstrophy through to epispadias. The anatomy in classic bladder exstrophy, where the genital tubercle in males is often separated from the outer genital folds (that form the scrotum) by a bridge of skin, suggests that the mesenchyme may have migrated aberrantly between the genital tubercle and the outer genital folds, disrupting the urethral development and leaving a deficiency in the abdominal wall above the genital tubercle (Fig. 9.4a).

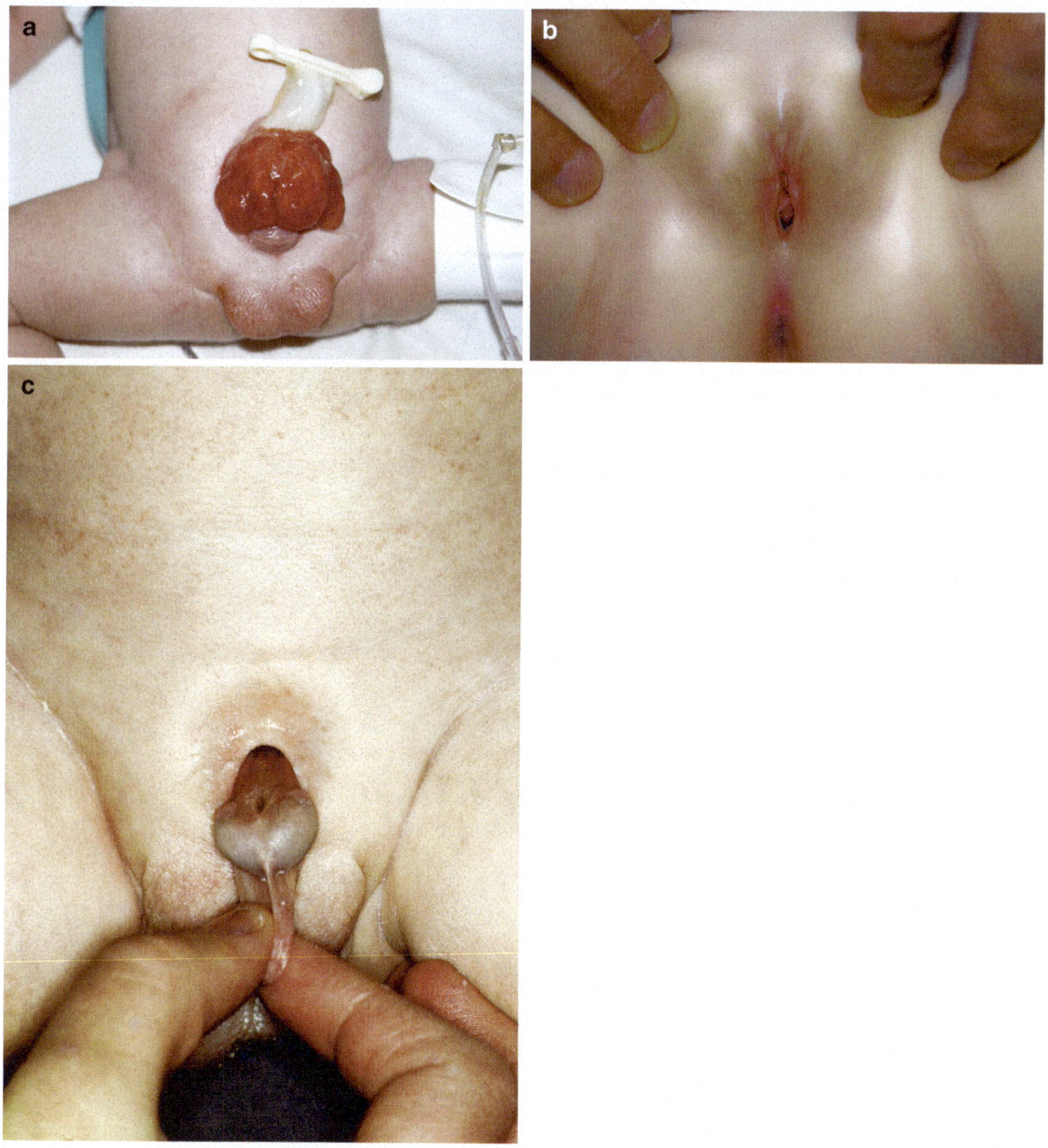

Fig. 9.4 (**a**) Classic bladder exstrophy, with deficiency of the anterior abdominal wall and the anterior wall of the bladder and urethra. (**b**) Epispadias in a girl showing a bifid clitoris. (**c**) Epispadias in a boy showing the open urethral plate exposed on the dorsal surface of the penis

Epispadias is a less severe variant where confusion with other DSD is less likely, although in girls the clitoris may be bifid (Fig. 9.4b), while in boys the urethra and penis are atypical (Fig. 9.4c).

9.5 Perineal Anomalies

Perineal development includes not only the urogenital tracts, but also the hindgut, so that atypical development may affect all three tracts and their respective external openings (Holschneider and Hutson 2006). One characteristic anomaly in this category is an anorectal malformation with a cutaneous fistula in the male, which is usually within the median raphe. The anatomy in boys with a recto-bulbar urethral fistula is potentially ambiguous, as the anomalous connection between the terminal hindgut and the bulb or anterior urethra is often associated with non-fusion of the hemi-scrotal folds, producing a bifid scrotum (Fig. 9.5a).

In females with anorectal malformations, the fistula is most commonly in the vestibule, leading to variable degrees of dysmorphogenesis of the introitus. The absence of an obvious anal opening, however, is a clear sign of a non-hormonal anomaly of embryogenesis (Fig. 9.5b).

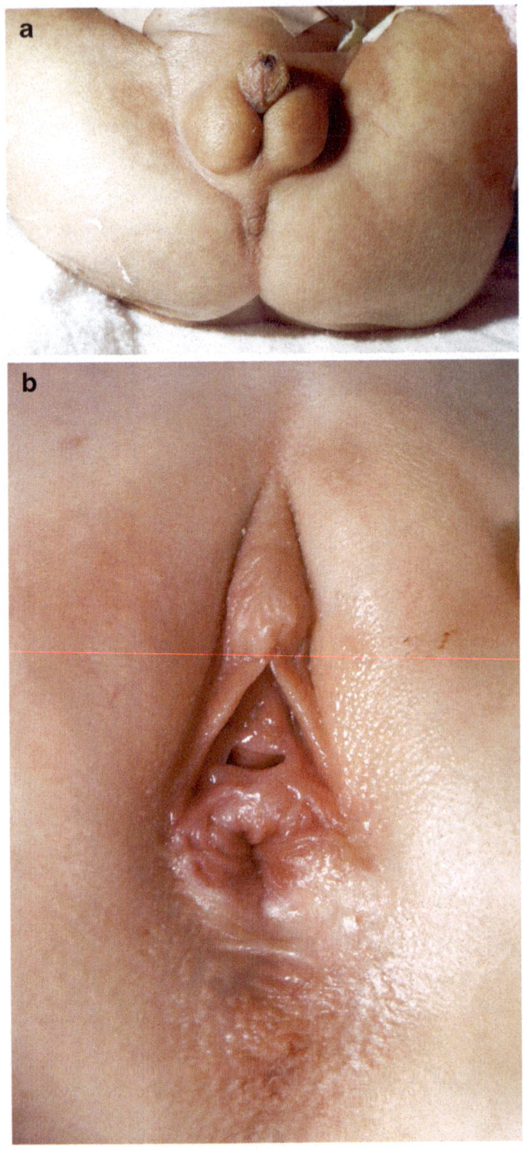

Fig. 9.5 (**a**) Anorectal malformation in a boy with a recto-bulbar fistula. The bifid scrotum is quite characteristic of this variation. (**b**) Anorectal malformation in a girl with a vestibular fistula distorting the genital anatomy

In some foetuses, the genital variation is secondary to compression of the foetus *in utero*, with pressure atrophy of variable genital and perineal structures. An example of this is a baby presenting with chordee of the penis associated with not only less ventral growth of the penile shaft but also an atypical urogenital opening, hypoplastic hemi-scrotum with an ipsilateral absent testis. Although this child could be mistaken to have mixed gonadal dysgenesis or ovotesticular DSD, careful inspection of the external genitalia demonstrates features that are not consistent with a urogenital sinus or hormonal DSD. Extrinsic pressure from the heel of the child onto the perineum may cause this anomaly with additional clues being the urethral meatus at the tip of the glans, an opening on the ventral surface which may look like a pressure sore or a urethral fistula after hypospadias repair, and careful palpation may reveal an atrophic nubbin in the hemi-scrotum consistent with ischaemic atrophy of the testis. Examination under anaesthesia may show that the heel of the child fits perfectly into the perineum (even at 6 years of age!) (Fig. 9.6). Extrinsic compression of the embryo or foetus is well described by Stephens and is discussed in detail in (Stephens et al. 2002).

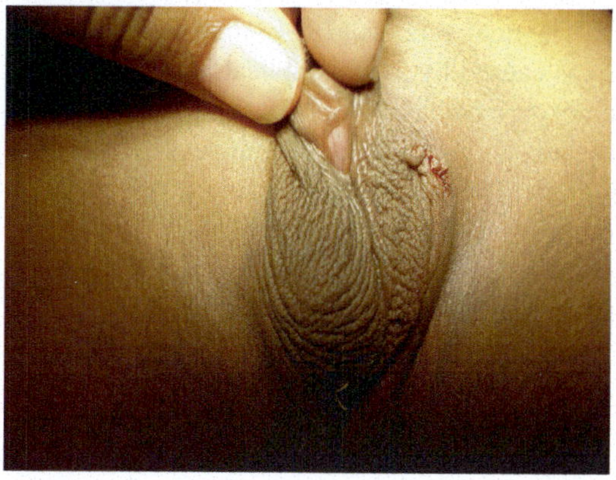

Fig. 9.6 Pressure sore over the urethra in a boy causing an atypical urethral opening initially thought to be a urogenital sinus. The boy had secondary chordee caused by scarring from the ischaemic necrosis of the urethra, as well as atrophy of the left testis. The right heel could be folded to fit perfectly into the perineum over the atypical urethral opening

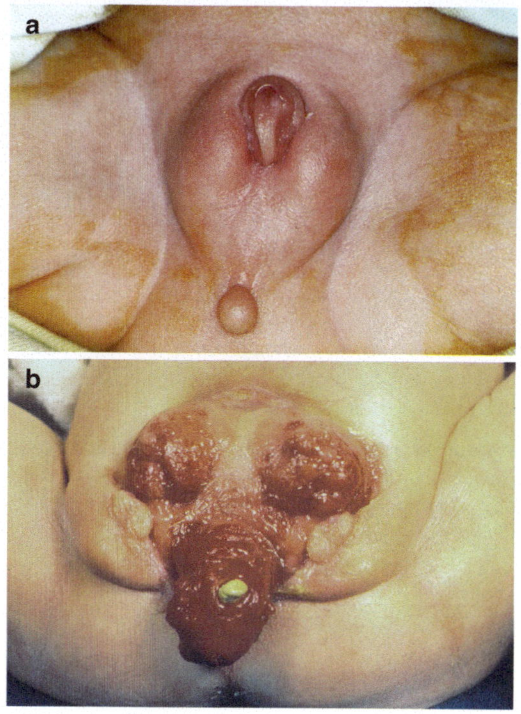

Fig. 9.7 (**a**) Cloacal anomaly with a tiny opening in the genital folds associated with overgrowth and stretching of the clitoral foreskin secondary to urinary obstruction. This has led to significant distortion of the external genitalia. (**b**) Cloacal exstrophy in a baby showing the exposed bowel mucosa centrally and bladder mucosa laterally. The partially concealed external genitalia are widely separated

9.6 Cloacal Maldevelopment

The cloaca is the endodermally derived common cavity for the anorectum and urogenital tracts. Failure of development of the posterior portion of the cloaca along with incomplete separation of the urogenital tracts may lead to persistence of the primitive cloacal cavity at birth. In female infants, this means all three tracts—urinary, genital and gastrointestinal—exit through a common opening. This anomaly may distort the external genital development and lead to ambiguity in appearance. This is particularly the case if the external opening is very small so that the genital folds appear fused, secondary to atypical early development, rather than androgen-induced fusion. The cloacal opening may be so small that it causes urinary obstruction with enlargement of the clitoral hood in a manner similar to distal urinary obstruction in a boy with phimosis. On physical examination, however, the erectile tissue is not enlarged; only the skin is stretched by the urinary blockage to create a phallus-like structure.

The key to recognition of this non-hormonal DSD is the very short introitus or pin-hole opening in the genital folds in a baby with an absent anus (McMullin and Hutson 1991) (Fig. 9.7a).

Arrested development at the cloacal stage in association with abnormal mesodermal development in the lower abdominal wall causes the rare cloacal exstrophy. This is associated with an unfused pelvic ring and exposure of the dysplastic midgut or hindgut on the surface between the bladder mucosal plate on each side. The genitalia are distorted and widely separated into two halves (Fig. 9.7b). Not unexpectedly, there are frequently multiple other developmental variations in the baby, which may impact on the plan of management. The obvious involvement of all the pelvic organs and the abdominal wall means that these infants are easily distinguished from hormonal DSD.

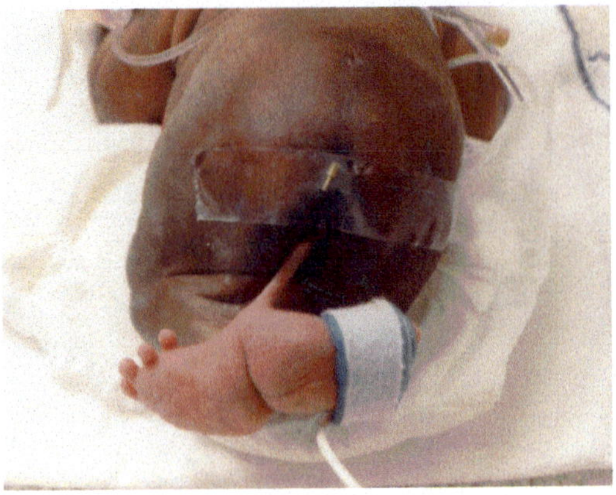

Fig. 9.8 Severe caudal regression in the rare anomaly of sirenomelia, leading to atypical external genital development (Reproduced with permission from Stanton et al. (2003))

There are two other rare conditions of the pelvis and perineum that lead to atypical external genitalia. The first of these is so-called "caudal regression", where regulatory signals controlling growth of the lower half of the embryo are deranged. The most severe variant of this is sirenomelia, where the legs are fused like a mermaid. In this well-described but extremely rare condition, the umbilical artery is a single vessel given off by the mid-abdominal aorta, which inhibits all distal growth by "vascular steal". In one such case that we have seen, the pelvic organs were absent, apart from the gonads, which were supported by ovarian arteries arising from the upper aorta above the abnormal umbilical artery. The anus was absent, the genital folds were rudimentary, and the urinary tract drained via a single dysplastic ureter directly onto the perineum (Fig. 9.8) (Stanton et al. 2003).

The final, rare anomaly of the external genitalia is caused by partial duplication of the caudal embryo, which is a form of incomplete conjoined twinning. There is little confusion with more common DSD, and management involves either removal of one half of the organs or joining the duplicated structures together, depending on the precise anatomy.

References

Bernardini L, Gimelli S, Gervasini C, et al. Recurrent microdeletion at 17q12 as a cause of Mayer-Rokitansky-Kuster-Hauser (MRKH) syndrome: two case reports. Orphanet J Rare Dis. 2009;4:25.

Grimbizis GF, Gordts S, Di Spiezio Sardo A, et al. The ESHRE-ESGE consensus on the classification of female genital tract congenital anomalies. Gynecol Surg. 2013;10(3):199–212.

Holschneider A, Hutson JM. Anorectal malformations in children. Berlin: Springer; 2006.

Leung AK, Robson WL, Tay-Uyboco J. The incidence of labial fusion in children. J Paediatr Child Health. 1993;29(3):235–6.

McMullin N, Hutson J. Female pseudohermaphroditism in children with cloacal anomalies. Pediatr Surg Int. 1991;6:56–9.

Morcel K, Camborieux L, Guerrier D. Mayer-Rokitansky-Kuster-Hauser (MRKH) syndrome. Orphanet J Rare Dis. 2007;2:13.

Norris JE, Elder CV, Dunford AM, et al. Spontaneous resolution of labial adhesions in pre-pubertal girls. J Paediatr Child Health. 2018;54(7):748–53.

Srinivasan J, McDougall P, Hutson JM. When is 'intersex' not intersex? A case of penile agenesis demonstrates how to distinguish non-endocrine disorders in neonates with genital anomaly. J Paediatr Child Health. 2003;39(8):629–31.

Stanton MP, Penington EC, Hutson JM. A surviving infant with sirenomelia (mermaid syndrome) associated with absent bladder. J Pediatr Surg. 2003;38(8):1266–8.

Stephens FD, Smith ED, Hutson JM. Congenital anomalies of the kidney, urinary and genital tracts. London: Martin-Dunitz; 2002.

10 Multiple Malformation Syndromes in DSD

Aurore Bouty and John M. Hutson

Some patients with DSD present with associated anomalies outside of the genital system, which make their overall management more complex. This chapter describes the most common syndromes and their genetic cause.

As per a previous review (Hutson et al. 2014), we have divided these syndromes into (a) 'hormonal DSD'", where the genetic variation is responsible for a perturbation of gonadal development or hormonal action and (b) 'non-hormonal DSD'.

10.1 Hormonal DSD

10.1.1 Gonadal Dysgenesis

Gonadal dysgenesis is the result of mutations in genes that control the development of the gonads. Dysgenetic gonads carry a considerable risk of transformation into both benign (gonadoblastoma) and malignant (dysgerminoma) gonadal germ cell tumours, in particular in the presence of a Y chromosome (Wolffenbuttel et al. 2016).

10.1.1.1 WAGR Syndrome (OMIM #194072)

Most cases are due to a *de novo* deletion of 11p13, a region including the *WT1* gene. WAGR is a rare syndrome. The key features are *W*ilms tumour, *A*niridia, *G*enitourinary anomalies and developmental *R*etardation (W-A-G-R). Ocular manifestations are due to the close relationship of *WT1* and *PAX6*. 46, XY patients present with dysgenetic testes and atypical genitalia or even female phenotype, while their 46, XX counterparts have completely female external genitalia. However, investigations in these girls can reveal streak ovaries and a bicornuate uterus. Affected individuals have a high frequency of cataracts and glaucoma (>50%), as well as a high risk of recurrent tonsillitis and glue ears (Fischbach et al. 2005). They may develop end-stage renal disease (Breslow et al. 2000) and have a high incidence of congenital diaphragmatic hernia (Scott et al. 2005).

10.1.1.2 Denys-Drash Syndrome (OMIM #194080) (Fig. 10.1)

This is another syndrome related to sporadic mutations in *WT1* (Shapiro et al. 2007). Testicular

A. Bouty (✉)
Department of Urology, The Royal Children's Hospital, Melbourne, VIC, Australia

Murdoch Children's Research Institute, Melbourne, VIC, Australia
e-mail: aurore.bouty@rch.org.au

J. M. Hutson
Department of Urology, The Royal Children's Hospital, Melbourne, VIC, Australia

Murdoch Children's Research Institute, Melbourne, VIC, Australia

Department of Paediatrics, University of Melbourne, Melbourne, VIC, Australia
e-mail: John.hutson@rch.org.au

J. M. Hutson et al. (eds.), *Disorders|Differences of Sex Development*,
https://doi.org/10.1007/978-981-13-7864-5_10

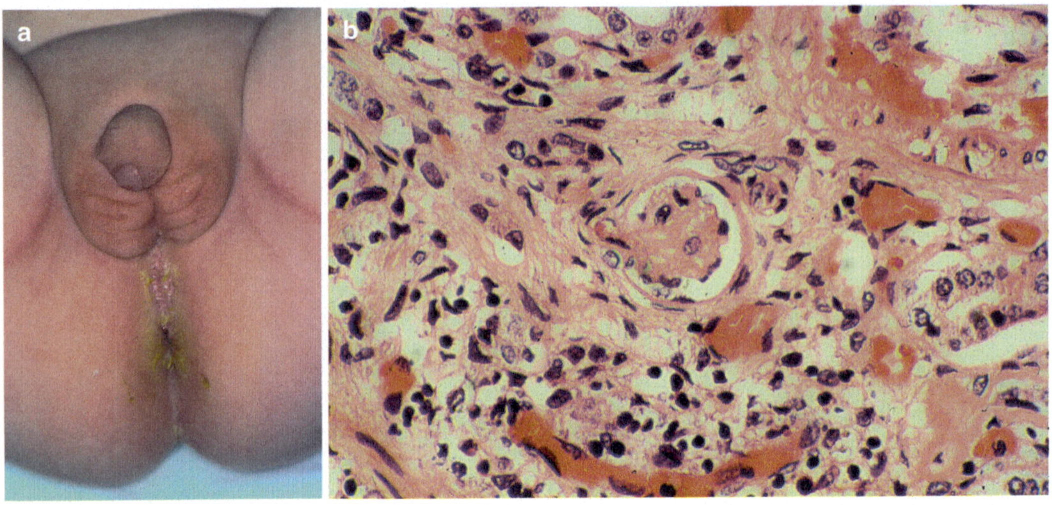

Fig. 10.1 (**a**) Genitalia in a baby with 46,XY DSD and Denys-Drash syndrome. (**b**) Glomerulosclerosis in the same infant which led to renal failure at 9 months of age

dysgenesis leads to inadequate levels of androgens and (Fig. 10.1) partial-to-complete undervirilization with female phenotype. Associated atypical development of the metanephros results in mesangial sclerosis that leads to early end-stage renal disease (Nso Roca et al. 2009). End-stage renal disease can also be related to the increased risk of Wilms tumour (75% of patients), requiring nephrectomy (Millar et al. 2017). Other haematopoietic malignancies (Rampal and Figueroa 2016) and congenital diaphragmatic hernia might also be more frequent than in the general population (Antonius et al. 2008).

10.1.1.3 Frasier Syndrome (OMIM #136680)

Frasier syndrome is closely related to Denys-Drash syndrome but involves a different mutation in *WT1*. This mutation in intron 9 is usually dominantly inherited (Ezaki et al. 2015). The gonadal dysgenesis is severe and 46, XY foetuses present with bilateral streak gonads and female phenotype. Therefore the risk of gonadal tumour is particularly high (higher than in Denys-Drash). However the risk of end-stage renal disease is lower, as the glomerular sequalae can affect only some areas of the kidney (Gwin et al. 2008).

10.1.1.4 Hand-Foot-Genital Syndrome (OMIM #140000)

HOXA13 is thought to be involved in the precise determination of the site of genital ridge formation. Mutations in this gene have been described in patients presenting limb malformations and urogenital defects. The latter include variations in Müllerian duct fusion in females and hypospadias of various severities in males.

10.1.1.5 Alpha-Thalassaemia/Mental Retardation Syndrome, X Linked (OMIM #301040)

Mutations in the *ATRX* gene (OMIM #300032), located at Xq21.1, result in a dysfunctional helicase, a chromatin-remodelling enzyme. The syndrome affects 1–10 in 1 000,000 live births (Gibbons 2006). In 46, XY foetuses, the presence of only one X chromosome does not allow for gene function compensation, and testicular development is disrupted in 80% of the cases. Gonads are dysgenetic or streak and the external genitalia can be atypical or present a female phenotype. Along with facial dysmorphism and intellectual disability, alpha-thalassaemia and skeletal anomalies, including short stature, and microcephaly are present. Renal and cardiac anomalies can be associated and many children have severe gastro-oesophageal reflux (Ausio et al. 2003; Gibbons 2006).

10.1.1.6 Opitz G/BBB Syndrome (OMIM #300000)

There are two forms, type 1, X linked, and type 2, related to a dominantly inherited deletion in 22q11.2 (Robin et al. 1995). Type 1 form is due to mutations in the *MID1* gene. Both cannot be differentiated clinically. The phenotype includes facial dysmorphism with hypertelorism, hypospadias with bifid scrotum and cryptorchidism, laryngo-tracheo-oesophageal cleft, cardiac malformations and intellectual disability. Anorectal malformation can also be present. Severe forms can exhibit brain midline anomalies, such as agenesis of the corpus callosum, and renal malformation. In carrying females, only hypertelorism is present (Robin et al. 1996).

10.1.1.7 Turner Syndrome

Turner syndrome is one of the most common genetic variants, affecting 1 in 2000–2500 liveborn females. Genotype varies from complete loss of one X chromosome to mosaicism with or without Y chromosome. The genotype-phenotype correlation is still currently poorly understood. Although the phenotype varies widely, the most common features are short stature and cardiac (hypertension, bicuspid aortic valve, coarctation of the aorta) and renal anomalies (horseshoe or pelvic kidney) (Gawlik 2015). All women with Turner syndrome are at increased risk of aortic dissection and require long-term cardiology follow-up (Cramer et al. 2014). In addition, they have dysgenetic gonads with primary ovarian failure or premature ovarian insufficiency. Those with an XY mosaicism have an increased risk of malignancy in their streak gonads. Therefore, it is recommended to perform bilateral gonadectomies for those gonads with no fertility or endocrine potential and a high risk of tumours (Coyle et al. 2016).

10.1.1.8 Complete Gonadal Dysgenesis (Swyer Syndrome) (OMIM #400044)

This is a complete gonadal dysgenesis in patients with 46, XY karyotype. Several mutations have been reported to be responsible: *SRY* (Wang et al. 2018), *NR5A1* (Rehkamper et al. 2017) or *MAP3K1* (Granados et al. 2017) among many others. The most common presentation is at adolescence with primary amenorrhea and tall stature in completely phenotypically female patients (Michala et al. 2008). However, with the current widespread use of antenatal karyotype, more cases are now diagnosed at a younger age, when there is a discrepancy between the 46, XY karyotype and female phenotype at birth. The presence of Y material associated with completely dysgenetic intraabdominal gonads significantly increases the risk of gonadal germ cell tumour. Bilateral prophylactic gonadectomy is recommended in complete gonadal dysgenesis as by definition, there is absent endocrine or fertility potential (Wolffenbuttel et al. 2016) (See Chap. 7).

10.1.2 Hypogonadism

Hypogonadism might be secondary to altered hypothalamic or pituitary function (hypogonadotrophic hypogonadism) or to primary testicular failure, with raised gonadotrophins. Gonadotrophin deficiency in 46, XY foetuses leads to smaller than typical penile length (previously termed 'micropenis') and cryptorchidism, but anatomically normal penis, as its development as part of initial masculinization is thought to be regulated by placental human chorionic gonadotrophin.

10.1.2.1 Klinefelter Syndrome

This form of hypogonadism affects 1 in 500–2000 males. Most common karyotype is 47, XXY but other variants have been reported (Fruhmesser and Kotzot 2011). Occasionally the diagnosis is made at birth in a neonate with variations in penile and scrotal development with undescended testes (Lee et al. 2007). Subsequently learning difficulties and behavioural problems may arise (Groth et al. 2013). At adolescence a 47,XXY boy may present with delayed and incomplete pubertal development, with small testes and gynaecomastia (Hutson et al. 2014). However diagnosis is most commonly made later, during investigation for infertility. As testicular function declines with time, fertility preservation can be performed by extracting viable sperm at puberty (Aksglaede and Juul 2013; Rives et al. 2013); however this is also feasible in young adulthood and to date, earlier intervention has not been shown to increase the chance of sperm retrieval (Shalender and Robert 2020). Adolescents and young adults are also prone to extra-gonadal germ-cell tumours, such as in the mediastinum or retroperitoneum, as well as diabetes mellitus, hypothyroidism and other auto-immune disorders (Aksglaede et al. 2013).

10.1.2.2 Noonan Syndrome (OMIM #163950)

Noonan syndrome occurs in 1 in 1000–2500 live births and is associated with short stature, facial dysmorphism and congenital heart defects (90%) as well as hypogonadism. Several genes have been implicated in the aetiology but they are all related to the RAS-MAPK pathway, known as RASopathies (Arroyo-Carrera et al. 2016). While boys have small and undescended testes, girls typically have normal puberty and fertility (Hutson et al. 2014). LEOPARD syndrome is a variant of Noonan syndrome and is characterized by multiple lentigines.

10.1.2.3 Kallman Syndrome (OMIM #308700)

This is a form of hypogonadotrophic hypogonadism, where the gonadal deficiency is secondary to hypothalamic dysfunction. Males are more commonly affected than females and may present with smaller penis and cryptorchidism in infancy or delayed puberty in adolescence. Associated variations in development or agenesis of the olfactory bulbs can lead to anosmia. Genetic aetiology of the syndrome is heterogeneous, with several genes identified, such as *FGF17*, *IL17RD*, *DUSP6*, *SPRY4* or *FLRT3* (Hutson et al. 2014).

10.1.2.4 CHARGE Syndrome (OMIM #214800)

*C*oloboma, *H*eart disease, *A*tresia of the choanae, *R*etardation of growth and/or development, *G*enital hypoplasia and *E*ar abnormalities are the features of CHARGE syndrome. Most patients present with hypogonadotrophic hypogonadism. The syndrome is due to loss-of-function, dominantly inherited mutations in the *CHD7* gene, which encodes the chromodomain helicase DNA-binding protein 7 (Moccia et al. 2018).

10.1.2.5 Prader-Willi Syndrome (OMIM #176270)

This is a form of hypogonadism in which both the hypothalamus and the gonads might be atypical and that can affect both males and females. Genital variations include smaller penile size, scrotal hypoplasia and small, undescended testes in boys, while clitoral and labial hypoplasia may be present in girls. Delayed onset or progression of puberty is common and sex hormone replacement therapy may be indicated from adolescence. Affected infants are usually hypotonic. Despite initial feeding difficulties, hyperphagia and obesity are common in late childhood and adolescence. Nearly all affected individuals have developmental delay. This is a human-imprinting disorder, with 75% of cases exhibiting a *de novo* deletion of paternal chromosome 15q11-q13 and the rest showing maternal disomy of chromosome 15 (Cheon 2016).

10.1.2.6 Congenital Adrenal Hypoplasia (OMIM #300200)

This is a rare syndrome usually caused by a mutation in the *NT0B1* gene, located on the X chromosome. It presents as a male infant with atypical genitalia that will develop adrenal insufficiency and hypogonadotrophic hypogonadism (Hutson et al. 2014).

10.1.2.7 Rubinstein-Taybi Syndrome (OMIM #180849)

This syndrome presents as broad thumbs and hallux, microcephaly, wide nasal bridge and a downward slant to the eye. Genital anomalies secondary to hypogonadism are common, in particular cryptorchidism. Two types of the syndrome exist. Type 1 is characterized by a heterozygous mutation in the CREB-binding protein gene (*CREBBP*), located on chromosome 16p13. Type 2 shows a heterozygous mutation in the *EP300* gene on chromosome 22q13 (Hutson et al. 2014).

10.1.2.8 Axenfeld-Rieger Syndrome (OMIM #180500)

The main features of this syndrome are malformations of the anterior chamber of the eye and iris. Additionally, genital variations such as hypospadias are secondary to pituitary dysfunction. This syndrome is a rare autosomal disorder resulting from a variety of mutations in some genes that encode transcription factors, such as *PITX2*, *FOXC1* and *PAX6* (Hutson et al. 2014).

10.1.2.9 Deletion 4p Syndrome

Also known as Wolf-Hirschhorn syndrome, deletion of the short arm of chromosome 4 results in hypospadias and cryptorchidism, associated with hypertelorism, abnormal nose, with or without cleft lip and palate, microcephaly and preauricular skin tag (Hutson et al. 2014).

10.1.2.10 Fraser Syndrome (OMIM #219000)

This rare autosomal recessive syndrome, also known as cryptophthalmos-syndactyly syndrome, occurs in 1 in 600,000 live births. Cryptophthalmos and renal agenesis are usually diagnosed antenatally and atypical genitalia are present in 13% of patients. Most cases result from a mutation in *FRAS1*, *FREM2* or *GRIP1* (Saleem and Siddiqui 2015).

10.1.3 Abnormal Cholesterol Metabolism (Fig. 10.2)

Smith-Lemli-Opitz (SLOS; OMIM #270400) occurs in 1 in 20,000–60,000 live births and is more common in Caucasians (Porter 2008). Patients present with facial dysmorphism, microcephaly, developmental delay, poor growth and generalized hypotonia. Genitalia in 46, XY foetuses vary from minor hypospadias and/or cryptorchidism to ambiguity or even female phenotype.

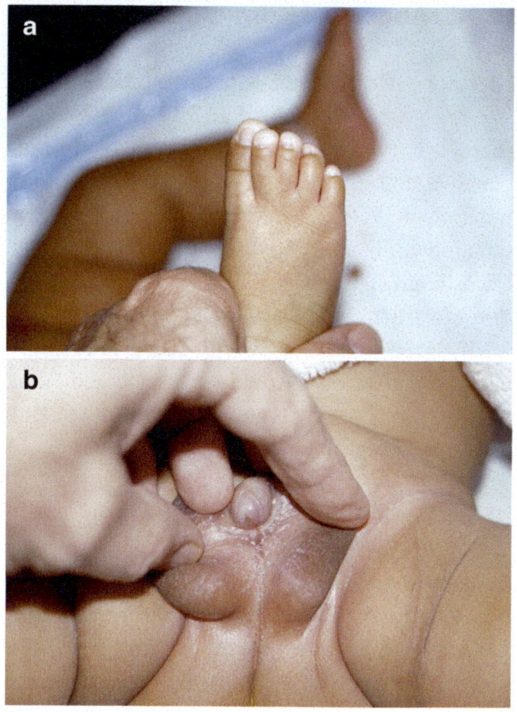

Fig. 10.2 (**a**) Partial syndactyly of second and third toes in a boy with SLO syndrome. (**b**) Severe hypospadias with bifid scrotum in the same boy

Other common associations are cleft palate, syndactyly of the second and third toes, postaxial polydactyly and anomalies in internal organs (Fig. 10.2). Adrenal insufficiency may also arise (Porter 2008). The syndrome is due to a recessively inherited mutation in *DHCR7*, an enzyme implicated in cholesterol biosynthesis (Porter 2008).

10.1.4 Abnormal Steroid Metabolism

A rare form of congenital adrenal hyperplasia, where both 46, XY and 46, XX patients exhibit abnormal genital development, exists. Association of skeletal anomalies, including craniosynostosis, raises the possibility of Antley-Bixler syndrome (OMIM #201750). The impaired cortisol biosynthesis is caused by combined deficiency of both 17α-hydroxylase and 21-hydroxylase, as a result of P450 oxidoreductase deficiency (Idkowiak et al. 1993).

10.1.5 Abnormal Hormonal Function

10.1.5.1 Robinow Syndrome (OMIM #180700 and 268310)

There are two forms of Robinow syndrome, recessive and dominant. The former is due to a mutation in *ROR2*, while the latter is due to a mutation in *Wnt5a*. Both are implicated in the downstream signalling of *INSL3*. Patients present with dwarfism with shortened forelimbs and brachydactyly, associated with facial anomalies and hypoplasia of the male external genitalia, with micropenis and cryptorchidism (Soman and Lingappa 2015).

10.1.5.2 Aarskog-Scott Syndrome (OMIM #305400)

Also known as faciogenital dysplasia, features are similar to those of Robinow syndrome, in particular vertebral anomalies, hypertension, anomalies of the fingers and atypical genitalia (hypospadias, shawl scrotum with undescended testes). In addition, patients have an increased risk of congenital heart disease (Volter et al. 2014). This is an X-linked disorder, due to a wide range of mutations in *FGD1* (Volter et al. 2014). Females might have milder manifestations.

10.2 Non-hormonal DSD

10.2.1 Affecting Internal Genitalia

Development of both mesonephric (Wolffian) and paramesonephric (Müllerian) ducts can be affected in non-hormonal DSD.

10.2.1.1 Wolffian Duct Anomalies

Failure of caudal migration of the Wolffian duct to reach the cloaca results in agenesis of the vas deferens (Shaw and Renfree 2014). As the ureteric bud also originates from the caudal Wolffian duct, this also leads to agenesis of the ipsilateral ureter and kidney.

This can arise in two common situations—firstly, in the male equivalent of the Mayer-Rokitansky-Küster-Hauser syndrome, where the agenesis of the Wolffian duct is unilateral. Secondly, male patients with congenital bilateral agenesis of the vas deferens (OMIM #277180) usually have a mutation of the *CFTR* gene, even if the complete phenotype of cystic fibrosis might be lacking (Sharma et al. 2014).

10.2.1.2 Müllerian Duct Anomalies

Mayer-Rokitansky-Küster-Hauser Syndrome

There are two forms of MRKH syndrome. Type 1 (OMIM #277000) does not usually present with associated developmental variations. Only the caudal part of the Müllerian ducts is affected, which leads to absence of the uterus and upper part of the vagina but normal lower vagina and external genitalia. It has an incidence of 1 in 4500 women.

Type 2 accounts for one-fifth of cases and present with associated anomalies, in particular ipsilateral renal agenesis. Women with MRKH can also demonstrate atypical cervico-thoracic somite development (altered development of the pronephros and other structures of the genital ridge, cervical vertebrae anomalies). The incidence of cardiac anomalies is also increased.

Several genes have been implicated or suspected to be responsible for the two forms but the aetiology remains largely unknown (Fontana et al. 2017; Ledig and Wieacker 2018).

Herlyn-Werner-Wunderlich Syndrome

This multiple malformation syndrome is closely related to MRKH. It is characterized by uterus didelphys and a blind hemivagina, associated with ipsilateral renal agenesis (Noviello et al. 2018). No specific genetic aetiology has been found so far.

10.2.2 Affecting External Genitalia

Primary atypical development of the external genitalia might be an isolated finding but is more often part of a regional defect of development of the lower abdominal wall, perineum or pelvis.

10.2.2.1 Prune Belly Syndrome (OMIM #100100)

This affects both the external genitalia and lower abdominal wall. It is characterized by a triad of symptoms: hypoplasia and agenesis of the anterior abdominal wall musculature, severe dilatation of the urinary tract and bilateral intraabdominal testes. Although it can affect both sexes, it is more common in males (Kheir et al. 2017). Associated anatomical variations are found in 60% of cases (e.g. cardiac and orthopaedic). The aetiology of the syndrome remains largely unresolved (Boghossian et al. 2018) but is likely to be caused by transient urethral obstruction during sexual development in the 10–15-week-old foetus (Beasley et al. 1988).

10.2.2.2 Lower Abdominal Wall Defects

When the two-dimensional embryonic disc folds into three dimensions, the lower abdominal wall is formed by fusion of the ectodermal folds caudal to the developing umbilicus. Ingrowth of the lateral plate mesoderm between the developing coelomic cavity and the ectoderm forms the musculature of the anterior abdominal wall and contributes to the ventral wall of the urogenital tracts between the cloacal membrane and the umbilicus.

Failure of this process has a number of repercussions on the external genitalia associated with the bladder exstrophy-epispadias complex (BEEC). Patients present with low umbilicus, absence of the rectus abdominis muscles and absence of the ventral bladder and urethral walls, associated with pubic diastasis, incomplete fusion and/or development of the genital tubercle and foreshortened perineum. Research to uncover the aetiology of BEEC is happening, with limited conclusions so far (von Lowtzow et al. 2016), but abnormalities in *P63* have been suggested (Cheng et al. 2006).

10.2.2.3 Perineum Defects

In the early embryo, the developing gastrointestinal, genital and urinary tracts join into a common cavity, the cloaca. The development of the urogenital membrane will separate the urinary and genital tracts. Neonates with an anorectal malformation can present with atypical genitalia, which can produce apparent genital ambiguity. Associated anomalies in other systems may exist and the more common forms are *V*ertebral anomalies, *A*norectal malformation, *C*ardiac defects, *T*racheo-oesophageal fistula with or without o*E*sophageal atresia, *R*enal anomalies and *L*imb deformities (VATER or VACTERL). Girls present with associated genital tract malformation (vaginal septum, uterus didelphys or bicornuate) in 10–60% of the cases (Breech 2010).

In neonates with absent genital tubercle, also known as aphallia, the urethra connects to the anterior anal canal. A scrotum might be present but an atypical scrotum with absence of the midline raphe is usually associated with severe renal dysplasia and poor prognosis. The genetic variant responsible has yet to be determined. A number of surgical approaches have been suggested to repair the malformation (Gabler et al. 2018).

Association of an anorectal malformation and a penoscrotal transposition with hypospadias is found in 13q deletion syndrome (OMIM #602553) (Garcia et al. 2006).

10.2.2.4 Cloacal Anomalies

In females, cloaca is a particular form of anorectal malformation, where the primitive cloaca persists. The gastrointestinal, genital and urinary tracts drain into a common cavity (Wood et al. 2018). Even more severe is the association of a vesico-intestinal fissure, known as cloacal exstrophy. The development of the lower abdominal wall, pelvis and perineum is disturbed, leaving an open lower abdominal wall, with an exposed mucosal plate made of the colon centrally and the two hemibladders on each side. Renal and Müllerian structural variations are common (Suson et al. 2016).

10.2.2.5 Caudal Regression Syndrome

This syndrome is characterized by a heterogeneous group of caudal anomalies of the trunk that might include agenesis of the vertebral column and spinal cord and anorectal and genitourinary anomalies (Kumar et al. 2017). Maternal diabetes mellitus is a well-recognized risk factor.

10.2.2.6 Sirenomelia

Sirenomelia, also known as 'mermaid syndrome', is secondary to a severe anomaly of the abdominal aorta below the renal arteries that forms a single umbilical artery. The failure of normal vasculature development leads to absence of the pelvic organs supplied by the internal iliac arteries and fusion of the lower limbs. Both internal and external genitalia are absent or underdeveloped, but the gonads are usually preserved because their blood supply originates above the abnormality (Ramphul et al. 2018).

DSD can be associated with numerous malformations outside of the genital system. Detailed physical examination can pinpoint subtle developmental differences that can orientate the diagnosis. Development of genetic knowledge allows precise diagnosis in an increasing number of cases and will likely in the future allow better counselling of the families for their affected child and their siblings.

References

Aksglaede L, Juul A. Testicular function and fertility in men with Klinefelter syndrome: a review. Eur J Endocrinol. 2013;168(4):R67–76.

Aksglaede L, Link K, Giwercman A, et al. 47,XXY Klinefelter syndrome: clinical characteristics and age-specific recommendations for medical management. Am J Med Genet C Semin Med Genet. 2013;163C(1):55–63.

Antonius T, van Bon B, Eggink A, et al. Denys-Drash syndrome and congenital diaphragmatic hernia: another case with the 1097G > a(Arg366His) mutation. Am J Med Genet A. 2008;146A(4):496–9.

Arroyo-Carrera I, Solo de Zaldivar-Tristancho M, Martin-Fernandez R, et al. RIT1: a novel gene associated with Noonan syndrome. Rev Neurol. 2016;63(8):358–62.

Ausio J, Levin DB, De Amorim GV, et al. Syndromes of disordered chromatin remodeling. Clin Genet. 2003;64(2):83–95.

Beasley S, Bettenay F, Hutson JM. The anterior urethra provides clues to the aetiology of prune belly syndrome. Pediatr Surg Int. 1988;3(169):172.

Boghossian NS, Sicko RJ, Giannakou A, et al. Rare copy number variants identified in prune belly syndrome. Eur J Med Genet. 2018;61(3):145–51.

Breech L. Gynecologic concerns in patients with anorectal malformations. Semin Pediatr Surg. 2010;19(2):139–45.

Breslow NE, Takashima JR, Ritchey ML, et al. Renal failure in the Denys-Drash and Wilms' tumor-aniridia syndromes. Cancer Res. 2000;60(15):4030–2.

Cheng W, Jacobs WB, Zhang JJ, et al. DeltaNp63 plays an anti-apoptotic role in ventral bladder development. Development. 2006;133(23):4783–92.

Cheon CK. Genetics of Prader-Willi syndrome and Prader-Willi-like syndrome. Ann Pediatr Endocrinol Metab. 2016;21(3):126–35.

Coyle D, Kutasy B, Suyin KH, et al. Gonadoblastoma in patients with 45,X/46,XY mosaicism: a 16-year experience. J Pediatr Urol. 2016;12(5):283 e281–7.

Cramer JW, Bartz PJ, Simpson PM, et al. The spectrum of congenital heart disease and outcomes after surgical repair among children with turner syndrome: a single-center review. Pediatr Cardiol. 2014;35(2):253–60.

Ezaki J, Hashimoto K, Asano T, et al. Gonadal tumor in Frasier syndrome: a review and classification. Cancer Prev Res (Phila). 2015;8(4):271–6.

Fischbach BV, Trout KL, Lewis J, et al. WAGR syndrome: a clinical review of 54 cases. Pediatrics. 2005;116(4):984–8.

Fontana L, Gentilin B, Fedele L, et al. Genetics of Mayer-Rokitansky-Kuster-Hauser (MRKH) syndrome. Clin Genet. 2017;91(2):233–46.

Fruhmesser A, Kotzot D. Chromosomal variants in Klinefelter syndrome. Sex Dev. 2011;5(3):109–23.

Gabler T, Charlton R, Loveland J, et al. Aphallia: a review to standardize management. Pediatr Surg Int. 2018;34(8):813–21.

Garcia NM, Allgood J, Santos LJ, et al. Deletion mapping of critical region for hypospadias, penoscrotal transposition and imperforate anus on human chromosome 13. J Pediatr Urol. 2006;2(4):233–42.

Gawlik A. Management of turner syndrome. Eur Endocrinol. 2015;11(2):100–1.

Gibbons R. Alpha thalassaemia-mental retardation, X linked. Orphanet J Rare Dis. 2006;1:15.

Granados A, Alaniz VI, Mohnach L, et al. MAP3K1-related gonadal dysgenesis: six new cases and review of the literature. Am J Med Genet C Semin Med Genet. 2017;175(2):253–9.

Groth KA, Skakkebaek A, Host C, et al. Clinical review: Klinefelter syndrome–a clinical update. J Clin Endocrinol Metab. 2013;98(1):20–30.

Gwin K, Cajaiba MM, Caminoa-Lizarralde A, et al. Expanding the clinical spectrum of Frasier syndrome. Pediatr Dev Pathol. 2008;11(2):122–7.

Hutson JM, Grover SR, O'Connell M, et al. Malformation syndromes associated with disorders of sex development. Nat Rev Endocrinol. 2014;10(8):476–87.

Idkowiak J, Cragun D, Hopkin RJ, et al. Cytochrome P450 oxidoreductase deficiency. In: Adam MP, Ardinger HH, Pagon RA, et al., editors.

GeneReviews® [Internet]. Seattle (WA): University of Washington, Seattle; 1993–2020.

Kheir AEM, Ali EMA, Medani SA, et al. Prune belly syndrome: a report of 15 cases from Sudan. Sudan J Paediatr. 2017;17(1):42–8.

Kumar Y, Gupta N, Hooda K, et al. Caudal regression syndrome: a case series of a rare congenital anomaly. Pol J Radiol. 2017;82:188–92.

Ledig S, Wieacker P. Clinical and genetic aspects of Mayer-Rokitansky-Kuster-Hauser syndrome. Med Genet. 2018;30(1):3–11.

Lee YS, Cheng AW, Ahmed SF, et al. Genital anomalies in Klinefelter's syndrome. Horm Res. 2007;68(3):150–5.

von Lowtzow C, Hofmann A, Zhang R, et al. CNV analysis in 169 patients with bladder exstrophy-epispadias complex. BMC Med Genet. 2016;17(1):35.

Michala L, Goswami D, Creighton SM, et al. Swyer syndrome: presentation and outcomes. BJOG. 2008;115(6):737–41.

Millar AJW, Cox S, Davidson A. Management of bilateral Wilms tumours. Pediatr Surg Int. 2017;33(7):737–45.

Moccia A, Srivastava A, Skidmore JM, et al. Genetic analysis of CHARGE syndrome identifies overlapping molecular biology. Genet Med. 2018;20(9):1022–9.

Noviello C, Romano M, Nino F, et al. Clinical and radiological findings for early diagnosis of Herlyn-Werner-Wunderlich syndrome in pediatric age: experience of a single center. Gynecol Endocrinol. 2018;34(1):56–8.

Nso Roca AP, Pena Carrion A, Benito Gutierrez M, et al. Evolutive study of children with diffuse mesangial sclerosis. Pediatr Nephrol. 2009;24(5):1013–9.

Porter FD. Smith-Lemli-Opitz syndrome: pathogenesis, diagnosis and management. Eur J Hum Genet. 2008;16(5):535–41.

Rampal R, Figueroa ME. Wilms tumor 1 mutations in the pathogenesis of acute myeloid leukemia. Haematologica. 2016;101(6):672–9.

Ramphul K, Mejias SG, Ramphul-Sicharam Y. Mermaid syndrome: a case report in Mauritius. Cureus. 2018;10(2):e2210.

Rehkamper J, Tewes AC, Horvath J, et al. Four novel NR5A1 mutations in 46,XY gonadal dysgenesis patients including frameshift mutations with altered subcellular SF-1 localization. Sex Dev. 2017;11(5–6):248–53.

Rives N, Milazzo JP, Perdrix A, et al. The feasibility of fertility preservation in adolescents with Klinefelter syndrome. Hum Reprod. 2013;28(6):1468–79.

Robin NH, Feldman GJ, Aronson AL, et al. Opitz syndrome is genetically heterogeneous, with one locus on Xp22, and a second locus on 22q11.2. Nat Genet. 1995;11(4):459–61.

Robin NH, Opitz JM, Muenke M. Opitz G/BBB syndrome: clinical comparisons of families linked to Xp22 and 22q, and a review of the literature. Am J Med Genet. 1996;62(3):305–17.

Saleem AA, Siddiqui SN. Fraser syndrome. J Coll Physicians Surg Pak. 2015;25(Suppl 2):S124–6.

Scott DA, Cooper ML, Stankiewicz P, et al. Congenital diaphragmatic hernia in WAGR syndrome. Am J Med Genet A. 2005;134(4):430–3.

Shalender B, Robert DO. Fertility considerations in adolescent klinefelter syndrome: Current Practice Patterns J Clin Endocrinol Metab. 2020;105(4):e1918–20.

Shapiro O, Welch TR, Sheridan M, et al. Mixed gonadal dysgenesis and Denys-Drash syndrome: urologists should screen for nephrotic syndrome. Can J Urol. 2007;14(6):3767–9.

Sharma H, Mavuduru RS, Singh SK, et al. Heterogeneous spectrum of mutations in CFTR gene from Indian patients with congenital absence of the vas deferens and their association with cystic fibrosis genetic modifiers. Mol Hum Reprod. 2014;20(9):827–35.

Shaw G, Renfree MB. Wolffian duct development. Sex Dev. 2014;8(5):273–80.

Soman C, Lingappa A. Robinow syndrome: a rare case report and review of literature. Int J Clin Pediatr Dent. 2015;8(2):149–52.

Suson KD, Inouye B, Carl A, et al. Congenital renal anomalies in cloacal exstrophy: is there a difference? J Pediatr Urol. 2016;12(4):207 e201–5.

Volter C, Martinez R, Hagen R, et al. Aarskog-Scott syndrome: a novel mutation in the FGD1 gene associated with severe craniofacial dysplasia. Eur J Pediatr. 2014;173(10):1373–6.

Wang X, Xue M, Zhao M, et al. Identification of a novel mutation (Ala66Thr) of SRY gene causes XY pure gonadal dysgenesis by affecting DNA binding activity and nuclear import. Gene. 2018;651:143–51.

Wolffenbuttel KP, Hersmus R, Stoop H, et al. Gonadal dysgenesis in disorders of sex development: diagnosis and surgical management. J Pediatr Urol. 2016;12(6):411–6.

Wood RJ, Reck-Burneo CA, Dajusta D, et al. Erratum to "cloaca reconstruction: a new algorithm which considers the role of urethral length in determining surgical planning" [YJPSU 53/1 (2018) 90-95]. J Pediatr Surg. 2018;53(3):582–3.

The Foetus

11

David Amor and Chloe A. Hanna

Prenatal tests for genetic conditions and congenital anomalies are part of routine pregnancy care in most settings. Screening tests, for example ultrasound and maternal serum screening for trisomy 21, are typically offered to all pregnant women, including those at low risk. In contrast, diagnostic tests such as chorionic villus sampling (CVS) and amniocentesis are more commonly undertaken where a pregnancy has been identified as being at increased risk, for example due to screening test results or family history.

The range of conditions that can now be detected by these technologies means that conditions previously unrecognised *in utero* are now being identified. It can be difficult for individuals to fully understand the extent of potential diagnoses and genetic variations that may be identified when undertaking this screening. Frequently individuals have no prior knowledge about these conditions and are confronted with challenging decisions while trying to digest complex medical information and uncertainty. Due to the many ways in which genetic variations present (affect someone), it may be difficult for clinicians to predict the long-term health outcomes for a given individual.

This applies across a wide range of potential diagnoses including DSD.

Adequate support and access to a full range of relevant information is crucial. Genetic counsellors and geneticists have an important role here (see Chap. 21). Additionally, access to support groups as well as clinicians who are involved in the care of infants, children and adults with the identified conditions may be appropriate.

11.1 Prenatal Diagnosis

Chorionic villus sampling (CVS) and amniocentesis can be used to obtain diagnostic samples that can be used for traditional cytogenetic analysis, chromosome microarray analysis and specific gene testing for monogenic disorders where the family gene variant is known. CVS testing

D. Amor (✉)
Department of Neurodisability and Rehabilitation, The Royal Children's Hospital, Melbourne, VIC, Australia

Murdoch Children's Research Institute, Melbourne, VIC, Australia

Department of Paediatrics, University of Melbourne, Melbourne, VIC, Australia

Victorian Clinical Genetics Services, Melbourne, VIC, Australia
e-mail: david.amor@mcri.edu.au

C. A. Hanna
Department of Gynaecology, The Royal Children's Hospital, Melbourne, VIC, Australia

Murdoch Children's Research Institute, Melbourne, VIC, Australia
e-mail: chloe.hanna@rch.org.au

J. M. Hutson et al. (eds.), *Disorders|Differences of Sex Development*,
https://doi.org/10.1007/978-981-13-7864-5_11

allows first trimester diagnosis using foetal tissue obtained from chorionic villi, can be performed from 11 weeks' gestation and carries a risk of miscarriage of ~1 in 500; in contrast, amniocentesis cannot be performed until 15 weeks' gestation and carries a lower risk of miscarriage of ~1 in 1000 (Akolekar et al. 2015). Foetal DNA circulating in the maternal blood can also be used for prenatal testing. This 'Non-Invasive Prenatal Testing' (NIPT) is particularly useful for the diagnosis of foetal sex and sex chromosome status; however, it is important to note that false-positive and false-negative results occur (Bianchi et al. 2015). A diagnosis of DSD in a newborn baby has become more common through the use of NIPT where a baby's sex chromosomes identified in the NIPT are discordant with the genital phenotype at birth (Richardson et al. 2017).

Foetal ultrasonography can provide additional prenatal diagnostic information. Ultrasound determination of foetal sex is unreliable prior to 12 weeks' gestation, but after 13 weeks' gestation, it is accurate in 99–100% of cases with typical external genital development (Odeh et al. 2009). Genital variations may be detected by ultrasound, but accuracy of diagnosis will depend on the severity of the variation. In some cases, foetal MRI may help to delineate the genital anatomy (Nemec et al. 2011).

DSD may also be diagnosed prenatally in pregnancies that have not previously been identified as being at increased risk. Chromosomal DSD are frequently diagnosed by CVS, amniocentesis or NIPT, as an incidental finding in pregnancies that are being tested primarily because of concern about an increased risk of Down syndrome. In the case of Turner syndrome, the detection of ultrasound markers such as nuchal oedema or cardiac malformation may also trigger chromosome testing in the foetus. When genital variation is detected at prenatal ultrasound, the differential diagnosis is broad and should trigger further investigation including chromosome microarray, FISH for SRY and careful ultrasound scanning for additional structural variation (Pajkrt et al. 2008; Chitty et al. 2012). In a 46,XX foetus, the most likely diagnosis is congenital adrenal hyperplasia, whereas in a 46,XY foetus, the differential diagnosis is broader and includes androgen insensitivity syndrome, 46,XY gonadal dysgenesis, testosterone biosynthesis defects, complex hypospadias and rare syndromes such as Smith–Lemli–Opitz syndrome and campomelic dysplasia. Atypical genitalia may be accompanied by other ultrasound abnormalities, including anomalies of the urinary system, and are associated with a number of chromosome disorders. Finally, the presenting finding may be discordance between chromosome sex at NIPT/CVS/amniocentesis and the appearance of genitalia on prenatal ultrasound (or when the baby is born). Such discordance may indicate the diagnosis of a DSD such as androgen insensitivity syndrome (AIS) (Bianca et al. 2009) or gonadal dysgenesis (Mazza et al. 2003).

Some couples who are at increased risk of having a child with a DSD, based on family history, will elect to have prenatal diagnosis. Exploration of how this testing would alter their decision making is clearly important. If specific antenatal testing is to be undertaken on families suspected of having a history of DSD, depending on the condition, knowledge of both the exact nature of the DSD and genetic variation is a prerequisite.

11.2 Preimplantation Genetic Testing

Preimplantation genetic testing (PGT) (also known as preimplantation genetic diagnosis [PGD]) was developed for couples at high risk of having a child with a genetic disorder, as an alternative to prenatal diagnosis and selective abortion. The number of PGT cycles performed each year is rising, and the number of PGT-conceived children now numbers in the tens of thousands. PGT commences with couples undergoing IVF treatment, using standard procedures to collect oocytes through ovarian hyperstimulation, followed by IVF techniques such as intra-cytoplasmic sperm injection (ICSI) and *in vitro* embryo culture. Embryos are most commonly biopsied on day 5 after fertilization (blastocyst stage), at which stage the embryo comprises approximately 100 cells. For genetic analysis of biopsied cells, cytogenetic techniques have now been replaced by molecular techniques, most commonly involving whole genome amplification followed by microarray or next generation sequencing (NGS). Chromosome microarray and NGS can both be used to generate a low resolution 'molecular karyotype' of the embryo and can identify whole chromosome aneuploidies and moderate-sized deletions and duplications. When PGT is performed for the diagnosis of single gene disorders, biopsied cells can be tested for specific DNA variants using DNA fragments that have been amplified by PCR; however, many laboratories now use an approach that utilises data from single nucleotide polymorphism (SNP) microarrays to generate a 'genetic fingerprint' that can be used for linkage analysis. Following successful diagnosis of the embryos, unaffected embryos are either transferred into the womb or frozen for possible future use. Approximately 50% of embryos transferred result in a clinical pregnancy.

Preimplantation genetic tests can be designed for virtually any inherited monogenic disorder or chromosome disorder, including many DSD, and PGT has been reported for congenital adrenal hyperplasia (van Rij et al. 2011) and androgen insensitivity syndrome (Harper et al. 2010). Although PGT is an attractive option for many families, the relatively high cost precludes some families from accessing the technology.

References

Akolekar R, Beta J, Picciarelli G, et al. Procedure-related risk of miscarriage following amniocentesis and chorionic villus sampling: a systematic review and meta-analysis. Ultrasound Obstet Gynecol. 2015;45(1):16–26.

Bianca S, Cataliotti A, Bartoloni G, et al. Prenatal diagnosis of androgen insensitivity syndrome. Fetal Diagn Ther. 2009;26(3):167–9.

Bianchi DW, Parsa S, Bhatt S, et al. Fetal sex chromosome testing by maternal plasma DNA sequencing: clinical laboratory experience and biology. Obstet Gynecol. 2015;125(2):375–82.

Chitty LS, Chatelain P, Wolffenbuttel KP, et al. Prenatal management of disorders of sex development. J Pediatr Urol. 2012;8(6):576–84.

Harper JC, Coonen E, De Rycke M, et al. ESHRE PGD Consortium data collection X: cycles from January to December 2007 with pregnancy follow-up to October 2008. Hum Reprod. 2010;25(11):2685–707.

Mazza V, Ottolenghi C, Di Monte I, et al. Early prenatal diagnosis of recurrent 46,XY partial gonadal dysgenesis. Prenat Diagn. 2003;23(9):716–21.

Nemec SF, Kasprian G, Brugger PC, et al. Abnormalities of the penis in utero—hypospadias on fetal MRI. J Perinat Med. 2011;39(4):451–6.

Odeh M, Granin V, Kais M, et al. Sonographic fetal sex determination. Obstet Gynecol Surv. 2009;64(1):50–7.

Pajkrt E, Petersen OB, Chitty LS. Fetal genital anomalies: an aid to diagnosis. Prenat Diagn. 2008;28(5):389–98.

Richardson EJ, Scott FP, McLennan AC. Sex discordance identification following non-invasive prenatal testing. Prenat Diagn. 2017;37(13):1298–304.

Van Rij MC, Gielen M, Lulofs R, et al. Profiles and motives for PGD: a prospective cohort study of couples referred for PGD in the Netherlands. Hum Reprod. 2011;26(7):1826–35.

The Neonate with Atypical Genitalia

12

John M. Hutson and Aurore Bouty

12.1 Introduction

A baby with atypical genitalia, and the unexpected uncertainties in relation to sex of rearing that this may bring, can be a significant source of distress for parents and families. Now, in the era of antenatal testing, a baby born with a phenotype that does not match the chromosome complement of the antenatal testing may also provoke the same confusion and concerns. Clinicians are challenged with coming to an accurate and speedy diagnosis, so that issues such as appropriate sex of rearing and likely future outcomes or uncertainties can be discussed openly with the family. The difficulty for clinicians is that DSD are rare and often complicated, which may make the clinical diagnosis difficult. To be able to diagnose these conditions, it is important to understand the basic developmental steps in sexual differentiation, which have been described in the chapter pertaining to embryology (see Chap. 3). Here, we briefly recapitulate the essential features of the development upon which the rules for clinical diagnosis are based.

Male and female embryos have similar internal genitalia until about 7–8 weeks of development. The key structure in the urogenital ridge is the regressing mesonephros, with its associated duct structures in the lateral edge of the ridge and the developing gonad on its antero-medial surface. The mesonephric or Wolffian duct develops first as the excretory duct of the primitive renal tract. The paramesonephric duct or Müllerian duct develops as an invagination of the peritoneum in the lateral edge of the urogenital ridge near the cranial end of the gonad and then migrates to the cloaca, crossing the Wolffian duct to become fused with the contralateral Müllerian duct (see later).

Testes development begins at about 8 weeks, with the production of anti-Müllerian hormone (AMH) and androgen. Under the exocrine action of androgens secreted down the Wolffian duct, it differentiates into epididymis cranially, vas deferens in the middle section and gives 2 buds which form the seminal vesicle and ureter caudally. The high concentration of testosterone within the duct obviates the need for conversion to dihydrotestosterone.

J. M. Hutson (✉)
Department of Urology, The Royal Children's Hospital, Melbourne, VIC, Australia

Murdoch Children's Research Institute, Melbourne, VIC, Australia

Department of Paediatrics, University of Melbourne, Melbourne, VIC, Australia
e-mail: john.hutson@rch.org.au

A. Bouty
Department of Urology, The Royal Children's Hospital, Melbourne, VIC, Australia

Murdoch Children's Research Institute, Melbourne, VIC, Australia
e-mail: aurore.bouty@rch.org.au

J. M. Hutson et al. (eds.), *Disorders|Differences of Sex Development*,
https://doi.org/10.1007/978-981-13-7864-5_12

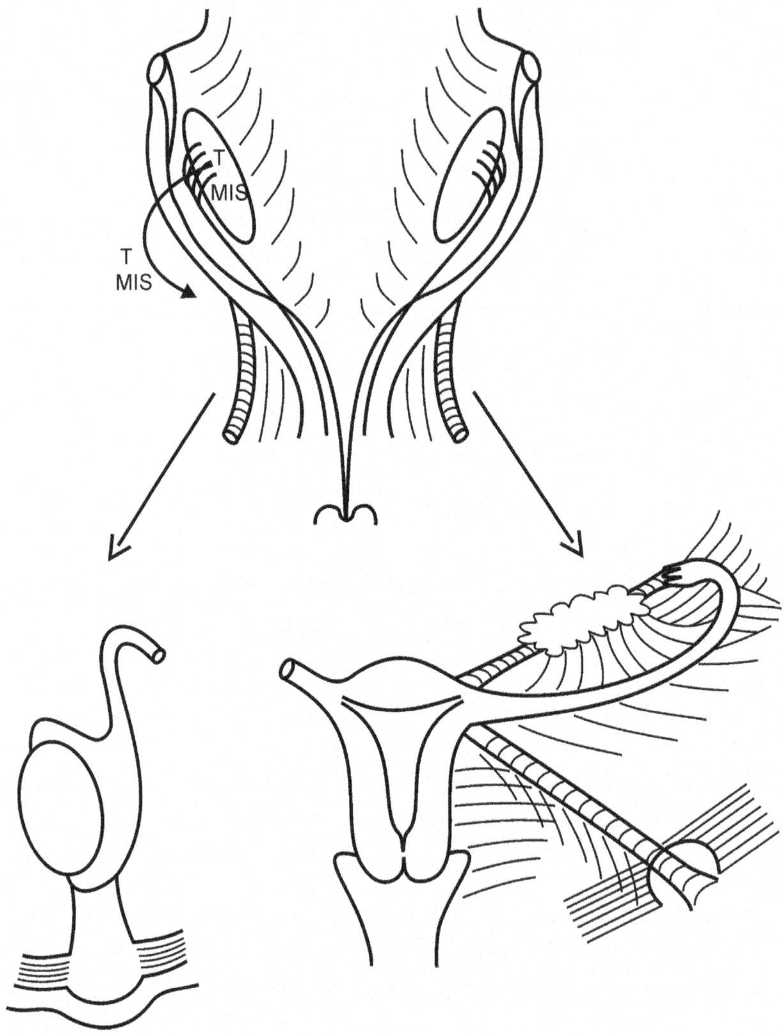

Fig. 12.1 Undifferentiated urogenital tracts at 7 weeks of gestation, showing gonad with adjacent Wolffian and Müllerian ducts. Caudally, there is an extra fold extending from the urogenital ridge to the anterior abdominal wall: the genito-inguinal ligament or gubernaculum. Male development is shown on the right side of the embryo, where testosterone and AMH (also known as Müllerian inhibiting substance (MIS)) are secreted by the developing testis and pass in an exocrine manner down the Wolffian duct to masculinise the Wolffian duct itself and cause regression of the adjacent Müllerian duct. By 12–15 weeks of gestation, the epididymis has formed from the proximal Wolffian duct, and the gubernaculum has undergone the 'swelling reaction,' in response to INSL3, which enables the enlarged gubernaculum to hold the testis near the inguinal region as the abdomen of the foetus enlarges. The cranial suspensory ligament has regressed in response to testosterone. On the left side, absence of male hormones triggers Wolffian duct regression, while the Müllerian duct develops into Fallopian tube, uterus and upper vagina. The regressing mesonephros leaves the ovary on a mesentery, which persists cranially as the suspensory ligament and laterally as the broad ligament. The gubernaculum elongates in proportion to growth to become the ligament of the ovary and the round ligament, which ends just outside the external inguinal ring

Secretion of AMH down the Wolffian duct causes regression of the adjacent Müllerian duct, which would, in the absence of this hormone, form the Fallopian tube, uterus and the upper vagina (Fig. 12.1). The lower third of the vagina is derived from endoderm of the urogenital sinus that is stimulated to grow into the vaginal plate by the arrival of the Müllerian ducts to produce the sino-vaginal bulb. Development of the vaginal plate is inhibited by circulating androgens

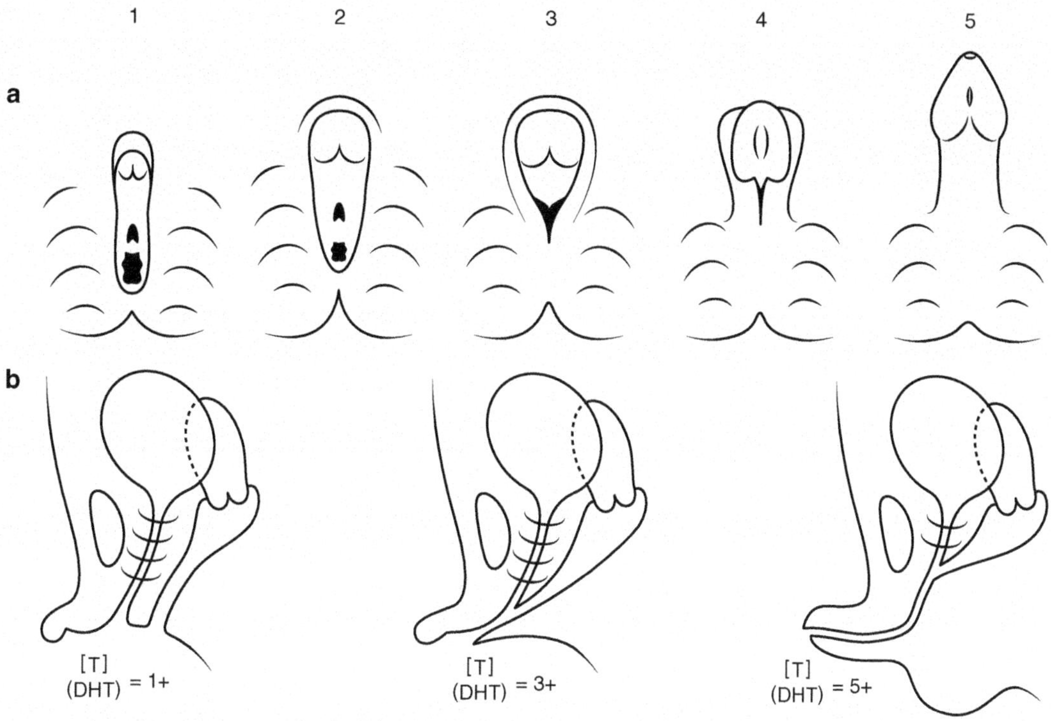

Fig. 12.2 (**a**) The Prader classification of the degree of virilisation of the external genitalia is from 0 (complete/typical female) to 5 (complete/typical male appearance). Prader 1 is clitoromegaly alone with normal introitus. Prader 2 is clitoromegaly and a funnel-shaped urogenital opening showing two orifices (urethra and vagina). Prader 3 is more virilised where only one opening is visible inside the urogenital sinus. Prader 4 is more masculinised still, where the opening is on the proximal shaft of the enlarged phallus. Prader 5 is where the opening is on the glans of the enlarged phallus. The increasing virilisation from 1 to 5 is directly related to levels of androgens the foetus is exposed to, and also inversely related to the degree of regression of the developing lower vagina. (**b**) The regression of the lower part of the vagina is directly related to the amount of androgens present and the degree of external genital virilisation

(after conversion to dihydrotestosterone—DHT), and therefore the degree of lower vaginal development is inversely related to the amount of androgens (i.e. DHT) to which the foetus is exposed (Fig. 12.2).

With differentiation of the testes at approximately 8 weeks of development, the amount of testosterone circulating in the bloodstream in an endocrine manner is relatively small because the total number of Leydig cells is still small. This has led to some special adaptations to increase the relative concentration of hormones into the active endocrine range. To virilise the internal genitalia, the hormones are secreted in an exocrine manner down the Wolffian duct, thereby exposing the ducts to very high local concentrations. This is an ipsilateral effect, hence in DSD wherethere is only one functioning testis, this effect is evident only on the side of that testis. To virilise the external genitalia, a different strategy is used, with conversion of circulating testosterone into dihydrotestosterone (DHT) (Fig. 12.3). The external genitalia require DHT because the serum concentration of testosterone itself is too low. Some actions of testosterone on sexual dimorphism of the brain, for example, are thought to be mediated by conversion of testosterone to oestrogen (Lombardo et al. 2018). The net effect of conversion of testosterone to another steroid metabolite is to increase the effective endocrine concentration so that it can act on the receptors in the remote target organs significantly.

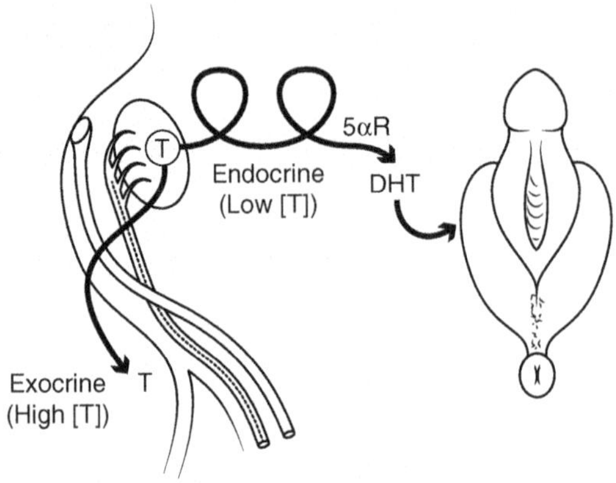

Fig. 12.3 The internal ducts respond to exocrine secretion of testosterone and AMH down the mesonephric (Wolffian) duct at high concentrations of both hormones. By contrast, the external genitalia are exposed to serum testosterone levels that are too low for normal endocrine function, probably related to the minute size of the developing testis. Conversion of testosterone to dihydrotestosterone (DHT) by the enzyme 5-alpha reductase overcomes the low levels, as DHT binds 5–10 times more tightly to the androgen receptor. This increases the effective androgen concentration 5–10 fold at this crucial time for external genital development

The testicular Leydig cells also produce insulin-like hormone 3 (INSL3), which stimulates development of the genito-inguinal ligament, or gubernaculum. Growth of the gubernaculum in the transabdominal phase of testicular descent is likely to be augmented by the action of AMH, which is thought to produce shortening of the gubernacular cord. This leads to a very tight relationship between production of AMH and the first phase of testicular descent (Fig. 12.1). The second phase of testicular descent, from the inguinal region to the scrotum, is regulated by androgens, which not only act to some extent locally but also indirectly via the genitofemoral nerve. The nerve releases the neuropeptide—calcitonin gene-related peptide (CGRP)—from its sensory nerve endings that supply the groin and scrotum to provide a concentration gradient for migration of the gubernaculum to the scrotum (Fig. 12.4).

Production of the enzyme 5-α reductase-2 enables conversion of testosterone to DHT in the external genitalia. DHT binds approximately 5–10 times more avidly to the androgen receptor than testosterone itself. DHT stimulates development of the external genitalia with growth of the genital tubercle and development of the male anterior urethra until it opens on the tip of the glans penis. It also stimulates fusion of both the inner and outer genital folds, the latter forming the scrotum. Finally, circulating androgens stimulate development of the posterior urethra to form the prostate and, at the same time, prevent development of the vaginal plate into the lower vagina.

Sexual dimorphism of the external genitalia is effectively completed by 12–15 weeks of gestation; however the phallus continues to grow in response to androgens throughout pregnancy. The initial production of testosterone between 8 and 12 weeks is probably controlled by chorionic gonadotrophin (hCG), but after this time, the foetal hypothalamus and pituitary takeover the regulation of androgen production (Fig. 12.5). Later in foetal development, the role of DHT becomes less important as the testes enlarge and the amount of testosterone produced increases. During this time, descent of the testes in response to testosterone and closure of the processus vaginalis occur, both under the combined action of testosterone and calcitonin gene-related peptide (CGRP) released by the genitofemoral nerve.

With a good understanding of typical development, the most likely underlying functional variation (diagnosis) in babies with a genital anatomical variation can be predicted using a set of rules (Low and Hutson 2003). These 'rules' outlined later predict the most common scenarios; however, as with all rules, exceptions may apply, and hence thorough diagnostic workup (targeted based on the most likely scenario and extended as needed should results not be consistent) remains important.

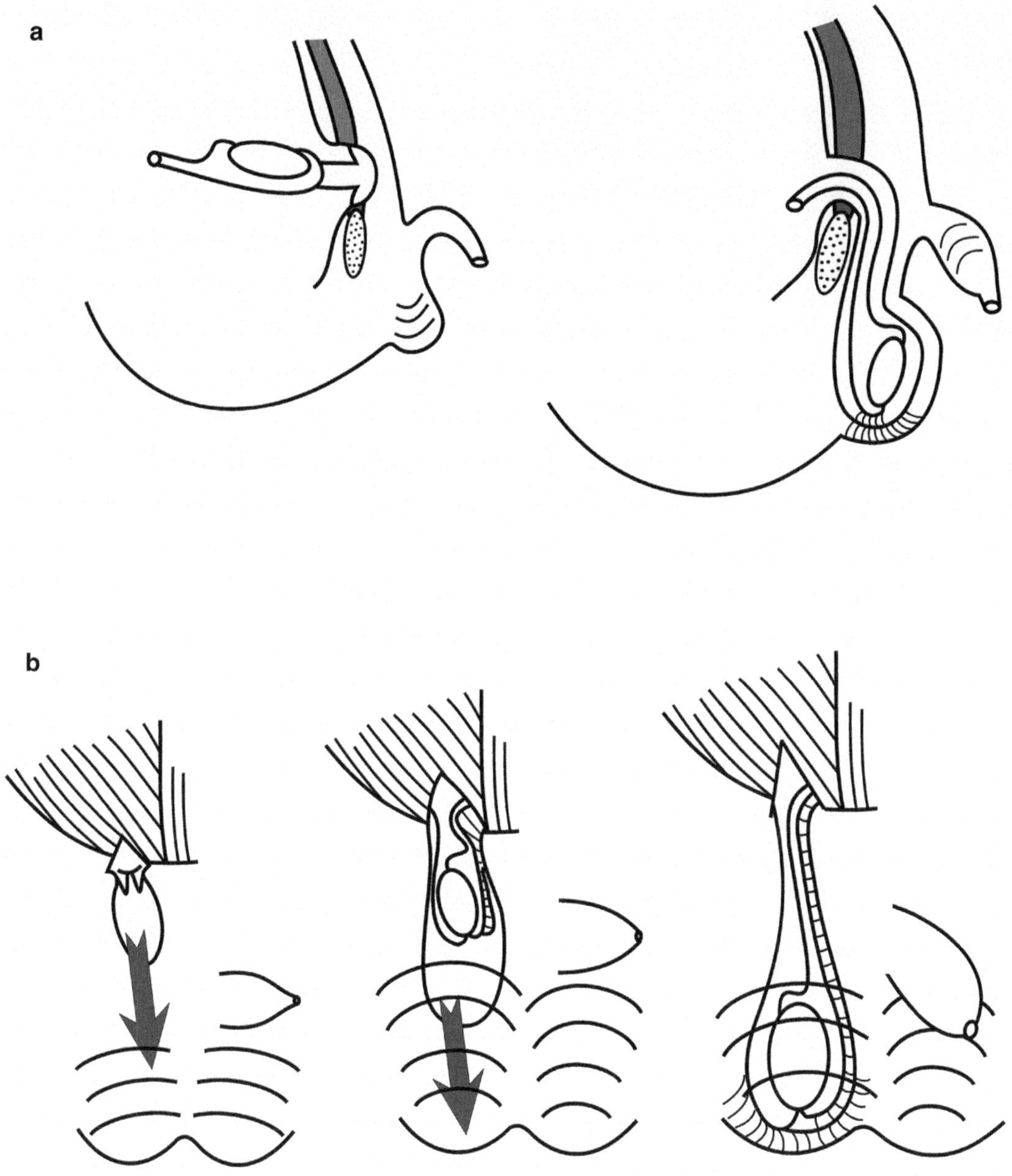

Fig. 12.4 The last morphological phase of sexual differentiation is descent of the testis. The first phase of so-called transabdominal descent occurs between 8 and 12–15 weeks of development, with enlargement of the gubernaculum ('swelling reaction'), which holds the testis nearer to the groin than the ovary in response to INSL3. (**a**) At the end of the first phase, the testis is anchored to the future inguinal canal as the processus vaginalis develops inside the gubernaculum. During the inguinoscrotal phase (25–35 weeks), the gubernaculum migrates to the scrotum, by mechanisms not yet fully understood, allowing the processus to elongate inside it so the testis can reach the scrotum within an extension of the peritoneal cavity. This is shown in sagittal section. (**b**) Viewed from the front, the gubernaculum, the end of which is gelatinous mesenchyme, migrates across the pubis and into the scrotum, within which it then becomes secondarily attached. The proximal *processus vaginalis* obliterates, leaving the testis inside a satellite peritoneal cavity within the hemi-scrotum

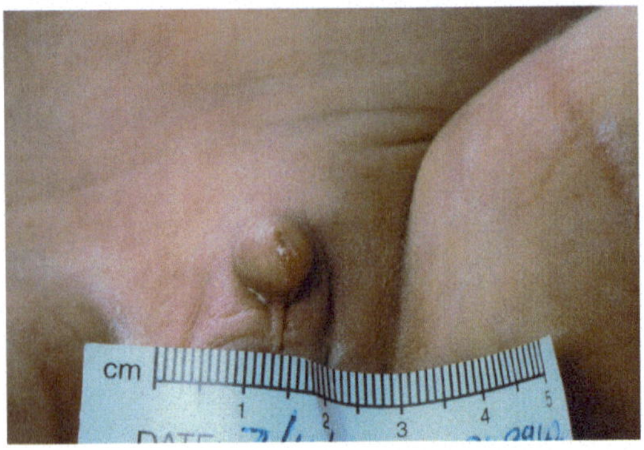

Fig. 12.5 The external genitalia respond to androgens between 8 and 12–15 weeks of development for virilisation, and beyond that no further virilisation of the urethra and labio-scrotal folds occurs. The phallus, by contrast, can grow in response to androgens right up to delivery. Early androgen production is autonomous and/or stimulated by placental hCG, until about 15 weeks, when the foetal hypothalamic-pituitary axis takes over regulation of testicular function. Baby boys with hypothalamic or pituitary insufficiency, therefore, have typical male external genital development but may have a smaller penile and an empty scrotum (undescended testes)

12.2 Diagnostic Rules and Clinical Significance

A summary of diagnostic rules and their clinical significance is found in Table 12.1

1. Testes produce the required hormones for gonadal descent, resulting in testicular descent through the abdominal wall and into the scrotum, whereas ovaries do not. The presence of a palpable gonad, therefore, almost invariably indicates the presence of testicular tissue on that side. With the discovery of *SRY* and its original attribution as the 'testis-determining gene,' it was previously thought that palpable testicular tissue invariably implied (Lopez-Hernandez et al. 2018) the presence of the *SRY* gene somewhere in the genome (Fig. 12.6). While this is still most commonly the case, it is, however, now recognised that testicular tissue can also (albeit rarely) arise without *SRY*, such as in 46,XX testicular or ovotesticular DSD arising as a result of increased expression of 'pro-testis' genes such as *SOX9* (or indeed *SOX3* and *SOX10*) or reduced expression of 'pro-ovarian' genes such as *WNT4* or *RSPO1* (Grinspon and Rey 2016). Although the ovary does not 'descend' like a testis, prolapse of an ovary into an inguinal hernia can occur, but this is extremely rare in the first week of life (Li et al. 2015).
2. As AMH is likely to control shortening of the gubernacular cord, as well as Müllerian duct regression, testicular descent is tightly linked to Müllerian duct regression. When two palpable testes are present, this means that there will be no uterus. When a single testis is palpable, it indicates that there should be a Wolffian duct on the ipsilateral side, but there should be no Müllerian duct on that side. In the absence of either palpable gonad, the gonadal and ductal status remains unknown.
3. The presence of the uterus indicates the absence of typical AMH function between 8 and 12 weeks of development, which most commonly relates to lack of typically functioning Sertoli cells (Fig. 12.7). This means that the testes are either missing or very dysgenetic. In the presence of normal testicular descent and male sexual development, it indicates the absence of AMH or its receptor in the rare syndrome of persistent Müllerian duct syndrome.
4. Regulation by male hormones of the internal genitalia is exocrine and hence is confined to the side that contains a testis/testicular tissue (see Chap. 3, Fig. 3.3) (Tong et al. 1996; Ben-Meir and Hutson 2005). This can be seen in the gonadal asymmetry that occurs in ovotesticular DSD and in 45,X/46,XY mixed gonadal dysgenesis, where the Wolffian duct is only present on the side of the testis, and the ipsilateral Müllerian duct is absent, due to the local exocrine action of both testosterone and AMH.
5. Circulating androgens from an adrenal gland or other sources are insufficient to allow development of the male internal genitalia. This means that even in babies with very marked external genital virilisation in CAH, there is no preservation of the Wolffian duct (Fig. 12.3), and Müllerian structures are present.

Table 12.1 The diagnostic significance of gonadal position and presence of uterus in babies with atypical genitalia

Gonadal position	Uterus	Predicted diagnosis	Comments
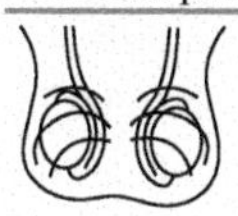 2 testes, fused scrotum	Absent	• Typical male	Expected karyotype XY Rarely, in PMDS, uterus and tubes are present
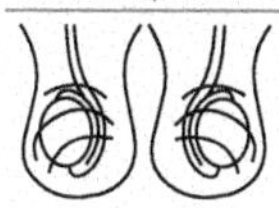 2 testes, bifid scrotum	Absent	• Undervirilized XY	Ovotesticular DSD with bilateral ovotestes possible but less likely; ovotestes are likely to be maldescended
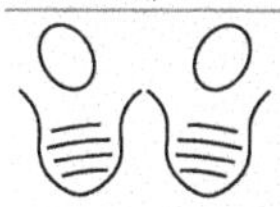 2 testes, both high, bifid under developed scrotum	Likely absent	• Undervirilized XY • Ovotesticular DSD with ovotestes • XY gonadal dysgenesis (dysplastic testes)	
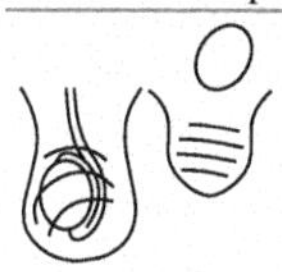 Bilateral palpable gonads, *asymmetrical* descent	Hemiuterus likely present	• Ovotesticular DSD with 1 testis, 1 ovotestis, ovary ± hernia	MGD with 1 testis, 1 streak gonad may present with a hernia mistaken as a palpable groin gonad
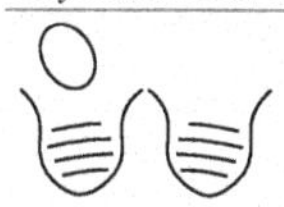 Gonadal *asymmetry*, only 1 palpable gonad	Hemiuterus likely present	• Ovotesticular DSD with 1 testis, 1 ovary/ovotestis • MGD with 1 testis, 1 streak gonad	
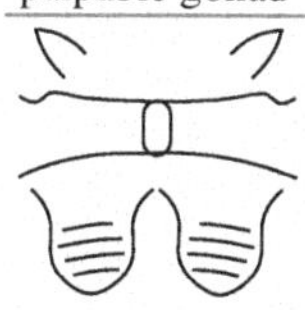 No palpable gonads, external rings open	Absent Present	• Undervirilized XY • XY gonadal dysgenesis • Ovotesticular DSD with 1 testis, 1 ovotestis or 2 ovotestes	An open external ring when gonads are non-palpable will be a clue to the presence of a high testis
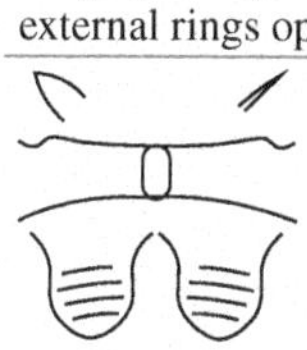 No palpable gonads, *asymmetry* with 1 ring open, 1 closed	Hemiuterus likely present	• Ovotesticular DSD with ovary, ovotestis • MGD with undescended testis, streak gonad	XX karyotype with normal steroid profile likely to suggest Ovotesticular DSD
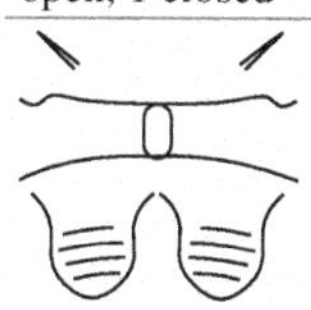 No palpable gonads, both external rings closed	Likely present	• Virilized XX • XY gonadal dysgenesis	Predict XX karyotype and raised 17 OHP

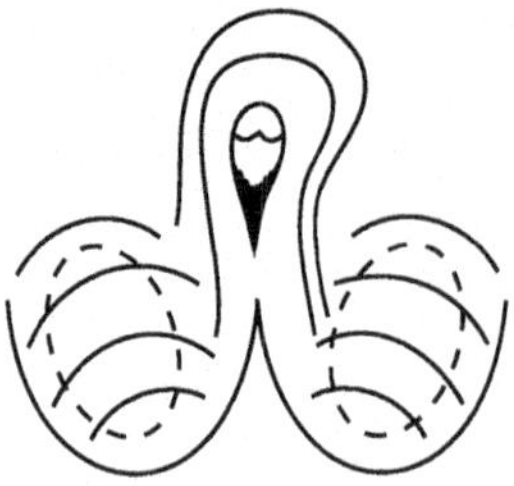
Palpable gonad
≡ Testicular tissue
≡ SRY present
≡ Absent ipsilateral Müllerian duct

Fig. 12.6 If gonads are palpable in the labio-scrotal folds or groin, it can be generally assumed that they have testicular tissue in them. In addition, it can be predicted that the ipsilateral Müllerian duct will be absent, as transabdominal testicular descent and Müllerian duct regression are very tightly linked

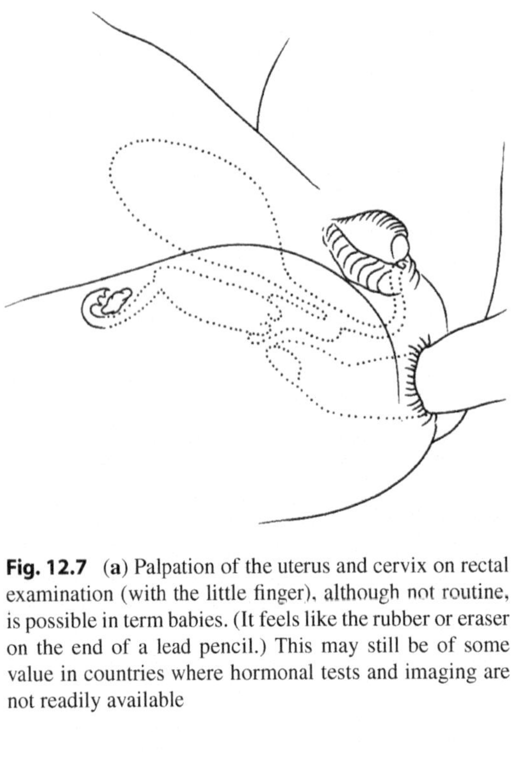

Fig. 12.7 (**a**) Palpation of the uterus and cervix on rectal examination (with the little finger), although not routine, is possible in term babies. (It feels like the rubber or eraser on the end of a lead pencil.) This may still be of some value in countries where hormonal tests and imaging are not readily available

6. External virilisation is directly proportional to the amount of androgen activity (Fig 12.2a). Any enlargement of the clitoris, even in an otherwise phenotypical female, indicates foetal exposure to androgens. The genotype in this case may be either 46,XX with virilisation (due to excess adrenal androgen production or exposure to external androgens) or 46,XY with lower levels of androgen production or function.
7. The degree of external masculine development is inversely proportional to the degree of lower vaginal development (Fig. 12.2b). In a baby with genital variation, the greater the degree of external virilisation, the shorter will be the length of the vagina.
8. Circulating androgens only virilise the external genitalia (except for the phallus) between 8 and 12 weeks of development (Fig. 12.5). Absence of androgens beyond this time leads to less penile growth and undescended testes in a baby with otherwise typically completely formed male external genitalia. This is seen in individuals when the gonadotrophin production is low, such as in those with atypical pituitary development. Androgen deficiency between 8 and 12 weeks leads to an unfused scrotum, but androgen deficiency after this time only prevents growth of the penis. The phallus can and does respond to androgens throughout pregnancy. An enlarged phallus without fusion of the scrotum or a masculine urethra indicates exposure to androgens only in the second half of pregnancy.

9. Use of the word *hypospadias* assumes the affected infant is a boy and should only be diagnosed at birth (without investigation) when both testes are fully descended into a fused scrotum (Fig. 12.8) (Tong et al. 1996). Typical male sexual development of the rest of the external genitalia demonstrates that this boy has a variation of the penis and urethra but not a global DSD. Failure of either typical urethral development or scrotal fusion in association with undescended testes in a baby with 46,XY karyotype is a sign of more significant under-virilisation in early embryogenesis, and hence these babies should be considered to have a DSD and investigated accordingly.
10. Genital differences caused by non-endocrine mechanisms (Fig. 12.9) have physical variations that lie outside the spectrum of development between male and female. Such examples include cloacal anomaly, cloacal exstrophy, bladder exstrophy, vaginal atresia, and penile agenesis (see Chap. 9).

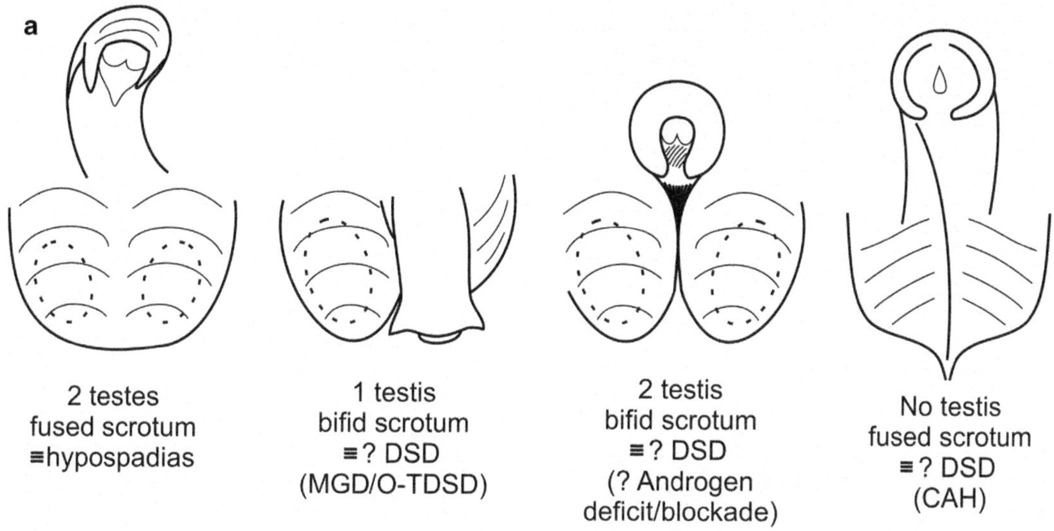

Fig. 12.8 (**a**) A diagnosis of 'hypospadias' should only be made after excluding patients with DSD. A safe rule is to assume that simple hypospadias is present *only* when there is a fused scrotum containing two testes. Babies with a single palpable gonad may have MGD or ovotesticular DSD; those with a bifid scrotum containing palpable gonads may have defects in androgen production or action; those with no palpable gonads may be males with undescended testes or females with significant virilisation (Prader 4–5) due to CAH. (**b**) A newborn genetic female with congenital adrenal hyperplasia (21-hydroxylase deficiency) with an empty 'scrotum' and trivial 'hypospadias.' The absence of gonads differentiates this clinical picture from a male with simple hypospadias and must trigger the early assessment of chromosomes (karyotype/FISH for Y material) as well as 17-OH progesterone and additional confirmatory tests of adrenal function (done from day 3 of life onwards to avoid maternal hormonal interference)

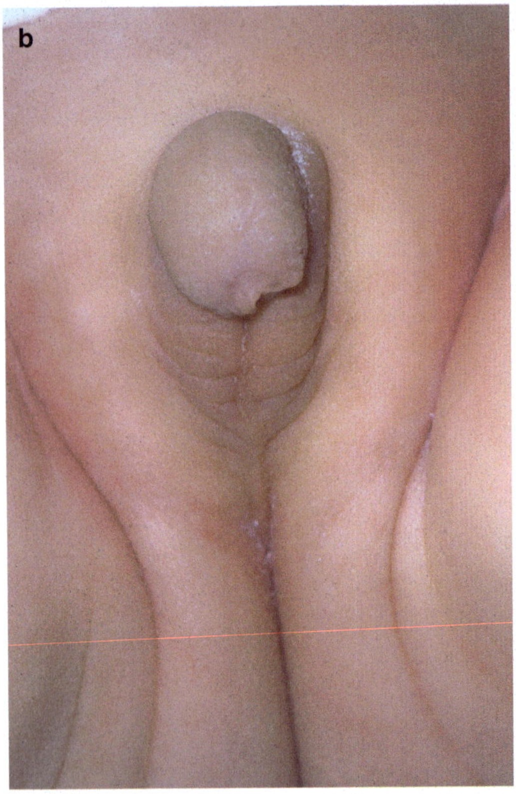

Fig. 12.8 (continued)

12.3 Clinical Approach to a New Baby with Atypical Genitalia

12.3.1 History

A careful history may reveal maternal steroid ingestion, an androgen-producing tumour with symptoms of maternal virilisation or a positive family history of a DSD.

12.3.2 Clinical Examination

Using the ten rules described earlier, it is usually possible to determine the likely underlying cause, or produce a very short differential diagnosis to guide further evaluations. In some instances, the baby has a genital appearance which is in-between typical male and typical female. The phallus is larger than a typical clitoris, but smaller than a penis (Oberfield et al. 1989; Phillip et al. 1996). The first step is to document the degree of masculine development. One such approach is with use of the semi-quantitative Prader scale which is a 6-point scale from 0 (typical female appearance) to 5 (typical male appearance). This gives a reasonably accurate estimation of the amount of androgen exposure between 8 and 12 weeks of development when the examiner estimates the degree of urethral fusion and labio-scrotal fusion (but not the size of the phallus). It also indicates the likely amount of lower vaginal regression. Recently, Ahmed and Rodie (2010) have suggested a modified scale known as the external masculinisation score (EMS) which is more detailed in its descriptors/scoring system. The Prader scale is less useful later in childhood, as postnatal exposure to androgens may allow the phallus to grow significantly.

The site of the urogenital opening should be identified. The labio-scrotal folds on either side of the urogenital opening should be gently parted, as this enables the examiner to inspect the urogenital sinus (Fig. 12.10). The funnel-shaped opening is characteristic of DSD but rare in children with simple hypospadias, where the opening is usually smaller than a normal urethral meatus in a male. Where a funnel-shaped opening is present, it can be helpful to inspect the cranial end of the funnel for mucosal tags with a slightly bluish colour, which indicates the presence of the hymen, and confirms that a vagina is present.

The next step is to determine whether or not there are gonads present, by palpation of the inguinoscrotal folds and the inguinal region. Palpable gonads are almost always testes. The exceptions are ovo-testicular DSD where the gonad may be an ovo-testis. It is possible for ovaries to prolapse into an inguinal hernia, but this is a rare presentation in a newborn female with typical external genitalia, although it can occasionally be seen in girls with uterovaginal agenesis (Kimberley et al. 2012), so, in general, this possibility can be discarded at this age (Hutson 2015). A palpable testis also indicates absence of the uterus/Müllerian structures on that side. There are three possible scenarios: (1) in the first instance, both gonads are palpable and symmetrical. This occurs in babies that have XY chromosomes and have formed testes, but there has been

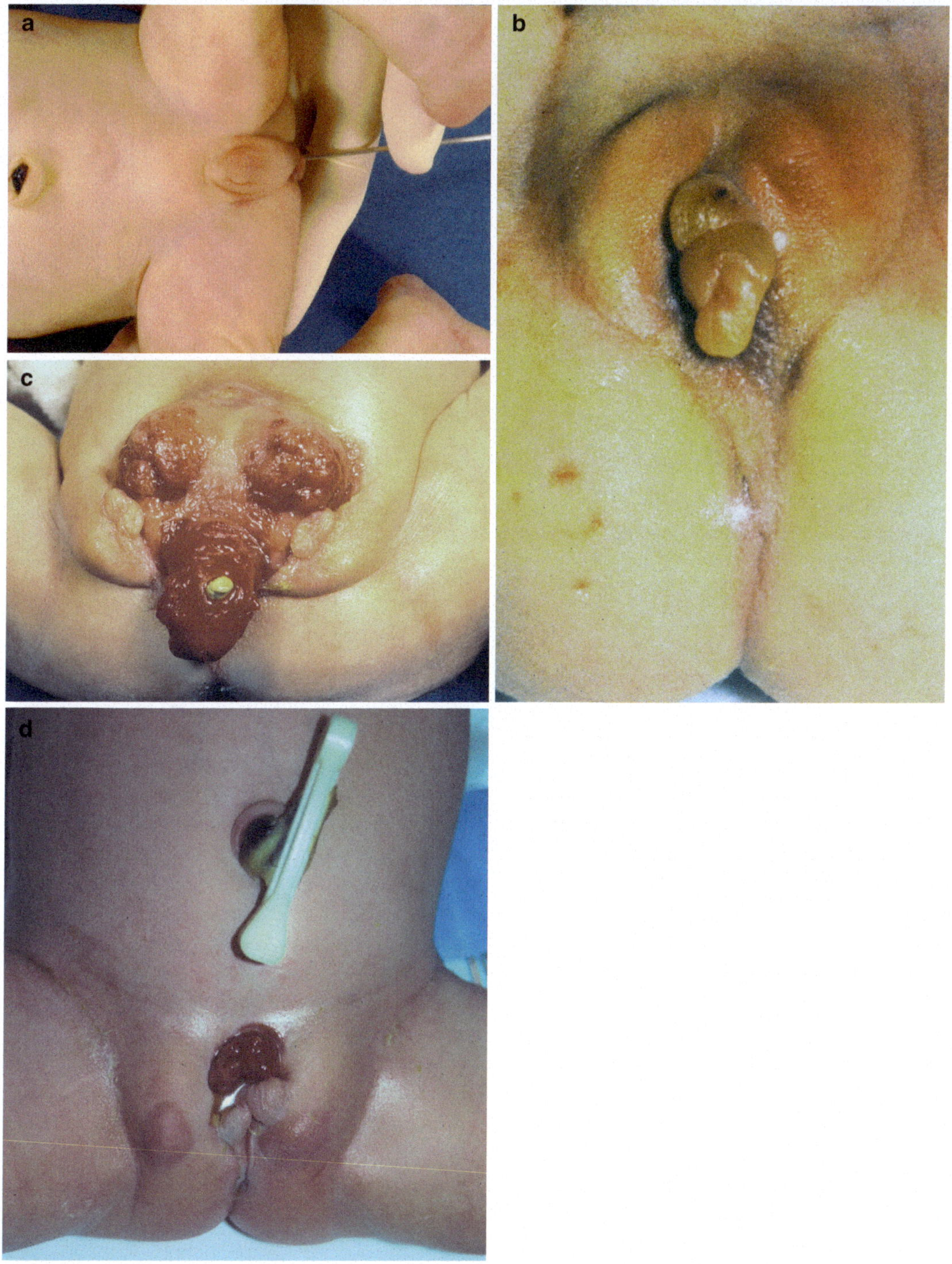

Fig. 12.9 Atypical external genitalia caused by non-endocrine mechanisms. (**a**) Penile agenesis; (**b**) Cloacal anomaly; (**c**) Cloacal exstrophy; (**d**) Bladder exstrophy

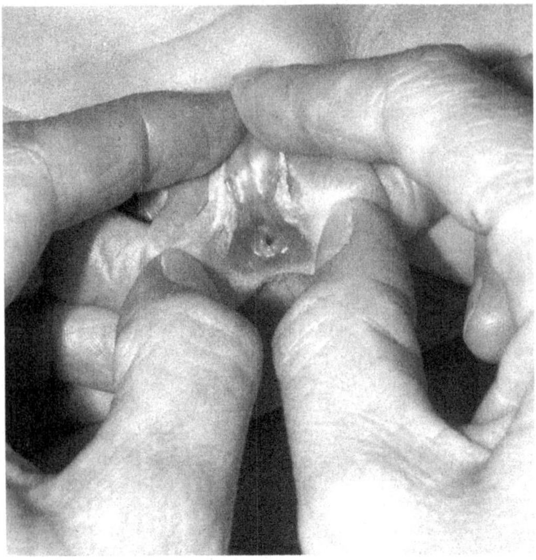

Fig. 12.10 The labio-scrotal folds can be gently parted to demonstrate the funnel-shaped urogenital sinus. If a hymen is present at the apex of the funnel, it will appear as slightly bluish mucosal tags

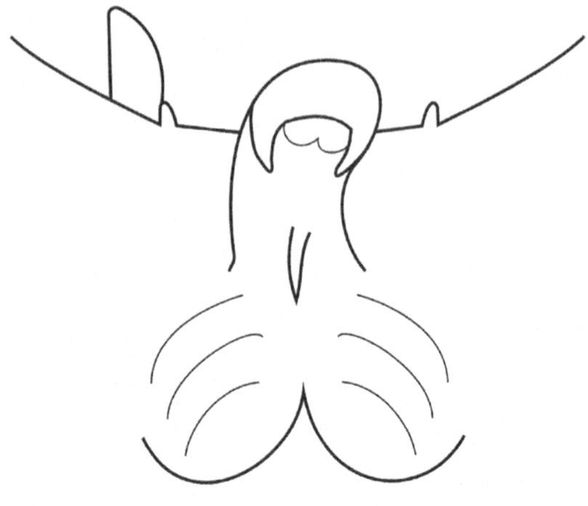

Fig. 12.11 When no gonad is palpable in the genital folds, the external inguinal area needs careful examination. If the external inguinal ring, as shown on the patient's left side, is closed, then a testis in the canal is very unlikely. By contrast, if a triangular defect is palpable, indicating that the external ring is open (seen on the right), then it is very likely that the inguinal canal contains a testis

inadequate testosterone production (gonadal dysgenesis) or action. (2) In the second instance, only one gonad is palpable. This indicates that at least one testis is present, although the other gonad may be an ovary, an ovo-testis or a dysgenetic/streak gonad. Gonadal asymmetry is very characteristic of ovo-testicular DSD and 45,X/46,XY mixed gonadal dysgenesis. (3) In the third instance, both gonads are impalpable, and in this circumstance, the status of the gonads and the internal genital ducts cannot be predicted. Further information on whether or not a testis is present can be obtained by very careful palpation of the external inguinal ring. If there is a testis within the inguinal canal the external inguinal ring is nearly always open and is palpated as an inverted V-shaped defect in the external oblique aponeurosis adjacent to the pubic tubercle. By contrast, when the external inguinal ring is closed, it is much more likely that there is no testis on that side at all, and that the internal anatomy is more typical female (Fig. 12.11). There may be ovaries or extremely dysplastic testes/gonads. This latter situation must trigger immediate investigation to rule out the potentially life-threatening situation of severe virilising (and hence salt losing) CAH in a 46,XX infant.

One should now look for other clues on general physical examination. The degree of pigmentation of the genital skin should be noted, as hyperpigmentation is seen in CAH, from the excess of melanocyte-stimulating hormone (MSH) production. This arises as 21-hydroxylase deficiency results in reduced cortisol production, which, in turn, triggers higher levels of adrenocorticotrophic hormone (ACTH) production. ACTH is derived from pro-opiomelanocortin (POMC), which is also the precursor for MSH, hence hyperpigmentation is often present in conditions characterised by persistently higher levels of ACTH production. The presence of dysmorphic features may indicate a multiple malformation syndrome, particularly in the presence of palpable gonads (see Chap. 10). Signs of a systemic illness should also be sought, as this may indicate a metabolic problem, such as evolving adrenal insufficiency, although this does not normally become clinically apparent until 1–2 weeks of age. The presence of other anatomical anomalies in the perineum, such as imperforate anus, suggests a morphological anomaly unrelated to abnormal hormones (see Chap. 9).

12.4 Investigations

12.4.1 Ultrasonography

Ultrasound scanning is widely available and has the advantages of using no ionising radiation as well as being reasonably quick and easy to perform. The main role of an ultrasound scan is to identify whether anticipated organs or structures are present and whether they have a typical appearance. These structures include the bladder, kidneys, adrenals and uterus, and they may occasionally identify ovaries or testes and their location. Transabdominal images should be obtained with transverse and sagittal orientation. A linear 9–13 MHz probe will produce excellent images of pelvic structures.

Ideally, the patient should be kept warm and wrapped to decrease movement and distress. A scan is done through a full bladder to assess the pelvic structures. It should be noted that even in experienced hands, visualisation of neonatal ovaries and testes can be difficult. Failure to identify organs on ultrasound should not therefore be interpreted as 'confirmation' of their absence but rather should prompt further additional investigation (e.g. hormonal testing to assess for the presence of functioning ovarian/testicular tissue). It is therefore important to explain to parents that findings on ultrasound are 'only one piece of the puzzle' that may help to better understand the origins of their baby's variation.

Hernanz-Schulman et al. (2002) demonstrated that in the neonatal period, ultrasound scanning has a sensitivity of 94% and specificity of 98% in detecting a uterus, the average length of the uterus being 3.2 cm ± 0.5 cm, thickness 1.4 cm and volume 3 cubic cm (Blask et al. 1991). An endometrial stripe was identified in 98%. Allowing for more experienced sonographers to perform the study is thought to improve accuracy further.

As maternal and placental hormones are still present, these lead to a relatively larger size of the neonatal uterus and ovaries, compared with later in infancy (Haber and Mayer 1994), and they are therefore relatively easy to demonstrate. Cervical length and width are often double in size compared with the fundus. Later on, during infancy, the proportion of cervix to uterine body changes to 1:1, with the uterine shape becoming tubular until just before puberty.

An echogenic endometrial stripe is also identified in the first few weeks, and fluid may be seen in the endometrial cavity as a normal finding (Garel et al. 2001; Stranzinger and Strouse 2008) (Fig. 12.12a, b). A typical male ultrasound scan will demonstrate the bladder anteriorly and rectum posteriorly with no uterus in the axial plane (Fig. 12.13a).

The ovaries have a mean volume of 1 cm^3, and follicles are generally visible; however, sonography is unlikely to demonstrate the tubes (Banerjee et al. 1992; Cohen et al. 1992) (Fig. 12.12c).

In assessing for testes, a scan is made from the level of the kidneys to the labio-scrotal folds. These should be homogeneous structures with no cysts or follicles (Figs. 12.13 and 12.14). Ultrasound scanning may also demonstrate an intra-abdominal testis; however, it is often not successful in detecting intra-abdominal testes due to their small size and overlying pelvic/abdominal structures (Fig. 12.15). Perineal views can also be performed to demonstrate a view of the urethra (Fig. 12.13b).

Ultrasonography is also useful to assess for associated developmental renal variations such as a solitary kidney, obstruction, duplex kidney and crossed fused renal ectopia (Ogilvy-Stuart and Brain 2004).

Additional structures such as paramesonephric (Müllerian) or mesonephric (Wolffian) duct remnants and hydro-metrocolpos may also be encountered (Fig. 12.16). Most cases of hydrometrocolpos are associated with a urogenital sinus or cloacal malformation.

Common artefacts encountered include overdistension of the bladder, leading to a markedly inferiorly displaced uterus, making identifying the whole organ difficult in the sagittal plane, with the axial plane being more successful in this situation. An empty bladder also makes identifying the uterus difficult. Identifying the rectum also assists in locating the uterus. In addition, bowel gas as well as bony structures may lead to artefacts.

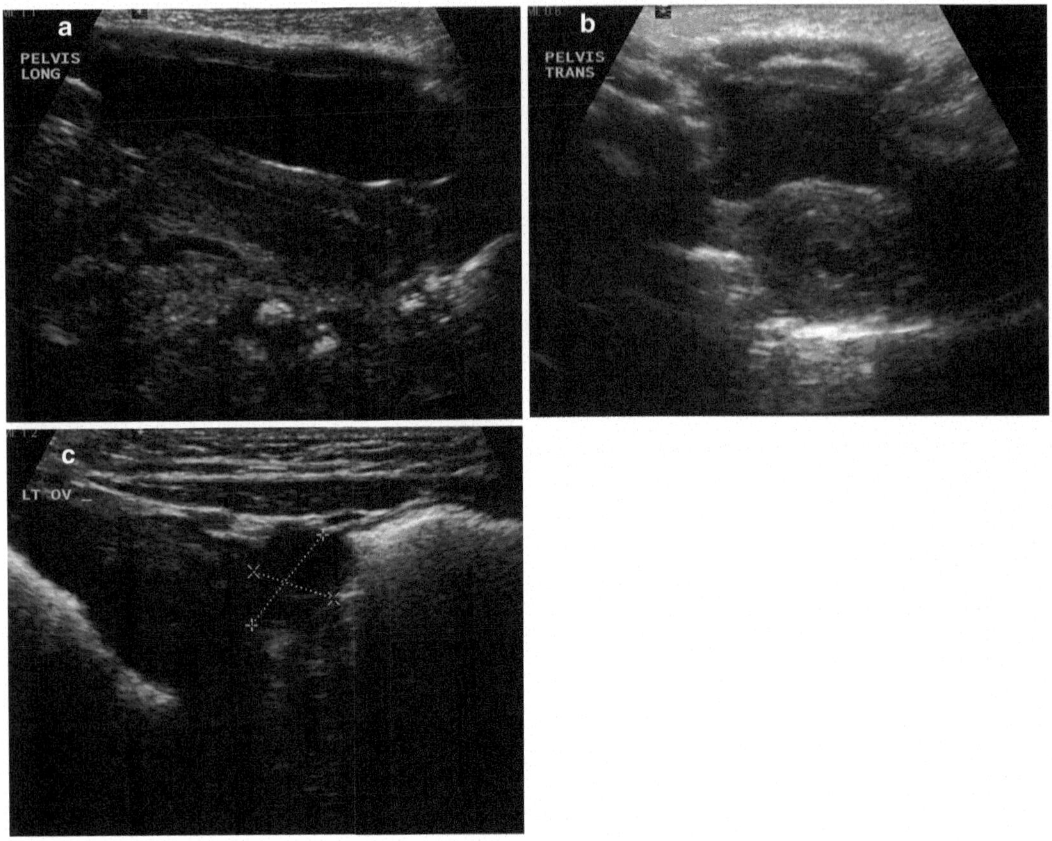

Fig. 12.12 Female Pelvic Ultrasound: (**a**) Sagittal view demonstrates the uterus. Note echogenic endometrial stripe and rectum posteriorly. (**b**) Transverse image through bladder and uterus. (**c**) Ovary with follicles identified

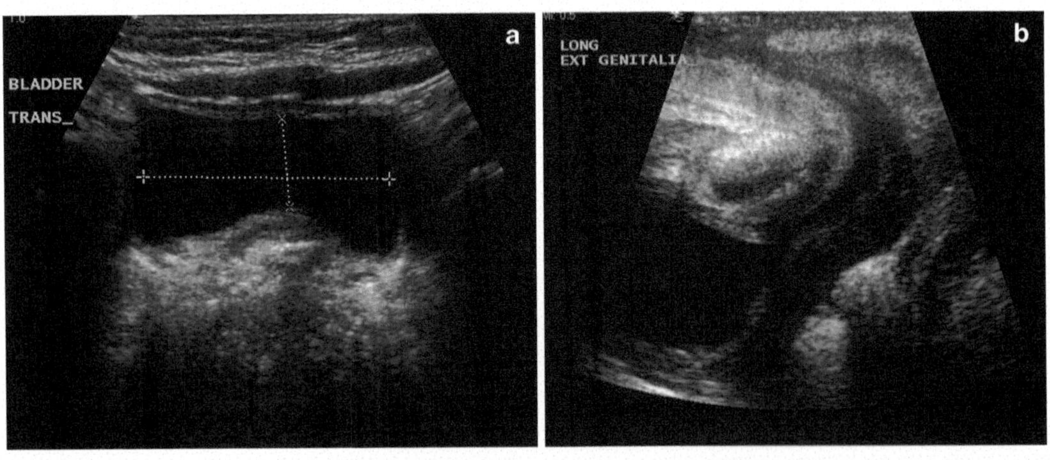

Fig. 12.13 Male Pelvic Ultrasound (**a**) Transverse view—note bladder and rectum with no evidence for a uterus. (**b**) Perineal view demonstrates a long urethra. Note pubic symphysis

In ovo-testicular DSD, ultrasound scanning of the ovo-testes may show focal cystic areas amongst heterogeneous tissue with the cystic areas corresponding to ovarian tissue (Eberenz et al. 1991).

In complete androgen insensitivity syndrome (CAIS), ultrasonography demonstrates typically formed testes, which are most often located in the inguinal region or in the inguinal canal, as well as absence of a uterus (indicating typical Sertoli cell function and AMH production *in utero*) (Gambino et al. 1992) (Fig. 12.17).

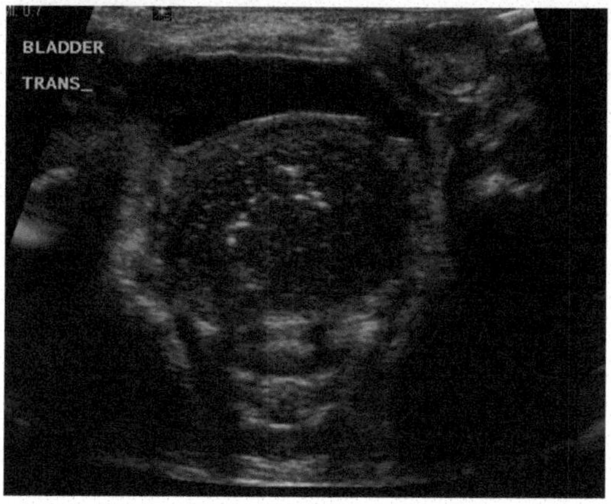

Fig. 12.14 Transverse ultrasound of male pelvis demonstrates bladder, distended rectum and no uterus. Note undescended testis with no evidence for follicles

12.4.1.1 Congenital Adrenal Hyperplasia

Ultrasonography is an ideal imaging modality used to assess for possible congenital adrenal hyperplasia (CAH). Most commonly, this is 21-hydroxalase deficiency (90%) (Oppenheimer et al. 1983). As 75% of CAH have the salt-wasting variety, they are vulnerable to circulatory collapse if not diagnosed early (Oppenheimer et al. 1983), and therefore ultrasound scanning can play an early role in assessing for this, although biochemical confirmation of CAH subtype, with genetic testing if hormonal testing does not yield easily interpretable results, is important.

In 46,XX CAH, the sonographer will be able to identify a typically appearing uterus and ovaries; however, the adrenal appearance will differ (Kutteh et al. 1995). A newborn's adrenal glands

Fig. 12.15 (**a**) Pelvic ultrasound: Sagittal image demonstrates an intra-abdominal testis. (**b**) Ultrasound Image demonstrates testis within labio-scrotal folds. (**c**) Ultrasound image: transverse view though atypical genitalia demonstrates labio-scrotal folds and a phallic structure but does not advance exact diagnosis. (**d**) Normal testis in inguinal canal

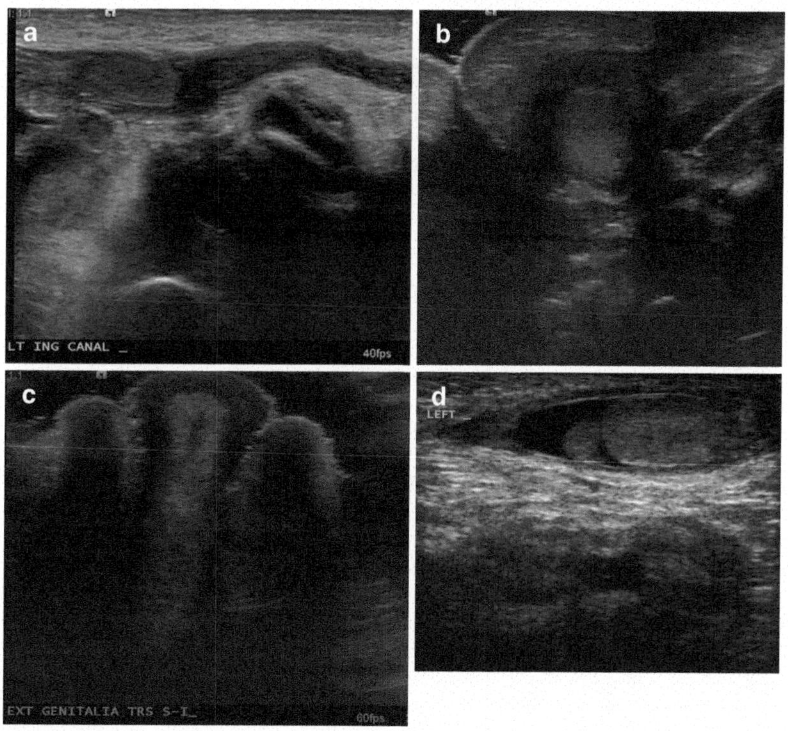

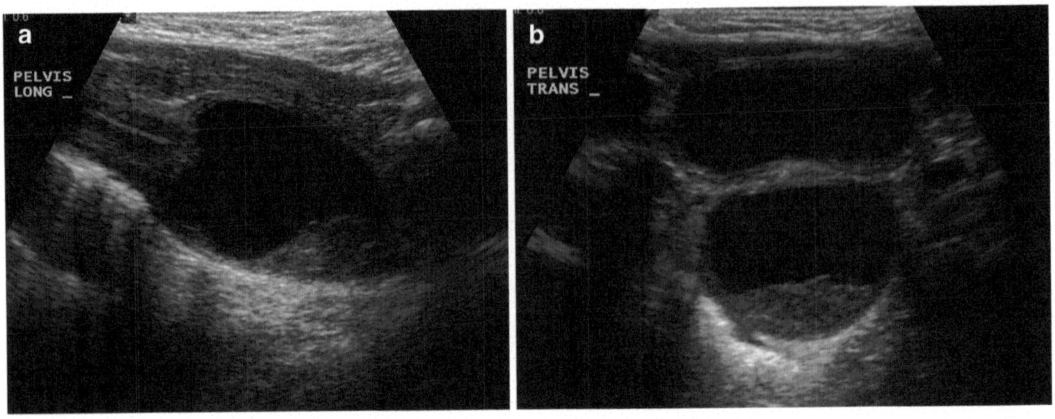

Fig. 12.16 Ultrasound images of hydro-metrocolpos. (**a**) Sagittal view shows uterus/endometrium and haemorrhagic debris. (**b**) Transverse view of hydro-metrocolpos

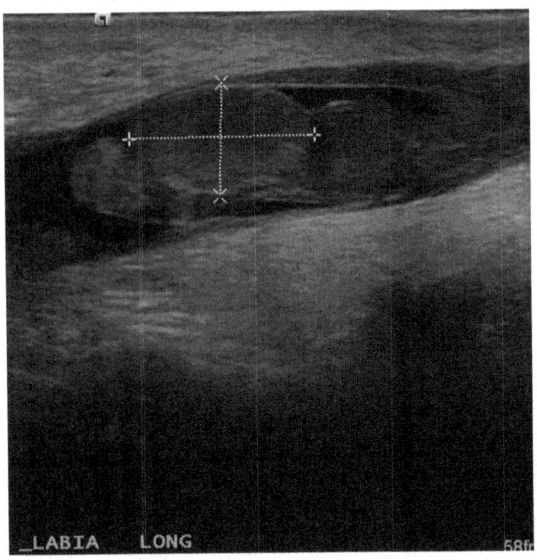

Fig. 12.17 Ultrasound in patient with CAIS. Note testis within patent *processus vaginalis*. These structures were contained in what was clinically thought to be labia

are routinely large relative to the older child's and therefore easier to identify. Adrenal glands should hence be identified in all newborns. The normal adrenals resemble a triangle or inverted Y, and they have a central echogenic stripe representing the medulla surrounded by a peripheral hypoechoic rim of the cortex (Avni et al. 1993) (Fig. 12.18).

The appearance of the echogenic medullary stripe is not altered in CAH. The exact size of the adrenal gland is difficult to measure due to the multi-planar nature of the gland. However, if the adrenals have a coiled appearance with a convoluted, cerebriform appearance, then this is highly specific for CAH (Oppenheimer et al. 1983; Sivit et al. 1991; Al-Alwan et al. 1999) (Fig. 12.19). The adrenal glands of CAH also have a generally bulky appearance compared to usual (Hernanz-Schulman et al. 2002).

The above-mentioned adrenal gland sonographic findings are very common in untreated CAH, but once treatment with adrenal hormone replacement therapy is commenced, the adrenal glands revert to a more typical size and shape; the axial plane being more successful in this situation.

12.4.2 Genitogram

Radiographic studies of the lower genito-urinary tract (genitography/sinugram) may assist in establishing the diagnosis in neonates with atypical genitalia. A genitogram is a study using fluoroscopy after catheterisation of the bladder and injection of contrast via the catheter to outline the bladder and Müllerian remnant if present. The findings on these studies range from a typical micturating cysto-urethrogram (MCU)-like appearance (despite atypical genitalia clinically) to complex anatomical variations (Fig. 12.20a–c).

The sinugram/genitogram technique includes utilising a sterile technique and ensuring there

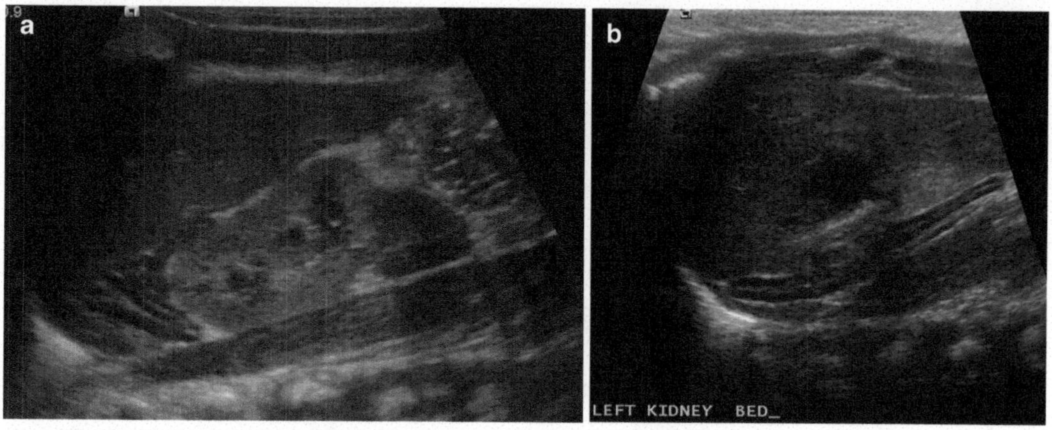

Fig. 12.18 Normal adrenal ultrasound: (**a**) Note hypoechoic cortex and hyperechoic medulla. Note the lack of a fine, coiled cerebriform appearance. (**b**) Ultrasound of renal bed demonstrates 'lying down adrenal,' which is demonstrated with agenesis of the kidney

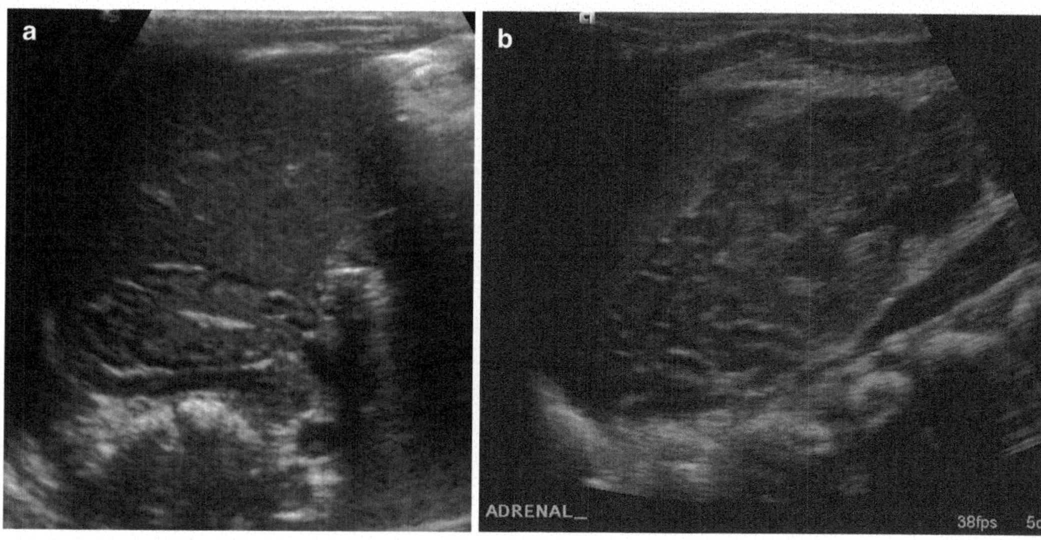

Fig. 12.19 Ultrasound suprarenal region in CAH: (**a**) Note enlarged appearance to the adrenal gland with increased number of gyrations giving a coiled, cerebriform appearance. (**b**) Transverse image demonstrates cerebriform appearance of CAH

are at least two catheters available prior to starting the procedure.

The radiologist should identify the number of perineal openings and then catheterise the urethra with a small catheter and fill the bladder with non-ionic contrast as per a routine MCU. This part of the examination will assess bladder position, communication with surrounding structures, fistulae, residual paramesonephric (Müllerian) or mesonephric (Wolffian) duct structures, vesicoureteric reflux and possible uterine indentation on the bladder.

Often, a urogenital sinus is identified, which is a common terminal channel for the anterior urethra and posterior Müllerian remnant pouch. This usually empties at the base of the genital tubercle. This is suspected if there is a single perineal opening. A voiding study may outline all

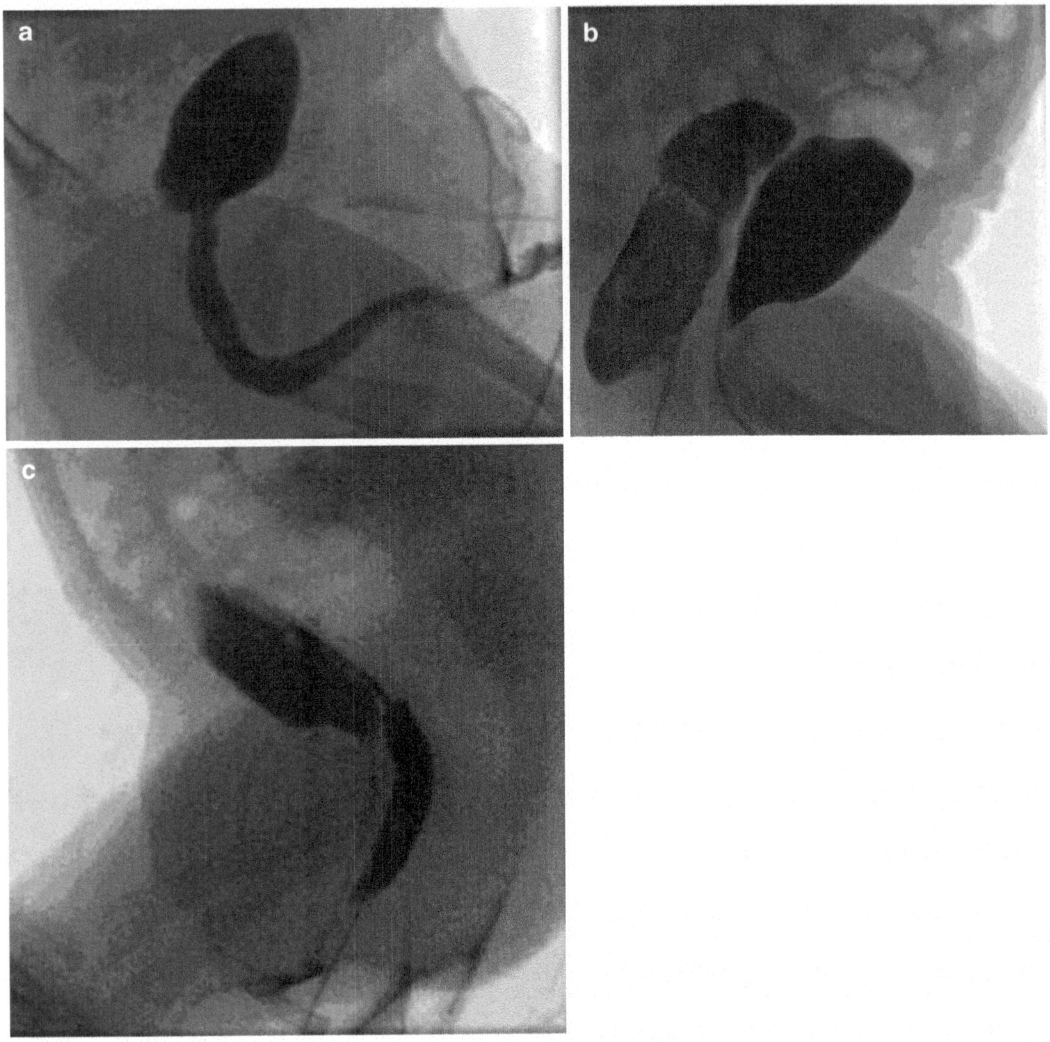

Fig. 12.20 Male sinugram: (**a**) The bladder is catheterised, and during micturition, there is no Müllerian remnant demonstrated or vesicoureteric reflux. Male-type urethra opacified. (**b**) Male sinugram: In this case rectal contrast was also injected to outline the rectum and its relationship to the bladder. (**c**) Female sinugram: Contrast outlines the bladder anteriorly. Second catheter is in the vagina with contrast outlining the vaginal cavity. An endometrial cavity is also outlined. Note indentation of the uterus on the posterior aspect of the bladder

structures; otherwise, other techniques can be used after the cystogram portion to opacify the Müllerian remnant and urogenital sinus.

When the baby urinates, the urethral length can be assessed and the presence or absence of a urogenital sinus and communication into the Müllerian remnant can be determined. If the remnant is opacified, then its size can be documented and sometimes contrast demonstrated passing into the uterine cavity (Fig. 12.21a) or Fallopian tubes (Fig. 12.21b). Evidence for cervical indentation on the vaginal cavity may also be observed.

If there is no urination or if the Müllerian remnant has not filled, then there are other options to opacify the genital tract:

1. Place a second catheter and try to position this into the Müllerian remnant and then instil contrast directly into it to outline its contour (Fig 12.22a).

   Or

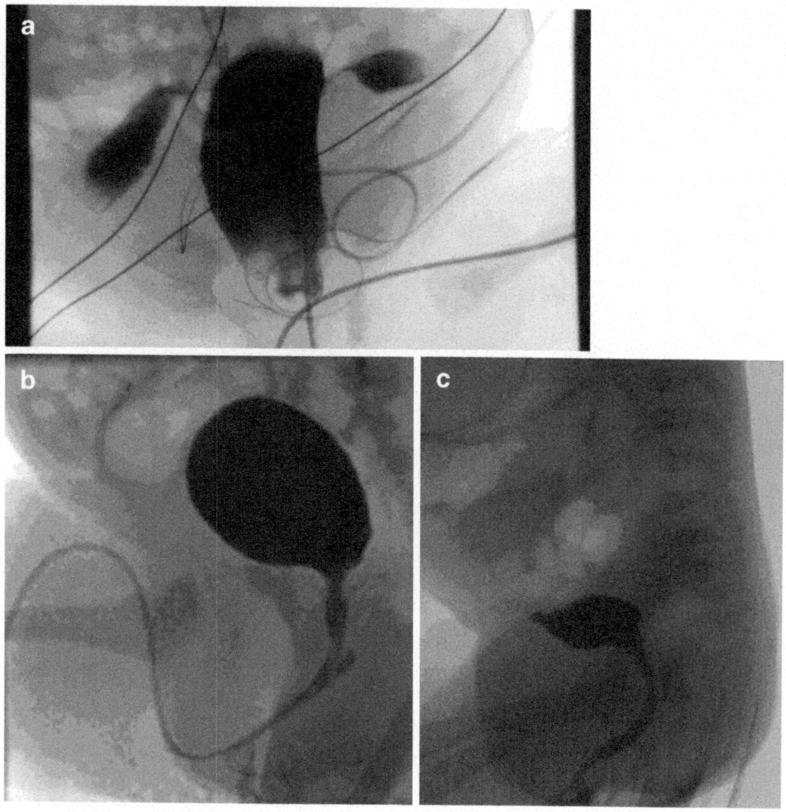

Fig. 12.21 Sinugram: (**a**) AP view demonstrates the vaginal cavity with spill of contrast into the Fallopian tubes confirming their presence. (**b**) Oblique projection demonstrating a small Müllerian duct remnant. (**c**) Lateral projection demonstrates small Müllerian duct remnant

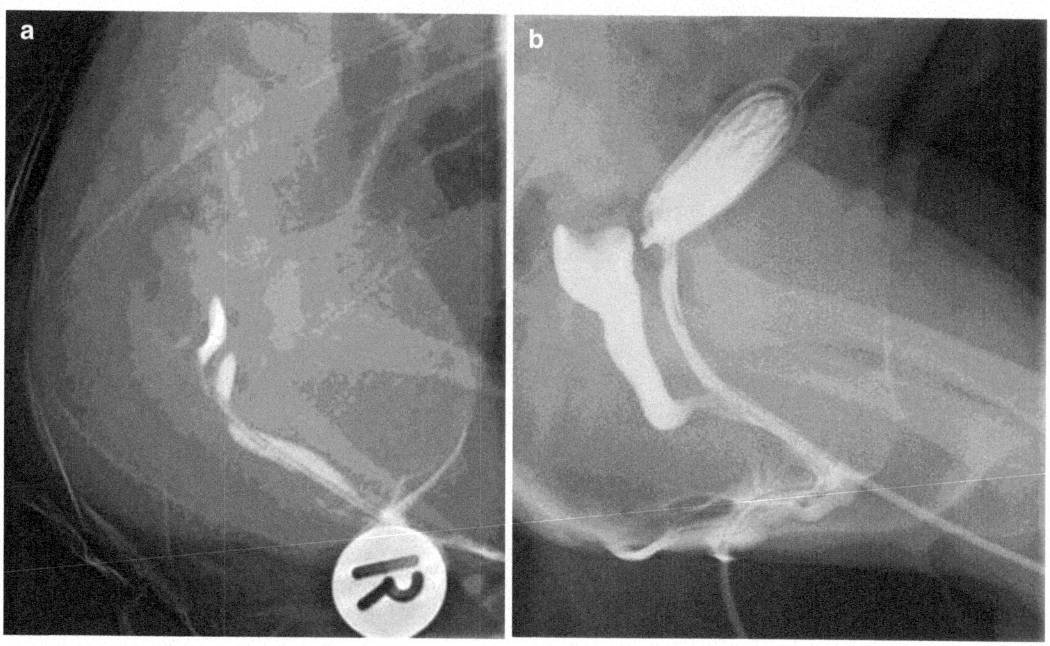

Fig. 12.22 (**a**) A metallic marker can be placed on the perineum to assist in outlining the perineal opening when assessment of urethral length is required. (**b**) Lateral projection demonstrates two catheters *in situ*—opacifying bladder, urogenital sinus and vagina. Note cervical indentation on the upper vagina

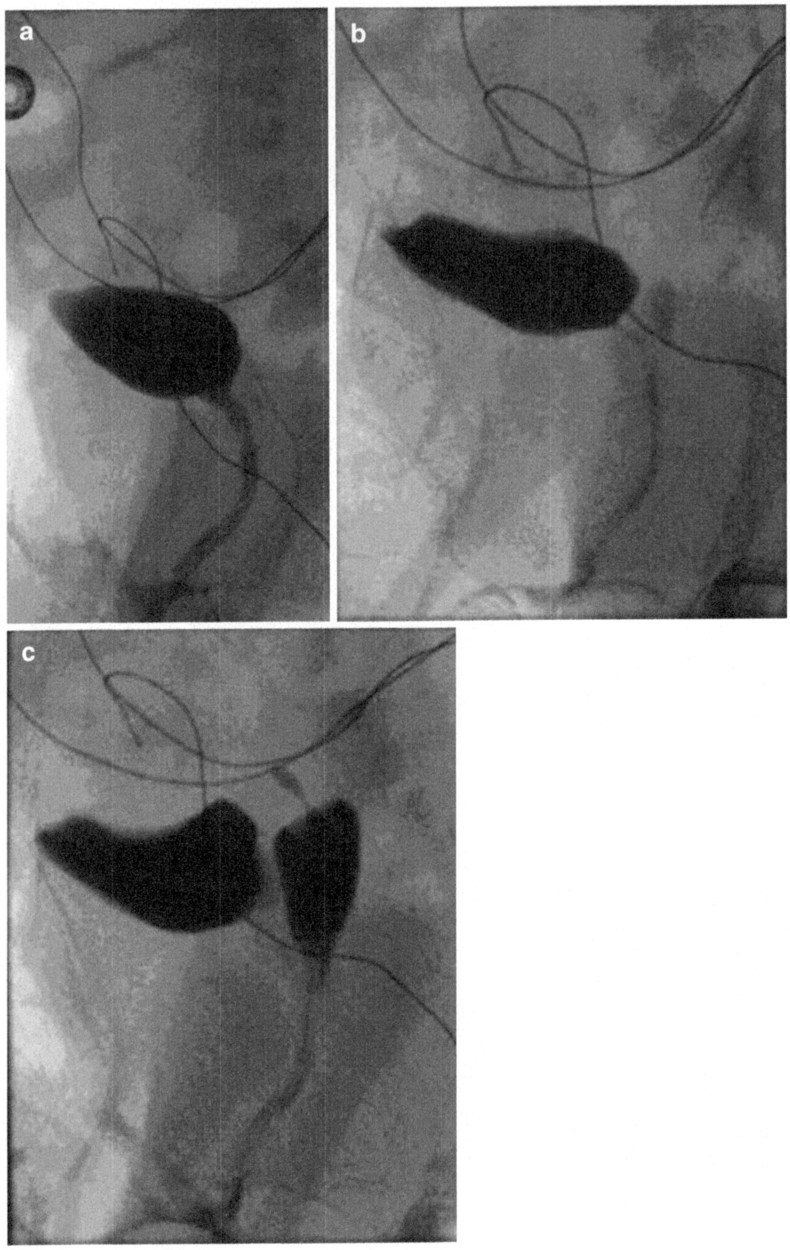

Fig. 12.23 Sinugram: Series demonstrates initial filling of the bladder (**a**) small amount of contrast just entering the urogenital sinus. (**b**) Later images reveal filling of a vaginal cavity (**c**) and subsequent contrast passing into the endometrial cavity of the uterus

2. Withdraw the first catheter slowly, while injecting contrast to opacify the Müllerian remnant (Fig 12.22b) using the same strategy as in a retrograde urethrogram.

   Antero-posterior (AP) and lateral films including long urethral view should be obtained.

The radiologist may need to perform a retrograde study if the catheter can only be advanced into the distal urethra by placing a catheter into the urethra and injecting while observing the contrast pass in a retrograde fashion through the urethra and fill the bladder and perhaps other structures. The study may show a cervical impression on the vaginal cavity if a uterus is present, and there is generally a uterine indentation on the bladder also (Fig. 12.22b). The cervical imprint may not be present if the vagina is under-filled, or there is a very small uterus. Minor anomalies such as small Müllerian duct remnants

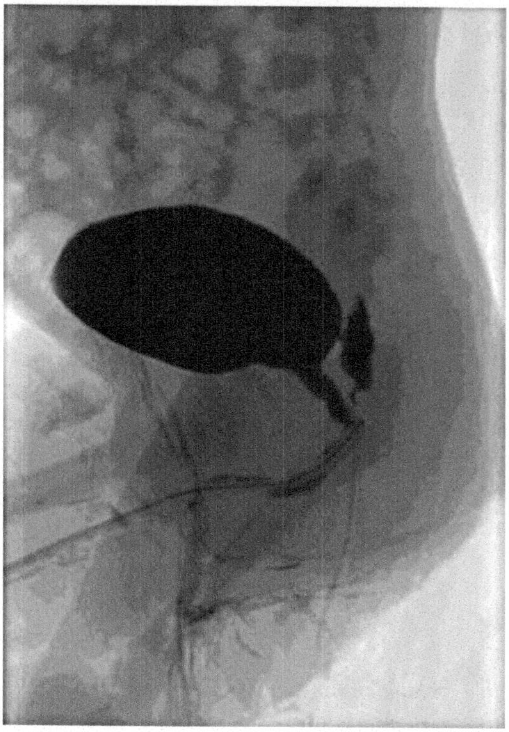

Fig. 12.24 Sinugram—demonstrates the catheter has been withdrawn out of the contrast-filled bladder in order to opacify a small Müllerian duct remnant

to small vaginal remnants can be outlined (Figs. 12.21b, c, 12.23 and 12.24).

The urogenital sinus may be very short or long. The length of the urogenital sinus and level of insertion of the vagina into the urogenital sinus are good indicators of the degree of virilisation. A metallic marker may be placed on the perineum to assist in estimating the urethral/urogenital sinus length (Fig. 12.22a). The abdominal radiograph in these patients may also demonstrate additional findings and should be evaluated as well, particularly for non-hormonal causes of genital anomaly.

12.4.3 Magnetic Resonance Imaging and Computerised Tomography

In some European countries, MRI is routinely used to assess atypical genitalia in patients with DSD; however, elsewhere, it is usually a second-line test that may assist the clinician if the other imaging modalities are unhelpful.

The advantages of MRI include the ability to image in multiple planes without radiation, high contrast of the soft tissues and its relatively non-invasive scanning.

This modality can assess for Müllerian structures which may consist of a single fused uterus or two separated uterine horns, functional endometrial tissue, vaginal obstruction/duplication/absence, ovaries and identification of the kidneys, but it has a low sensitivity in identifying small rudimentary horns and also for clarifying obstructions.

The technique will vary from institution to institution; however, a general protocol will provide all the required information:

(a) Phased array or surface coils to allow highest resolution.
(b) Coronal T1- and T2-wide full view including kidneys and ovaries.
(c) Fast Spin Echo T2 (sagittal) is excellent for anatomy of the uterus and vagina and also to determine their relationship to the rectum and bladder (Fig. 12.25).
(d) The axial plane is used for ovaries, lower uterine segment and cervix.
(e) The vagina is best seen on T2 axial slices (Hata et al. 1989).

In the neonatal period, as a consequence of oestrogen stimulation, the uterine fundus is usually larger than the cervix, and there will be a high T2 signal in the endometrium. Hydro-metrocolpos can also be visualised (Gambino et al. 1992). After 4–6 weeks, these features revert to the typical prepubertal appearance. Vaginal epithelium in the newborn is a well-developed thick structure and also has a high signal on T2 (Cohen et al. 1993) (Fig. 12.26).

Multi-planar images can confirm the absence of a uterus if undertaken in the early neonatal time period and demonstrate intra-abdominal or inguinal testis (Gambino et al. 1992).

Both testes and immature, non-cystic ovaries have intermediate signal on T1 and high signal on T2. Gonads often show an outer rim of medium-intensity signal, which helps distinguish them from lymph nodes.

In 45,X/46,XY, mixed gonadal dysgenesis MRI may be useful to detect streak or dysgenetic gonads and characterise internal structure.

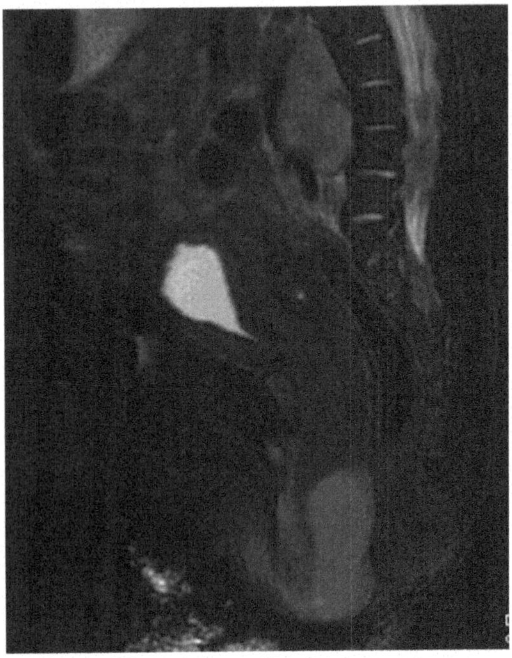

Fig. 12.25 MRI Sagittal T2 image demonstrates bladder, uterus and rectum

12.4.4 Endoscopy

On occasions, the genitogram fails to demonstrate a vaginal opening, and it is necessary to perform a cystoscopy. In children where the vagina is present, its opening into the urinary tract is heralded on endoscopy by small mucosal folds which represent the hymen. These folds may flutter in the current of water perfusing the cystoscope and often look like seaweed or an anemone underwater. The opening of the vagina is always in the centre of these folds, and it can be demonstrated by the insertion of a ureteric catheter. The size of the cavity can be determined by direct measurement or by injection of contrast medium and fluoroscopy.

12.4.5 Laparoscopy (See Chap. 17)

This investigation is not required in most cases, as the external anatomy, complemented by an ultrasound of the internal genitalia and hormonal investigations, is usually diagnostic. Laparoscopy is most useful diagnostically in patients with 45,X/46,XY mixed gonadal dysgenesis or ovo-testicular DSD, where it may be necessary to biopsy the gonad, and to determine the precise anatomy of the internal genital ducts. This is particularly true if there is a

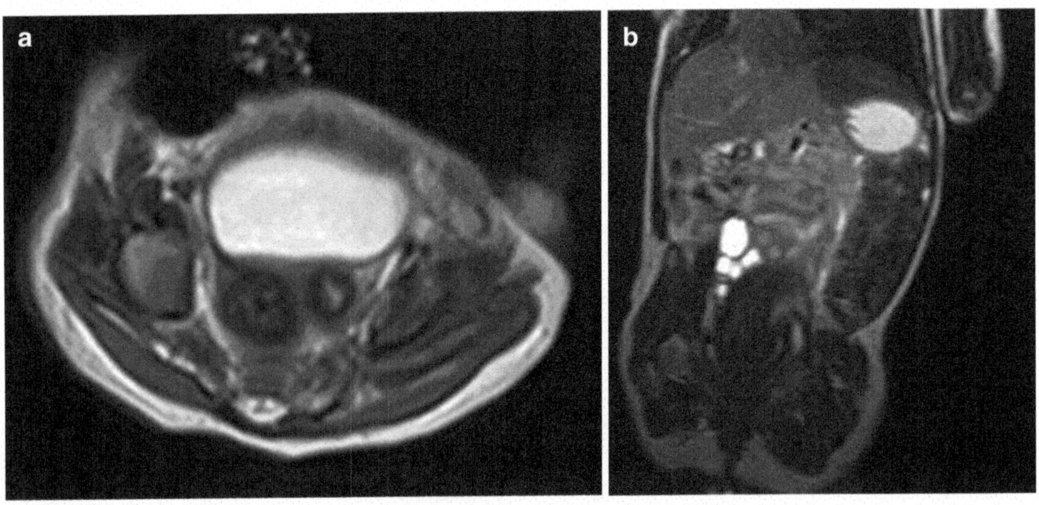

Fig. 12.26 MRI: (**a**) Transverse T2 image, (**b**) Coronal T2—demonstrates uterus/endometrial cavity. (**c**) Sagittal T2 image showing normal anatomy, and (**d**) Transverse T2—inguinal gonads and uterus

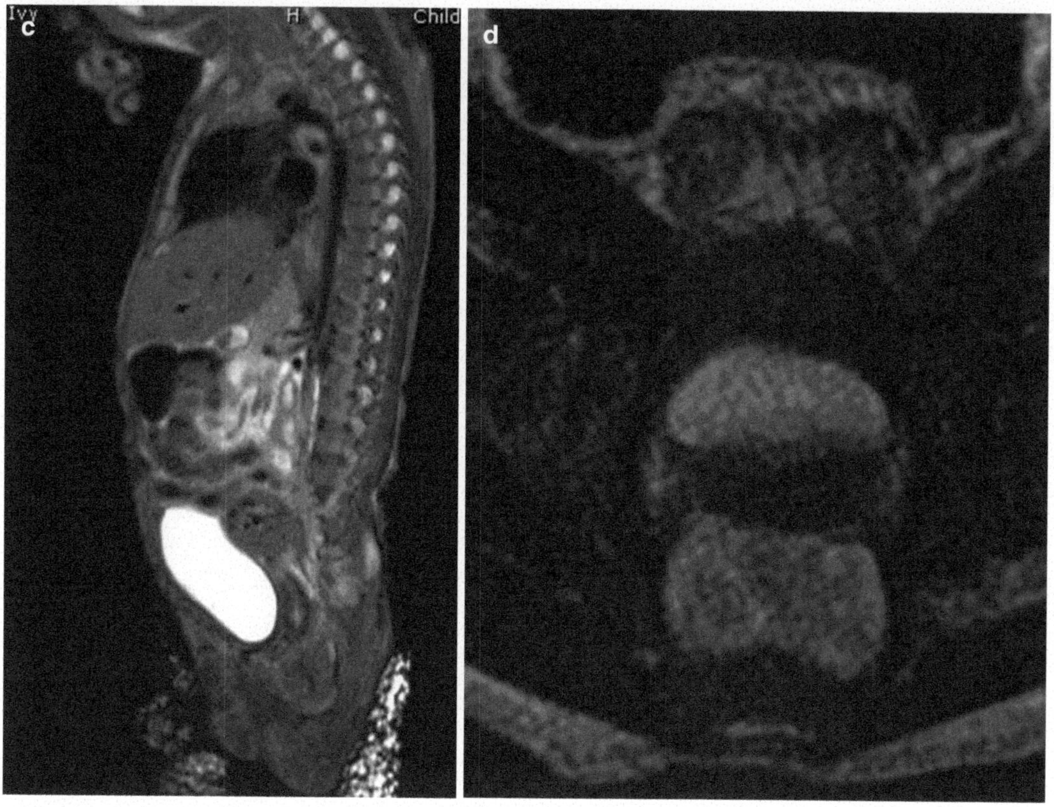

Fig. 12.26 (continued)

hemi-uterus and single fallopian tube. The details of laparoscopic management are given in Chap. 17.

12.4.6 Initial Laboratory Investigations

Investigations such as a karyotype, fluorescent *in situ* hybridisation (FISH) for Y, 17-OH progesterone and urinary steroid profile should be performed if the clinical picture suggests the baby may have CAH (e.g. virilisation of external genitalia but no palpable gonads). It should be noted that normal urea, electrolytes and creatinine (UEC) and glucose results in the early days of life do not exclude CAH, as electrolyte abnormalities are typically not evident until closer to 1 week of age, and hypoglycaemia is not universal. Other hormone levels, including serum testosterone (Leydig cells), AMH (Sertoli cells) and LH and FSH (pituitary) will help to assess gonadal function if tested during the window of mini-puberty. The serum ratio of testosterone/DHT may be useful to distinguish between the overlapping clinical pictures seen in 5-alpha reductase type-2 deficiency and androgen resistance due to partial androgen insensitivity syndrome (PAIS); however, it should be noted that the DHT immunoassay is problematic and may yield confusing results. Urgent fluorescent *in situ* hybridisation (FISH) to detect Y chromosome sequences will indicate whether a Y chromosome is present. A full karyotype will be required to distinguish chromosomal and aneuploidy DSD.

Depending on initial results, or outside of the mini-puberty period, an hCG-stimulation test may be needed to determine the presence of androgen-producing testicular tissue and the ratio of T/DHT. An ACTH stimulation test will help to document any steroid biosynthesis anomaly in the testis or adrenal gland. A 24-h urine collection permits a full steroid profile for defects in steroid biosynthesis by the use of gas chromatography and mass spectrometry.

Additional specific genetic screening may be helpful to identify variants in genes known to be associated with DSD. In tandem with our increasing knowledge of the genetics of DSD, the availability of more specific genetic testing with DSD gene panels or on exome sequencing is also increasing and in time, as associated costs reduce, may become more commonplace (Dong et al. 2016; Eggers et al. 2016; Kim et al. 2017). This, along with prospectively collated data on clinical course and outcomes, will help to improve our knowledge of genotype-phenotype correlations as well as typical progress over time in specific genetic variations and ultimately improve the information and care we can provide to affected individuals.

Acknowledgments We acknowledge with thanks to Murray Bartlett, who contributed to the first edition.

References

Ahmed SF, Rodie M. Investigation and initial management of ambiguous genitalia. Best Pract Res Clin Endocrinol Metab. 2010;24(2):197–218. https://doi.org/10.1016/j.beem.2009.12.001.

Al-Alwan I, Navarro O, Daneman D, et al. Clinical utility of adrenal ultrasonography in the diagnosis of congenital adrenal hyperplasia. J Pediatr. 1999;135(1):71–5.

Avni EF, Rypens F, Smet MH, et al. Sonographic demonstration of congenital adrenal hyperplasia in the neonate: the cerebriform pattern. Pediatr Radiol. 1993;23(2):88–90.

Banerjee AK, Clarke O, MacDonald LM. Sonographic detection of neonatal hydrometrocolpos. Br J Radiol. 1992;65(771):268–71.

Ben-Meir DB, Hutson JM. The anatomy of the caudal vas deferens in patients with a genital anomaly. J Pediatr Urol. 2005;1(5):349–54.

Blask AR, Sanders RC, Rock JA. Obstructed uterovaginal anomalies: demonstration with sonography. Part II. Teenagers. Radiology. 1991;179(1):84–8.

Cohen HL, Bober SE, Bow SN. Imaging the pediatric pelvis: the normal and abnormal genital tract and simulators of its diseases. Urol Radiol. 1992;14(4):273–83.

Cohen HL, Shapiro MA, Mandel FS, et al. Normal ovaries in neonates and infants: a sonographic study of 77 patients 1 day to 24 months old. AJR Am J Roentgenol. 1993;160(3):583–6.

Dong Y, Yi Y, Yao H, et al. Targeted next-generation sequencing identification of mutations in patients with disorders of sex development. BMC Med Genet. 2016;17:23.

Eberenz W, Rosenberg HK, Moshang T, et al. True hermaphroditism: sonographic demonstration of ovotestes. Radiology. 1991;179(2):429–31.

Eggers S, Sadedin S, van den Bergen JA, et al. Disorders of sex development: insights from targeted gene sequencing of a large international patient cohort. Genome Biol. 2016;17(1):243.

Gambino J, Caldwell B, Dietrich R, et al. Congenital disorders of sexual differentiation: MR findings. AJR Am J Roentgenol. 1992;158(2):363–7.

Garel L, Dubois J, Grignon A, et al. US of the pediatric female pelvis: a clinical perspective. Radiographics. 2001;21(6):1393–407.

Grinspon RP, Rey RA. Disorders of sex development with testicular differentiation in SRY-negative 46,XX individuals: clinical and genetic aspects. Sex Dev. 2016;10(1):1–11.

Haber HP, Mayer EI. Ultrasound evaluation of uterine and ovarian size from birth to puberty. Pediatr Radiol. 1994;24(1):11–3.

Hata K, Nishigaki A, Makihara K, et al. Ultrasonic evaluation of the normal uterus in the neonate. J Perinat Med. 1989;17(4):313–7.

Hernanz-Schulman M, Brock JW 3rd, Russell W. Sonographic findings in infants with congenital adrenal hyperplasia. Pediatr Radiol. 2002;32(2):130–7.

Hutson JM, Kearsey I. "Is the ovary in an inguinal hernia 'descended' like a testis or not". J Pediatr Surg, 2015;51(7):1197–200.

Kim JH, Kang E, Heo SH, et al. Diagnostic yield of targeted gene panel sequencing to identify the genetic etiology of disorders of sex development. Mol Cell Endocrinol. 2017;444:19–25.

Kimberley N, Hutson JM, Southwell BR, et al. Vaginal agenesis, the hymen, and associated anomalies. J Pediatr Adolesc Gynecol. 2012;25(1):54–8.

Kutteh WH, Santos-Ramos R, Ermel LD. Accuracy of ultrasonic detection of the uterus in normal newborn infants: implications for infants with ambiguous genitalia. Ultrasound Obstet Gynecol. 1995;5(2):109–13.

Li R, Vannitamby A, Meijer J, et al. Postnatal germ cell development during mini-puberty in the mouse does not require androgen receptor: implications for managing cryptorchidism. J Urol. 2015;193(4):1361–7.

Lombardo MV, Auyeung B, Pramparo T, et al. Sex-specific impact of prenatal androgens on social brain default mode subsystems. Mol Psychiatry. 2018:1–14.

Lopez-Hernandez B, Mendez JP, Coral-Vazquez RM, et al. Duplication of SOX9 associated with 46,XX ovotesticular disorder of sex development. Reprod Biomed Online. 2018;37(1):107–12.

Low Y, Hutson JM. Rules for clinical diagnosis in babies with ambiguous genitalia. J Paediatr Child Health. 2003;39(6):406–13.

Oberfield SE, Mondok A, Shahrivar F, et al. Clitoral size in full-term infants. Am J Perinatol. 1989;6(4):453–4.

Ogilvy-Stuart AL, Brain CE. Early assessment of ambiguous genitalia. Arch Dis Child. 2004;89(5):401–7.

Oppenheimer DA, Carroll BA, Yousem S. Sonography of the normal neonatal adrenal gland. Radiology. 1983;146(1):157–60.

Phillip M, De Boer C, Pilpel D, et al. Clitoral and penile sizes of full term newborns in two different ethnic groups. J Pediatr Endocrinol Metab. 1996;9(2):175–9.

Sivit CJ, Hung W, Taylor GA, et al. Sonography in neonatal congenital adrenal hyperplasia. AJR Am J Roentgenol. 1991;156(1):141–3.

Stranzinger E, Strouse PJ. Ultrasound of the pediatric female pelvis. Semin Ultrasound CT MR. 2008;29(2):98–113.

Tong SY, Hutson JM, Watts LM. Does testosterone diffuse down the wolffian duct during sexual differentiation? J Urol. 1996;155(6):2057–9.

DSD Later in Childhood

13

John M. Hutson and Sonia R. Grover

13.1 Introduction

When the external genitalia are atypical at birth, a diagnosis of DSD is usually suspected immediately, particularly if the appearance is really intermediate between typical male and typical female. There are situations, however, when initial presentation is much later in childhood. This occurs in two special circumstances. The first is when the external genital variation is so subtle that it escapes immediate attention at delivery and at the new-baby examination. The second situation is where the external genitalia appear typically formed, yet when events lead to the internal genitalia being examined, they are then found to be discordant with expectation. The common surgical scenarios are described in Table 13.1 and are discussed later. In a third major group of conditions, the DSD is recognised when the child develops precocious puberty. A recent review describes these clinical scenarios (Kearsey and Hutson, 2017).

13.2 Inguinal Hernia

Failure of the *processus vaginalis* to obliterate, leading to inguinal hernia, is a common occurrence requiring surgery in infancy. Because of testicular descent, the frequency in males is about tenfold higher than in females. In the latter, there is often a sliding hernia of peritoneum being pulled into the sac by pressure from the prolapsed bowel loops. As the attachment of the broad ligament to the lateral pelvic wall is close to the internal inguinal ring, the ovary (with adjacent Fallopian tube) is commonly found in the hernial sac. The anatomy demonstrates that this is not normal descent of the gonad, as seen in boys, as the ligament of the ovary, which is homologous with the cranial end of the gubernacular cord in males, passes back inside the inguinal canal to the uterine fundus. By contrast, in males, the gubernaculum attaches the caudal testis and epididymis directly to the bottom of the hernial sac (Fig. 13.1).

J. M. Hutson (✉)
Department of Urology, The Royal Children's Hospital, Melbourne, VIC, Australia

Murdoch Children's Research Institute, Melbourne, VIC, Australia

Department of Paediatrics, University of Melbourne, Melbourne, VIC, Australia
e-mail: john.hutson@rch.org.au

S. R. Grover
Department of Gynaecology, The Royal Children's Hospital, Melbourne, VIC, Australia

Murdoch Children's Research Institute, Melbourne, VIC, Australia

Department of Paediatrics, University of Melbourne, Melbourne, VIC, Australia
e-mail: Sonia.grover@rch.org.au

J. M. Hutson et al. (eds.), *Disorders|Differences of Sex Development*,
https://doi.org/10.1007/978-981-13-7864-5_13

Table 13.1 Surgical presentations of DSD during childhood

Clinical scenario	Likely DSD
1. Inguinal hernia	
Female with hernia containing testis	CAIS, GD
Male with hernia containing ovo-testis	O-T DSD
Male with hernia containing uterus	PMDS
Male with absent vas deferens	Cystic fibrosis/Rokitansky sequence
2. Cryptorchidism	
Uterus found with testis	PMDS
Ovo-testis	O-T DSD
Streak gonad ± Fallopian tube	MGD, GD
3. Laparoscopy	
Atypical/absent ovaries	GD, Turner syndrome
Absent uterus/fallopian tube	Rokitansky sequence/MRKH
4. Hypospadias	
Absent/atypical testis	O-T DSD, MGD
5. Cystoscopy	
Cavity in posterior urethra	46,XY DSD with retained Müllerian remnant

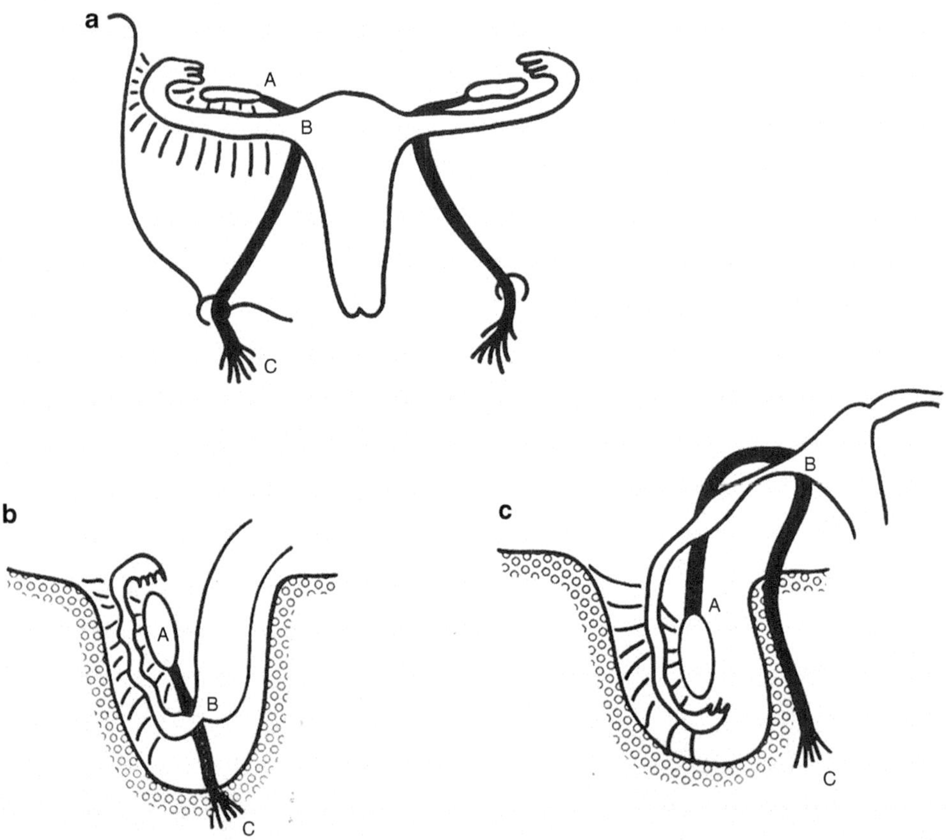

Fig. 13.1 (**a**) Schema showing normal anatomical arrangement of gubernaculum in a female, with proximal ligament of ovary attached to caudal pole of the ovary (A). The gubernaculum in the mid-region (B) is attached to the Fallopian tube where it joins the uterus. The distal gubernaculum forms the round ligament and ends just outside the inguinal canal (C). (**b**) If the ovary was normally descended in an inguinal hernia, the gubernacular attachments (A–B–C) would all be in alignment. (**c**) However, when ovaries are found inside an inguinal hernia sac, the gubernacular attachments show that the peritoneum has been pulled into the sac, so that the cranial, not the caudal, pole of the ovary comes out first, as the gubernaculum is not attached directly to the lower sac (A–C), as it would be in a male

13.2.1 DSD Identified at Herniotomy in Girls: Complete Androgen Insensitivity Syndrome

In 46,XY DSD caused by completely non-functional androgen receptors (complete androgen insensitivity syndrome—CAIS), the child has a typical female external genitalia phenotype. In addition, because the Müllerian ducts are fully regressed, the vagina is slightly shorter than normal and has a blind ending. The testes are the only internal genitalia, and they commonly reside inside the hernial sac in the inguinal region. The epididymis and vas deferens are absent in CAIS, as they require androgenic function for development. The gubernaculum (or genito-inguinal ligament) is more prominent than normal for the child's age and attaches the testis directly to the caudal end of the hernial sac (Fig. 13.2a, b). The migration phase of the gubernaculum to the scrotum is absent, as this requires androgens (Hutson 1985, 1986).

Are there any clues to the diagnosis before operation? In CAIS, the lack of functional androgen receptors means that the negative feedback on the hypothalamic-pituitary axis is absent, so that pituitary stimulation of the testes is increased. This leads to increased growth of the testes, which can be visibly larger than normal (Fig. 13.2a). Palpation of the enlarged gonad in the hernial sac may allow a preoperative diagnosis of CAIS to be suspected. If CAIS is suspected on the operating table, vaginoscopy can be performed to confirm the absence of a cervix at the top of the vagina. Opening the hernial sac will confirm a testis without a normal adjacent epididymis but with a prominent, gelatinous gubernaculum, which is the persistent "swelling reaction" of the first phase of testicular descent (androgens are needed to cause involution of the swelling reaction) (Fig. 13.2b).

Management depends on the timing of recognition of the DSD relative to the operation. Not uncommonly, this variation is only suspected intraoperatively when testes are found in a phenotypically female child who presented with a hernia. When confronted with this unexpectedly, a sensible approach is to biopsy the gonads and replace them within the abdomen and complete the inguinal herniotomy as planned. Photographs of the gonads are extremely useful for documentation and help in providing a full explanation to the family. Gonadal excision is not indicated and decisions around this should be left to a later date. Current evidence suggests that the risk of malig-

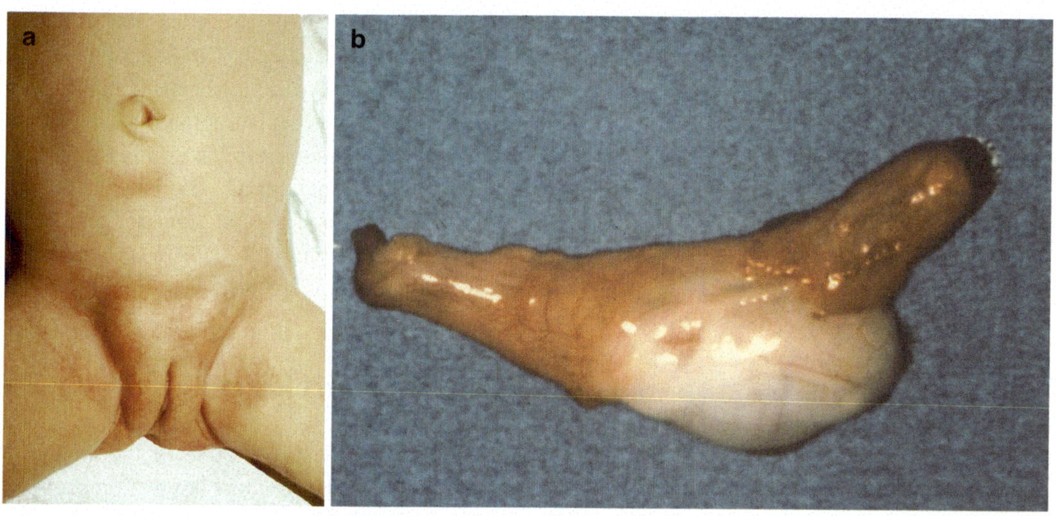

Fig. 13.2 (**a**) Inguinal hernia in a female infant with CAIS. The visible masses are the testes (which are enlarged because of lack of negative feedback on the hypothalamus) and the persisting enlarged swelling reaction of the gubernaculum. (**b**) Excised gonad in CAIS showing testis (with absent epididymis) and persistence of the swelling reaction in the gubernaculum. Excision of the testes is no longer performed in childhood due to recognition of the exceedingly low malignancy risk and the benefits of leaving the testes to produce endogenous hormones

nancy is very low prior to puberty (see Chap. 7). Discussion with the individual regarding the options of either monitoring the testes (with ultrasound, if the testes are now intra-abdominal) versus orchidectomy can be undertaken when the individual is older. It is now recognised that the potential benefits of endogenous hormone production exceed the risk of malignancy. Leaving the testes *in situ* allows normal induction of female puberty by aromatisation of the higher androgens into oestrogens, while the risk of testicular tumour is extremely low until after puberty, and even then it is not very high (Cassio 1990). Newer data assessing the risk of germ cell tumour development in AIS are emerging, although precise factors that influence risk in a given individual remain to be further defined (see Chap. 7).

Caution needs to be taken in distinguishing girls with CAIS from girls with MRKH. Inguinal hernias are more common in MRKH syndrome (Oppelt et al. 2006; Khen-Dunlop et al. 2007), where the uterus will also be absent and vagina may be absent or the length reduced.

13.2.2 DSD Found at Herniotomy in Boys

Several different anomalies of genital tract development can present first at inguinal herniotomy in an otherwise typical-looking boy (Table 13.1).

A common problem is the inability of the surgeon to identify the vas deferens during isolation of the hernial sac, raising the question of whether the vas is either truly absent or it has been transected accidentally. A simple way to resolve this issue at open herniotomy is to stretch open the internal inguinal ring (which by definition is away from where the initial dissection of the spermatic cord has been done), so that the intra-abdominal vas deferens can then be identified easily if it is present. If the herniotomy is done laparoscopically, then the surgeon will notice that there is no vas deferens exiting through the internal inguinal ring.

Absence of the vas deferens is seen in two conditions: the Rokitansky sequence and cystic fibrosis (CF). In the Rokitansky sequence, the Wolffian duct migration to the embryonic cloaca is deficient, leading to absence of the vas deferens to a greater or lesser extent. If there was complete agenesis of the Wolffian duct, then the ipsilateral epididymis will also be absent. Müllerian duct migration to the cloaca stops at the same level, as there is no guidance without the Wolffian duct, but as the Müllerian ducts regress, their caudal deficiency is concealed. By contrast, the ipsilateral ureteric bud cannot form if the caudal Wolffian duct is missing, leading to agenesis of the ipsilateral kidney. Confirmation of the Rokitansky sequence can be obtained by renal ultrasound to show a single, contralateral kidney. During laparoscopy, the surgeon may observe that the ipsilateral ureter is absent if the boy has the Rokitansky-sequence anomaly.

The second genital variation associated with unexpected absence of the vas deferens at inguinal herniotomy is a variant of the CF gene (Sung and Hutson 2003). Bilateral congenital absence of the vas deferens (BCAVD) occurs in males carrying variants in the CF gene, some of whom may have clinical features of cystic fibrosis, but most appear otherwise completely normal, with no chronic lung disease or pancreatic enzyme deficiency. In these boys, the anomaly is always bilateral, and the renal ultrasound is normal (Sung and Hutson 2003).

Rare occurrences of DSD identification during herniotomy include the finding of an ovotestis rather than a typical testis inside the hernial sac, or the presence of a Fallopian tube and small uterus in a boy presumed to have simple cryptorchidism and inguinal hernia. The latter situation is one of the common presentations for persistent Müllerian duct syndrome (PMDS), which is described in detail in the next section.

13.3 Cryptorchidism

Failed testicular descent is one of the common features of DSD, but in most boys, it presents as an isolated difference in a baby with no other obvious variation. This is also the rare presentation for PMDS, where there is an impalpable undescended testis (uni- or bilateral) in the presence of completely normal virilisation of the external genitalia. Where there is a palpable mass in the inguinal region, it can be a unilateral cryptorchid testis with attached Fallopian tube and infantile uterus, also known as "*hernia uteri inguinalis*." An alternative finding is that the inguinal mass turns out to be both testes within the tunica vaginalis along with uterus and tubes, which is one of the presentations of transverse testicular ectopia (Fig. 13.3). In these cases, the gubernaculum is abnormally elongated so that the testes and internal genitalia ducts can be delivered easily right out of the abdominal wound in a way not possible in either typical males or females (Hutson et al. 1987; Hutson and Lopez-Marambio 2017). This increased mobility may also lead to torsion of the genital tracts with loss of both testes, a situation that is well described in PMDS (Josso et al. 1993).

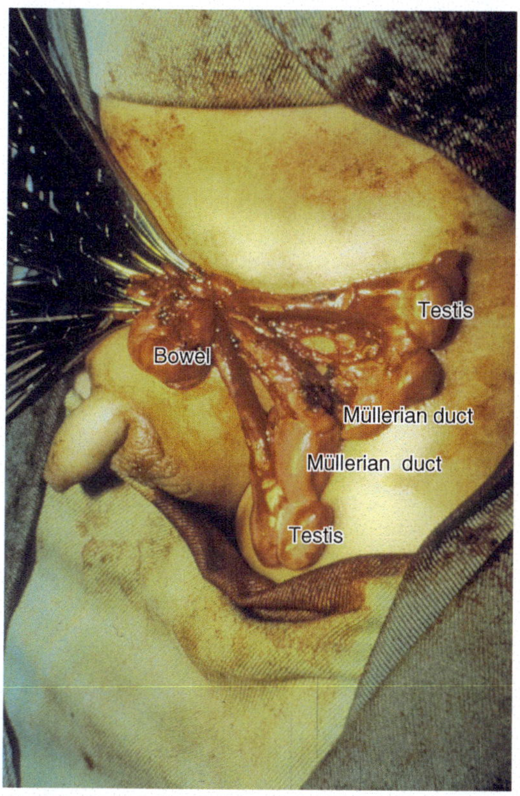

Fig. 13.3 Transverse testicular ectopia as part of persistent Müllerian duct syndrome (PMIDS), presenting with inguinal hernia (containing two testes, uterus and tubes) and cryptorchidism (Reproduced with permission from Hutson et al. (1987))

Where unilateral cryptorchidism is associated with hypospadias and bifid scrotum, there is a high possibility that the undescended gonad may be an ovo-testis or even an ovary (in ovo-testicular DSD), or an undifferentiated streak gonad (in 45,X/46,XY mixed gonadal dysgenesis). Once a DSD has been identified, then appropriate management of the child including endocrine work up will be required. Usually male sex of rearing will be retained, and the impalpable gonad and genital ducts (if present) will be managed accordingly.

13.4 DSD Found at Laparoscopy

Laparoscopic examination of the internal genitalia may be a planned procedure. This would not only be the case for individuals with 46,XY DSD, who have a female phenotype with presumed streak or dysgenetic gonads, but also for those with sex chromosome DSD with 45,X/46,XY Turner syndrome, where some sex chromosome mosaicism is present (Turner-Ullrich variant). In both of these cases, the dysgenetic streak gonads need to be removed because of the risk of malignancy in Y-chromosomal cells (see also Chap. 7, 8 and 17).

In some individuals, however, atypical internal genitalia may be found unexpectedly during laparoscopic surgery for other problems. Genital anomalies in phenotypic girls include absent uterus or streak gonads, while in boys there may be genital duct anomalies, such as absent vas deferens or the presence of uterus/Fallopian tube (PMDS). Genital duct anomalies are seen in females with the Rokitansky sequence, and as in boys, the surgeon should check to see if the ipsilateral ureter is missing, indicating Mayer-Rokitansky-Küster-Hauser syndrome type 2.

One difficulty in infancy is that the uterus may be so small that it may be missed on laparoscopy, particularly if the anatomy is distorted by other pathology. The child may be labelled as having uterine agenesis, when at puberty there is normal commencement of menses.

13.5 DSD Found with Hypospadias

Hypospadias is a variation of development of the penis, where the urethral meatus is on the ventral surface of the penis, rather than at the tip of the glans. Implicit in the name is the assumption that the baby is a boy. In some instances of hypospadias the baby actually has a DSD. In such cases, there is more distal hypospadias (perineal/penoscrotal urethral opening), atypical development of the scrotum and/or testicular descent which should alert the medical attendant that the baby is likely to have a more complex disorder than simple "hypospadias" alone (Tong et al. 1996).

So when is "hypospadias" not hypospadias, but a possible DSD? A useful rule of thumb for this is to only use "*hypospadias*" as the initial diagnosis when the scrotum is typically fused and contains two testes. Any variant of scrotal fusion or gonadal descent in a baby with apparent hypospadias needs referral and investigation for a DSD. Such babies may have gonadal dysgenesis or ovo-testicular DSD, or they may be significantly virilised females with 21-OH deficiency CAH (Prader 4–5) (Scheffer et al. 1988).

If an older infant presents for management of their "hypospadias", full investigation is required if the scrotum is bifid or testes are not fully descended. Tests should include hormonal studies and karyotype, as well as a urogenital sinugram ± cystoscopy, as deemed appropriate.

13.6 DSD Found at Cystoscopy

Occasionally, the diagnosis of DSD will not be made until cystoscopy is done in a baby with "hypospadias" and bifid scrotum. The Müllerian remnant opening has several characteristic appearances. In some children, there is a visible opening somewhere between the bulb of the urethra and the site of the verumontanum in a male, through which a ureteric catheter or the cystoscope itself can be passed (Fig. 13.4). Another typical appearance is to find mucosal folds or polyps in the posterior urethra that look like seaweed floating underwater. This is the hymen, and the vaginal opening will always be found in the middle of these folds. The size of the retained Müllerian remnant will depend on the degree of virilisation in these children, who are most likely to have 46,XY DSD.

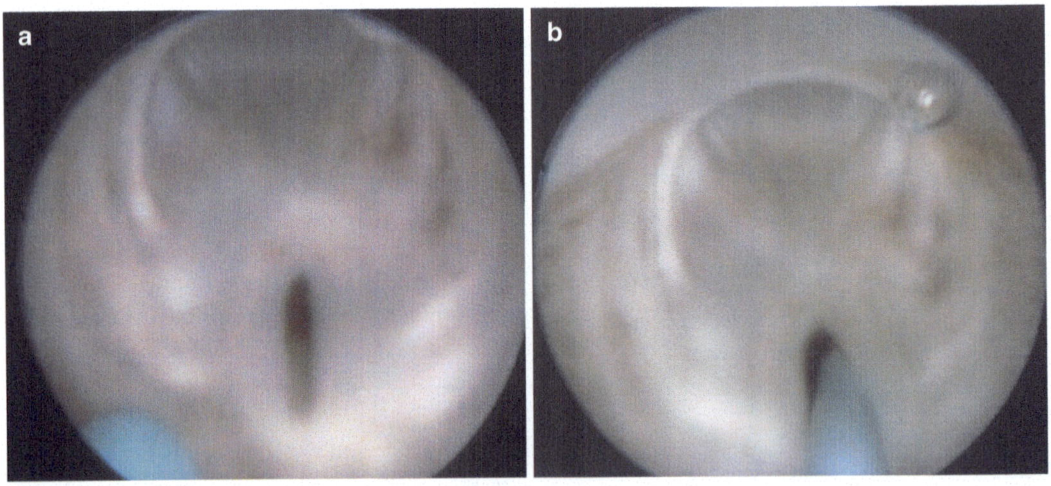

Fig. 13.4 (**a**) Cystoscopic appearance of persisting Müllerian remnant opening into the posterior urethra. (**b**) Ureteric catheter passed through opening to measure length of retained Müllerain remnant

13.7 Precocious Puberty

One presentation for DSD that is not discovered incidentally at surgery is precocious puberty. The child presents with progressive signs of secondary sex characteristics as well as a recent growth spurt. The diagnosis may be hypothalamic, pituitary or gonadal disorders or tumours, but in the context of slightly atypical external genitalia, it is most commonly 46,XX DSD with CAH (see Chap. 16).

Acknowledgments With thanks and acknowledgement to Professor Garry L. Warne AM who was one of the authors of this chapter in edition 1.

References

Cassio A. Incidence of intratubular germ cell neoplasia in androgen insensitivity syndrome. Acta Endocrinol. 1990;123:416–22.

Hutson JM. A biphasic model for the hormonal control of testicular descent. Lancet. 1985;2(8452):419–21.

Hutson JM. Testicular feminization: a model for testicular descent in mice and men. J Pediatr Surg. 1986;21(3):195–8.

Hutson JM, Lopez-Marambio FA. The possible role of AMH in shortening the gubernacular cord in testicular descent: A reappraisal of the evidence. J Pediatr Surg. 2017;52(10):1656–60.

Hutson J, Chow C, Ng W. Persistent müllerian duct syndrome with transverse testicular extopia. an experiemnt of nature with clues for understanding testicular descent. Pediatr Surg Int. 1987;2:191–4.

Josso N, Cate RL, Picard JY, et al. Anti-Müllerian hormone: the Jost factor. Recent Prog Horm Res. 1993;48:1-59.

Kearsey I, Hutson JM. Disorders of sex development (DSD): not only babies with ambiguous genitalia. A practical guide for surgeons. Pediatr Surg Int. 2017;33(3):355–61. https://doi.org/10.1007/s00383-016-4036-5. Epub 2016 Dec 18.

Khen-Dunlop N, Lortat-Jacob S, Thibaud E, et al. Rokitansky syndrome: clinical experience and results of sigmoid vaginoplasty in 23 young girls. J Urol. 2007;177(3):1107–11.

Oppelt P, Renner SP, Kellermann A, et al. Clinical aspects of Mayer-Rokitansky-Kuester-Hauser syndrome: recommendations for clinical diagnosis and staging. Hum Reprod. 2006;21(3):792–7.

Scheffer I, Hutson J, Warne G, et al. Extreme virilisation in patients with congenital adrenal hyperplasis fails to induce descent of the ovary. Pediatr Surg Int. 1988;3:165–8.

Sung V, Hutson JM. A novel way to diagnose cystic fibrosis in the neonate with a bowel obstruction and possible meconium ileus. J Paediatr Child Health. 2003;39(9):720.

Tong SY, Donaldson K, Hutson JM. When is hypospadias not hypospadias? Med J Aust. 1996;164(3):153–4.

14 The Adolescent or Young Adult with DSD

John M. Hutson and Sonia R. Grover

14.1 Introduction

Most patients with DSD present at birth, in infancy or early childhood when genital anatomy is noted to be atypical. However, there is a group where the presentation of a significant DSD is delayed until teenage years or young adulthood. The conditions can be subdivided into two broad groups, depending on the sex of rearing (Tables 14.1, 14.2 and 14.3). Co-ordinated team management is important to ensure that the psychological as well as the physical issues are addressed (Liao et al. 2010) (see Chap. 20).

Table 14.1 Presentations of DSD at puberty/young adulthood in phenotypic females

Clinical scenario	Likely DSD
1. Precocious puberty	46, XX DSD with untreated CAH
2. Virilisation at puberty	Severe under-virilisation in 46,XY DSD with PAIS, androgen synthesis defects or 5α RD2
3. Enlarging, tender swelling in groin	Inguinal testes enlarging in early adolescence in CAIS/ severe PAIS/17βHSD3 with Müllerian agenesis and testes in the inguinal hernias
4. Delayed puberty	Gonadal dysgenesis/ Hypothalamic-pituitary disorders
5. Primary amenorrhoea	Müllerian duct/vaginal agenesis CAIS
6. Deficient secondary sex characters	(a) Turner syndrome (b) Deficient axillary/pubic hair with CAIS
7. Cyclical abdominal pains ± pelvic mass	Müllerian tract anomalies/ Unilateral Müllerian duct agenesis/atresia (Rokitansky sequence)
8. Problems with sexual intercourse	Micro-perforate vaginal septum/Müllerian agenesis
9. Infertility	Müllerian agenesis Late-onset CAH
10. Secondary amenorrhoea	Mosaic Turner syndrome/ other causes of POI

J. M. Hutson (✉)
Department of Urology, The Royal Children's Hospital, Melbourne, VIC, Australia

Murdoch Children's Research Institute, Melbourne, VIC, Australia

Department of Paediatrics, University of Melbourne, Melbourne, VIC, Australia
e-mail: john.hutson@rch.org.au

S. R. Grover
Department of Gynaecology, The Royal Children's Hospital, Melbourne, VIC, Australia

Murdoch Children's Research Institute, Melbourne, VIC, Australia

Department of Paediatrics, University of Melbourne, Melbourne, VIC, Australia
e-mail: sonia.grover@rch.org.au

J. M. Hutson et al. (eds.), *Disorders|Differences of Sex Development*,
https://doi.org/10.1007/978-981-13-7864-5_14

Table 14.2 Presentations of DSD at puberty/young adulthood in phenotypic males

Clinical scenario	Likely DSD
1. Cyclical haematuria	46,XX DSD CAH Prader 4–5 raised as male
2. Abdominal/pelvic mass with absent testis	Chromosomal DSD 45,X/46,XY MGD with retained streak gonad and tumour
3. Deficient/failed pubertal development	Gonadal dysgenesis Partial AIS Hypothalamic—pituitary axis disorders Klinefelter syndrome 47,XXY
4. Infertility	Anatomical anomalies of vas deferens

Table 14.3 DSD presenting in adolescence in phenotypic females

	Condition	Presentation
46,XY DSD	Complete AIS	Primary amenorrhoea No axillary/public hair
46,XY DSD	Partial AIS (with female phenotype)	Primary amenorrhoea Some axillary/pubic hair
46,XY DSD	Complete gonadal dysgenesis (Swyer)	Absent puberty Pelvic mass
46,XY DSD	Complete/partial testosterone synthesis defects (e.g. 17β-HSD3 deficiency)	Unexpected virilisation
45,X 45,X/46,XY	Turner syndrome	Delayed puberty or delayed menarche. (Presence of Y chromosome indicates risk of germ cell cancer—with potential for presentation with pelvic mass)
46,XX DSD	Non-classical CAH 21-OH deficiency Or 11β-OH deficiency	Hirsutism Infertility
46,XX DSD	Müllerian agenesis	Primary amenorrhoea (In developing countries potential for presentation with primary infertility)

14.2 Phenotypic Females

There are numerous disorders of the hypothalamic-pituitary-gonadal axis that cause precocious puberty, but they are usually associated with completely typical female external genitalia. These conditions are not the subject of this chapter, but, rather, we focus on those diagnoses where sexual development is atypical. The most important condition is congenital adrenal hyperplasia (CAH) in a girl with minimal virilisation (Prader-Willi 1–2) where the minor genital differences went unnoticed at birth, female sex was assigned and no treatment given.

14.2.1 Precocious Puberty

Severe salt-wasting forms of CAH usually presents at 1–3 weeks of age with adrenal crisis (often in the second or third week after birth), or more severe virilisation, so the delayed presentation of CAH in late childhood or early adolescence with precocious puberty is likely to be in the less severe non-salt-wasting forms.

14.2.2 Virilisation at Puberty

Many rare conditions can present with virilisation of an individual at puberty. Usually, they are manifestations of 46,XY DSD with severe under-virilisation prenatally, so female sex of rearing occurred without any concerns about sexual development. Partial androgen insensitivity syndrome (PAIS) has usually been diagnosed earlier in infancy, but less obvious genital virilisation may have gone unnoticed in some patients, who then develop some further clitoral enlargement at puberty.

Variations in androgen biosynthesis quite often present with virilisation at puberty. Prenatally, the atypical enzyme was unable to produce enough androgens to trigger typical virilisation. At puberty, however, the growth of the testis is significant, and now, the amount of testosterone produced is sufficient to trigger some virilisation. A deficiency in 17β-hydroxysteroid dehydrogenase-3 (17βHSD-3) (OMIM no. 264300) is the most common anomaly in testosterone biosynthesis that causes 46,XY DSD. Patients with 17βHSD-3 deficiency have a range of presentations, depending on the severity of the enzyme dysfunction. There may be clitoral enlargement (Fig. 14.1), excess body hair, excess body odour or more severe virilisation with development of a more typically masculine body shape or even gender change to a male role (George et al. 2011).

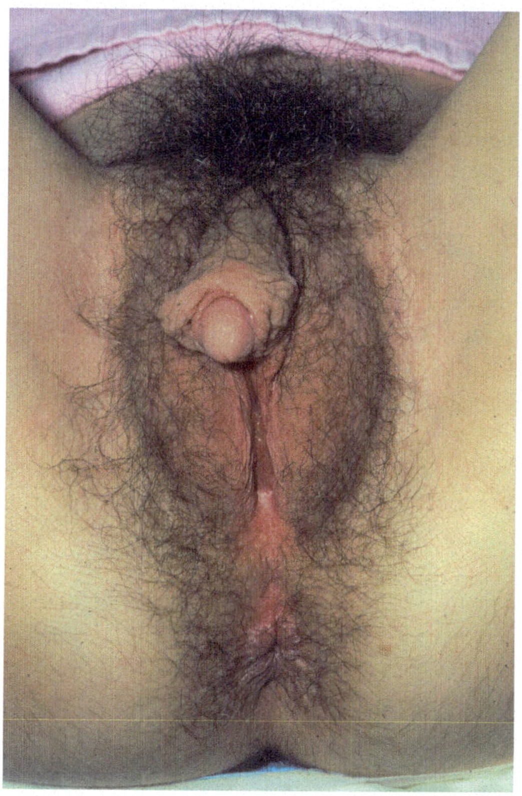

Fig. 14.1 Clitoromegaly in a pubertal girl with 46, XY DSD and 17β HSD-3 deficiency. Excess androgen exposure is only recent with the onset of puberty. The introitus is otherwise normal because the level of androgen production in utero was too low to cause labial/midline fusion. There are no testes descended into the labia

One classic situation of female-to-male change at puberty is in 5α-reductase-2 deficiency, although this will usually be already known in infancy because of atypical genitalia (Imperato-McGinley et al. 1974). At puberty, there is further virilisation, but usually there is no gynaecomastia, and pubic, axillary and facial hair is reduced. The typical masculine hairline recession at the temple is absent. On rectal examination, the prostate is deficient.

14.2.3 Groin Lump

Because the first phase of testicular descent is independent of androgenic function, those adolescents with 46,XY DSD caused by androgen blockade or deficiency may first present at puberty with enlargement of inguinal testes. At birth, the testes are usually in the inguinal canal or just outside the external ring, and at puberty, their growth may lead to tender masses palpable in the groin, which initially might be mistaken for an incarcerated hernia (Fig. 14.2) Absence of other secondary sex characteristics or some minor enlargement of the clitoris would usually alert the clinician to the diagnosis (Ahmed et al. 2000).

A slightly shortened vagina in association with the groin lumps may lead to the impression of a diagnosis of complete androgen insen-

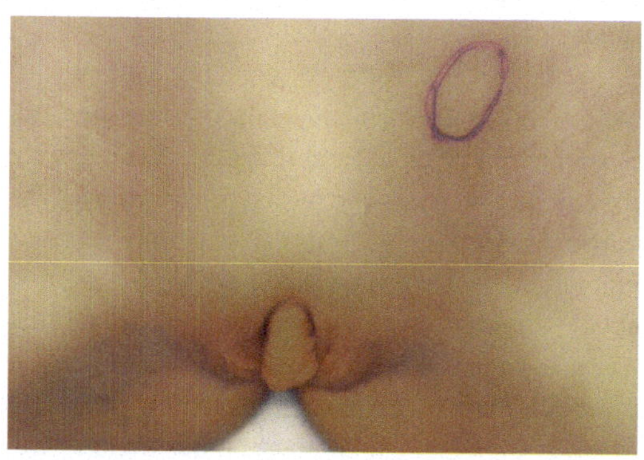

Fig. 14.2 A girl with PAIS, where clitoral enlargement and tender groin lump (marked on skin) was first noticed when pubertal development was delayed

sitivity syndrome (CAIS), but great caution is needed as there is a higher rate of inguinal hernias reported in girls with vaginal agenesis (Oppelt et al. 2006; Khen-Dunlop et al. 2007). Confirmation of these diagnoses with appropriate further testing is essential.

14.2.4 Delayed Puberty

Where there is complete gonadal dysgenesis with either XX or XY chromosomes (e.g. 46,XY DSD with complete gonadal dysgenesis (previously known as Swyer syndrome), or 46, XX complete gonadal dysgenesis), the external phenotype is typical female and the internal genitalia are concordant, although the uterus remains prepubertal and small. In both circumstances, there is delayed onset of pubertal development with primary amenorrhoea. Ultrasonography will confirm the underdeveloped female genital tract, and the gonads will be completely undescended and commonly non-functional streaks. Care is needed in interpreting the ultrasound reports in the presence of gonadal dysgenesis, as the uterus will be a very small structure due to the lack of oestrogen stimulation. Ultrasonography, MRI and even laparoscopy findings have incorrectly reported "no uterus" in these young women. Hormone levels will show absent oestradiol and increased plasma FSH and LH. Gonadectomy will be required, usually by laparoscopy, for 46,XY complete gonadal dysgenesis because of the significantly elevated cancer risk (see Chap. 7).

In the 46,XX form of gonadal dysgenesis, there may be sensorineural hearing loss present in about 10% of cases, and this is associated with an autosomal recessive inheritance when it is known as Perrault syndrome. Distinction between premature ovarian insufficiency (POI) is not always clear if ovarian insufficiency or failure has occurred early. Investigation needs to cover other potential causes for POI, including Fragile-X testing, and autoantibodies looking for evidence of an autoimmune origin for the ovarian failure.

14.2.5 Primary Amenorrhoea

Some patients with 46,XX chromosomes and normal ovaries on ultrasonography will have complete or partial agenesis of the Müllerian ducts and vagina. In its simplest form, this may be an imperforate hymen that was not diagnosed with mucocolpos postnatally and is now re-presenting with haematocolpos (see below for cyclic abdominal pain).

In more complex forms, the vagina and/or uterus may be absent, so that there is no haematometrocolpos. In girls with these Müllerian anomalies, the remainder of pubertal development including axillary and pubic hair is typical.

It is not uncommon for the Müllerian agenesis to be the last of a series of previously diagnosed problems to be recognised, and a careful review for the other anomalies is often instructive. Renal anomalies are reported in up to 40% of girls, with unilateral renal agenesis making up half of these anomalies, consistent with the Rokitansky sequence. Associated skeletal anomalies are also reported in 10% of girls (Creatsas 2009), and up to 10% of girls with vaginal agenesis will have evidence of having their Müllerian anomalies as part of the Klippel-Feil syndrome (where there is fusion of cervical vertebrae) (Willemsen 1982), or part of MURCS association (Müllerian agenesis, Renal agenesis, Cervicothoracic Somite anomalies).

The combination of cardiac anomalies and particular hand anomalies is Holt-Oram syndrome (HOS). The association between this and vaginal agenesis has been reported (Fakih et al. 1987; Ulrich et al. 2004). Likewise, the combination of cardiac, hand and orofacial clefting is known as the velo-cardio-facial syndrome (VCFS) (Cheroki et al. 2006). For both of these conditions, there is evidence that there may be recognised gene mutations. For HOS, the mutations are in the gene coding for T-box transcription factor TBX5 located on chromosome 12q24 (Böhm et al. 2008) and for VCFS, the VCFS region of chromosome 22q11.1. Efforts to further delineate potential genetic mutations in Müllerian anomalies with these conditions, where there is a known genetic mutation by the searching for major deletions or duplications in these regions, has failed to show any abnormality (van Lingen et al. 1998; Cheroki et al. 2006; Drummond et al. 2008; Hofstetter et al. 2008).

The clinical distinction between CAIS and Müllerian agenesis, where both patients will have typical breast development, is the recognition of the scant pubic and axillary hair in the former. Nevertheless, the presence of other adolescent issues such as an eating disorder or participation in high-level athletics or sporting competition will impact on hypothalamic hormone production and peripheral adipose tissue conversion of testosterone to oestrogens. Thus, breast development, pubic hair and axillary hair may be influenced by factors other than the DSD and may make a clinical diagnosis difficult.

14.2.6 Secondary Sex Characteristics

Limited secondary sex characteristics are seen in most cases of 45,X DSD with Turner syndrome (TS) and other causes of streak ovaries. Gonadal failure can be complete, but in many young women with TS and other causes of POI, the gonadal failure may be post-pubertal, yet premenarchal. Specific reduction in pubic and axillary hair is seen in 46,XY DSD with CAIS and can be the presenting complaint.

14.2.7 Cyclical Abdominal Pain

Müllerian duct development is normally associated with caudal fusion to create the uterus and vagina. Failure of this fusion produces a double vagina but normally no interruption in menstrual flow. However, in some circumstances, the bifid genital tract is associated with ipsilateral absence of the kidney and lower ipsilateral vagina and will present with an obstructed hemi-vagina at the onset of puberty. This is a characteristic presentation for the Rokitansky embryological anomaly (Masse et al. 2009; Acien et al. 2010; Takagi et al. 2010).

Transverse vaginal septa may consist of a thick membrane across the vagina which obstructs menstrual outflow. The loss of a larger segment of the vagina is usually considered a vaginal atresia with these segments extending over 4–6 cm.

Cervical agenesis can occur in association with vaginal agenesis, where the entire lower Müllerian tract is absent, but a uterus, or one or both uterine horns, may be present, or alternatively, there can be an isolated absence of the cervix in the presence of a normal uterus and normal vagina. There have been several reports of successful anastomoses of the uterus without a cervix to the vagina (Deffarges et al. 2001).

The terminology around rudimentary uterine horns is confusing, particularly now that uterine horns with an absent cervix are successfully being anastomosed and positive pregnancy outcomes reported (Deffarges et al. 2001). In general, rudimentary uterine horns represent varying degrees of Müllerian agenesis and can occur with or without a corresponding unicornuate uterus. The rudimentary horn can be communicating or non-communicating (with the corresponding unicornuate uterus), and cavitated or non-cavitated, depending on whether the process of canalisation of the Müllerian structure has occurred. In the absence of canalisation, there is no cyclic pain, and the detection may be incidental on imaging or at surgery, or alternatively, an ectopic pregnancy into this horn may occur (Jayasinghe et al. 2005).

The non-communicating-cavitated horn usually leads to presentation with increasing dysmenorrhoea (where there is a corresponding unicornuate normal system). The cavitated horn without a corresponding unicornuate uterus will have its presentation as cyclic abdominal pain in an individual with primary amenorrhoea.

These conditions, where the uterus is present, but there is atypical development of the vagina or cervix, are not generally considered DSD, presumably, as the diagnosis does not usually challenge the fertility potential of the young woman, and there are no other features of atypical sex development. The definitions are still unclear, as those women who have their rudimentary uterine horns removed, or those who have their uterine horn in the setting of cervical agenesis removed, are in the same clinical predicament as those with uterine agenesis.

14.2.8 Difficulties with Sexual Intercourse

Some women with transverse septa have micro-perforations or tracts through the septum, and do not present with cyclic pain and a haematocolpos, but rather with pain or difficulty with sexual intercourse. Examination with a speculum reveals a smooth upper vagina with no evidence of a cervix—but with a history of regular menses. An ultrasound scan, particularly at the time of menstruation, will clarify the findings and help to define the thickness of the septum. Although other conditions with a slightly shorter vagina, such as vaginal agenesis or CAIS, may have symptoms associated with sexual activity, they are not usually the presenting symptoms for these DSD.

14.2.9 Infertility

Some young women with vaginal and/or uterine agenesis will present with primary infertility—with their diagnosis of primary amenorrhoea having been ignored or unrecognised. This occurs most frequently in developing countries where marriage occurs in the mid-teens, and the issue of primary amenorrhoea has not been addressed. In this case, the vagina may be normal—due to sexual activity having resulted in the creation of the vagina with a pressure dilator effect.

In the young woman presenting with infertility, hirsuitism and oligomenorrhoea need to be considered for the diagnosis of late-onset CAH or non-classical CAH. There may be no other evidence of virilisation. Measurement of serum 17-OH progesterone will allow this diagnosis to be made.

14.2.10 Secondary Amenorrhoea

Gonadal failure related to TS may be delayed. This is more likely in young women with the mosaic form of TS or one of the iso-chromosome variations. Additionally, women with POI may present with secondary amenorrhoea associated with ovarian failure. High FSH and low oestradiol will be found. The uterine volume will reduce in size with increasing duration of the secondary hypo-oestrogenic state. A low AMH will also be present, confirming the low or absent ovarian follicle reserve.

14.3 Males

14.3.1 Haematuria

Blood in the urine is caused by a range of urinary tract disorders, but rarely, this may be the presentation for 46, XX DSD with CAH, where the degree of virilisation was so great that the baby was raised as a boy. At puberty, which is often precocious, masculinisation is present with secondary short stature. Despite the high androgens, the female internal genital tract persists (in the absence of AMH) and responds to oestrogens from the ovary. Menstruation then leads to cyclical haematuria until the diagnosis is made.

14.3.2 Abdominal/Pelvic Tumour

This may be the presentation of 45,X/46, XY with mixed gonadal dysgenesis where the streak gonad has been left in the abdomen and then has become malignant. Although this seems an unlikely scenario, an intra-abdominal streak gonad may be missed if laparoscopy has not been performed, and an inguinal exploration reveals no testis in a boy with "hypospadias" and one descended testis. In this case, it may have been assumed that the testis was "vanishing", following perinatal torsion. Gonadoblastoma is the usual neoplasm in the dysgenetic gonad containing a Y-chromosomal cell line, and adolescence is a frequent time of presentation, although gonadoblastoma is sometimes already present in infancy (Cools et al. 2006).

14.3.3 Altered Pubertal Development

Limited pubertal virilisation is caused by a range of conditions, from XY gonadal dysgenesis and PAIS through to hypothalamic disorders and primary mixed chromosomal DSD (aneuploidy), such as 47,XXY Klinefelter syndrome.

14.3.4 Infertility

Some DSD have no atypical phenotype or physiology in childhood, but present later in life with male infertility. It is not the intention to provide an exhaustive description here, but several conditions will be highlighted that relate to the vas deferens. In complete bilateral agenesis of the vas deferens (CBAVD), pubertal development is normal, and the man may present to an infertility clinic because of inadequate ejaculate (Stern 1997). This condition is now recognised to be caused by mutations in the cystic fibrosis gene (Δ508) which codes for a chloride channel protein in the cell membrane. These men have none of the other features of cystic fibrosis (CF), although boys with clinical CF all have atresia of the caudal epididymis and vas deferens (Plyler et al. 2019), which can be confirmed by absence of the caudal epididymis and vas deferens, but a normal head of the epididymis on physical examination.

The distal connections of the vas deferens into the ejaculatory duct and associated seminal vesicles are nearly always abnormal in patients with inadequate androgen production or insensitivity. As the Wolffian duct is developing between 8–12 weeks of gestation, it must be exposed to adequate androgen levels to continue differentiating. Where the androgen effects are impaired, it is its distal end which undergoes involution, leaving a near-normal epididymis and proximal vas, but a blind-ending distal vas deferens. Often when there is concomitant deficiency of AMH, the caudal Müllerian duct is preserved and the distal vas deferens enters into a hypoplastic Müllerian remnant (Ben-Meir and Hutson 2005). Normal maturation and transport of sperm is interrupted and the "plumbing" variation almost always leads to infertility. Fortunately, assisted reproductive technology can bypass this anomaly in some patients who have viable spermatogonia in their testis or epididymis.

14.4 Imaging

14.4.1 Imaging in Girls During Late Childhood and Early Adolescence

Appreciating the impact of oestrogens on the size of Müllerian structures is very important when attempting to interpret the findings in girls during childhood and early adolescence. Under oestrogenic influence, the Müllerian structures are usually readily identified and where there is an endometrium present, a well-defined endometrial stripe will be visible. In the absence of oestrogen, the uterine structures are small and the endometrial strip may not be apparent at all.

Thus, an MRI and ultrasound scan performed in this older age group, particularly in girls presenting with primary amenorrhoea, need careful interpretation. If the teenager is also pre-pubertal, the uterus will still be a very small structure on MRI and ultrasound and can easily be missed or considered a rudimentary structure. Great care is needed in assuming the absence of the uterus and vagina in a pre-pubertal girl when no oestrogen exposure has occurred. This includes girls with 46,XY gonadal dysgenesis, 46,XX gonadal dysgenesis or hypothalamic hypogonadism, who may all have incorrect reports of absent Müllerian structures.

Clarification of the Müllerian structures in girls with complex anomalies such as cloaca can also be challenging and often joint meetings between radiologists and gynaecologists will be useful. In general, in the post-pubertal girl with a complex anomaly, presenting with pain, thick-walled pelvic (although potentially abdominal) structures which are fluid filled (blood) will be the uterus. If there is a relatively thinner-walled, blood-filled space below this then this will be the vagina. The cervix may not be readily identifiable—apart from some potential hour-glass narrowing. The presence of a thin walled blood-filled space below the uterus implies that the cervix is present. A fluid-filled structure, often snake like in shape, with internal septations is likely to be a haematosalpinx. Additionally, a complex mass representing an ovary with endometriomas may also be present. In girls with cloacal anomalies, the presence of obstructed Müllerian components often does not correlate with the presence or absence of renal anomalies.

Acknowledgements With acknowledgement of Prof. Garry L. Warne AM, who contributed to the first edition.

References

Acien P, Galan F, Manchon I, et al. Hereditary renal dysplasia, pulmonary hypoplasia and Mayer-Rokitansky-Kuster-Hauser (MRKH) syndrome: a case report. Orphanet J Rare Dis. 2010;5:6.

Ahmed SF, Khwaja O, Hughes IA. The role of a clinical score in the assessment of ambiguous genitalia. BJU Int. 2000;85(1):120–4.

Ben-Meir DB, Hutson JM. The anatomy of the caudal vas deferens in patients with a genital anomaly. J Pediatr Urol. 2005;1(5):349–54.

Böhm J, Heinritz W, Craig A, et al. Functional analysis of the novel TBX5 c.1333delC mutation resulting in an extended TBX5 protein. BMC Med Genet. 2008;9(88)

Cheroki C, Krepischi-Santos AC, Rosenberg C, et al. Report of a del22q11 in a patient with Mayer-Rokitansky-Kuster-Hauser (MRKH) anomaly and exclusion of WNT-4, RAR-gamma, and RXR-alpha as major genes determining MRKH anomaly in a study of 25 affected women. Am J Med Genet A. 2006;140(12):1339–42.

Cools M, Drop SL, Wolffenbuttel KP, et al. Germ cell tumors in the intersex gonad: old paths, new directions, moving frontiers. Endocr Rev. 2006;27(5):468–84.

Creatsas G. Creatsas modification of Williams vaginoplasty: more than 20 years experience. Fertil Steril. 2009;92(6):e61.

Deffarges JV, Haddad B, Musset R, et al. Utero-vaginal anastomosis in women with uterine cervix atresia: long-term follow-up and reproductive performance. A study of 18 cases. Hum Reprod. 2001;16(8):1722–5.

Drummond JB, Reis FM, Boson WL, et al. Molecular analysis of the WNT4 gene in 6 patients with Mayer-Rokitansky-Kuster-Hauser syndrome. Fertil Steril. 2008;90(3):857–9.

Fakih MH, Williamson HO, Seymour EQ, et al. Concurrence of the Holt-Oram syndrome and the Rokitansky-Kuster-Hauser syndrome. A case report. J Reprod Med. 1987;32(7):549–50.

George MM, Sinha S, Mamkin I, et al. Isolated mild clitoral hypertrophy may reveal 46,XY disorders of sex development in infancy due to 17betaHSD-3 defect confirmed by molecular analysis. Gynecol Endocrinol. 2011;27:890–4.

Hofstetter G, Concin N, Marth C, et al. Genetic analyses in a variant of Mayer-Rokitansky-Kuster-Hauser syndrome (MURCS association). Wien Klin Wochenschr. 2008;120(13-14):435–9.

Imperato-McGinley J, Guerrero L, Gautier T, et al. Steroid 5alpha-reductase deficiency in man: an inherited form of male pseudohermaphroditism. Science. 1974;186(4170):1213–5.

Jayasinghe Y, Rane A, Stalewski H, et al. The presentation and early diagnosis of the rudimentary uterine horn. Obstet Gynecol. 2005;105(6):1456–67.

Khen-Dunlop N, Lortat-Jacob S, Thibaud E, et al. Rokitansky syndrome: clinical experience and results of sigmoid vaginoplasty in 23 young girls. J Urol. 2007;177(3):1107–11.

Liao LM, Tacconelli E, Wood D, et al. Adolescent girls with disorders of sex development: a needs analysis of transitional care. J Pediatr Urol. 2010;6(6):609–13.

van Lingen B, Reindollar R, Davis A, et al. Further evidence that the WT1 gene does not have a role in the development of the derivatives of the müllerian duct. Am J Obstet Gynecol. 1998;179(3):597–603.

Masse J, Watrin T, Laurent A, et al. The developing female genital tract: from genetics to epigenetics. Int J Dev Biol. 2009;53(2-3):411–24.

Oppelt P, Renner SP, Kellermann A, et al. Clinical aspects of Mayer-Rokitansky-Kuester-Hauser syndrome: recommendations for clinical diagnosis and staging. Hum Reprod. 2006;21(3):792–7.

Plyler ZE et al. Mechanisms of Development. 2019;155: 15–26.

Stern RC. The diagnosis of cystic fibrosis. N Engl J Med. 1997;336(7):487–91.

Takagi H, Matsunami K, Imai A. Uterovaginal duplication with blind hemivagina and ipsilateral renal agenesis: review of unusual presentation. J Obstet Gynaecol. 2010;30(4):350–3.

Ulrich U, Schrickel J, Dorn C, et al. Mayer-von Rokitansky-Kuster-Hauser syndrome in association with a hitherto undescribed variant of the Holt-Oram syndrome with an aorto-pulmonary window. Hum Reprod. 2004;19(5):1201–3.

Willemsen WN. Combination of the Mayer-Rokitansky-Kuster and Klippel-Feil syndrome--a case report and literature review. Eur J Obstet Gynecol Reprod Biol. 1982;13(4):229–35.

Ethical Principles for the Management of DSD

15

Lynn Gillam

15.1 Introduction

Making decisions about the management of children and adolescents with DSD can be ethically complex and socially fraught, as well as medically challenging. The ethical complexities of decision-making about medical treatment and management of children and young people with DSD are reflected in the contention about terminology. It is hard to even name the topic of the discussion without implying some sort of ethical position. "DSD" is used in this chapter with the intention of being value-neutral and could be read as "Difference of Sex Development" (a term preferred by some advocates, along with the similar "Variations of Sex Characteristics") or "Disorder of Sex Development", which is the current medical nomenclature. The use of the word "disorder" is strongly opposed by many advocates because of the negative connotations of the word "disorder" (Feder and Karkazis 2008; Davis 2013), and clinicians are increasingly also avoiding this expression (Schweizer et al. 2017; Bessiene et al. 2018).

Decisions about infants and older children with DSD are made today against a backdrop of dissatisfaction and anger of some adults with DSD (Daaboul and Frader 2001) and concerns about the insufficient information and lack of opportunities for considered decision-making given in the past to parents of infants with DSD (Chase 1998; Groveman 1998). The view has been put forward that no genital surgery should be performed until the child is old enough to understand the situation and make his or her own decision (Diamond 1998). This view is strongly argued by advocates for the rights of intersex people (Carpenter 2016; Ammaturo 2016). There has also been considerable debate in the medical and ethics literature about the management of DSD, which addresses issues such as ethical failings of past medical practice, informed consent, the right of parents to make decisions about surgery for infants when the consequences are so far-reaching and fundamental to personal identity, and whether children should be surgically altered to suit the norms of societies which happen to see gender only in stereotypical binary terms (Reiner 1998; Hester 2004; Spriggs and Savulescu 2006; Karkazis 2008).

Given this level of ethical and social complexity, great care and sensitivity is vital when making treatment decisions in individual cases. It is also vital, however, not to be paralysed by complexity. A decision pathway which takes account of complexity but does not get lost in it is needed. In this chapter, we propose a set of seven ethical principles on which to base treatment decisions

L. Gillam (✉)
Children's Bioethics Centre, The Royal Children's Hospital, Melbourne, VIC, Australia

Murdoch Children's Research Institute, Melbourne, VIC, Australia

Department of Paediatrics, University of Melbourne, Melbourne, VIC, Australia
e-mail: Lynn.Gillam@rch.org.au

J. M. Hutson et al. (eds.), *Disorders|Differences of Sex Development*,
https://doi.org/10.1007/978-981-13-7864-5_15

for DSD. These principles were the basis for a resolution of the Fifth World Congress on Family Law and Children's Rights in 2009 in Halifax on the medical and surgical management of infants and children with DSD (2009).

The ethical principles which we put forward are substantive rather than related to the process for decision-making. They assume that conditions for good ethical decision-making, such as the procedural and process matters outlined by Wiesemann et al., are already in place (Wiesemann et al. 2010). These principles specify the considerations which ought to be taken into account by clinicians when making significant management decisions, especially in the absence of clear medical evidence to direct such decisions. The ethical principles set out in this chapter are relevant to all forms of DSD, and to all the ethically significant decisions that clinicians make in relation to children and young people with DSD. These include decisions about surgery, hormone therapy, sex of rearing and what information and explanation is given to children and their parents about the DSD and the medical treatment. Surgery may be considered for a number of reasons—to alter the appearance of the genitalia, to improve urogenital function or to reduce cancer risk. These reasons invoke different ethical principles, so different types of surgeries need to be considered separately. These principles can be understood as describing, in precise terms, the nature of clinicians' basic ethical obligation, which is to act so as to promote the well-being and interests of the child or young person in this situation, taking into account the views and wishes of the parents and of the child or young person. The first six principles relate specifically to infants, so are not formulated to include the views of the child with DSD. Decision-making for children who are able to have and express views, and may even have decisional competence themselves as mature minors, is much more ethically complicated, and we do not cover all the issues but provide some general comments on the important principle of considering the views of the older child or young person.

In addition to uncertainty regarding long-term medical and psychosocial outcomes of the various management options, there is a need to consider the family situation and social context, including prevailing views about gender, sexuality and fertility. Views on these matters have changed considerably over time in the Western world, and continue to change. Views also vary between cultures. Making well-considered and ethically sound decisions is very important, as poor decision-making can lead to significant distress for the individual with DSD later in life (Schutzmann et al. 2009).

15.2 Methodology

These ethical principles for management of infants with DSD were formulated by a process of dialogical analysis of clinicians' reasoning in particular cases (Gillam et al. 2010), in relation to established principles of bioethics (Beauchamp and Childress 2009). This was led by the ethicist in our team (LG), in systematic consultation with the clinicians (GW and JH). This process was a practical implementation of John Rawls' concept of reflective equilibrium as a method for building ethical theory (Rawls 1972). The crucial feature of reflective equilibrium is that it gives as much weight to individual ethical judgements in particular cases as it does to abstract moral theory, provided those judgements are made by those well placed to decide. Ethical principles for a particular clinical situation, in Rawls' approach, are not simply derived from more general moral theory but are built up by considering individual case judgements in constant reference to normative moral theory.

Using reflective equilibrium as a method means that we started from "first principles", so to speak, rather than with the existing bioethics and sociology literature about DSD and the ethics of genital surgery. The analytic process focuses on judgements of expert clinicians in actual individual cases, and drawing inferences about generalisable principles that explain these judgements, and are consistent with moral theory at a relatively high level of abstraction. It does not focus on arguments put forward by ethicists, philosophers and others about the ethics of approaches to management and treatment of DSD in general terms. Hence, this chapter does not refer directly to that literature. However, as would be expected, there are clear similarities between the principles proposed here and some of the arguments in the literature. The substance of each of our individual principles is not necessarily novel. What is novel is the process by which they were derived, and intended comprehensiveness as a set which identifies all the relevant ethical considerations for decision-making in particular cases.

In the following sections, we set out the principles which we identified as arising from the reflective equilibrium process and give an account of their scope and theoretical ethical foundations. For each principle, we identify the specific clinical features which need to be taken into account and provide key questions to aid in application of the principle. Application of principles of course requires clinicians to be aware of and use best-available current evidence about outcomes of various surgical procedures. The principles in themselves do not specify a decision about an individual child, or about all children with a particular diagnosis. Evidence is always needed; since the available evidence will increase and improve in quality over time, it is possible for ethical decisions to evolve over time. Whenever more than one ethical principle is involved, there will inevitably be tension between them in some circumstances, so weighing and balancing between principles will also be needed. Finally, we discuss the advantages of working with an articulated set of principles, rather than relying solely on the professional and ethical judgement of individual clinicians in their particular circumstances.

15.3 Ethical Principles for DSD

The primary ethical consideration in any form of medical treatment for children is the well-being (physical, psychological and social, both short and long term) of the child (Friedman 1998). The other issue of major ethical importance is the parents' wishes. Generally, parents are entrusted with the responsibility of making medical decisions for their children in order to best promote their well-being in this broad sense (Pinnock and Crosthwaite 2005). However, when parents' wishes are likely to result in significant harm to a child (social, emotional or physical), consideration of the child's well-being takes precedence. This is sometimes known as the harm principle and is well established in ethics and law (Diekema 2004). In situations where the factors are complex and difficult to weigh up, and where future outcomes are difficult to predict, parents' wishes may be at variance with doctors' recommendations, without constituting clear harm to the child. In these situations, the parents' wishes should be respected (Dresser 2003; Jonas 2007) as falling within the Zone of Parental Discretion (Gillam 2015). As children get older and become more able to understand their medical condition and its impacts, increasing ethical weight also attaches to the child's wishes and preferences (Friedman 1998). These wishes and preferences may be in tension with both the parents' wishes and medical views, making the situation even more ethically complex. However, in the context of DSD, significant decisions about sex of rearing and genital surgery may have to be made whilst the child is very young (noting that a decision against surgery counts as one of the decisions that could be made, rather than a non-decision).

For infants and young children with DSD, the fundamental ethical question relates to the potential harms a child is exposed to because of the particular DSD which the child has, and what courses of action will adequately prevent or reduce these risks, allowing the child to have a high level of well-being over their lifetime. The following principles address that question by providing a specification in this particular context of the fundamental values of beneficence and non-maleficence (Beauchamp and Childress 2009).

The principles we propose are:

1. Minimising ***physical risk*** to child.
2. Maximising ***psychosocial well-being***.
3. Preserving potential for ***fertility***.

4. Preserving or promoting capacity to have satisfying ***sexual experiences***.
5. Leaving ***options open for the future***.
6. Respecting the ***parents' wishes*** and beliefs.
7. Taking into account the ***views of the child***.

15.4 Basis and Application of the Principles

It is clearly not always possible to fulfil every principle or right to the maximum degree. The nature of the DSD and the social environment into which the child has been born may make this impossible. It then becomes a matter of seeking to balance and weigh up the various principles in relation to the options available in the situation. The aim is to find the option that is the closest fit with the principles overall. This task requires clarity about the basis for each of principles and what they are intended to encompass.

15.4.1 Minimise Physical Risk

Depending on which DSD the child has, there may be a range of risks to the child's physical well-being in the short and long term. These typically include risks of malignancy, osteoporosis, adrenal crisis and urinary passage obstruction (Gozzi et al. 2005; Cools et al. 2006; Falhammar et al. 2007; Nabhan and Eugster 2007).

The questions to be asked in considering this ethical principle are as follows:

1. How much harm would be done to the child if the risk is eventuated? Would it mean loss of life, damage to an organ or body system or less serious physical consequences? This is the magnitude aspect of risk.
2. To what extent could this harm or damage be corrected after it occurred?
3. How likely is it that the harm will occur? This is the probability aspect of risk.
4. What measures are available to reduce the risk?
5. How successful would the proposed measures be in reducing both the probability and magnitude of the risk, in comparison to other measures?
6. Do the risk-reduction measures carry their own risks or known negative consequences, and if so, are these less than the magnitude and probability of the risks that the measures are meant to protect against?

The answers given to these questions will vary depending on the nature and severity of the condition at hand, and on the medical care that is available to the child in that particular setting. For example, the risks associated with not removing a gonad are lower if the gonad is palpable in the scrotum, rather in the abdominal cavity (Hughes et al. 2006). It is also possible that the answers will change in the future, as more evidence is acquired and new techniques and drugs are developed.

15.4.2 Maximise Psychosocial Well-being

There a number of factors that could have a negative impact on the psychosocial well-being of a child (and later adult) with a DSD. These are not typically within the control of clinicians but are important for clinicians to be aware of and take account of when making recommendations about medical treatment. The factors that clinicians need to take account of include:

1. The unpredictable nature of future gender identity. There is always a chance that the sex of rearing chosen on the basis of best match with anatomy, hormones, chromosomes and fertility, will later be rejected by the adolescent or adult, potentially leading to gender dysphoria, depression or other mental health problems (Meyer-Bahlburg 2005).
2. The possibility that a child will not be accepted by parents in the sex of rearing that would usually be recommended by doctors on the basis of medical considerations. This could lead to impaired bonding between parent and child, with associated negative consequences.

3. Possible social or cultural disadvantage to children with DSD who are born and raised in particular cultural settings. Decisions about sex of rearing may have particular implications in particular social circumstances. Parents may have concerns about reduced opportunities for marriage or intimate relationships or reduced opportunity for meaningful employment and capacity to earn an income (Warne and Bhatia 2006), which lead them to prefer a particular sex of rearing.
4. Risk of social isolation, restrictions or difficulties, for example, caused by embarrassment or social stigma associated with having genitalia which do not match the gender in which the person lives.
5. The possibility that the later adolescent or adult will feel regret or distress at interventions done on their bodies when they were young and unable to have or express a view.

These factors can be seen as psychosocial risk factors, with all the questions relevant to physical risk, also applying. For all risks, consideration must be given to the magnitude and probability of the risk, and the extent to which it can successfully be reduced, either by the medical management options available or by other types of support or intervention.

This process raises two difficulties. One is the present (and perhaps continuing) lack of solid evidence for making such assessments of risk—there will always be a risk that the child or later adult with a DSD will feel a disjunction between their body and their gender identity. A child with a DSD may later identify as intersex, but also may identify as male or female. Statistical predictions of adult gender identity based on the nature of the DSD will never be fully accurate. The second difficulty is the intangible nature of comparisons between physical and psychosocial risk. For example, it is not at all clear how to decide whether it is worse for a child to be at a risk of malignancy in the future or at risk of distress in the future due to having their gonads removed as a child. This is where personal and professional judgement and a good understanding of the family's social and cultural context are necessary. It is also a place where the parents' views might be given particular weight, as an authoritative source on the values held by their family or community. As the child becomes older and more able to form and express a view, increasing weight should also be put on the child's perspective. Children may have quite strong and settled views about their gender identity, for example, when they are still quite young, and well before they have general decision-making capacity as a mature minor. There is no evidence which can definitively adjudicate on the comparative weighting of risks, since it is ultimately a matter of the value that people place on the various aspects of life.

15.4.3 Preserving Potential for Fertility

Fertility is listed here as a separate ethical consideration because it has both physical and psychosocial components, and also because of its unique and fundamental significance in human life, across all cultural settings (as evidenced by the inclusion of the right to found a family in the UN Declaration on Human Rights). Infertility is both a physical dysfunction (which does not itself cause morbidity or mortality) and potentially a major psychosocial harm, depending on the importance attached to fertility by the individual concerned in their own social and cultural context. Fertility is a complex socially mediated concept and may relate to a number of different physical states, including the following:

1. Having ovaries or testes.
2. Having viable gametes, and, hence, having the possibility of having one's own genetic children, whether conceived naturally or by assisted reproductive technologies.
3. Having the physical capacity for one's gametes to produce pregnancy as a result of sexual intercourse, hence being able to "have children naturally".
4. Being able to carry a pregnancy, whether or not the foetus has been produced by one's own gametes.

The key question is what courses of action offer the best chance of preserving the potential for fertility in a way that is likely to be meaningful for this person in adulthood. One ethical complexity likely to be raised by this principle is that courses of action which give the best chance of preserving fertility may bring with them higher risks of physical harm, such as malignancy—risks which could be removed at the cost of losing the chance for fertility. Again, the relative weighting of these considerations cannot be scientifically determined, since they depend on subjective meanings and values. It is important to keep in mind that the subjective values which are relevant are those of the person with DSD, not those of the clinician. Parents' values will be an important consideration here, but even they will not be able to predict the values their child will grow up to have, and will have to make a "best guess". This is problematic even for older children and adolescents who will be able to understand the issue and articulate a view: the attitude of a 15-year-old to fertility may be very different from that of the same person at 25. Erring on the side of protecting fertility is a reasonable position, given that such a high proportion of adults in all settings value it so strongly, but the specificities of individual situations must always be considered.

15.4.4 Preserving or Promoting Capacity to Have Satisfying Sexual Experiences

Capacity for having satisfying sexual relations is arguably just one aspect of psychosocial well-being which has already been dealt with earlier. It is listed separately here because it can assume overwhelming importance in adulthood, becoming the foundation for all other aspects of psychosocial well-being, rather than one aspect among many (Cousineau and Domar 2007). Again, this is a complex matter which involves values and interpretations, and not simply medical facts.

The key and contested issue is what counts as "satisfying" in terms of sexual experiences. Two obvious biomedical markers would be physical ability to experience orgasm and for some, physical ability to engage in penetrative vaginal intercourse. Again, however, this is a matter of individual preferences and values. For example, penetrative vaginal intercourse is likely to be valued much less by people with DSD who have an exclusively homosexual orientation. In general, medicine cannot stipulate a best way to have sex. Nevertheless, if these two physical capacities are preserved by the preservation of the relevant tissue, or enhanced by reconstructive surgery, this at least provides the physical basis for the satisfying psychosexual experience. For example, one reason for retaining all the tissue in an enlarged clitoris is that any surgery to reduce the size of the clitoris carries some risk of damaging sensory nerves and hence impairing the capacity for sexual response.

15.4.5 Leaving Options Open for the Future

Options for the future can be left open in a number of ways in relation to surgery for infants with DSD, including the following:

1. Not removing gonadal tissue even if it appears non-functional, to allow for the possibility that in the future, advances in medical technology may provide an option for fertility in those previously considered infertile.
2. Performing surgery in such a way that it leaves open the possibility of further surgery to change the assigned sex later on.
3. Delaying surgery which could be left until later in medical terms, or is purely for appearance reasons, so that the child or adolescent can have input into decisions affecting their body.

Leaving options open for the future is an ethically important consideration in general, in relation to children (Davis 1997). In the context of DSD, it is important for two reasons. Firstly, it recognises the uncertainty inherent in decisions about sex of rearing and genital surgery. Knowing that things may not work out as expected or intended, the ethically responsible course is to take this into account when making decisions, and where possible allow scope for change of mind or change of the individual's circumstances or wishes. This is a strategy for meeting the ethical obligation to minimise harm to the child and future adult, and maximise benefit.

Secondly, leaving options open for the future provides a way to acknowledge and respect the rights of individuals to participate in or make decisions about their treatment. Infants are completely incapable of making any decisions for themselves, so this right cannot be directly respected at the time, but the infant with DSD will grow up to be a young person, who has preferences, values and plans for their life. It is important to note, however, that leaving options open for the future is presented here as one ethical principle in a set of six. Our framework does not give it overriding status, or accord more weight to it than to the other principles. The ethical importance of leaving options open is to be considered alongside the principles of minimising physical risk, maximising psychosocial well-being, preserving fertility and promoting the capacity for satisfying sexual relations. It may turn out to be a principle which cannot be fully adhered to in a decision which must take account of multiple, potentially competing factors.

15.4.6 Respecting the Parents' Wishes and Beliefs

This principle is the most controversial, both in its wording and weighting. There are widely differing views on how much parents' wishes ought to be regarded as determinative. This difference of opinion can be seen in the final wording resolution of the Fifth World Congress on Family Law and Children's Rights, where "respect parents' wishes" was changed to "consider parents' wishes". Parents' wishes and beliefs are ethically significant for at least two reasons. Firstly, they are closely implicated in the child's psychosocial well-being. How the child feels about him- or herself is very strongly influenced by the parents' attitudes and behaviours, and the parent-child relationship is the basis of the child's overall well-being. In addition, the parents are the most knowledgeable about the family and social environment in which the child will be raised, and they have the best sense of how others around the child will react to him or her, now and in the long term. For example, in a culture that does not allow infertile females to marry and which offers males more legal rights, freedom and privileges than females, a 46,XY child with ambiguous genitalia might be considered to have better chances of economic independence and a good quality of life if raised male than as an infertile female, even if the genitalia have a predominantly female appearance. This thinking does not endorse the social norms of that culture but does accept them as a reality for that family and child. Secondly, parents have a primary ethical responsibility to protect and promote their children's interests, and they have a right to be allowed to carry out this responsibility (Gillam 2015). On this understanding, the parents' wishes matter because parents have a moral claim to be the decision-makers for the child by virtue of their parental role, and not just because they are likely to be well placed to make a good decision (McDougall et al. 2016).

However, this right is not absolute. As mentioned earlier, the accepted foundational ethical principle of paediatric healthcare is that the child's interests are paramount, and that parents' decisions should be overridden if it is likely that they will cause significant harm to the child. By listing "respect for parent's wishes" as an ethical principle alongside other ethical principles, these guidelines allow for the possibility that if the other ethical considerations point strongly enough against what the parents want, then it would be ethically appropriate to go against their wishes. Respecting parents' wishes does not necessarily mean doing whatever the parents want, but it always involves taking the parents' wishes (and the beliefs they are based on) seriously and according them moral weight. It also involves interacting in a respectful way with parents, even when their beliefs and values are radically different from those of the treating clinicians.

Our framing of "respecting parents' wishes" as one among a number of prima facie principles is potentially controversial. There are two possible types of objections: (1) that we give too little weight to the views of parents, and (2) that we give too much.

In relation to objection (1), some clinicians may hold a view that, where DSD are concerned, parents' wishes are paramount and should always be followed. This may be based on an ethical belief, for example, that on matters of such personal importance as the gender and identity of their children, parents should have ultimate authority (even if they do not have absolute moral authority in other medical situations, such as life-saving blood transfusions for children of Jehovah's Witness parents).

Others may endorse objection (2), believing that parents' wishes are always secondary to considerations of the best interests of the child, or perhaps are not relevant at all. This position would amount to the claim that nothing significant is added to appropriate ethical deliberation by including the parents' wishes and beliefs. This would mean that everything that ought to be considered in relation to the well-being and interests of the child can be fully covered by the other principles. This position is contrary to the usual view about the discretion and latitude rightfully owed to parents (Daaboul and Frader 2001). It also seems to underestimate the extent to which the infant's future well-being, especially psychosocial well-being, depends on its relationship with its parents. Assigning a sex of rearing contrary to the parents' wishes, and making related decisions about surgery, has the potential for serious negative consequences for the child. For example, parents may strongly reject advice to raise a 46,XX child with ambiguous genitalia as female, if their strong belief is that the child is a boy. The difficulties for this child and family if doctors assign a female sex of rearing in the face of the parents' view are likely to be enormous.

15.4.7 Consider the Views of Children and Adolescents

The thoughts, feelings and wishes of the older child or young person with a DSD matter ethically for two reasons: promoting the psychosocial well-being of the child and respecting the developing autonomy of the child or young person.

In relation to psychosocial well-being, much of the concern about psychosocial risk relates to how the child will be seen by others and by himself/herself. Is the child distressed or embarrassed by their body, or by others' reactions to their body? If bodily changes are occurring due to puberty, how are they reacting to those changes? The child's thoughts and feelings about this are highly relevant to decisions about medical treatment even from quite a young age. Children also begin establishing a gender identity early on, and their feelings about their bodies are strongly shaped by what gender they perceive themselves to be. So from about the age of 3 onwards, children's thoughts and feelings are ethically relevant in making assessments of what would promote or hinder their psychosocial well-being, and whether a medical intervention (e.g. clitoral reduction surgery) would be ethically appropriate. This does not mean that children should be directly asked if they want surgery, nor that their views about surgery would be definitive; simply that their thoughts, feelings, ideas and preferences should be taken into account.

In relation to respect for developing autonomy, it is only later that the children develop sufficient cognitive capacity to understand and consider for themselves the issues involved in medical treatment decisions. This capacity develops slowly over time and comes at different ages in different children. No firm age cut-offs can be set, and individual assessment is required. Once the child has started to develop this capacity, it is ethically appropriate to respect this developing capacity for autonomy by involving them in discussion or decision-making in ways appropriate to their developmental stage. The nature of this involvement, and the ethical weight that should be accorded to child or young person's view (Buchanan Allen and Brock 1998) will increase over time. Some young people may develop a high level of decision-making before the age of 18, sufficient to be regarded as fully competent "mature minors" who can make independent decisions and consent to treatment on their own behalf. This might occur by the age of 15 or 16 years, but again, there is no defined age limit. Unless a child or young person is a mature minor, their wishes about medical treatment should not be taken as determinative but should be taken seriously alongside other ethical considerations. The consent of a mature minor to medical treatment would be ethically definitive in theory, though parents' wishes at this stage are still very important. Disagreement between a mature minor and their parents about medical treatment such as genital surgery would be a significant ethical dilemma (Ross 1997)—best managed with specialist clinical ethics consultation and legal advice.

15.5 Using Ethical Principles in Clinical Practice

These ethical principles can be used in a number of ways. Perhaps the most obvious use is by individual clinicians in their own thinking and decision-making about their patients. The principles could also be used to frame a discussion with parents, to help them understand their child's situation and the factors that need to be thought about when deciding on gender of rearing and any surgery (Gillam et al. 2011). A third use is in a formal process of clinical ethics review. This is the practice that we have set in place at our own centre, The Royal Children's Hospital Melbourne. After a trial period where all new cases of DSD were routinely referred for review by the Clinical Ethics Response Group (CERG), which provides clinical ethics case consultation services for the hospital (Gold et al. 2011), we formulated a process where ethics referral is made in cases which have characteristics which indicate greater-than-usual ethical complexity. The clinical ethics discussion takes place after a diagnosis has been made or confirmed, appropriate investigations and assessments have been completed and a management plan formulated in consultation with the parents, and individual, if old enough to participate (Fig. 15.1). The clinical ethics meeting is attended by the multidisciplinary treating team, and members of the CERG, including the clinical ethicist and others trained in ethics. At the meeting, a discussion guide based on the principles set out in this chapter is used (Fig. 15.2) to both give some structure to the discussion and make sure that all ethically relevant aspects are fully considered. This process is organised so that there is minimal or no delay for the parents and individual. Ideally, CERG is notified when an individual first presents, some days to weeks in advance of time when a management plan will be available to discuss. In any case, the CERG is able to convene at 24–48 hours of notice. The process is not bureaucratic in the way that research ethics is—there is no application form, and lengthy documentation is not required. Clinicians complete a short pro forma referral which asks for the same information that would normally be provided when making a referral to a consultant for specialist clinical advice (Fig. 15.3). There is a process in place to deal with a situation where ethical concerns are raised and cannot be resolved at that meeting. This involves a higher level of ethical review within the hospital, and possible referral to a court if the concerns cannot be resolved, or if there is significant on-going disagreement between parents and Fig. 15.3 the treating team.

The reason for this process of clinical ethics review is to ensure that we have a robust and comprehensive decision-making process in an area of clinical practice where decisions have life-long implications for the personal identity of individuals and evidence for long-term outcomes is sketchy. Treatment for DSD is a contested, emotive field that, in Australia at least, is subject to legal scrutiny. In this context, there are benefits to individuals, families and clinicians in having a transparent and formal (and fully documented) decision-making process explicitly guided by ethical principles.

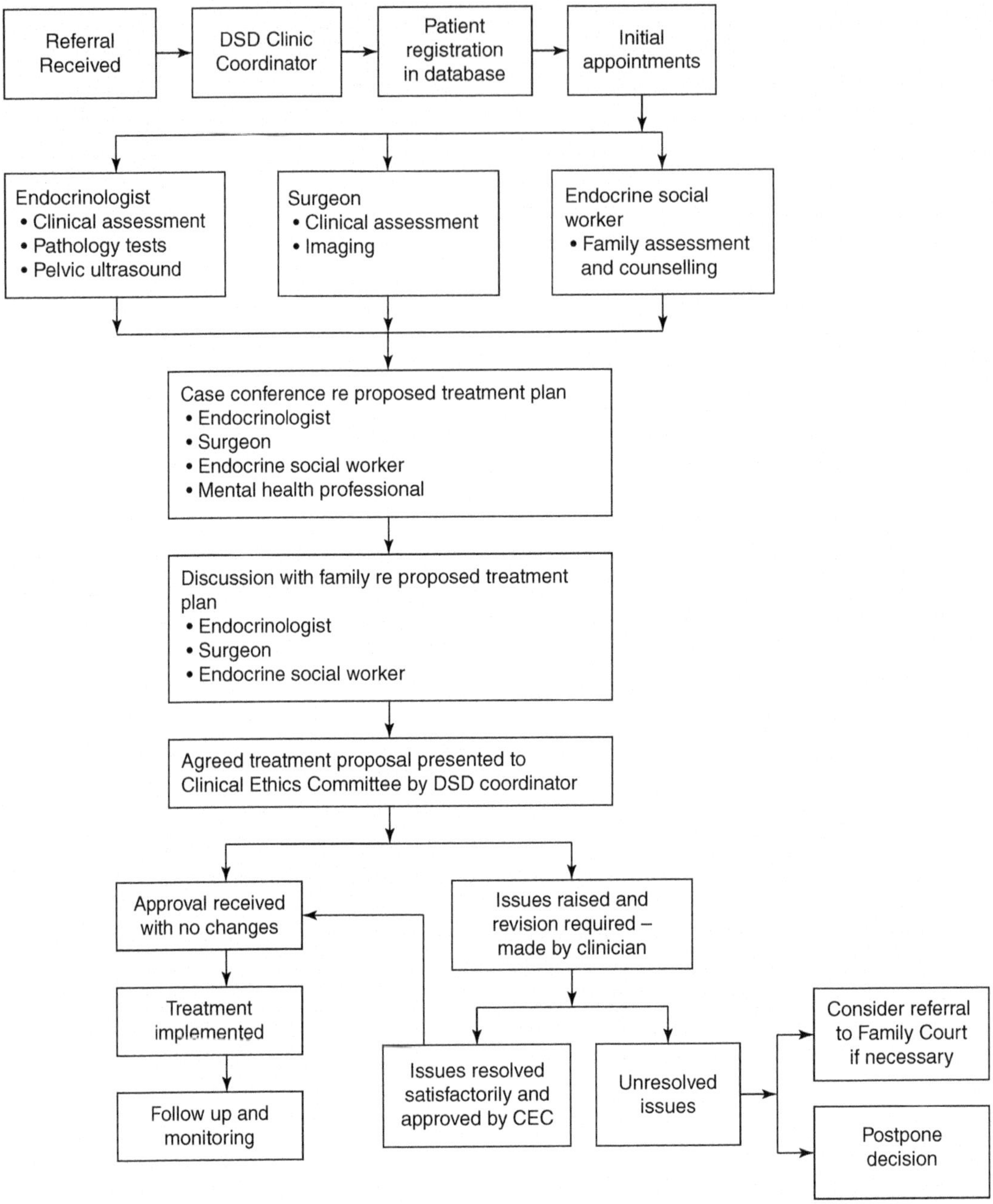

Fig. 15.1 Pathway for clinical ethics review of proposed treatment plan for a child with a DSD

ETHICAL PRINCIPLE	COMMENTS RE THIS CASE
Minimise ***physical risk*** / promote physical ***well-being***	
Promote psychosocial ***well-being***	
Preserve potential for ***fertility***	
Preserve or promote capacity to have satisfying ***sexual experiences***	
Leave ***options open for the future***	
Consider ***views and wishes of child*** – give increasing weight as child approaches decisional capacity – if adolesecent has decisional capacity (ie is mature minor) give same weight as would be given to wishes of adult patient	
Respect the ***parents' wishes*** and beliefs (but do not regard as fully determinative)	

Fig. 15.2 CERG discussion guide: Ethical principles for use in consideration of child with a DSD

Clinical Ethics Meeting Request

1. Child's name:

2. Referring clinician:

3. Timeline: how soon is Clinical Ethics meeting needed
   Eg 1-2 days 5-10days

4. Date/s suggested for clinical ethics meeting (please provide at least 2 alternatives. Friday afternoons are one preferred option):

5. Treating team members who will attend meeting:

Proposed Management Plan

1. Child's name, DOB and UR

2. Treating clinician/s

3. Diagnosis (indicate uncertainty, if relevant)

4. Brief history:
   a. Medical
   b. Social/family, including cultural or religious aspects that are relevant

5. Brief overview of discussions held with
   a. parents
   b. child/young person (if relevant)
   c. other family members (if relevant)

6. Proposed gender of rearing and rationale (inc. factors on which the decision was based)

7. Proposed management plan with rationale (inc. factors on which the decision was based), including
   a. Any proposed surgery, and rationale
   b. Any proposed medication, and rationale
   c. Proposed psychosocial support and follow-up for family

8. Parents' and child's (if relevant) views on proposed gender of rearing and management plan

9. Any particular ethical questions concerns or issues identified by treating team

Fig. 15.3 Referral of a child with a DSD for clinical ethics review

15.6 Conclusion

These principles provide a systematic approach to decision-making in a medically complex field. They are general enough to be applicable to any individual case, are not condition specific and are not specific to the current state of medical knowledge and technical capacity. The principles are flexible and do not constitute hard and fast rules. However, they are specific enough to give some direction about priorities in decision-making. A systematic ethical approach is useful in a number of ways, both in the clinical setting and beyond. A set of agreed ethical principles embodies accepted standards of practice. It provides a framework to guide comprehensive consideration of all factors relevant to decision-making, whether this is done by individual clinicians a multi-disciplinary team or by a clinical ethics committees. Ethical principles can also assist in clinical practice, especially in training of junior doctors and others involved in management, and in discussing treatment with parents. More broadly, a set of ethical principles provides clarity in an emotive, contested field. It may identify enough neutral or common ground with advocacy groups to enable more constructive dialogue, rather than conflict. It forms the basis for explaining clinical practice to people in the community, especially the affected community, and gives a tangible demonstration that decisions are not taken lightly. It also provides professional guidelines to refer to in legal proceedings, government inquiries and the like, which can depersonalise issues by putting them in a broader professional context.

Acknowledgements With thanks and acknowledgements to the authors who had been involved in the first edition of this chapter: Dr. Jacqueline Hewitt, Professor Garry L. Warne AM.

References

Beauchamp TL, Childress JF. Principles of biomedical ethics. Oxford: Oxford University Press; 2009.

Bessiene L, Lombes M, Bouvattier C. Differences of sex development (DSD): controversies and challenges. Ann Endocrinol (Paris). 2018;79(Suppl 1):S22–30.

Buchanan Allen E, Brock DW. Deciding for others: the ethics of surrogate decision making. Cambridge: Cambridge University Press; 1998.

Carpenter M. The human rights of intersex people: addressing harmful practices and rhetoric of change. Reprod Health Matters. 2016;24(47):74–84.

Chase C. Surgical progress is not the answer to intersexuality. J Clin Ethics. 1998;9(4):385–92.

Cools M, Drop SL, Wolffenbuttel KP, et al. Germ cell tumors in the intersex gonad: old paths, new directions, moving frontiers. Endocr Rev. 2006;27(5):468–84.

Cousineau TM, Domar AD. Psychological impact of infertility. Best Pract Res Clin Obstet Gynaecol. 2007;21(2):293–308.

Daaboul J, Frader J. Ethics and the management of the patient with intersex: a middle way. J Pediatr Endocrinol Metab. 2001;14(9):1575–83.

Davis G. The power in a name: diagnostic terminology and diverse experiences. Psychology & Sexuality. 2013;5(1):15–27.

Diamond M. Intersexuality: recommendations for management. Arch Sex Behav. 1998;27(6):634–41.

Diekema DS. Parental refusals of medical treatment: the harm principle as threshold for state intervention. Theor Med Bioeth. 2004;25(4):243–64.

Dresser R. Standards for family decisions: replacing best interests with harm prevention. Am J Bioeth. 2003;3(2):54–5.

Falhammar H, Filipsson H, Holmdahl G, et al. Fractures and bone mineral density in adult women with 21-hydroxylase deficiency. J Clin Endocrinol Metab. 2007;92(12):4643–9.

Feder EK, Karkazis K. What's in a name? The controversy over "disorders of sex development". Hast Cent Rep. 2008;38(5):33–6.

Friedman RL. Children, families and health care decision-making. Oxford: Clarendon Press; 1998.

Gillam L. Fifty years of paediatric ethics. J Paediatr Child Health. 2015;51(1):8–11.

Gillam LH, Hewitt JK, Warne GL. Ethical principles an essential part of process in DSD care. Horm Res Paediatr. 2011;76(5):367–8.

Gold H, Hall G, Gillam LH. The role and function of a paediatric clinical ethics service - experiences at the Royal Children's Hospital, Melbourne. J Paediatr Child Health. 2011;47:632–6.

Gozzi TG, Harris NP, McGown IN, et al. Autopsy diagnosis of 21-hydroxylase deficiency CAH in a case of apparent SIDS. Pediatr Dev Pathol. 2005;8(3):397–401.

Groveman SA. The Hanukkah bush: ethical implications in the clinical management of intersex. J Clin Ethics. 1998;9(4):356–9.

Halifax Resolutions from http://www.lawrights.asn.au/index.php?option=com_content&view=article&id=76&Itemid=109 2009.

Hester JD. Intersex(es) and informed consent: how physicians' rhetoric constrains choice. Theor Med Bioeth. 2004;25(1):21–49.

Hughes IA, Houk C, Ahmed SF, et al. Consensus statement on management of intersex disorders. Arch Dis Child. 2006;91(7):554–63.

Jonas M. The baby MB case: medical decision making in the context of uncertain infant suffering. J Med Ethics. 2007;33(9):541–4.

Karkazis K. Fixing sex. Intersex, medical authority and lived experience. Durham, NC: Duke University Press; 2008.

Meyer-Bahlburg HF. Introduction: gender dysphoria and gender change in persons with intersexuality. Arch Sex Behav. 2005;34(4):371–3.

Nabhan ZM, Eugster EA. Upper-tract genitourinary malformations in girls with congenital adrenal hyperplasia. Pediatrics. 2007;120(2):e304–7.

Pinnock R, Crosthwaite J. When parents refuse consent to treatment for children and young persons. J Paediatr Child Health. 2005;41(7):369–73.

Rawls J. A theory of justice. Oxford: Oxford University Press; 1972.

Reiner WG. Special issue. J Clin Ethics. 1998;9(4): 337–420.

Ross LF. Health care decision making by children - is it in their best interest? Hast Cent Rep. 1997;27(6)

Schutzmann K, Brinkmann L, Schacht M, et al. Psychological distress, self-harming behavior, and suicidal tendencies in adults with disorders of sex development. Arch Sex Behav. 2009;38(1):16–33.

Schweizer K, Brunner F, Gedrose B, et al. Coping with diverse sex development: treatment experiences and psychosocial support during childhood and adolescence and adult well-being. J Pediatr Psychol. 2017;42(5):504–19.

Spriggs M, Savulescu J. The ethics of surgically assigning sex for intersex children. In: Benatar D, editor. Cutting to the core: exploring the ethics of contested surgeries. Lanham, MD: Rowman & Littlefield; 2006.

Warne G, Bhatia V. Intersex, east and west. In: Sytsma S, editor. Ethics and intersex. Dordrecht: Springer; 2006. p. 183–205.

Wiesemann C, Ude-Koeller S, Sinnecker GH, et al. Ethical principles and recommendations for the medical management of differences of sex development (DSD)/intersex in children and adolescents. Eur J Pediatr. 2010;169(6):671–9.

16 Medical Management of DSD

Michele A. O'Connell, John M. Hutson, and Sonia R. Grover

16.1 Introduction

The medical approach to the management of children with DSD has undergone significant changes in recent years. Successful prediction of outcomes has previously been limited by incomplete understanding of underlying genetics, aetiology or pathogenesis and hence natural history. While our understanding is continuously improving and scientific publications in this area have increased significantly since the 2005 consensus meeting, optimal management is still limited by a lack of good-quality longitudinal studies to inform an evidence-based practice. Uncertainties remain in a number of areas, including how best to quantify risk of germ cell malignancy for an individual, optimal timing of surgical interventions if these are considered appropriate and predicting the potential for future gender dysphoria in a given individual. Past practices were also weak in relation to disclosure of diagnoses to affected individuals and parents. The distress caused by this was compounded by implications of secrecy and shame surrounding DSD as well as inadequate access to psychological support.

Research has been driven by the need to improve outcomes for children with DSD and has focussed on understanding underlying genetic mechanisms. It has also yielded improved methods for diagnostic testing. The ability to identify androgen receptor gene mutations in patients with androgen insensitivity syndrome (AIS), for example, has made both carrier detection and prenatal diagnosis possible (Hughes and Deeb 2006). In recent years, more comprehensive targeted DSD gene panels have been shown to significantly increase the diagnostic capability in those with DSD, with one large study of a research panel incorporating 64 DSD genes yielding a likely genetic diagnosis in 43% of 278 individuals with 46,XY DSD (Eggers et al. 2016). Previously, the rates of clinical molecular genetic

M. A. O'Connell (✉)
Department of Endocrinology and Diabetes, The Royal Children's Hospital, Melbourne, VIC, Australia

Murdoch Children's Research Institute, Melbourne, VIC, Australia
e-mail: Michele.Oconnell@rch.org.au

J. M. Hutson
Department of Urology, The Royal Children's Hospital, Melbourne, VIC, Australia

Murdoch Children's Research Institute, Melbourne, VIC, Australia

Department of Paediatrics, University of Melbourne, Melbourne, VIC, Australia
e-mail: john.hutson@rch.org.au

S. R. Grover
Department of Gynaecology, The Royal Children's Hospital, Melbourne, VIC, Australia

Murdoch Children's Research Institute, Melbourne, VIC, Australia

Department of Paediatrics, University of Melbourne, Melbourne, VIC, Australia
e-mail: Sonia.grover@rch.org.au

J. M. Hutson et al. (eds.), *Disorders|Differences of Sex Development*,
https://doi.org/10.1007/978-981-13-7864-5_16

diagnosis were reported at 13% (Lux et al. 2009). Incorporation of such gene panels into clinical practice will help with provision of an accurate diagnosis as well as assisting in medical management. Diagnosis-based outcome studies that have been completed have led to an improved understanding of the potential pathway or journey for an affected individual. This has added greater perspective to some of the contentious debate between the medical profession and some patient advocacy groups, regarding issues such as genital surgery. Multidisciplinary care and open disclosure of diagnosis have become the norm in many countries, and expanding this to all countries and cultures will be important. The availability of psychosocial support is improving. Improved understanding of DSD is contributing to improved patient care. At the same time, it is also clear that there is still much to learn, and a great deal of more research is needed.

The potentially significant impact upon both children and their families of a DSD diagnosis warrants particular attention from their physician, who carries the responsibility for practising evidence-based medicine combined with empathy, cultural sensitivity and compassion. The first half of this chapter will highlight areas in which there has been recent progress and the evidence available to inform the care of children with DSD.

The definition and diagnostic terminology used in relation to DSD were reviewed at an international consensus meeting jointly hosted in 2005 by the European Society for Paediatric Endocrinology (ESPE) and the Lawson Wilkins Pediatric Endocrine Society (LWPES). The ensuing consensus statement dealt not only with terminology, but also with management concepts and future research directions (Hughes et al. 2006).

Further outcome-based evidence relating to specific genetic aetiologies of DSD is required in order to improve care. Until evidence from such research has been produced, the 'next best' approach is management by multidisciplinary teams (MDT) with experience and expertise in DSD and who are willing to follow consensus guidelines. It is accepted, however, that consensus guidelines may become outdated as new information becomes available, and they cannot universally account for the individual nuances of a particular situation. Reasons for consideration of divergence of management approach from such guidelines should therefore be openly discussed amongst the MDT and in age-appropriate terms with the child or adolescent; documentation to reflect these discussions and decisions is also important.

16.2 Classification System

The diagnostic terms that came out of the 2005 Chicago consensus meeting were designed to eliminate the more confusing and stigmatising elements of the previous classification lexicon. They were confusing because a number of different terms and definitions could be used to describe a particular diagnosis. An individual with 46,XY DSD, for example, could be termed an under-virilised male or an under-masculinised male, regardless of whether he/she had a variation in gonadal development or androgen synthesis or action (Table 16.1). In addition, earlier terms such as 'hermaphrodite' were no longer considered appropriate, while others such as 'intersex' were considered pejorative by many. As noted in Chap. 1, however, there is no universally agreed or preferred terminology, and many affected individuals feel 'DSD' is unnecessarily pathologising.

Table 16.1 Summary of new terminology

Title	Previous terminology
Disorders of sex development	Intersex
46,XY DSD	Male pseudohermaphrodite Under-virilised male Under-masculinised male
46,XX DSD	Female pseudohermaphrodite Virilised female Masculinised female
Ovo-testicular DSD	True hermaphrodite
46,XY complete gonadal dysgenesis	XY female XY sex reversal
46,XX testicular DSD	XX male XX sex reversal

Adapted from Hughes et al. (2007)

DSD is defined as any congenital condition in which development of the chromosomal, gonadal or anatomic sex is atypical. This is a definition that encompasses a wide spectrum of disorders. Taken literally, it includes all types of hypospadias, ambiguous genitalia, sex reversal, Turner and Klinefelter syndromes and a range of variations such as vaginal and uterine agenesis, cloacal exstrophy and bladder exstrophy.

The conditions fall into three diagnostic groups based on peripheral blood karyotype: 46,XY DSD, 46,XX DSD and sex chromosome aneuploidy DSD. Aneuploidy DSD refers to conditions in which there is an atypical number of sex chromosomes, such as 47,XXY Klinefelter syndrome, 45,X Turner syndrome, 45,X/46,XY mixed gonadal dysgenesis and 46,XX/46,XY chimerism,. Within each of these karyotypic groups are three sub-groups of DSD defined by aetiology. These are gonadal dysgenesis, abnormal hormone synthesis or action and syndromic causes. An outline of the specific causes of DSD is represented in Table 16.2.

The 2005 classification system has made a significant improvement for reporting of medical outcomes, in that it creates structure and definitions that are suitable for universal use, and although terminology remains contentious, the DSD classification system has eliminated previously used odious terminology such as 'true hermaphrodite' or 'pseudohermaphrodite'. Nevertheless, in the opinion of the authors, the diagnostic structure is still imperfect and may benefit from future refinement. The diagnostic stem relates to peripheral blood karyotype, but pathologists frequently group diagnoses according to gonadal development because their concern is in defining the future risk of malignancy.

16.3 Clinical Diagnosis

The most common presentation of DSD is with atypical genitalia in the newborn. However, as outlined in previous chapters, DSD may also present later—in infancy, childhood, at puberty or even in adult life. The true incidence of DSD is unknown. Penile hypospadias affects up to 1:150 male births, Klinefelter syndrome up to 1:500 male births and Turner syndrome 1:2500 female births (Nielsen and Wohlert 1990; March of

Table 16.2 Summary of new diagnostic structure

	46,XY DSD	46,XX DSD	Aneuploidy DSD (e.g. Klinefelter syndrome XXY, Turner syndrome X, Mosaic X/XY)
Abnormal gonadal development	Partial gonadal dysgenesis Mixed gonadal dysgenesis Complete gonadal dysgenesis Ovo-testicular DSD Testicular regression syndrome Denys-Drash, Frasier and WAGR syndromes	Partial gonadal dysgenesis Complete gonadal dysgenesis Testicular DSD Ovo-testicular DSD Denys-Drash, Frasier and WAGR syndromes	Partial gonadal dysgenesis Mixed gonadal dysgenesis Complete gonadal dysgenesis Ovo-testicular DSD
Abnormal androgen action	*Poor androgen synthesis or action* *Androgen biosynthesis defect* 17β-Hydroxysteroid dehydrogenase deficiency, 5α-reductase-2 deficiency, lipoid adrenal hyperplasia *Androgen insensitivity* Androgen insensitivity syndrome (partial, severe or complete)	*Androgen excess* *Increased synthesis* Congenital adrenal hyperplasia	
Syndromic and non-hormonal	Cloacal exstrophy, simple hypospadias	Cloacal exstrophy, vaginal agenesis	

Modified from Achermann and Hughes (2008)

Dimes 2001). It is estimated that variations in genital appearance at birth requiring genetic and endocrine investigation occur with an incidence of 1 in 4500 births (Hamerton et al. 1975; Sax 2002; Thyen et al. 2006). A review of a large referral clinic caring for children with DSD (excluding distal penile hypospadias, Klinefelter and Turner syndromes and children with multiple congenital abnormalities) found that presentation in infancy accounted for 71% of referrals (Parisi et al. 2007). Extrapolating from the above data and applying the broadest interpretation to the definition, the surprisingly frequent incidence approximates 1 in 280 live births. The frequency of more severe forms of DSD, excluding less severe hypospadias, Klinefelter and Turner syndromes could approximate 1:2600.

The neonate with atypical genitalia should have specialist medical evaluation as soon as possible, as 21-OH deficiency CAH, the most common cause of such a DSD is potentially life threatening. In addition, the birth of an infant with atypical genitalia may present unexpected difficulties for the parents, who may find responding to well-meaning enquiries from family and friends challenging at a time when they themselves may be feeling bewildered and unsure about what to say (see Chap. 19). The potential for a clinician or other health professional to add to their distress and cause psychological harm through ill-prepared comments and poor advice is very real.

The parents should be reassured that although they may have never encountered or heard of DSD, they are not uncommon and are a normal variation. Since genital appearance may be discordant with the underlying sex (eg 46,XX CAH), it may be best to delay any announcement about the child's sex of rearing until they have heard the outcome of a multidisciplinary specialist assessment and the result of all investigations and have had a chance to be involved in discussions as to what is best for their child. The team of specialists would usually include a paediatric endocrinologist, urologist/surgeon and a psychologist or other mental health/family support worker. It should be explained that informed decisions should be made about such an important issue as sex of rearing, and it is best to wait for specialist review and investigation results. The family should be reassured that all clinicians involved appreciate the urgency in achieving an optimally assigned sex and kept up to date with results of investigations and their meaning.

While a final decision with regards to the baby's sex is awaited, we recommend that health professionals should avoid referring to the infant as 'he' or 'she' and should instead refer to the neonate as 'your baby' or the more general, 'they'. A member of the multidisciplinary team, usually the paediatric endocrinologist, would explain the process of sex differentiation and its potential variations using simple diagrams—some excellent options are available online at https://www.rch.org.au/endo/differences-of-sex-development/. The family should be reassured that the examination and investigations will give important information that will help to determine the optimal sex of rearing of the child. The family should have daily medical and review and support.

The mother should be asked about any prenatal exposure to androgens or endocrine disrupters, if she experienced any virilisation during pregnancy, whether or not there is a family history of infant death or infertility and about consanguinity.

Examination of the infant includes a thorough general physical examination, including ascertainment of any dysmorphic features (see Chap. 12). The stretched length of the phallus, measured from the symphysis pubis, and its circumferential girth are recorded. The mean stretched penis length of −2.5 SD in full-term males is reported as 2.6 cm for Caucasian, 2.5 cm for Indian and 2.3 cm for Chinese infants (Cheng and Chanoine 2001). The position of the urethral opening, which can be on the dorsal or ventral surface of the phallus, or in the perineum, is precisely recorded. Palpable gonads outside the inguinal canal or in the labio-scrotal folds will usually be testes, but ovaries can rarely be found in this superficial position. The anogenital distance (Holschneider and Hutson 2016), and the degree of rugosity and pigmentation of the labio-scrotal tissue are additional markers of virilisation. The degree of external genitalia virilisation of a 46,XX infant can be graded using the Prader classification (see Fig. 7.1 in Chap. 7).

Appropriate first-line investigations of an infant with atypical genital appearance include an urgent request for fluorescent *in situ* hybridisation (FISH) to detect Y chromosome material, as well as a full karyotype. A pelvic ultrasound scan should also be requested for determination of internal genitalia. It should be noted that the accuracy of this investigation is highly dependent on the skill and experience of the sonographer and the availability of small probes. The measurements of serum electrolytes, 17-OH-progesterone, testosterone, follicle-stimulating hormone and luteinising hormone also constitute baseline investigations that may be considered; optimal timing of investigations relative to post-partum hormonal variations (gonadotrophins) and to avoid maternal contamination (17-OHP) are important to consider. Serum anti-Müllerian hormone (AMH) is also recommended (Rey et al. 1999) as a marker of Sertoli cell function. While this test is increasingly available, standardised age-appropriate reference ranges are lacking. Further investigation is determined by the results of expert assessment and initial investigations. These may include the hCG stimulation test to examine the presence of functional androgen-producing testicular tissue. The adrenocorticotrophic hormone (ACTH) stimulation test can outline a steroid hormone biosynthetic defect affecting adrenal gland as well as testicular function. Urinary steroid profiling by gas chromatography and mass spectrometry can outline the level of any enzyme defect in steroid synthesis pathways, ideally using a 24-h urine collection. Detailed visualisation of the internal genitalia is performed using magnetic resonance imaging in some centres, particularly in Europe. A urogenital sinugram is only rarely needed to outline the anatomy of the lower genital tract (see Chap. 12). Gonadal biopsy to exclude pre-malignant or frankly malignant changes is indicated in most infants with Y chromosome material and atypical genitalia (see Chap. 8 section 8.2.1 for further discussion). It should be noted that the absence of premalignant cells in the dysgenetic testis of an infant does not preclude this problem later; a second biopsy after the onset of puberty is recommended. Molecular genetic testing for specific gene mutations is more widely available and increasingly requested. Diagnostic algorithms are available to guide the use of these investigations (Leon et al. 2019; Brown and Warne 2005), but despite the increasing sophistication of investigation strategies, it is the widespread experience that many infants with 46,XY DSD will be left without a precise aetiological diagnosis.

It must be noted that DSD present in many guises, not only with atypical genitalia. They sometimes masquerade as precocious puberty, pubertal delay or primary amenorrhoea, or development of contra-sexual secondary sex characteristics, and clinical suspicion should remain present (see Chaps. 13 and 14 for details).

16.4 Common Causes

The three most common diagnoses where a DSD is caused by a gonadal or hormonal variation are congenital adrenal hyperplasia (CAH), androgen insensitivity syndrome (AIS) and mixed gonadal dysgenesis (MGD), with these diagnoses comprising 32–47% of all children with DSD caused by variations in hormone production or effects (Al-Agha et al. 2001; Joshi et al. 2006; Thyen et al. 2006; Parisi et al. 2007; Bhullar et al. 2011) (Table 16.3). The small fraction of these disorders in the broader diagnostic group is due to the difficulty of accurate diagnosis in many cases. Here, we briefly outline the specific management of the three most common diagnoses.

16.4.1 46,XX DSD: Congenital Adrenal Hyperplasia (CAH) Due to 21-Hydroxylase Deficiency

CAH occurs when an enzyme defect in the steroid-producing pathway of the adrenal gland leads to glucocorticoid and often also mineralocorticoid deficiency (salt-wasting CAH). In a gland with CAH, steroid precursors that accumulate proximal to the step involving altered enzymatic function

Table 16.3 Diagnostic breakdown of reported DSD cohorts

Authors	Country	Cohort size	Study population	Common diagnoses
Parisi et al. (2007)	United States	250	Children with DSD assessed by hospital gender team (excluding Klinefelter and Turner syndrome and multiple congenital abnormality patients)	CAH 14% AIS 10% MGD 8%
Thyen et al. (2006)	Germany	80	Infants with ambiguous genitalia	CAH 18% AIS 16% MGD 9%
Al-Agha et al. (2001)	Australia	51	Infants with ambiguous genitalia	CAH 31% AIS 10% MGD 6%
Bhullar et al. (2011)	Melbourne	199	All children aged 0–10 years identified with DSD using consensus statement	Perineal hypospadias 34% CAH 22% Exstrophy 14%
Joshi et al. (2006)	India	109	Infants with ambiguous genitalia	CAH 28% AIS 15% 5ARD 12%

CAH congenital adrenal hyperplasia, *AIS* androgen insensitivity syndrome, *MGD* mixed gonadal dysgenesis, *5ARD* 5α-reductase deficiency

are instead redirected or channelled along the sex steroid pathway, leading to over-virilisation of a female child.

Every infant with atypical genitalia should be assumed to have salt-wasting CAH due to 21-hydroxylase deficiency until proven otherwise. Failure to make this diagnosis in a timely manner may potentially have a fatal outcome. A provisional diagnosis of CAH in the child with ambiguous genitalia can be made on clinical grounds: although there may be atypical genital appearance, the infant, being genetically 46,XX with ovaries, will not have palpable external gonads. In addition, the skin is likely to be hyperpigmented due to the effects of excessive ACTH and related peptides. She will have a uterus. The degree of pigmentation of the skin may be hard to judge, as there is natural variation due to racial background. Examination under sunlight or white light rather than yellow incandescent light is essential. Newborn infants with salt-wasting CAH are not initially dehydrated nor do they have electrolyte disturbance. Clinically significant salt depletion is typically seen towards the end of or after the first week of life, when most babies have left hospital and are at home. In the first week, the only metabolic disturbance that might occur is hypoglycaemia (which is not invariable but may also go unrecognised).

Newborn screening (NBS) for 21-OH deficiency CAH is being undertaken in progressively more countries (Torresani and Biason-Lauber 2007) and has recently been approved for addition to the NBS program in Australia. It is based on measurement of 17-hydroxyprogesterone in heel-prick dried blood samples collected on days 2–3 of life. In these countries, the first contact the paediatrician has with an infant with CAH may be a referral from the screening laboratory. Importantly, the presence of genital variations cannot be relied upon to guarantee an early diagnosis of CAH, even in countries with a highly resourced medical system. In the Texas CAH screening program, nearly 70% of cases were not clinically suspected, including 20% of females and 99% of males with CAH (Therrell et al. 1998). Newborn screening for CAH has reduced mortality, adrenal crises and incorrect sex of rearing (Torresani and Biason-Lauber 2007).

A clinical suspicion of CAH, or referral from a screening laboratory, should be followed by careful clinical assessment, looking for features that would confirm the diagnosis. Family history should seek evidence consistent with autosomal recessive inheritance. Symptoms that may be present after the first week include persistent vomiting, listlessness, poor feeding and reduced urine output, indicating dehydration. Infants with CAH are at risk of seizures due to hypoglycaemia or hyponatraemia and also of cardiac arrest due to extreme hyperkalaemia.

Confirmation of the diagnosis involves requesting an urgent serum 17-Hydroxyprogesterone (17-

OHP) assay, which, in optimal circumstances, can be completed within several hours. Blood for a karyotype and rapid FISH test for Y-chromosome material should be collected. In most cases of classical CAH (a baby girl born with ambiguous genitalia), a greatly elevated 17-OHP result makes the diagnosis easy. If the clinical suspicion is strong and the 17-OHP result is borderline, an ACTH stimulation test will provide a definitive answer. In addition, we recommend collecting urine for steroid analysis to confirm that the CAH is due to 21-Hydroxyase deficiency and not one of the less common varieties, such as 11β-Hydroxylase deficiency. Other essential tests are serum electrolytes and urea (looking for a low sodium, a high potassium and normal or only slightly high urea) and blood glucose. Genetic analysis of CYP21A2 gene is also widely available, although associated costs may limit its routine uptake in some settings

The treatment of an infant with salt-wasting CAH should be provided in a centre of excellence where there is a team approach to management. We strongly recommend early contact with and transfer to such a centre. If the diagnosis is initially suspected based on atypical genital appearance at birth, then this should occur within the early postnatal days, although preferably timed to avoid separation of mum and baby (i.e. once mum is ready for discharge post delivery); if diagnosis is at time of clinical salt wasting then transfer following emergency resuscitation. The paediatric endocrinologist can advise treatment with either oral or intravenous hydrocortisone (parenteral route is typically preferred in unwell children), rehydration and fludrocortisone. The endocrinologist and MDT would also provide education for the parents, using resource material that is available on the internet and which can be downloaded from the website https://www.rch.org.au/endo/differences-of-sex-development/. The risk of adrenal crisis during inter-current illness and how to prevent it must be clearly understood by the family. A mental health professional can support the family in accepting the unexpected appearance of their baby's genitalia as a natural variation and, where relevant, in managing the associated implications of a lifelong medical condition such as CAH (see Chaps. 19 and 20). The paediatric surgeon/urologist member of the DSD team will also assess the baby and review imaging and other investigations to determine the degree of genital variation. For girls with evidence of more significant antenatal androgen exposure (e.g. a high urogenital confluence—Prader 3+) the potential role for surgical interventions should be discussed. This should include open discussion about the more contentious aspects such as optimal timing of surgery and the option to defer until the girl is old enough to be involved in the decision (see Chap. 17). Genetic counselling about the recurrence risk and availability of future prenatal genetic diagnosis and treatment should be made available (see Chap. 21). Prenatal dexamethasone treatment has been offered to prevent the development of genital virilisation in an affected female foetus; however, there are many unknowns in relation to this practice, and some concerns (e.g. on outcomes in unaffected males who were exposed *in utero*) have been reported. It is therefore recommended that it should only be offered and undertaken as part of a well-designed longitudinal research study.

Following discharge from hospital, it is likely that the child would be followed up by a paediatric endocrinologist often in conjunction with a local paediatrician. Treatment is monitored using a combination of clinical measures (height, weight, blood pressure and general examination) and biochemical test results. Repeated genital examination throughout childhood and beyond has been highlighted as a source of significant distress by many affected individuals. Historically, this practice was established as means of monitoring androgen exposure and effect, but as this information can be obtained by other means, routine genital examination is not recommended. Optimal biochemical sampling schedules vary. Our routine practice is 3-monthly collection of an early morning blood sample (delaying taking the morning dose of steroid medications until after the blood collection, hence recognising that this may be a longer than typical interval), for serum 17-OHP and renin/plasma renin activity (PRA). Other centres use other approaches such as dry blood spot 17-OHP profiling across a 24-h period, which may become more easily available with increasing use of tandem mass spectrometry. Additional tests may include occasional checks using 24 h urinary pregnanetriol as well as assessment of bone age as a surrogate for androgen exposure (and to assist with interpretation of growth) in school-age children and adolescents.

The aims of treatment are (1) good general health without adrenal crises, (2) normal linear growth, (3) avoidance of obesity, unwanted virilisation, Cushingoid features and hypertension and (4) appropriate sexual development for age. This is generally achieved using hydrocortisone as the preferred glucocorticoid, in a dose of 10–15 mg/m^2/day in three divided doses. In all patients who had electrolyte disturbance in infancy or with persistently elevated PRA, fludrocortisone should be added. For approximately first 3–4 months of life, the typical infant diet is low in salt and all infants' kidneys are relatively insensitive to aldosterone. Levels of PRA and aldosterone in the blood are higher at this time than later in childhood. Infants with salt-wasting CAH are therefore relatively resistant to the effects of fludrocortisone until 3–4 months of age. In addition to needing doses of fludrocortisone that would usually be used in adults (0.1–0.3 mg/day), they typically require a dietary sodium chloride supplement (on average, 2–3 mmol/kg per day) to avoid hyponatraemia and hyperkalaemia (Mullis et al. 1990). At around 3 months, the kidneys develop greater sensitivity to the effects of mineralocorticoids and salt excretion falls. Blood pressure may rise abruptly at this time and requires close monitoring. Once the transition to greater sensitivity has occurred, the salt supplement can be ceased and dose of fludrocortisone can usually be reduced to ~0.05–0.1 mg/day.

The hydrocortisone dose should be adjusted to achieve a 3-monthly 17-OHP result <70 nmol/L. While a 17-OHP level of 70 nmol/L is far from normal (hence, many clinicians may have an upper target of ~50 nmol/L), it is unlikely to be associated with clinical hyper-androgenism, and control of androgen secretion is the true aim (Hughes 1988). Some clinics prefer to monitor serum Δ^4-androstenedione levels instead of or in addition to 17-OHP. Complete suppression of 17-OHP (tested after an appropriate timeframe [~8 h] from the previous dose) likely means hydrocortisone dosing is excessive which may negatively impact linear growth and may result in the child becoming frankly cushingoid. Plasma renin activity (PRA) or renin levels should be maintained in the normal range and the dose of fludrocortisone is adjusted up and down to achieve this target.

The risk of adrenal crisis is greatest in children under the age of 4 years. Parents should be issued with a letter of introduction that can be used in the event of an emergency. It should clearly state that the child urgently requires hydrocortisone by injection (2–3 mg/kg body weight; or 50–100 mg/m^2 stat IM or IV) if she presents with vomiting, diarrhoea or dehydration, also, if she suffers significant injury, for example, a fracture, or requires surgery under general anaesthetic (Donald et al. 1993). It is common practice to teach parents how to administer IM hydrocortisone and to provide them with an injection of hydrocortisone to have on hand in case of emergency, so that they are never disempowered.

One quarter of girls with classical CAH have the non-salt-wasting form and have a very low risk of adrenal crisis (New 1998). Treated adequately from infancy, their development is the same as that for girls with the salt-wasting form.

A study of girls aged 10–13y with classical and non-classical CAH reported no differences between groups in gender identity or cognitions, although male gender-role behaviour and activities (e.g. tomboy behaviour) were more common in those with classical CAH (Berenbaum et al. 2018). Diversity of gender identity and sexuality is more common in CAH girls and women. Rates of gender dysphoria (Razzaghy-Azar et al. 2017) and same sex attraction (Meyer-Bahlburg et al. 2008) are reported as higher than the background population; the reasons for this are likely multifaceted but exposure to higher levels of androgen (prenatally and often postnatally) may play a role. An appreciation of this is helpful in supporting teenagers with CAH. Fertility is impacted to a variable degree in women with CAH, especially the salt-losing form, although this is treatable. Referral during early adolescence to a gynaecologist experienced in CAH management is important, so that discussions around an individual's genital/vaginal variation and its potential impact, if any, on future sexual function can take place. In addition, open discussions around possible interventions to allow the use of tampons and penetrative sexual activities may be appropriate and should be introduced and discussed in more detail, should this be something that the girl herself wishes to pursue. The endocrinologist's role is to ensure that hormonal balance is optimised. Once linear growth is complete, a longer acting steroid replacement such as daily or twice-daily prednisolone may be considered in place of tds hydrocortisone. Although not very commonly used in paediatrics, older girls (who have reached final height) with menstrual irregularity may achieve a more regular pattern if they are treated with once-daily dexamethasone (Young and Hughes 1990). Occasionally, in an adolescent or adult patient, it may be difficult using any form of oral steroid to achieve adequate control of hyper-androgenism, without causing cushingoid features and excessive weight gain. In this situation, there may be a place for considering bilateral laparoscopic adrenalectomy (Ogilvie et al. 2006), although in practice, this is infrequently undertaken. Hormone replacement using much lower doses is usually possible once the requirement to suppress adrenal androgens has been removed. Bilateral adrenalectomy may also improve fertility. Some women with CAH have psychosexual difficulties, and rates for avoidance of sexual activity have previously been reported as higher than those for the general population (May et al. 1996); in contrast a more recent systematic review of women with CAH who had undergone genital surgery reported most women are sexually active, although rates of discomfort were high and levels of satisfaction were variable (Almasri et al. 2018) (see Chap. 20). Of note a recent case series of four individuals with 46XX CAH and significant virilisation at birth such that sex was assigned male, has reported male gender identity and sexual attraction to women in all four, with satisfactory sexual function reported by the two who had partners (Apóstolos et al. 2018).

16.4.2 46,XY DSD: Androgen Insensitivity Syndrome (AIS)

Androgen insensitivity syndrome was first described in 1953 (Morris 1953). In the *complete* form (CAIS), a person with a 46,XY karyotype and testes is born a phenotypic female. At puberty, breast development occurs and body shape is female, but little or no body hair develops and menstruation does not happen due to an absence of the Müllerian structures (including the uterus), which regressed *in utero* under the influence of AMH from the testes. The testes, which may be located superficially in the inguinal area, grow during puberty and may be a source of pain or discomfort. The risk of malignant change is very low prior to puberty, and even after puberty, the risk is thought to be 0.8%–2% (Cools et al. 2006). Newer data in a cohort of adolescents and adults with genetically proven AIS (median age 17.5years) have shown earliest pre-malignant changes (pre-GCNIS) only in gonadal tissue from prophylactic gonadectomies (14% of CAIS and 10% of PAIS samples), with no GCNIS or TGCT reported (see 7.6.1.1 for further discussion). Factors that influence progression from pre-GCNIS remain to be elucidated but it appears rates of this occurrence are low. There has been considerable debate about performing gonadectomy in CAIS in recent years, but it appears evident that there is no universal medical reason for this to occur before puberty. Leaving the testes *in situ* allows natural breast development to occur under the influence of endogenous oestradiol, produced from aromatisation of higher circulating levels of testosterone. If the testes can be monitored by palpation, potentially biopsied, and studied with ultrasound, it is debatable that removal is required at all, but lifelong surveillance to detect cancer is essential (Nojima et al. 2004). As the testes are inside a patent processus vaginalis, it is important that the hernia has been repaired surgically if a decision to leave the testes *in situ* is made.

A minority of women with CAIS have vaginal hypoplasia (because of Müllerian duct regression) to a degree that makes penetrative intercourse difficult (Sarpel et al. 2005). For most women with CAIS, with adequate support and positive body image, penetrative sexual activity will be fine. For some, dilatation may be helpful if the girl or woman wishes to increase vaginal length, and only infrequently, surgery is required. Nevertheless, there is a significant difference in approaches to this internationally with some countries offering surgery earlier than others.

A person with the *partial* form of AIS (PAIS) is born with different degrees of genital variation, which may include ambiguity in appearance, underdevelopment of the penis or incomplete midline scrotal fusion. Virilisation at puberty is incomplete, despite considerable growth of the testes, and it is usual for breast development to occur in response to endogenous oestradiol (produced from aromatised testosterone). Parents may decide to raise an infant with atypical genitalia due to PAIS either as a boy or as a girl, depending on the overall appearance and perceived degree of androgen effect. If raised as a girl, previous practice has been to consider removal of the testes in childhood. Reasons to do this included removal of future risk of germ cell cancer as well as removal of future testosterone/androgen production (perceived to be 'unwanted' in someone being raised as female). The risk of seminoma and other germ cell cancers in PAIS testes is increased: previously documented at as high as 50% when the testes are intra-abdominal and 15% when the testes are outside the external inguinal ring (Cassio et al. 1990; Cools et al. 2006) although more recent data in a cohort with confirmed genetic variants and PAIS do not support these data and suggest rates of malignant change are lower (Cools et al. 2017). Removal of intra-abdominal testes, which cannot be brought to the inguino-scrotal area and are therefore difficult to monitor but have a higher malignant potential, has until recently been considered important; however the more recent data indicating lower rates of invasive disease than previously identified (Cools et al. 2017) have challenged this approach. In the absence of clear evidence based pathways, the pros and cons of such an intervention should be carefully discussed with the adolescent and his family. Optimal timing for this is unknown; however, malignancy occurring pre-pubertally is not typical; hence, deferral of decisions until puberty/early adolescence, when the young person can be involved in discussions as to possible outcomes and interventions and participate in the decision as to their preferred management plan, is thought to be appropriate where possible. Surgery for the purpose of removing a source of 'unwanted' future testosterone should no longer be considered routine. This is because suppression of endogenous testosterone that may ultimately be unwanted or incongruent with gender identity (in a 46,XY child with PAIS whose gender identity is congruent with an assigned female sex, for example) can be achieved with gonadotrophin-releasing hormone analogues at least temporarily, while decisions in relation to removal or otherwise of testes are discussed. This latter approach more closely aligns with the ethical principles outlined in Chap. 15. Gender dysphoria has been reported in as many as 25% of adults with PAIS, regardless of the initial assigned sex of rearing (Migeon et al. 2002a, b). Since future gender identity cannot be predicted in an infant with PAIS, leaving options open for the future when the individual themselves can decide on the optimal course is an important ethical consideration. If the testes are not removed, regular self examination of scrotal testes is recommended; after the onset of puberty, biopsy to assess for pre-malignant or malignant changes are found (Cools and Looijenga 2017; Muller and Skakkebaek 1984; von der Maase et al. 1987).

Androgen insensitivity affects all tissues, including the hypothalamus, and therefore in individuals with AIS, the negative feedback normally exerted by testosterone on LH secretion is impaired, resulting in higher levels of circulating LH. Serum testosterone levels are considerably higher than those found in men with typically functioning androgen receptors, and aromatisation to oestrogen is stimulated in the presence of high levels of gonadotrophins. Serum oestradiol levels thus exceed those found in post-pubertal males without AIS but are lower than those found in women during the menstrual cycle. The lack of any testosterone effect on bones and relatively lower levels of oestradiol expose women with CAIS to an increased risk of osteoporosis (Sobel et al. 2006). Spermatogenesis is absent in the testes because, although the local concentration of testosterone within the testis is high, as androgen action is required, the tubular response is inhibited (Yong et al. 2003; Hashmi et al. 2008).

AIS is an X-linked condition, associated with variants in the androgen receptor gene. Phenotypic variation is related to the type of gentice change present and the resulting alteration in the structure of the androgen receptor protein. In CAIS, the mutation results in an androgen receptor that is either absent or unable to bind any testosterone or dihydrotestosterone (DHT). Mutational analysis is commonly positive in patients with CAIS but may require sequencing of the entire gene if no gross deletion is detected. In people with a clinical diagnosis of PAIS, however, an androgen receptor gene mutation is found in only about 30% (De Bellis et al. 1994). Higher overall rates have been reported in more recent studies using massively parallel sequencing (MPS)-targeted DSD gene panels (Eggers et al. 2016). Hundreds of different AR gene mutations have been found in AIS, and structure-function relationships are complex (Gottlieb et al. 2004). In addition, over 70 androgen receptor-interacting proteins have been identified, and mutations in genes regulating these have been found in a small number of AR mutation-negative patients. Females who are carriers may show mild expression in that they tend to have less pubic hair than other women. The incidence of CAIS is reported to be about 1:20,000 (Hashmi et al. 2008).

16.4.3 Mixed Sex Chromosome (Aneuploidy) DSD: Mixed Gonadal Dysgenesis

Mixed gonadal dysgenesis (MGD) refers to asymmetrical gonadal development, with a developed gonad on one side and a dysgenic or streak gonad on the other. It is commonly associated with a mosaic karyotype and sex chromosome aneuploidy. The karyotype is usually 45,X/46,XY. Children with 45,X/46,XY mosaicism show considerable phenotypic variation, from completely male, through a range of genital variations to female. Some have features of Turner syndrome and most have short stature (Telvi et al. 1999). It should be noted that most individuals with a 45,X/46,XY mosaicism do not have MGD; the male phenotype was found in 95% of antenatally diagnosed cases, 27% of whom had histological evidence of gonadal dysgenesis (Chang et al. 1990). A uterus and Fallopian tubes can be present regardless of the gonadal sex and external genitalia. Gonadal dysgenesis manifests asymmetrically, but both testes may have some degree of dysgenesis with raised serum FSH levels at puberty, even though during childhood one gonad appeared normal.

Children with MGD are diagnosed in various ways: by antenatal screening of pregnancies, on clinical grounds in neonates with ambiguous/atypical genitalia, at investigation of delayed puberty or short stature, or when a child presents with a germ cell cancer. Examination findings may include only one palpable gonad, likely to be a testis; presence of both a (hemi-)uterus and a testis strongly suggests MGD. The diagnosis is made with a karyotype examination, imaging and direct visualisation of the internal genitalia laparoscopically and the subsequent histologic examination of the gonads (see Chap. 8).

The sex of rearing is usually concordant with the predominant external genital phenotype but can be difficult to determine in children who have true ambiguity of their genitalia. Investigations to delineate the anatomy and ascertain current and hence likely or possible future gonadal function are important. These will inform the detailed discussions with the family so that an informed decision can be made. The surgeon will then discuss the potential role for any surgical intervention and its optimal timing with the family. This may initially include gonadal biopsy to establish tissue type and stain for OCT 3/4 and c-kit ligand to help inform potential malignancy risk.

Children with MGD are reported to be at high risk of germ cell malignancy in all gonads left *in situ*. The precursor of malignancy in streak gonads is gonadoblastoma, found in approximately 25% of Y-positive streak gonads (Hughes et al. 2006), whereas in testes with differentiated tubules, cancer develops from Germ cell neoplasia *in situ* (Skakkebaek 1994). It is therefore recommended that any highly undifferentiated or streak gonads should be removed, as these organs will not have endogenous hormonal or fertility potential; hence, the potential malignancy risk can be mitigated without impacting on future function. The consideration to leave testes *in situ* in a male child, when the evidence indicates a high risk of malignancy, should be made in consultation with the family. They need to be both well informed and cognisant of the necessity for regular surveillance to prevent death from malignancy. They also need to understand that a retained dysgenic testis may also develop failure of Leydig and Sertoli cell function with time (Wikstrom and Dunkel 2008). Any retained testis should be one that is well differentiated and should be brought into the scrotum to where it can easily be palpated every 6 months and examined by ultrasonography each year. Testicular tumours often present as painless masses found on examination. Hydroceles may be associated with a testicular tumour and should prompt further investigation (Dorfinger et al. 1997). In addition, signs of precocious puberty or gynaecomastia on regular physical examination may indicate a functional gonadal tumour. Investigation of suspected tumour involves serum tumour markers such as β-hCG, α-fetoprotein, lactate dehydrogenase, an abdomino-pelvic CT or MRI and biopsy. It is recommended that biopsy should also be performed in all *in situ* gonads after the onset of puberty, and if pre-malignant histology is found, then sperm banking be offered prior to radiotherapy (Looijenga et al. 2007). In boys with a well-differentiated testis who are unable to produce an ejaculate sample, intraoperative sperm salvage procedures may be considered. Monitoring for the development of primary hypogonadism should form part of the follow-up in addition to the surveillance for malignancy. Delayed or slow pubertal progression or post-pubertal lethargy and poor libido may indicate hypogonadism.

Hormone replacement therapy is required in all females with MGD and in males who have either had bilateral gonadectomy or developed testicular failure (Warne et al. 2005a, b). The dose and commencement of sex hormone replacement is planned to maximise height potential and age appropriate development of secondary sex characteristics. Females are commenced on low-dose oestrogen supplementation with a schedule of increasing doses ~6 monthly over ~2 years. A progestin is usually added after approximately 2 years, or following the first breakthrough bleed. Testosterone replacement for those with a masculine gender identity can be given orally, by regular intramuscular injection or by transdermal patch. Prior to the commencement of sex steroid therapy, we recommend that all children should be included in the decisions around commencement of hormone replacement therapy and be fully informed as to the expected effects of treatment on secondary sex characteristics and other attributes. Psychological outcome has been evaluated in a small cohort of six MGD adolescents, with one female found to have gender dysphoria (Szarras-Czapnik et al. 2007). Screening questions in relation to gender diversity or possible gender dysphoria should be included in discussions, and if either is suspected, youth should have a more formal assessment of possible gender dysphoria with an experienced mental health clinician (see Chap. 20). All girls should be referred to a gynaecologist at puberty (see Chap. 18).

Bone mineral density and lipid profile may be adversely affected by inadequate sex hormone replacement resulting from insufficient dosing, its non-physiological effects or potentially non-compliance, and children should be monitored for these associated pathologies. We would suggest bone mineral densitometry in patients who have experienced fractures and lipid profile assessments at puberty and thereafter as necessary.

Some females with MGD, who have good uterine anatomy and access to oocyte donation, are able to carry a pregnancy. Sperm production is highly unlikely (Robboy et al. 1982).

16.5 Summary of Management Concepts During Childhood

It is widely accepted that the management of children with DSD should be performed by an experienced multidisciplinary team. In the absence of diagnosis-specific outcome studies, difficult management issues such as gender assignment are best approached through specialist and family consensus.

As described, many children do not receive an accurate aetiological diagnosis to explain their variation. In the absence of a definitive diagnosis, targeted care is impossible and management is best performed using the general guidelines and concepts currently accepted and described here.

Sex of rearing is influenced by many factors including diagnosis, prenatal androgen exposure, potential for spontaneous virilisation, potential for sexual function and fertility (acknowledging that the individual's future preferences in this regard cannot be known) and parental attitudes and cultural background. It is generally accepted that most females with CAH and those with CAIS should be reared female. Children with 46,XY DSD and limited external genital virilisation were commonly reared female in the past; however, they are now mostly reared male, as evidence shows satisfaction with sexual function and gender identity in adulthood (Warne et al. 2005a, b). Children with 5α-reductase-2 and 17-β hydroxysteroid dehydrogenase (17βHSD3) deficiencies represent a difficult group, as they are born with a female phenotype but virilise at puberty and often later identify as male (Imperato-McGinley et al. 1974; Gross et al. 1986). In the absence of strong evidence from outcome studies in other forms of DSD, decisions on optimal sex of rearing are made after detailed discussions both amongst a multidisciplinary team and with the child's family who should be fully informed in relation to potential outcomes. This should include uncertainties and areas of management where knowledge on natural history is limited and the family should be supported in accepting that future gender identity may differ from sex of rearing (acknowledging that this is the case for all children, whether a DSD is present or not). With this in mind, surgical interventions should be limited to include only procedures deemed medically necessary (e.g. removal of streak gonads with Y material) and where possible, structures such as hemi-uterus/Müllerian structures should be left *in situ* until the individual can decide at a later age whether this is appropriate for them.

Surgery for children with DSD should, wherever possible, be performed by paediatric urologists who are highly experienced in the techniques required for genital surgery (see Chap. 17). The surgeon is responsible for explanation of the entire surgical plan until adulthood and the potential difficulties with outcome. In Y-chromosome-positive children raised female, completely dysplastic gonads such as those in complete gonadal dysgenesis, have a high malignancy risk, and it is recommended that these should be removed in early childhood by either paediatric urologists or paediatric gynaecologists. At our centre, we have experience of finding histological evidence of dysgerminoma in dysplastic gonads of an 8-month-old 46,XY infant with complete gonadal dysgenesis (unpubl. data); hence, true malignant changes can occur early in life in this scenario. Where previously it has been recommended that testes should also be removed in children with androgen biosynthetic defects who are raised as girls, early surgery for this reason is increasingly deemed unnecessary. It is evident that this may indeed cause significant harm should the young person ultimately have a male/masculine gender identity, as testes with the potential for endogenous hormonal function would have been removed. Deferral at least until adolescence when the young person can participate in informed decision making is therefore considered optimal at our centre. If necessary to aid in this process, pubertal hormone production can be temporarily (and reversibly) 'blocked' with use of a GnRHa to remove any perceived urgency in the decision-making process. Assessment of gender identity is also important at this time, as high rates of gender dysphoria are reported. Whether these high rates are influenced by exposure to masculinising hormones at puberty cannot clearly be established from studies to date.

The testes of girls with CAIS, however, do not need removal prior to puberty due to their very low malignancy risk at this age (Cools et al. 2006). Discussion regarding the long-term follow-up and monitoring of these testes and regarding any potential removal can be delayed until after puberty. In 46,XY DSD children raised male, all streak gonads should be removed without delay, and any dysgenetic testes left *in situ* should have regular screening for malignancy. How best to image for screening is not well defined, but ultrasound (6–12 monthly) is most commonly undertaken at our centre, with MRI performed if any clinical or ultrasound suspicion of malignancy/atypical features. Fertility should be considered, with preservation of ovarian tissue, or sperm banking if required, although for many of these conditions, fertility is absent or significantly reduced.

Our long-term follow-up study of males who had had surgery for a DSD showed a high prevalence of persisting urological difficulties, including wetting (25%), spraying of urine (31%) and recurrent infections (25%) (see Chap. 23) (Warne et al. 2005a, b). In women with CAH, increased rates of urinary symptoms, including urge and stress incontinence have been reported, although uroflow studies are within normal range (Davies and Creighton 2004; Bogdanska et al. 2018). It is not clear whether these are a result of the surgery or virilisation of the pelvic floor.

Medical management involves ensuring that sex steroid replacement, if required, is given appropriately and includes pubertal induction. In addition, those children who proceed through spontaneous puberty continue to carry a risk for premature gonadal failure. The paediatrician should also ensure follow-up of problems associated with inadequate sex hormone replacement such as low bone mineral density and dyslipidaemia, and any known associated features of a given DSD (such as cardiac anomalies, vision or hearing defects in Turner syndrome). A group of syndromes caused by variants of a similar gene region share problems with renal and gonadal development and some carry high risk for Wilms tumours of the kidney as well as germ cell malignancy of the gonads. These disorders include Denys-Drash Syndrome, Frasier Syndrome and WAGR Syndrome (Jadresic et al. 1990) (see Chap. 10).

Finally, psychological support is recommended to be provided to the family at initial diagnosis and regularly for the affected child throughout their life. Disclosure should occur in stages appropriate to the developmental level of the child and begin from the age of 3 or 4 years. Parents should be supported with written and online resources outlining ways to approach this. Our current approach involves introduction of the concept of diversity in all aspects of life from an early age, such that diversity in physical appearance is one aspect of how people differ. Psychological support is particularly important at puberty and should include open screening questions relating to gender identity and more formal assessment of this where appropriate. This should occur universally but is particularly important where decisions in relation to sex of rearing were less clear, for example, in cases with ambiguity of genital appearance at birth. Psychological support of children with DSD and their families is arguably the most important aspect of care yet is commonly poorly resourced and hence lacking from a MDT. Access to peer support has been shown to be very beneficial in normalising variations in sex development and debunking previous assumptions in relation to how an individual might 'manage' or cope with their genital variation. Care to ensure that heteronormative assumptions are not imposed when establishing management pathways for a young child is also important.

16.6 Gender Dysphoria in Relation to DSD

As shown in a number of long-term outcome studies, some adults who had been surgically treated for a DSD as children develop gender dysphoria, that is, they feel a persistent and unpleasant insecurity about their gender identity (Cohen-Kettenis 2005a, b) (see Chap. 20). For some, the dysphoria is such that they actively seek medical or surgical intervention to support transition to living in their affirmed gender. The incidence of gender dysphoria varies. Most papers published to date have focussed on the small number of patients seeking a sex change and comparison between different DSD on the number who are simply unhappy about their own gender to a lesser degree, is currently not possible.

Overall it is thought that relatively few girls and women with classical CAH, treated with effective suppression of androgens from infancy, identify as male, but the number wishing to change gender from female to male rises if hyperandrogenism is allowed to exist for long periods during childhood, and it is more common to encounter this in developing countries (Warne and Raza 2008).

Gender dysphoria has also been reported following treatment for mixed gonadal dysgenesis, and it has been said that those raised male experience less psychopathology than those raised female (Szarras-Czapnik et al. 2007). This perhaps related to the fact that surgery to fashion male genitalia conserves all external tissues and thus preserves options for surgical review in the future, whereas feminising genitoplasty involves the removal of some genital skin and erectile tissues, making a later reversal more difficult. Findings such as these have resulted in calls for changes in practice such that irreversible surgical procedures that are not definitively medically warranted but rather are performed mostly with a view to creating a genital appearance that more closely aligns with that of typical male or female genitalia are only performed at an age when the individual themselves can be involved in giving informed consent for the procedure (Darlington Statement 2017).

In some particular conditions, overt gender dysphoria may become manifest in adolescence when this was not present or not anticipated earlier in childhood. This is well described in conditions such as 46,XY DSD due to 5α-reductase deficiency or 17-beta HSD deficiency (Cohen-Kettenis 2005a, b; Rosler 2006; Faienza et al. 2008), where children raised as female undergo virilisation in adolescence. This can be associated with early gender dysphoria and then complete gender identity transition to male (Maimoun et al. 2011), particularly in the context of ongoing exposure to male puberty hormones. In certain geographic locations, such as the Dominican Republic (Imperato-McGinley et al. 1974; Cai et al. 1996) and the highlands of Papua New Guinea (Imperato-McGinley et al. 1991), this phenomenon is common enough to have produced local cultural changes in these communities. The frequency of the conditions in these areas is related to higher rates of consanguinity. Recent evidence, however, suggests that 5α-reductase-2 deficiency may be more common than previously thought and may have been mistaken for PAIS in some patient cohorts (Maimoun et al. 2011). This underlines the importance of being as thorough as possible in establishing the diagnosis to inform gender assignment in infancy but also to be watchful for signs of gender dysphoria in early adolescents with all 46,XY DSD without a genetic diagnosis (Meyer-Bahlburg 2001, 2002; Meyer-Bahlburg et al. 2004). In affected individuals with an established female gender identity in whom virilisation occurs at puberty, the option to put further progression of masculinisation 'on hold' with GnRHa should be discussed. If female gender identity persists, discussions with the young person in relation to the potential for gonadectomy and female hormone replacement therapy can then occur without the perceived pressure of associated further irreversible masculinisation. As this latter approach is relatively novel, long-term outcome studies assessing its impact are lacking. Nonetheless, it is currently preferred to avoid early gonadectomy in those with androgen biosynthetic defects at our centre, as it more closely aligns with the ethical principle of leaving more options open for the future (see Chap. 15).

Amongst those with genetically confirmed PAIS treated at the Johns Hopkins Hospital in Baltimore, adult gender identity conformed in the majority to the initially assigned gender, but nearly 25% of adults surveyed expressed some degree of dissatisfaction with their gender, regardless of whether they had been raised as boys or girls (Migeon et al. 2002a, b). Evidence for potential factors that may have influenced this is lacking. Women with the complete form of AIS, on the other hand, do not demonstrate higher rates of gender dysphoria, despite having inguinal testes, an XY karyotype, and testosterone levels that are significantly higher than those of many males. This implies that the extent of gender dysphoria in those with varying DSD may therefore relate, at least in part, to androgen action in the brain.

16.7 Management During Transition to Adulthood

The transition in adolescence to the wider world of adulthood is a testing time even for youth without a DSD but considerably more complex for those with DSD. Here, we highlight the existential issues, as well as the major medical issues that need management in boys and girls, as they become men and women.

16.8 Existential Issues

Adolescents with DSD face a huge range of social and psychological issues in the context of their underlying variation. Many of these difficulties may originate from or be compounded by perceived societal pressure to 'conform' to a binary norm as well as low levels of awareness in the general population of the existence of differences in sex or genital characteristics or appearance, hence the potential for associated stigma in discussing such issues (Table 16.4). Adolescence can be a time of lower self-esteem and negative body image for many young people; this is also true of those with DSD. In recent years, advocacy groups have been more vocal in their calls for

Table 16.4 Existential issues for adolescents

Female	Male
Why me? Why am I different? Who am I? Is the introitus large enough for tampons? Is the introitus large enough for sex? Is my vagina large enough for sex? Do I have a womb? Will I have periods or not? Can I have children? Will I need 'IVF'? Will my ovaries get cancer? Do my ovaries need to be removed? What hormone treatment do I need? Does 'XY' mean I am a 'boy'? Who else can I talk to?	Why me? Why am I different? Who am I? Why is my penis small? Will my penis function normally for sex? Will girls laugh at me? Why are my testes small? Why don't I ejaculate? Will my testes get cancer? Why do I have so many urinary infections? Why is my urinary stream poor? Can I have children? Will I need 'IVF'? Who else can I talk to?

intersex variations/DSD to be viewed as part of the normal diversity of life, as the emphasis on 'disorder' or 'difference' is deemed unnecessarily pathologising. A driving force behind this desired change in emphasis is to reduce potential for stigma and shame that may be perceived in the context of a 'disorder' of sex development. Efforts to improve awareness of the relatively common frequency of DSD/intersex variations amongst the general population will also be important in this regard.

Historically, issues relating to clinical care have also had a negative impact. Where previously medical photographs and repeated genital examinations have reportedly been relatively commonly encountered, the negative impact of these on well-being and self-esteem is now well-recognised (Hughes et al. 2006; Jones et al. 2016), and these interventions are no longer routine. If a genital examination is deemed necessary, the importance of both clear explanation of its proposed purpose and ensuring appropriately informed consent is received for the examination is paramount. The young person should have the option for a support person to be present if desired, but medical students or additional observers should not be present. Similarly, discussions with trainee doctors or medical students are more appropriately held outside of a direct patient consultation. The importance of age-appropriate, and where possible, diagnosis-specific, information on an individual's underlying variation and its associated health or functional impacts (where relevant) is now well recognised. Open discussions that involve a young person in decisions that may arise in relation to their healthcare and options for medical interventions are a cornerstone of optimal contemporary care. The opportunity to discuss their diagnosis and to have psychological support as relevant to their age and developmental stage is also important. Engaging with peer support groups has also been described as positive by many with DSD/intersex variations, although such interactions are not universally appealing to adolescents and repeated offers for introductions or links may be warranted over time.

Girls with CAH may have some side effects of the steroid replacement therapy with excess weight, or even frank signs of Cushing syndrome if hydrocortisone doses have not been adjusted carefully enough; efforts to avoid this through regular monitoring as above are important. Girls with 46,XY DSD may experience unexpected and unwanted virilisation, which may induce significant anxiety if this is the first presentation of an underlying DSD. Retrospective reports of distress at diagnosis have been shown to be lower in those who felt well informed and well supported at the time of diagnosis or disclosure of their DSD (Gina Tolkien MDRP Uni Melb research 2018). Providing adequate reassurance, normalising the diversity and clearly explaining potential options for intervention (if desired and indicated) and the young person's role in a given decision-making process may therefore help to diminish distress or anxiety at this timepoint. As in childhood, psychological support is also recommended, although rates of uptake may be low, particularly when offered for the first time.

In many families, a child with a known DSD may have been brought up in a somewhat overly protective environment, albeit subconsciously. There may be parental concern about steroid treatment in CAH, or excessive secrecy about the child's underlying variation and anatomy, so that some DSD children may reach adolescence without ever going on a 'sleep-over' or a school camp. In this scenario, once the child reaches adolescence, their need for progressive independence comes into direct conflict with the parents' desire to maintain a protective 'cocoon'. As outlined above, age-appropriate disclosure and discussions around an individual's variation, starting from a young age (early primary school as developmentally appropriate) are now recommended (2006 Consensus and BSPED guidelines 2016).

Open, honest and well-informed communication from healthcare teams is very important at all stages but particularly when discussing their body and underlying variations with adolescents. It is important not to assume that information shared previously has been universally retained and understood. Poor or infrequent communication by professionals may mean adulthood arrives without the right background knowledge to enable them to be comfortable with themselves as individuals. In other circumstances, the medical management may have been adequate, but too focussed on the medical or anatomical issues, rather than helping the adolescent with ensuring general well-being (both medical and psychosocial) as well as appropriate understanding of their DSD. Feedback in recent decades from adults with DSD who grew up in a previous generation would suggest that counselling with adequate knowledge and moral support is one of the most important, but neglected, factors in the entire management plan for DSD patients. Sadly, the transition between childhood and adult life coincides with a transfer from paediatric to adult medical care, often creating a gap in the management plan at what is emerging as one of the most crucial times of psychological support.

Linking in with peer-support groups who can offer unique insights into lived experience with a given or similar DSD may help bridge some of these gaps in medical care and is routinely recommended. How best to approach and establish such links is not well known, however, but some families find 'reaching out' to a support group independently to be very confronting/challenging and may welcome a more direct introduction from a health professional.

Adolescence is a testing social environment, where long-term friendships may be disrupted by differences in personality and world view that in retrospect may appear trivial. Cliques form and reform almost continuously as adolescents mature; in some social environments, there may be a perception of severe consequences for anyone who is 'different'. For young women with Müllerian agenesis, or CAIS, the 'feeling different' can relate to the fact that they do not menstruate. Exploring the issues and role-playing potential responses should this discussion arise amongst friends is a useful step. 'Difference' can also be felt by those with a DSD due to a need for daily medications. In some scenarios (CAH), this medication is essential and potentially life-saving; for others (e.g. previously post gonadectomy in CAIS or PAIS), this may be surgically induced. In the latter groups in particular, the need for lifelong hormone replacement therapy, particularly if gonadectomy was performed at an age when the individual was too young to provide their own informed consent, has been reported to be associated with lower quality of life and adverse longer term outcomes (Jones et al. 2016). As such, delaying such interventions until the individual has had appropriate and comprehensive discussions relating to the pros and cons of a given intervention and has had the opportunity to provide fully informed personal (not parental) consent is now deemed preferable. This may involve gonadal surveillance given the increased risk of malignancy, although the latter is rare prior to puberty in AIS.

For those with a childhood diagnosis of complete gonadal dysgenesis where dysgenetic gonads are intra-abdominal and entirely non-functioning, hormone replacement therapy will not be iatrogenic but rather as a result of the inherent lack of hormone production from a non-functioning under-developed gonad. Given the higher rates of malignancy and reports of malignant change in gonads of affected toddlers, seeking parental consent to gonadectomy at a younger age is recommended. In such a scenario, open disclosure with the child and ultimately adolescent in relation to their underlying anatomy and DSD and the reason they need to have medication to induce and sustain pubertal development is important for wellbeing. If the diagnosis of gonadal dysgenesis is made due to presentation in adolescence with absent evidence of pubertal development, this too may have significant psychological impacts in terms of both the delay in the development of anticipated secondary sexual characteristics and the implications of their underlying difference in gonadal and internal genital development.

Being aware of the educational activities in which the adolescent with a DSD is participating is useful in terms of ensuring that they have the knowledge to cope with potentially challenging lessons. School classes on reproductive health and biology may pose confronting challenges as classrooms are told about chromosome and karyotypes of males and females in a rigid dichotomous/binary manner without any recognition of naturally occurring variations. This issue can extend to health and psychology classes discussing 'unusual cases' of DSD, where phenotype and karyotype are atypical.

Disclosure is a complex and multifaceted problem. Many individuals with DSD report inadequate knowledge regarding their diagnosis (Migeon et al. 2002a, b). On the other hand, others with DSD report the process of being told their diagnosis as traumatic—with many being able to describe in vivid detail even years later the circumstances of being told their diagnosis in a manner that is similar to those who experience post-traumatic stress disorders (Grover and Loughlin 2002). In young teenagers with DSD, care needs to be taken because as friendship groups change, the disclosure of personal information can be misused and potentially abused. On the other hand, older teenagers are likely to be developing close relationships and should be able to disclose to close friends and partners at least some of the details regarding their individual variation. Failure to do this suggests that the details are perceived as so frightening that they are 'worthy' of secrecy and the adolescent fears rejection. Identification of this degree of fear of disclosure in an adolescent is a clear indication of need for further discussion, education and referral for psychological support. Increasing efforts to improve broader access to education on DSD as a natural occurrence (e.g. in primary school discussions on anatomy or in high school biology classes) are ultimately aiming to reduce these perceptions, although social change such as this will take time. The pattern of discussion and disclosure of the adolescent's DSD diagnosis by parents and family members is an issue that needs to be explored. As they seek increasing autonomy and independence, they may feel uncomfortable with family members disclosing information about their diagnosis to others.

Working in the context of a multidisciplinary team enables various members to explore the young person's understandings. Although the medical records may not always make it clear what elements of the diagnosis have been explained in earlier consultations or what has been understood, asking the adolescent to explain to you as the clinician what they currently understand about their diagnosis is a useful process and ensures a clearer understanding.

Those adolescents who are same-sex attracted have historically been at higher risk of discrimination and bullying. For teens with a DSD, determining their sexual orientation in the context of their intersex variation and being accepting of themselves may pose additional challenges. All of these potential tensions indicate the need for specialised sexual counselling during and beyond this crucial period of adolescence, although, historically, this may not be well supported in the context of paediatric hospital settings. The need for and access to such services should nonetheless be considered when managing an adolescent with a DSD. Similarly, for those with genital variations who may wish to undergo surgical intervention (e.g. feminising genitoplasty in girls with CAH), allowing the adolescent time and privacy to explore these issues and the optimal timing for them is also important. In recent years, there has been a significant push from advocacy groups of affected individuals and Human Rights organisations to defer 'non-essential' surgeries that are performed largely to align a person's genital anatomy to that of a more typical male or female until an age when the young person can be involved in the decision and give fully informed personal consent to undergo such an intervention. It is likely that such a time would be adolescence, although the associated potential challenges for a young person to broach such decisions and how best to support them have not been well described in the literature and warrant further research.

In adolescents with DSD, where sex hormone replacement therapy is indicated at puberty (e.g. due to gonadal dysgenesis or ovarian insufficiency in Turner syndrome), seeking affirmation of an individual's gender identity and desire for secondary sex characteristics of their assigned sex is an important but not infrequently overlooked aspect of holistic medical care.

16.9 Medical Issues in Adolescence (Table 16.5)

Medical treatment of CAH through adolescence may be quite challenging, as pubertal growth makes the suppression of adrenal androgen production more difficult. Optimising the balance between too much cortisone, which might be associated with irregular menses and signs of Cushing syndrome and inadequate replacement, leading to increasing virilisation, may prompt some changes in strategy, such as a change to once-daily treatment with dexamethasone (Young and Hughes 1990). Recently, some groups have reported on the role of bilateral laparoscopic adrenalectomy as a way of lowering steroid replacement doses, as following adrenalectomy, it is no longer necessary to suppress the abnormal androgen production from the adrenal glands (Ogilvie et al. 2006). It is suggested that adrenalectomy also may improve the prognosis for fertility, although long-term follow-up studies after surgery are not yet available.

Table 16.5 Potential issues in adolescent males and females with DSD

Female	Male
Steroid hormone maintenance (CAH) Oestrogen/progesterone treatment Control of irregular periods Hemiuterus Streak ovary with Y chromosome (Turner syndrome) Vaginal agenesis (Rokitansky) Short vagina (CAIS) Introitoplasty/vaginoplasty ? Removal of testes in CAIS Donor oocyte source ? Surrogate pregnancy	Androgen supplements/ replacement Testicular biopsy to screen for CIS Penile augmentation/ erectile dysfunction Urethral stricture Recurrent UTIs Poor ejaculate Possible fertility options Recurrent epididymitis

For these adolescent females with streak or significantly dysplastic ovaries (e.g. in Turner syndrome), puberty may need to be induced with hormone treatment. The timing and rate of puberty induction has some flexibility—but ensuring that the young person feels adequate in their development with respect to their peers is an important issue. The protocols for pubertal induction vary widely, although the principle of beginning oestrogen replacement at a low dose and very gradually increasing the dose every 6 months is broadly used. Oral oestrogens, transdermal oestrogen patches or cream can be used. Adherence to prescribed medications may be optimised by ensuring the adolescent is well informed as to the reason for introducing hormonal medications and the expected associated physical health and well-being benefits. Where a uterus is present, progestogens will need to be added. This can be usually be initiated after the first spontaneous bleed has occurred, with the option of using progestogens continuously to avoid menstruation, or cyclically, using 10–14 days of progestogens monthly or in alternate months.

Assessing response to exogenous oestrogen therapy can be made through monitoring of breast growth and height. Bone density assessments (interpreted in the context of height and bone age) may also be useful to ensure optimal doses of oestrogen are being used. Given individual responses to different oestrogens, there is some benefit from trialling different oestrogen preparations and doses to ensure that the eventual oestrogen suits the individual. In general terms, the lowest clinically effective dose of an unconjugated oestrogen (e.g. oestrogen valerate) should be used in preference to a product containing ethinyloestradiol (often supraphysiological doses and higher side-effect profile). Likewise, when a uterus is present, assessment of uterine volume, uterine body versus cervical length and the development of an endometrial stripe all provide information that confirms appropriate maturation is occurring.

16.9.1 Oestrogens

The optimal dose of oestrogen for hormone replacement therapy in young women is not known. The doses of oestrogen that are recommended for the prevention of osteoporosis in women are derived from studies on postmenopausal women rather than on young women aiming to achieve optimal peak bone mass. For postmenopausal women, the following are the daily doses generally accepted as adequate for the maintenance of bone density: conjugated equine oestrogen 0.625 mg; oestradiol valerate 2 mg and piperazone oestrone sulphate 1.25 mg. As the attainment of peak mass is determined by several factors including exercise, calcium intake, genetics and 1, 25(OH)VitD, these factors also need to be optimised in young women, as well as oestrogen dose.

A few studies have been carried out to determine the optimal dosage of oestrogen for women with Turner syndrome. One study (Paterson et al. 2002) showed that ethinyloestradiol in the most commonly used doses leads to appropriate pubertal development but is insufficient to induce mature uterine shape or size in 50% of the population. A further study (McDonnell et al. 2003) of girls treated with a variety of synthetic and natural oestrogens reported more consistent uterine growth. Additionally, other work in women with TS has shown that spontaneous puberty versus induction of puberty was associated with the achievement of better bone density—with no differences in other factors including calcium intake and physical activity (Carrascosa et al. 2000). Likewise, studies in women with CAIS with and without gonadectomy have also demonstrated that many will fail to achieve optimal bone density (Marcus et al. 2000).

16.9.2 Progestogens

For women with DSD with a uterus, it is essential that progestogens be used. Choice of progestogen is largely determined by presence or absence of side effects. Administration can be oral, transdermal, intramuscular or intrauterine (levonorgestrel intrauterine system). Progesterone administration can be cyclic (e.g. medroxy progesterone acetate 10 mg daily for 14/7, Dydrogesterone 10 mg, 14 days per month) or continuous, for the achievement of amenorrhoea. There are no data on 'best' progestogen, although data on minimal dosage and duration are available to ensure prevention of endometrial hyperplasia (Warne et al. 2005a, b).

16.9.3 Fertility

For young women where a uterus is present, there is a possibility of carrying a pregnancy. For women with CAH, adequate control of adrenal hormones is necessary to optimise spontaneous or assisted ovulation and attainment of pregnancy. For girls with a unicornuate-uterus, such as in the context of ovo-testicular DSD or mixed chromosome DSD with mixed gonadal dysgenesis, referral to an experienced gynaecologist for advice is appropriate, although carrying a pregnancy will often be possible (potentially with use of a donor egg/embryo).

In girls with 'streak' or significantly dysplastic ovaries, another important issue is whether Y chromosome-containing cell lines are present as these are known to significantly increase the associated malignancy risk in a dysgenetic intra-abdominal gonad (Looijenga et al. 2007, 2010). Improvements in molecular and cytogenetics have shown that many children with 45,X Turner syndrome have some previously unrecognised 45,X/46,XY mocaicism, which predisposes the streak gonads to malignancy (Nishi et al. 2002). The current consensus for management is that these girls and young women should all have their karyotype tested on a sufficient complement of cells with modern molecular techniques to detect any occult mosaicism, and if identified, prophylactic laparoscopic removal of the dysgenetic ovaries is recommended (Cadeddu et al. 2001). Alternatively, if virilisation occurs in a girl thought to have 45,XO karyotype, examination of 2–3 tissues (eg buccal mucosa, skin in addition to peripheaarl blood) is recommended.

For girls with 46,XY DSD and intra-abdominal non-functioning gonads, a gonadectomy is usually recommended earlier in childhood because of the cancer risk in intra-abdominal dysgenetic gonads (Zielinska et al. 2007) (see Table 7.2 in Chap. 7). Where gonads are non-functioning, the benefit:risk ratio of this intervention is more straightforward as there is no hormonal or fertility related benefit to leaving the gonads in situ. As outlined previously, the situation for PAIS is a little less clear-cut, as, although malignancy risk is higher than in the general population, this risk is largely seen post-pubertally. As the testes in PAIS have the ability to produce hormones and will do so in higher than typical adolescent male levels (albeit with diminished peripheral response to these androgens), it may be preferable to defer a decision on removing those gonads until the affected individual can give informed consent as to his or her gender identity, wishes in relation to retention or removal of their gonads and thoughts on exogenous hormone replacement therapy to attempt to further masculinise (if male gender identity) or feminise (if female/feminine gender identity).

By contrast, for girls with CAIS, recent decades have been a time of significant controversy about whether the inguinal or intra-abdominal testes should be excised, as the cancer risk in early life appears to be much lower than that previously believed (Looijenga et al. 2007). In a previous generation, and still currently in many centres, gonadectomy is carried out in infancy or shortly after diagnosis of CAIS (Wisniewski et al. 2000). There is now a shift to delaying this at least until after pubertal development has occurred as a result of aromatisation of the excess androgens into oestrogen. Even then, evidence to on which to base decisions re timing of possible orchidectomy is limited and a recent international survey indicated that practices vary signficantly worldwide (Tack et al. 2018). The site of the testes in the girl with CAIS may influence this decision. For the girl with intra-abdominal testes, monitoring of the testes is necessary due to the perceived higher risk of malignant change. For the girl with testes in the groin, inguinal canal or labia, their presence may be the source of pain, particularly with sexual activity and this may influence her decision in relation to gonadectomy.

The other main medical issues for girls and young women with DSD relate to the gynaecological management of the introitus and the short or absent vagina and are discussed more fully in Chap. 18.

Future fertility in a young woman with no ovaries, but a normal uterus or a unicornuate-uterus may be achieved with the aid of assisted reproductive technology. Oocyte donation can be from related or non-related women. Although we are seeing parents of infants arranging to store oocytes in the bank for possible future use by their daughters, there are considerable ethical questions around this. Some countries do not allow the parent to be an egg donor due to the complexity of the young woman effectively carrying a pregnancy, that is, effectively her sister.

In girls with Turner syndrome, the ovary may initially contain ova prior to premature senescence and the resultant loss of fertility potential. In this circumstance, the ova may be harvested prior to this time and stored for subsequent use by the patient herself. Cryopreservation of ovarian tissue in this setting is being performed, but it has not yet become standard therapy. A number of outstanding issues remain relating to the timing of ovarian failure, which is quite variable and occurs in early childhood and whether harvesting ova from infant ovaries is feasible, let alone ethical. Although cryopreservation of ovarian tissue is now being undertaken regularly in the setting of onco-fertility with numerous pregnancies reported, none have been from ovarian tissue from a woman with gonadal dysgenesis. There are concerns regarding higher rates of problems in the early embryos from women with Turner syndrome (TS) (Bodri et al. 2006, 2009). An additional consideration is the increased pregnancy complication risks for women with TS. The overall pregnancy risks are thought to be

100-fold increased (Bodri et al. 2006), with reports of a 2% maternal mortality associated with aortic dissection (Karnis et al. 2003). Although those women with TS who have risk factors such as prior coarctation, bicuspid aortic valve or hypertension are clearly at higher risk, there is evidence that even those without any specific risk factors and who have pre-implantation and antenatal monitoring of their aortic root may still develop aortic root dissection (Karnis et al. 2003). These concerns do not apply to women with DSD who have a uterus and require donor oocytes due to non-functioning gonads that are not in the context of Turner syndrome.

In young women with Müllerian duct agenesis causing absent vagina and/or absent uterus, there is the possibility of a surrogate pregnancy, as the ovaries are usually normal (Sheean et al. 1989). Techniques for super-ovulation and harvesting of ova are now well established, and the major remaining barrier to this treatment is moral and ethical. This remains a controversial area, with debate about financial reimbursement for the woman carrying the pregnancy. However, as attitudes to assisted reproductive technologies evolve, this option is likely to become more frequently exercised. Furthermore, uterine transplant with successful pregnancy outcomes for women with MRKH has now been performed (Brannstrom 2018). In young women with 46,XX DSD and complex anomalies, fertility and the option of a pregnancy may be confounded by their other anomalies. Extensive previous surgery to correct bladder or cloacal exstrophy may result in pelvic adhesions and infertility. Assisted reproductive techniques can be used to overcome this. Renal function and stomas may pose additional pregnancy-related challenges, and the mode of delivery will need special consideration—including the risk to bladder and bowel sphincters with a vaginal delivery versus the challenge of a caesarean section in the presence of altered anatomy.

Genetic counselling for women with DSD who have fertility (CAH, vaginal agenesis—with surrogacy, bladder exstrophy and cloacal exstrophy) is important to allow the opportunity to discuss the risk of similar variations in the offspring.

16.9.4 Male

In many DSD patients raised as males, the dysgenetic testes may produce some androgens at puberty; first, it is difficult to predict beforehand whether this will be sufficient. Some boys may need full induction of puberty, while others may only need supplemental androgen treatment (Table 16.6).

Table 16.6 Currently available forms of testosterone in Australia

Product	Form	Mode of administration	Usual dose	Comment
Testosterone esters (Sustanon)	250 mg ampoule	Deep intramuscular injection	Adolescent: Start with 50–100 mg/month Adult: 250 mg 2–4 weekly	Peaks and troughs of hormone level may be symptomatic
Testosterone enanthate injection	250 mg ampoule	Deep IMI	Adolescent: Start with 50–100 mg/month Adult: 250 mg 2–4 weekly	Peaks and troughs of hormone level may be symptomatic
Testosterone undecanoate (Andriol)	40 mg capsule	Oral	Adolescent: 40 mg once or twice daily Adult: 80–120 mg twice daily	Efficacy variable
Testosterone undecanoate injection (Reandron 1000)	1000 mg in 4 mL	Deep IMI	Adult: 4 mL every 10–12 weeks	Delivers relatively constant hormone levels
Testosterone gel	10 mg/g, 5 g sachets	Transdermal gel	Adult men: 5 g applied at night, adjusted according to testosterone levels	Sexual partners may be exposed to effects of testosterone through contamination
Testosterone transdermal patches	2.5 and 5 mg patches	Transdermal patch	Adults: 2.5–7.5 mg/24 h	Skin irritation may arise

Once puberty is advancing, there needs to be consideration of whether the underlying testicular dysgenesis is likely to predispose to GCNIS and subsequent testicular cancer later in early adult life. A sensible plan is to recommend testicular biopsy in middle-to-late adolescence to determine whether GCNIS is present or not (Cools et al. 2006; Levin 2000; Hoei-Hansen et al. 2005). If the biopsy is negative, then regular surveillance with ultrasonography is probably sufficient. However, if GCNIS is identified, then a decision needs to be made about management. Attempts for retrieval of sperm at the time of the initial pubertal testicular biopsy may also be warranted and are increasingly being undertaken in scenarios where potential for reduced gonadal function in the context of an underlying DSD is likely. If an orchidectomy is deemed appropriate with the adolescent's fully informed consent, then insertion of prostheses along with full hormone replacement will be needed.

Young men with a smaller than typical penile size secondary to hormone deficiency/resistance, a primary isolated genetic anomaly, or associated with complete anterior abdominal wall defects (e.g. bladder exstrophy and cloacal exstrophy) may seek penile enlargement or substitution. In this scenario, however, reassurance about otherwise-normal sexual function may be sufficient. In men with penile agenesis or loss from trauma, a surgically created phallus is the only option (Ricketts et al. 2011).

Common problems in young men with DSD are the complications arising from hypospadias surgery (Jones et al. 2009). Where the urogenital sinus opens between the labioscrotal folds, there are increased risks of urethral stricture and meatal stenosis following construction of a very long neourethra from skin ± buccal mucosa. After hypospadias repair, the neourethra is relatively narrow, and during micturition, urine may be forced into the Müllerian remnant, causing progressive enlargement. The latter allows stasis to develop in the diverticulum with colonisation by bowel flora, leading to recurrent urosepsis.

Over the years, some boys have required formal vasectomy to prevent recurrent retrograde spread of faecal organisms to the epididymis. The vasectomy may only be required on one side, but in many boys, the Müllerian remnant itself needs to be excised to prevent urinary and/or epididymal chronic sepsis. Where this is needed, the vas deferens, if present, is nearly always found draining into the cavity, so that Müllerian remnant excision is tantamount to bilateral vasectomy. In the authors' view, this is usually appropriate management, as ejaculation is hardly ever normal if the vas is connected to a Müllerian remnant, as the seminal vesicles are abnormal, and there is chronic sepsis in the cavity. By contrast, disconnection of the Müllerian remnant from the posterior urethra may enhance fertility potential (albeit needing medical assistance) by protecting the epididymis from chronic sepsis, which would lead to the destruction of crucial storage and maturational functions for sperm.

Recently, we have begun disconnecting the Müllerian remnants from the male urethra laparoscopically without excision. This aims to avoid recurrent urosepsis and epididymitis in any remaining testis but preserve these structures should the individual wish to change gender later in life. Whether this is an advance in medical management remains to be seen but already seems to be an advance from an ethical perspective.

If the remaining testicular tissue is in a scrotal position and therefore functioning at the correct temperature (33 °C), and there is sufficient androgen function, then production of spermatozoa is possible.

Even if the plumbing of the vas deferens is abnormal as described above, aspiration of mature sperm from the epididymis or testis may allow fertilisation of an ovum. This technology holds promise for many young men with DSD and is a major advance compared with the bleak fertility prognosis in the past.

16.10 Holistic Care Through Adolescence (Table 16.7)

It is just over 60 years since Lawson Wilkins first described congenital adrenal hyperplasia (CAH) as a cause for genital variation in 1953 (Wilkins 1965). This triggered rapid advances in medical and surgical treatments for an expanding range of DSD but with not all treatments are equally successful. As in all areas of advancing knowledge,

Table 16.7 Holistic management through adolescence

Psychological counselling
Sexual counselling
Establishing appropriate adult transition
(a) Medical management
(b) Cancer screening
Support groups

Table 16.8 Useful websites for information on DSD

www.sgan.nhsscotland.com
www.sickkids.ca/childphysiology/cpwp/Genital/genitaldevelopment.htm
www.aisg.org/26_PARENTS.HTM#Books2
www.mrkh.org
www.youngwomenshealth.org
www.turnersyndrome.org.au
www.dsdguidelines.org
www.rch.org.au/cah_book/index.cfm?doc_id=1375

learning something new is by trial and error, and the management of DSD was no exception (Ahmed and Rodie 2010; Brain et al. 2010). As we have now had several waves of young adults emerge from different eras of medical treatment, we are just starting to appreciate the strengths and weaknesses of some therapies, mostly by feedback from the patients themselves.

The message from past patients is clear: holistic care that is medically sophisticated as well as non-judgemental and on-going through adolescence into adult life is needed. Psychosocial supports should be part of DSD care through childhood, adolescence and adulthood, with sexual counselling part of this. Importantly, there are relatively few places even in the developed world where there is formal transition to adult care by experts, for on-going medical and psychological treatment and cancer screening.

Perhaps, most importantly for the management of adolescents and young adults is the establishment of a number of patient support groups, where young people with DSD can meet peers with a similar variation. In the 1980s, support groups were established for parents of children with DSD, with the CAH Support Group being one of the first. Now what is occurring is networks of young adults with DSD, aided by informative websites (Table 16.8) as well as social media fora, which have enabled people with relatively rare conditions to meet others with the same variation.

16.11 Conclusions

As with other chronic diseases of childhood, the management of DSD continues to evolve. Improvements in diagnostic evaluations mean that there are now increasingly large numbers of adolescents and young adults with reasonably well-defined variations, although some are more commonly encountered than others and some are still rare or as yet undiagnosed. Medical and psychosocial management is advancing, but there remain deficiencies, particularly in supporting and empowering young people to assimilate and integrate knowledge in relation to their underlying condition and translate that, when appropriate, into making decisions in relation to their health and management pathways. Options for holistic and well-supported transition to adult centres with sufficient expertise and teams to provide optimal care are also limited, even in relatively well-resourced healthcare settings. Along with advances in molecular diagnosis, this is likely to be one of the major sites of improvement in care in the next decade.

Acknowledgements With thanks and acknowledgements to Prof Garry L. Warne AM and Dr. Jacqueline Hewitt who were involved in the first edition of this chapter.

References

Achermann JC, Hughes IA. Disorders of sex development. In: Larsen PR, Kronenbery HM, Melmed S, editors. Williams textbook of endocrinology. 11th ed. Philadelphia: Saunders; 2008.

Ahmed SF, Rodie M. Investigation and initial management of ambiguous genitalia. Best Pract Res Clin Endocrinol Metab. 2010;24(2):197–218.

Ahmed SF, Achermann JC, Arlt W, Balen A, Conway G, Edwards Z, Elford S, Hughes IA, Izatt L, Krone N, Miles H, O'Toole S, Perry L, Sanders C, Simmonds M, Watt A, Willis D. Society for Endocrinology UK guidance on the initial evaluation of an infant or an adolescent with a suspected disorder of sex development (Revised 2015). Clin Endocrinol (Oxf). 2016;84(5):771–88.

Al-Agha AE, Thomsett MJ, Batch JA. The child of uncertain sex: 17 years of experience. J Paediatr Child Health. 2001;37(4):348–51.

Almasri J, et al. Genital reconstructive surgery in females with congenital adrenal hyperplasia: a systematic review and meta-analysis. J Clin Endocrinol Metab. 2018;103(11):4089–96.

Apóstolos RAC, et al. Gender identity and sexual function in 46,XX patients with congenital adrenal hyperplasia raised as males. Arch Sex Behav. 2018;47(8):2491–6.

Berenbaum SA, Beltz AM, Bryk K, McHale S. Gendered Peer involvement in girls with congenital adrenal hyperplasia: effects of prenatal androgens, gendered activities, and gender cognitions. Arch Sex Behav. 2018;47(4):915–29.

Bhullar K, Grover S, Hutson J, Warne G, Loughlin E, Hewitt J. Spectrum of disorders of sex development in children aged 0-10 years. J Paed Adolesc Gynecol. 2011;24(2):e50.

Bodri D, Vernaeve V, Figueras F, et al. Oocyte donation in patients with Turner's syndrome: a successful technique but with an accompanying high risk of hypertensive disorders during pregnancy. Hum Reprod. 2006;21(3):829–32.

Bodri D, Guillen JJ, Schwenn K, et al. Poor outcome in oocyte donation after elective transfer of a single cleavage-stage embryo in Turner syndrome patients. Fertil Steril. 2009;91(4 Suppl):1489–92.

Bogdanska M, Morris A, Hutson JM, et al. Long-term urinary symptoms in adolescent and adult women with congenital adrenal hyperplasia. J Pediatr Urol. 2018;14(3):240.e241–5.

Brain CE, Creighton SM, Mushtaq I, et al. Holistic management of DSD. Best Pract Res Clin Endocrinol Metab. 2010;24(2):335–54.

Brannstrom M. Current status and future direction of uterus transplantation. Curr Opin Organ Transplant. 2018;23(5):592–7.

Brown J, Warne G. Practical management of the intersex infant. J Pediatr Endocrinol Metab. 2005;18(1):3–23.

Cadeddu JA, Watumull L, Corwin TS, et al. Laparoscopic gonadectomy and excision of müllerian remnant in an adult intersex patient. Urology. 2001;57(3):554.

Cai LQ, Zhu YS, Katz MD, et al. 5 Alpha-reductase-2 gene mutations in the Dominican Republic. J Clin Endocrinol Metab. 1996;81(5):1730–5.

Carrascosa A, Gussinye M, Terradas P, et al. Spontaneous, but not induced, puberty permits adequate bone mass acquisition in adolescent Turner syndrome patients. J Bone Miner Res. 2000;15(10):2005–10.

Cassio A, Cacciari E, D'Errico A, et al. Incidence of intratubular germ cell neoplasia in androgen insensitivity syndrome. Acta Endocrinol. 1990;123(4):416–22.

Chang HJ, Clark RD, Bachman H. The phenotype of 45,X/46,XY mosaicism: an analysis of 92 prenatally diagnosed cases. Am J Hum Genet. 1990;46(1):156–67.

Cheng PK, Chanoine JP. Should the definition of micropenis vary according to ethnicity? Horm Res. 2001;55(6):278–81.

Cohen-Kettenis P. Psychological long-term outcome in intersex conditions. Horm Res. 2005a;64(Suppl 2):27–30.

Cohen-Kettenis PT. Gender change in 46,XY persons with 5alpha-reductase-2 deficiency and 17beta-hydroxysteroid dehydrogenase-3 deficiency. Arch Sex Behav. 2005b;34(4):399–410.

Consensus statement Arch Dis Child 2006.

Cools M, Drop SL, Wolffenbuttel KP, et al. Germ cell tumors in the intersex gonad: old paths, new directions, moving frontiers. Endocr Rev. 2006;27(5):468–84.

Cools M, Wolffenbuttel KP, Hersmu R. Malignant testicular germ cell tumors in postpubertal individuals with androgen insensitivity: prevalence, pathology and relevance of single nucleotide polymorphism-based susceptibility profiling. Hum Reprod. 2017;32(12):2561–73. https://doi.org/10.1093/humrep/dex300.

Cools M, et al. Update on the Pathophysiology and Risk Factors for the Development of Malignant Testicular Germ Cell Tumors in Complete Androgen Insensitivity Syndrome. 2017;11(4):175–81. https://doi.org/10.1159/000477921.

Darlington Statement. Joint consensus statement from the intersex community retreat in Darlinghurst. Darlington Statement; 2017.

Davies MC, Creighton SM. Vaginal construction using sigmoid colon in children and young adults. BJU Int. 2004;94(7):1143–4.

De Bellis A, Quigley CA, Marschke KB, et al. Characterization of mutant androgen receptors causing partial androgen insensitivity syndrome. J Clin Endocrinol Metab. 1994;78(3):513–22.

von der Maase H, Giwercman A, Muller J, et al. Management of carcinoma-in-situ of the testis. Int J Androl. 1987;10(1):209–20.

Donald RA, Perry EG, Wittert GA, et al. The plasma ACTH, AVP, CRH and catecholamine responses to conventional and laparoscopic cholecystectomy. Clin Endocrinol. 1993;38(6):609–15.

Dorfinger K, Kratzik C, Madersbacher S, et al. Tumor markers in hydrocele fluids of patients with benign and malignant scrotal diseases. J Urol. 1997;158(3 Pt 1):851–5.

Eggers S, Sadedin S, van den Bergen JA, et al. Disorders of sex development: insights from targeted gene sequencing of a large international patient cohort. Genome Biol. 2016;17(1):243.

Faienza MF, Giordani L, Delvecchio M, et al. Clinical, endocrine, and molecular findings in 17beta-hydroxysteroid dehydrogenase type 3 deficiency. J Endocrinol Investig. 2008;31(1):85–91.

Gottlieb B, Beitel LK, Wu JH, et al. The androgen receptor gene mutations database (ARDB): 2004 update. Hum Mutat. 2004;23(6):527–33.

Gross DJ, Landau H, Kohn G, et al. Male pseudohermaphroditism due to 17 beta-hydroxysteroid dehydrogenase deficiency: gender reassignment in early infancy. Acta Endocrinol. 1986;112(2):238–46.

Grover SR, Loughlin E (2002) Recurring themes from psychotherapeutic group work leading to the development of a clinical practice checklist for women with intersex and related conditions. IX European Congress in Paediatric and Adolescent Gynaecology. Florence.

Hamerton JL, Canning N, Ray M, et al. A cytogenetic survey of 14,069 newborn infants. I. Incidence of chromosome abnormalities. Clin Genet. 1975;8(4):223–43.

Hashmi A, Hanif F, Hanif SM, et al. Complete androgen insensitivity syndrome. J Coll Physicians Surg Pak. 2008;18(7):442–4.

Hoei-Hansen CE, Rajpert-De Meyts E, Daugaard G, et al. Carcinoma in situ testis, the progenitor of testicular germ cell tumours: a clinical review. Ann Oncol. 2005;16(6):863–8.

Hughes IA. Management of congenital adrenal hyperplasia. Arch Dis Child. 1988;63(11):1399–404.

Hughes IA, Deeb A. Androgen resistance. Best Pract Res Clin Endocrinol Metab. 2006;20(4):577–98.

Hughes IA, Houk C, Ahmed SF, et al. Consensus statement on management of intersex disorders. Arch Dis Child. 2006;91(7):554–63. is 'consensus 2006'

Hughes IA, Nihoul-Fekete C, Thomas B, et al. Consequences of the ESPE/LWPES guidelines for diagnosis and treatment of disorders of sex development. Best Pract Res Clin Endocrinol Metab. 2007;21(3):351–65.

Imperato-McGinley J, Guerrero L, Gautier T, et al. Steroid 5alpha-reductase deficiency in man: an inherited form of male pseudohermaphroditism. Science. 1974;186(4170):1213–5.

Imperato-McGinley J, Miller M, Wilson JD, et al. A cluster of male pseudohermaphrodites with 5 alpha-reductase deficiency in Papua New Guinea. Clin Endocrinol. 1991;34(4):293–8.

Jadresic L, Leake J, Gordon I, et al. Clinicopathologic review of twelve children with nephropathy, Wilms tumor, and genital abnormalities (Drash syndrome). J Pediatr. 1990;117(5):717–25.

Jones BC, O'Brien M, Chase J, et al. Early hypospadias surgery may lead to a better long-term psychosexual outcome. J Urol. 2009;182(4 Suppl):1744–9.

Jones T, Hart B, Carpenter M. Intersex: stories and statistics. Cambridge: Open Book Publishers; 2016.

Joshi RR, Rao S, Desai M. Etiology and clinical profile of ambiguous genitalia an overview of 10 years experience. Indian Pediatr. 2006;43(11):974–9.

Karnis MF, Zimon AE, Lalwani SI, et al. Risk of death in pregnancy achieved through oocyte donation in patients with turner syndrome: a national survey. Fertil Steril. 2003;80(3):498–501.

Leon NY, Reyes AP and Harley VR. A Clinical Algorithm to diagnose differences of sex development. Lancet Diabetes Endocrinol. 2019;7(7):560–74.

Levin HS. Tumors of the testis in intersex syndromes. Urol Clin North Am. 2000;27(3):543–51, x.

Looijenga LH, Hersmus R, Oosterhuis JW, et al. Tumor risk in disorders of sex development (DSD). Best Pract Res Clin Endocrinol Metab. 2007;21(3): 480–95.

Looijenga LH, Hersmus R, de Leeuw BH, et al. Gonadal tumours and DSD. Best Pract Res Clin Endocrinol Metab. 2010;24(2):291–310.

Lux A, Kropf S, Kleinemeier E, et al. Clinical evaluation study of the German network of disorders of sex development (DSD)/intersexuality: study design, description of the study population, and data quality. BMC Public Health. 2009;9:110.

Maimoun L, Philibert P, Cammas B, et al. Phenotypical, biological, and molecular heterogeneity of 5alpha-reductase deficiency: an extensive international experience of 55 patients. J Clin Endocrinol Metab. 2011;96(2):296–307.

March of Dimes, M. A. C. D. P., and California Birth Defects Monitoring Program. Leading categories of birth defects. 2001.

Marcus R, Leary D, Schneider DL, et al. The contribution of testosterone to skeletal development and maintenance: lessons from the androgen insensitivity syndrome. J Clin Endocrinol Metab. 2000;85(3):1032–7.

May B, Boyle M, Grant D. A comparative study of sexual experiences. Women with diabetes and women with congenital adrenal hyperplasia due to 21-hydroxylase deficiency. J Health Psychol. 1996;1(4):479–92.

McDonnell CM, Coleman L, Zacharin MR. A 3-year prospective study to assess uterine growth in girls with Turner's syndrome by pelvic ultrasound. Clin Endocrinol. 2003;58(4):446–50.

Meyer-Bahlburg HF, Dolezal C, Baker SW, New MI. Sexual orientation in women with classical or non-classical congenital adrenal hyperplasia as a function of degree of prenatal androgen excess. Arch Sex Behav. 2008;37(1):85–99.

Meyer-Bahlburg HF. Gender and sexuality in classic congenital adrenal hyperplasia. Endocrinol Metab Clin North Am. 2001;30(1):155–71, viii.

Meyer-Bahlburg HF. Gender assignment and reassignment in intersexuality: controversies, data, and guidelines for research. Adv Exp Med Biol. 2002;511:199–223.

Meyer-Bahlburg HF, Gruen RS, New MI, et al. Gender change from female to male in classical congenital adrenal hyperplasia. Horm Behav. 1996;30(4):319–32.

Meyer-Bahlburg HF, Migeon CJ, Berkovitz GD, et al. Attitudes of adult 46, XY intersex persons to clinical management policies. J Urol. 2004;171(4):1615–9; discussion 1619.

Migeon CJ, Wisniewski AB, Brown TR, et al. 46,XY intersex individuals: phenotypic and etiologic classification, knowledge of condition, and satisfaction with knowledge in adulthood. Pediatrics. 2002a;110(3):e32.

Migeon CJ, Wisniewski AB, Gearhart JP, et al. Ambiguous genitalia with perineoscrotal hypospadias in 46,XY individuals: long-term medical, surgical, and psychosexual outcome. Pediatrics. 2002b;110(3):e31.

Morris JM. The syndrome of testicular feminization in male pseudohermaphrodites. Am J Obstet Gynecol. 1953;65(6):1192–211.

Muller J, Skakkebaek NE. Testicular carcinoma in situ in children with the androgen insensitivity (testicu-

lar feminisation) syndrome. Br Med J (Clin Res Ed). 1984;288(6428):1419–20.
Mullis PE, Hindmarsh PC, Brook CG. Sodium chloride supplement at diagnosis and during infancy in children with salt-losing 21-hydroxylase deficiency. Eur J Pediatr. 1990;150(1):22–5.
New MI. Diagnosis and management of congenital adrenal hyperplasia. Annu Rev Med. 1998;49:311–28.
Nielsen J, Wohlert M. Sex chromosome abnormalities found among 34,910 newborn children: results from a 13-year incidence study in Arhus, Denmark. Birth Defects Orig Artic Ser. 1990;26(4):209–23.
Nishi MY, Domenice S, Medeiros MA, et al. Detection of Y-specific sequences in 122 patients with Turner syndrome: nested PCR is not a reliable method. Am J Med Genet. 2002;107(4):299–305.
Nojima M, Taguchi T, Ando Y, et al. Huge seminoma developed in a patient with testicular feminization. J Obstet Gynaecol Res. 2004;30(2):109–12.
Ogilvie CM, Rumsby G, Kurzawinski T, et al. Outcome of bilateral adrenalectomy in congenital adrenal hyperplasia: one unit's experience. Eur J Endocrinol. 2006;154(3):405–8.
Parisi MA, Ramsdell LA, Burns MW, et al. A Gender Assessment Team: experience with 250 patients over a period of 25 years. Genet Med. 2007;9(6): 348–57.
Paterson WF, Hollman AS, Donaldson MD. Poor uterine development in Turner syndrome with oral oestrogen therapy. Clin Endocrinol. 2002;56(3):359–65.
Razzaghy-Azar M, Karimi S, Shirazi E. Gender identity in patients with congenital adrenal hyperplasia. Int J Endocrinol Metab. 2017;15(3):e12537.
Rey RA, Belville C, Nihoul-Fekete C, et al. Evaluation of gonadal function in 107 intersex patients by means of serum antimüllerian hormone measurement. J Clin Endocrinol Metab. 1999;84(2):627–31.
Ricketts S, Hunter-Smith DJ, Coombs CJ. Quality of life after penile reconstruction using the radial forearm flap in adult bladder exstrophy patients – technique and outcomes. ANZ J Surg. 2011;81(1–2):52–5.
Robboy SJ, Miller T, Donahoe PK, et al. Dysgenesis of testicular and streak gonads in the syndrome of mixed gonadal dysgenesis: perspective derived from a clinicopathologic analysis of twenty-one cases. Hum Pathol. 1982;13(8):700–16.
Rosler A. 17 Beta-hydroxysteroid dehydrogenase 3 deficiency in the Mediterranean population. Pediatr Endocrinol Rev. 2006;3(Suppl 3):455–61.
Sarpel U, Palmer SK, Dolgin SE. The incidence of complete androgen insensitivity in girls with inguinal hernias and assessment of screening by vaginal length measurement. J Pediatr Surg. 2005;40(1):133–6; discussion 136–7.
Sax L. How common is intersex? A response to Anne Fausto-Sterling. J Sex Res. 2002;39(3):174–8.
Sheean LA, Goldfarb JM, Kiwi R, et al. In vitro fertilization (IVF)-surrogacy: application of IVF to women without functional uteri. J In Vitro Fert Embryo Transf. 1989;6(3):134–7.
Skakkebaek NE. Management and biology of carcinoma in situ and cancer of the testis. Histopathology. 1994;25(1):97–8.
Sobel V, Schwartz B, Zhu YS, et al. Bone mineral density in the complete androgen insensitivity and 5alpha-reductase-2 deficiency syndromes. J Clin Endocrinol Metab. 2006;91(8):3017–23.
Szarras-Czapnik M, Lew-Starowicz Z, Zucker KJ. A psychosexual follow-up study of patients with mixed or partial gonadal dysgenesis. J Pediatr Adolesc Gynecol. 2007;20(6):333–8.
Tack LJW, et al. Management of gonads in adults with androgen insensitivity: an International Survey. Horm Res Paediatr. 2018;90(4):236–46.
Telvi L, Lebbar A, Del Pino O, et al. 45,X/46,XY mosaicism: report of 27 cases. Pediatrics. 1999;104 (2 Pt 1):304–8.
Thankamony A, Pasterski V, Ong KK, Acerini CL, Hughes IA. Anogenital distance as a marker of androgen exposure in humans. Andrology. 2016;4(4):616–25. https://doi.org/10.1111/andr.12156. Epub 2016 Feb 4.
Therrell BL Jr, Berenbaum SA, Manter-Kapanke V, et al. Results of screening 1.9 million Texas newborns for 21-hydroxylase-deficient congenital adrenal hyperplasia. Pediatrics. 1998;101(4 Pt 1):583–90.
Thyen U, Lanz K, Holterhus PM, et al. Epidemiology and initial management of ambiguous genitalia at birth in Germany. Horm Res. 2006;66(4):195–203.
Tonkin HG. Identifying resource needs for adolescents with differences of sex development. Medicine. Melbourne: University of Melbourne; 2018.
Torresani T, Biason-Lauber A. Congenital adrenal hyperplasia: diagnostic advances. J Inherit Metab Dis. 2007;30(4):563–75.
Warne GL, Raza J. Disorders of sex development (DSDs), their presentation and management in different cultures. Rev Endocr Metab Disord. 2008;9(3):227–36.
Warne G, Grover S, Hutson J, et al. A long-term outcome study of intersex conditions. J Pediatr Endocrinol Metab. 2005a;18(6):555–67.
Warne GL, Grover S, Zajac JD. Hormonal therapies for individuals with intersex conditions: protocol for use. Treat Endocrinol. 2005b;4(1):19–29.
Wikstrom AM, Dunkel L. Testicular function in Klinefelter syndrome. Horm Res. 2008;69(6):317–26.
Wilkins L. The diagnosis and treatment of endocrine disorders in childhood and adolescence. IL: Springfield; 1965.
Wisniewski AB, Migeon CJ, Meyer-Bahlburg HF, et al. Complete androgen insensitivity syndrome: long-term medical, surgical, and psychosexual outcome. J Clin Endocrinol Metab. 2000;85(8):2664–9.
Yong EL, Loy CJ, Sim KS. Androgen receptor gene and male infertility. Hum Reprod Update. 2003;9(1):1–7.
Young MC, Hughes IA. Dexamethasone treatment for congenital adrenal hyperplasia. Arch Dis Child. 1990;65(3):312–4.
Zielinska D, Zajaczek S, Rzepka-Gorska I. Tumors of dysgenetic gonads in Swyer syndrome. J Pediatr Surg. 2007;42(10):1721–4.

Surgical Management in DSD

17

John M. Hutson, Sonia R. Grover, and Aurore Bouty

17.1 Introduction

The surgical management of DSD is complex, and is best managed with a team approach. The number of surgeons involved in the team is relatively small, enabling them to maintain expertise. Diagnoses that are common can be managed by many different doctors, even if they are complex, as their frequency allows different practitioners to become competent by practice. By contrast, it is less appropriate for diagnoses which are both rare and complicated to be managed by clinicians who are not exposed to the clinical variations frequently enough to become experts in their management. One solution to this problem, which is occurring worldwide, is the development of specialised centres where rare, complicated DSD can be managed by a multidisciplinary team.

In our own hospital, individuals with DSD have been surgically managed by only 4–5 surgeons over 30 years (Hrabovszky and Hutson 2002); likewise, in Hanoi, only a small number of surgeons are involved in the feminising genitoplasty procedures undertaken in Vietnam (Grover 2010). In contrast, many papers reporting outcomes following feminising genitoplasties often fail to report the number of surgeons involved. Alizai et al. (1999) reported on 13 girls from 4 centres in the UK; Creighton et al. (2001) reported on 44 women, from all over the UK; Minto et al. (2003) on 39 women from all over the UK with all of these studies failing to mention the number of surgeons involved. Some studies do report the number of surgeons for the number of cases (Nordenskjold et al. 2008), where there were 10 different surgeons for the 18 patients. The concentration of expertise occurred earlier at our institution than at many other places and has allowed us to ensure that the surgery is undertaken by a surgeon with specific interest and expertise, which is likely to be one of the factors responsible for our positive outcomes as measured in both short-term

J. M. Hutson (✉)
Department of Urology, The Royal Children's Hospital, Melbourne, VIC, Australia

Murdoch Children's Research Institute, Melbourne, VIC, Australia

Department of Paediatrics, University of Melbourne, Melbourne, VIC, Australia
e-mail: john.hutson@rch.org.au

S. R. Grover
Department of Gynaecology, The Royal Children's Hospital, Melbourne, VIC, Australia

Murdoch Children's Research Institute, Melbourne, VIC, Australia

Department of Paediatrics, University of Melbourne, Melbourne, VIC, Australia
e-mail: sonia.grover@rch.org.au

A. Bouty
Department of Urology, The Royal Children's Hospital, Melbourne, VIC, Australia

Murdoch Children's Research Institute, Melbourne, VIC, Australia
e-mail: aurore.bouty@rch.org.au

J. M. Hutson et al. (eds.), *Disorders|Differences of Sex Development*,
https://doi.org/10.1007/978-981-13-7864-5_17

and long-term follow-up studies, examining cosmetic and anatomic outcomes (Lean et al. 2005) as well as genital sensation and patient satisfaction (see Chap. 24). Nevertheless, there have been a number of other practices that have been in place at our centre for many years, including the avoidance of genital examinations, and efforts to normalise the experiences of the children and adolescents which may have also contributed to these outcomes. Work undertaken specifically to explore whether surgical interventions impact on the psychosexual and cosmetic outcomes in women with DSD who have variations in their genital appearance did not indicate that feminising surgery itself had a positive or negative impact in a Dutch centre, although the number of surgeons involved or surgical techniques were not defined (Callens et al. 2012), and other potential contributing factors could not readily be measured. Regardless of the impact of other factors that may contribute to long-term outcomes, centralisation of specialised surgical services has been advocated by other centres in light of their own findings, where the quality of the outcome was found to be determined by the exact operative procedure (Nordenskjold et al. 2008).

The recent discussions by patient advocates and involving human rights organisations, the media and medical circles regarding the demand to limit surgery in this area is likely to be a direct consequence of a number of factors. These include changes over the past 30–50 years of the understanding of gender from dichotomous to a more fluid state; an improved understanding of the differing gonadal malignancy risk with different conditions (Spoor et al. 2018); and surgery being performed on children in centres by people with no special expertise in the area. Further to this, measuring outcomes of surgical treatment cannot be undertaken in isolation as other factors occurring during medical care, including repeated genital examination, medical photography (Creighton et al. 2002) and non-disclosure, all impact on self-esteem, body image and the long-term outcome.

It is easy to forget that congenital adrenal hyperplasia (CAH) was only discovered in 1953, and that surgical interventions began in the 1960s or 1970s. Not surprisingly, the first few cohorts of patients from the 1960s and the 1970s have had a mixed outcome, with many now as adults unhappy with the standard of their previous surgical management in childhood (Farkas and Chertin 2001). In some parts of the world, response to this has been to recommend that treatment should be delayed until adolescence, and this is particularly true in the UK and parts of Europe as well as the USA. Outcomes of girls and young women where surgery has been routinely deferred have not yet been reported but will be important. A more detailed discussion of the pros and cons of treatment in infancy is given in Chap. 15. In our centre our MDT discusses all possible pathways (medical management only or additional consideration of surgery) available for a given child or adolescent. Parents are also informed of the widespread debate in relation to surgical intervention on genitalia of children too young to give their own consent. The role of support groups and peer interaction is also discussed with families. If parents ultimately wish to proceed with surgical intervention and it is indicated for functional outcomes, we offer the option for early feminising genital surgery because our short-term and longer-term results support this practice, as described in Chap. 23 (Lean et al. 2005; Warne et al. 2005; Crawford et al. 2009; Bogdanska et al. 2018).

Our first long-term review of our patients was done in the 1980s, and this demonstrated many clinical practices that we subsequently avoided (Luthra and Hutson unpublished). When our first cohort of adult patients were interviewed, we found that many patients vividly remembered having genital examinations in later childhood, and they often found postoperative vaginal dilatations very distressing. We additionally realised that dilatations are actually completely unnecessary when surgery is done in infancy and are best left to adolescence, when the girl can decide if she wishes to undertake this herself. In addition, we found that the patients appreciated the follow-up by the surgeon involved in the reconstruction, as this enables them to discuss the anatomical details directly with the doctor who is familiar with their anatomy. If the patient is being raised as a girl, our adolescent gynaecologist is involved at a very early stage and will commonly assist at the surgery in infancy (see Chap. 18). This enables the transfer to gynaecological care in early adolescence to be much simpler, as the family has already met the gynaecologist and discussed the gynaecological issues earlier in childhood. The other major benefit of our first major review in the 1980s was the realisation that we needed an open disclosure policy with both the parents and the patients themselves. It became very clear that patients needed a low-key, matter-of-fact honest approach rather than being treated as abnormal or different in the presence of an assembly of medical students. This aspect of our psychological management is discussed at length in Chaps. 19 and 20.

Optimal timing of surgery, including genital surgery, is a topic that has changed substantially over time. With the improvement in anaesthetics, the age of surgery was progressively reduced so that by 2000–2002 surgery was undertaken in infants only a few months old. With some more recent data suggesting that there may be negative effects from general anaesthetics in younger infants, surgery is not performed in the first 6 months of age (Ing et al. 2012; Clausen et al. 2018). This also allows adequate time for the foetal androgen effects to reduce (although detailed research on these timelines have never been undertaken).

On the other hand, there are some data in males that report better body image and psychosexual outcomes when genital surgery is completed before the child is 2–3 years of age, independent of the anatomic or functional outcomes, implying that it is the recall of the surgical procedure that may be influencing outcomes (Mureau et al. 1995; Jones et al. 2009). There are no such data available in females, but there is reason to expect that the recalled experience of hospitalisation and surgery may have a negative impact.

There are some surgical conditions, for example, in those associated with cloacal anomalies, where some early surgery is essential due to the presence of urinary and/or bowel obstruction, and thus surgery is an emergency and life-saving.

17.2 Feminising Genitoplasty

The surgical management of individuals being raised as females includes the following principles:

1. Creation of a functional and typical female-looking introitus with labia minora and labia majora.
2. Vaginoplasty to provide a functional and adequate opening in the introitus for the vagina.
3. Reduction of the erectile tissue of the enlarged phallus with preservation of the glans and its neurovascular supply and ensure the presence of a clitoral hood.

The extensive debate that currently exists regarding the necessity of this surgery and the appropriate timing is discussed further in Chap. 15.

17.2.1 Clitoroplasty

The principal surgical procedure to manage enlargement of the clitoris until the 1960s was excision of the clitoris or clitoridectomy. This technique has continued in many parts of the world even till quite recently (Riepe et al. 2002). Unfortunately, amputation of the clitoris left a typical female-appearing introitus but removed a crucial organ for adult sexual function. This led to several new operations in the 1960s and 1970s (and again in the twenty-first century) to bury the clitoris in the mons. These procedures preserved neurovascular supply and function, and they produced a good cosmetic effect in early childhood but led to painful erection during sexual arousal in adult life. Such techniques have now been mostly abandoned for this reason. The next phase of development was reduction clitoroplasty, where part of the erectile tissue was removed with preservation of the glans. A number of different variations were described which aimed to preserve the dorsal neurovascular bundle but reduce the volume of the erectile tissue in the shaft of the clitoris (Schnitzer and Donahoe 2001).

In the early 1970s, Robert Fowler, who was the first surgeon in our department to have a special interest and expertise in the management of children with DSD, devised a novel operation for reduction clitoroplasty (Hutson et al. 1991). The principle of this technique is to reduce the girth of the clitoris by excision of some of the erectile tissue on the ventral surface, away from the nerve supply, after placing tourniquets around each corpus cavernosum. As the neurovascular bundles are on the dorsal surface of the shaft, the ventral surface can be trimmed without risk to blood supply or sensation. If the glans of the clitoris is enlarged, this is also partly excised in the coronal plane, and the dorsal half of the glans is then reconstituted into a cone. The clitoris is folded upon itself to create a hairpin bend so that the raw surfaces on the ventral surface of the corpora cavernosa are approximated by watertight suturing down each side. The position of the fold is arranged so that the glans will be placed just superficial and cranial to the bifurcation of the crura. This technique creates a typical-sized clitoris which is positioned (with a clitoral hood, see later) in a functional site. Because the dorsal surface of the clitoris has been left untouched, there is no interference with the neurovascular bundle, thereby avoiding ischaemic injury to the glans and also avoiding any risk of denervation of the glans. Given the positive long-term outcomes in terms of sensation as well as cosmetic and anatomic, this technique continues to be used with only minor modification nearly 40 years later (Lean et al. 2005).

Creation of labia minora occurs by using the entire skin of the shaft of the genital tubercle, which is divided in the midline and brought down on each side of the clitoris and newly formed introitus (Roberts and Hutson 1997). The inner layer of the skin lying over the clitoris is not excised so that it can be reused to constitute a hood over the clitoris. The detailed operative steps are described separately using Fig. 17.1a–p).

17.2.2 Vaginoplasty in the Setting of Virilised Genitalia

Creation of a functional vagina for menstrual outflow, tampon use and the potential for penetrative sexual activity is thought by most surgeons to be dependent upon the level of entry of the existing vagina into the common urogenital sinus. Many urologists recommend endoscopic examination and a retrograde urethrogram to identify the connection between the genital and urinary tracts. This has been done to establish whether the vagina enters the urogenital sinus distal or proximal to the external urethral sphincter. If the vagina was found to enter the urogenital sinus above the sphincter, then a more complex operation rather than a simple inverted V-Y vaginoplasty was thought to be necessary (Hendren 1998). Certainly, the distance of the vaginal opening from the surface is greater in babies with more marked virilisation, although in babies with CAH it is extremely rare for the vagina to enter the urethra above the sphincter, even when the Prader score is 4 or 5. This can be seen on the urogenital sinugram, where the connection is some distance from the urethral opening, but it is nearly always at or just above the junction between the anterior urethra and the posterior urethra (Marei et al. 2016). Thus, a flap vaginoplasty in all but the most severe anomalies has been undertaken at The Royal Children's Hospital (RCH) in almost all cases, as the distance from the lower end of the vagina to the skin is not very different between minor and more significant degrees of virilisation.

The inverted V-Y vaginoplasty is nearly always sufficient to correct the vaginal anatomy, especially in CAH. In our experience, it is important to insert the inverted V-flap of perineal skin well above the hymen on the posterior wall of the vagina. With androgen exposure during foetal development, the lower vagina becomes narrow, and if the flap is not inserted into the vagina above this narrow segment, it is likely to be associated with some narrowing of the lower vagina later in life. During infancy, the lower vagina is narrow for about a centimetre above the hymen in girls with CAH, so the flap is placed above this, with the apex of the flap in the vaginal cavity where there is invariably adequate width.

Some surgeons recommend commencement of vaginal dilatations a few weeks after surgery, but, as previously mentioned, we have deliberately avoided this, as regular dilatations are not only unnecessary in infancy but the process is very stressful for parents and any children old enough to understand what is happening. Although a perineal pull-through operation has been described for situations where the vagina is

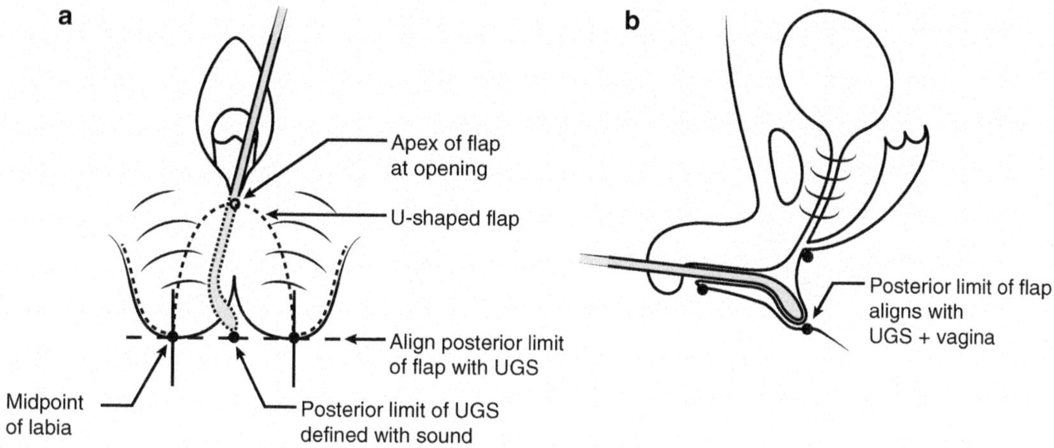

Fig. 17.1 Standard feminising genitoplasty as performed at The Royal Children's Hospital. (**a**) The key to identifying the skin landmarks for creating the incisions for a vaginoplasty. A urethral sound is passed into the urogenital sinus to identify the posterior limit of the urogenital sinus (UGS), which is running subcutaneously similar to the anterior urethra in a male. (**b**) The posterior limit of the sound is in alignment with the opening of the vagina in the urethra. (**c**) The skin is marked in the midline at the posterior limit as well as at the same level in the midpoints of the labioscrotal folds. The U-flap is marked as shown, with lateral extensions outlining the rounded edge of the labia in the skin crease, marking the attachment of Scarpa's fascia. (**d**) Although the length of the UGS may be long and increases in proportion to Prader score (A), the distance from the surface to the vaginal opening (B) remains relatively constant. (**e**) The UGS is divided in the midline to its posterior limit once the U-shaped skin flap has been raised. This exposes the hymen at the back of the urethra, allowing a small Foley catheter to be inserted into the vagina to provide traction. The midline incision in the UGS can now be continued through the hymen and up the posterior wall of the vagina until one reaches the dilated proximal vagina (the masculinised lower vagina is always too narrow). (**f**) The U-flap is sutured to the apex of the incision in the posterior vaginal wall, completing the vaginoplasty. The incisions for the clitoroplasty are shown. Importantly, the inner foreskin is left with the glans, so that the clitoral hood can be reconstructed later. The glans is otherwise circumscribed along the coronal groove, ventrally, and the incisions are extended to meet with the anterior ends of the UGS incisions, thus permitting complete mobilisation of the glans. (**g**) The shaft skin is divided in the midline up to nearly the base of the shaft and held with stays. The shaft is mobilised until the suspensory ligament (Z) is identified and divided. Anteriorly, the mucosal strip of the UGS, along with its attached corpus spongiosum (X), is mobilised off the front of the corpora cavernosa. There is a plane here which is almost completely avascular. The corpus spongiosum is lifted off until the bifurcation of the crura is reached (Y). (**h**) The subcutaneous tissue in front of the symphysis pubis is divided to expose the symphysis itself (W). (**i**) A right angle forceps is inserted under the corpora in the midline superiorly, and using palpation for guidance, the tip of the forceps is brought through anteriorly, allowing vascular loops to be placed around each corpus cavernosum. This provides vascular control of the entire shaft. (**j**) The anterior surface of the glans and shaft is excised under tourniquet control. The amount of glans and erectile tissue removed varies, depending on the original severity of virilisation. (**k**) The glans is reconstituted with 6/0 interrupted sutures, leaving the raw surfaces of the corpora still exposed. (**l**) The clitoris is folded over so that the raw surfaces are approximating each other, and then sutured together down each side with a continuous watertight suture of 6/0 or 5/0. This will join the fascia at the base of the shaft (just above the bifurcation with the coronal groove area of the shaft. (**m**) The clitoris is now reconstructed with a conical glans of appropriate size and shape, and a hairpin shaft. The vascular loops should be released at this time to ensure haemostasis. (**n**) The hairpin fold is now attached to the periosteum of the symphysis pubis with two sutures, being careful not to anchor it so tightly that the dorsal clitoral arteries are occluded at the hairpin fold. (**o**) The shaft skin is reattached to the shaft, with a deep suture (B $\rightarrow$ B^2) and a superficial suture ($A^1 \rightarrow A^2$), joining the pubic skin at the apex of the foreskin flaps to the inner layer of the foreskin over the glans. The UGS mucosa and corpus spongiosum is reattached under the tip of the glans. Finally, the shaft and foreskin flaps are brought down on each side of the now open UGS, joining C^1 to C^2. Once the medial side of each flap has been attached to the glans, UGS mucosa and side of the vaginoplasty U-flap, the lateral side required suture, between the shaft flaps (future labia minora) and the labia majora. Starting anteriorly, the suture picks up each skin edge as well as the deep soft tissues, to pull in the suture line to create a fold between labia minora and majora. (**p**) Finally, the posterior edge of the labia majora needs trimming, as appropriate. Excision of the redundant posterior labial skin, which is often wrinkled and pigmented, and suture of the edges in two layers to create rounded labia posteriorly, along the line of attachment of Scarpa's fascia. A deep layer of sutures ensures that there is not major wound breakdown when the superficial skin stitches are resorbed

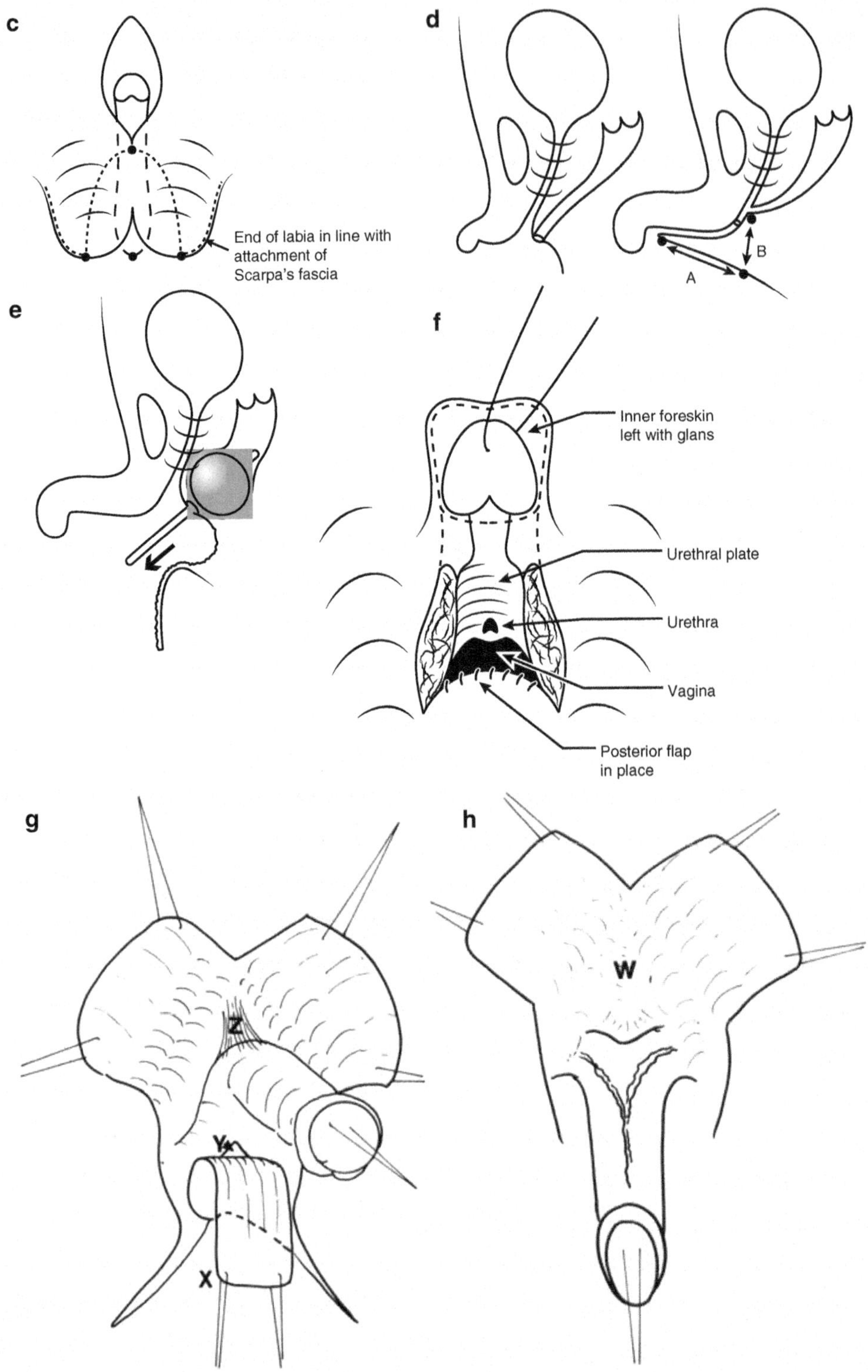

Fig. 17.1 (continued)

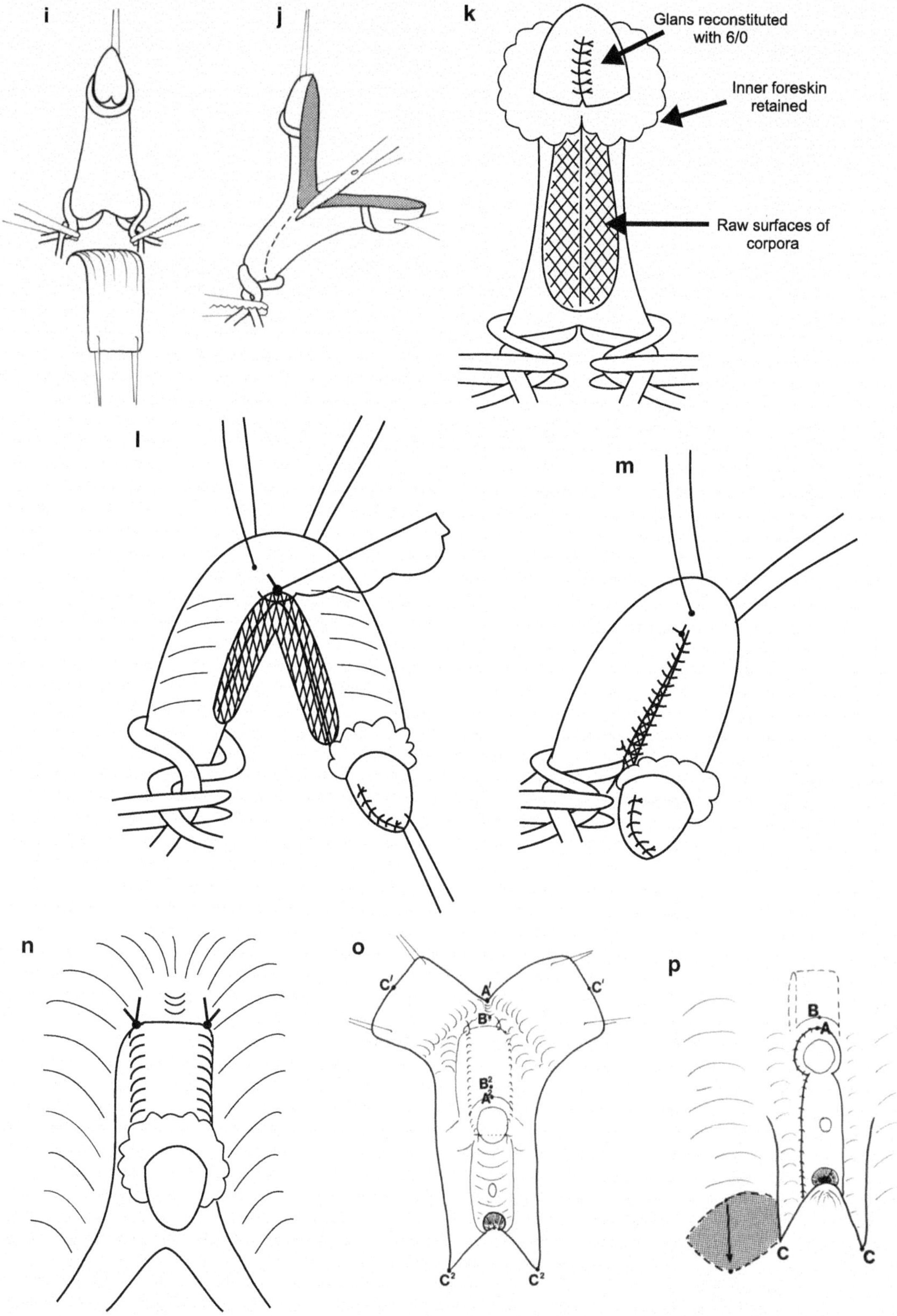

Fig. 17.1 (continued)

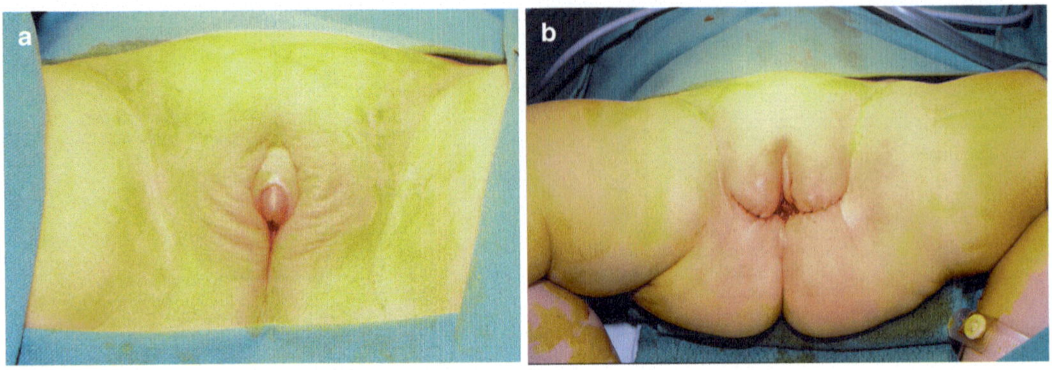

Fig. 17.2 Preoperative (**a**) and immediate post-operative (**b**) appearance in a patient with Prader 2–3 virilisation. These images are historical. Of note, surgical intervention would not be performed for such a presentation nowadays

entering very high in the posterior urethra (Hendren and Atala 1994), in our experience, this is extremely rare and such operations are mostly not required. These more extensive procedures may also contribute to more denervation of the genital tissues and thus alter sensation. In Chap. 23, we describe our medium- and long-term results using the standard method originally developed by Robert Fowler, with our immediate results shown in Fig. 17.2.

Passerini-Glazel (1989) has described an operation for reconstruction of the vagina using the skin of the urogenital sinus inverted back inside and anastomosed to the opening of the vagina, which is occasionally useful. Pena has also described surgical reconstruction of the high vagina using a posterior sagittal approach dividing the anorectum after a temporary colostomy (Pena et al. 1992; Pena and Hong 2003). This approach has enthusiastic advocates as well as critics. In some very complicated cases, the vagina is so rudimentary that surgical reconstruction, particularly in infancy, should be deferred until a definitive operation can be done once in adolescence. These procedures are discussed in Chap. 18.

17.3 Masculinising Genitoplasty

Reconstruction of the genitalia for male gender of rearing depends on the following principles:

1. Hypospadias repair.
2. Orchidopexy.
3. Correction of the bifid scrotum and of the prepenile position of the scrotum.
4. Separation of retained Müllerian duct structures from the urethra.
5. Excision of any gonadal tissue at risk of malignancy.

As in girls, there has been some discussion regarding the appropriate timing of procedures to correct genital variations.

The principles of hypospadias repair are the same as that elsewhere in urology, with correction of chordee, rearrangement of the skin using Byars' flaps, as described by Smith (1981, 1983), or grafting of a future urethral tube as described by Manzoni et al. (2004) and Bracka (2011). The various techniques do not need to be discussed at length here as standard techniques are used, and these are described in urology texts. In those with a pre-penile, bifid scrotum, transposition of the scrotal skin to the perineum may be performed as part of a hypospadias repair, or at a separate operation. Most patients with a hypospadias of this degree require a two-stage operation; scrotal transposition would usually be done at the same time as creation of the urethra. A number of these children also present with a Müllerian remnant, also called prostatic utricle. If the Müllerian remnant is left *in situ* at the time of hypospadias repair, the creation of the urethra may cause significant back-pressure on the passage of the urine such that the Müllerian remnant will fill with urine on micturition. This is likely to lead to recurrent urinary tract infections and may predispose to break down of the hypospadias repair. Disconnection of the Müllerian remnant from the posterior urethra has therefore been advocated but the issue is still debated (Hester and Kogan 2017; Mostafa et al. 2018).

Recently, management of the retained Müllerian remnant has been done laparoscopically, with either excision at the posterior wall of the urethra or ligation and division of the remnant, but with the structures left *in situ*. This has been done to maintain all options for the future, in case the individual wishes female gender later in childhood or adolescence. This strategy is too new to have any long-term follow-up results on its efficacy, but this will require confirmation that retention of female internal genital ducts does not predispose the boy to increased risk of female genital tract pathology.

Where resection is selected as the treatment option (recurrent urinary tract infections or epididymo-orchitis, for example), the genital remnant can often be excised via the perineum, as the confluence with the distal common urogenital sinus is frequently quite close to the perineal skin. Complete excision is possible up to the connection with the vas deferens, which usually drains into the cranial end of the cavity. Alternatively, submucosal resection, leaving the muscular wall *in situ*, can also be done easily, which decreases the risk of anterior rectal wall injury. The latter can be prevented by periodic insertion of a finger into the rectum during the surgery to palpate the anterior wall to estimate the proximity of the dissection plane to it.

17.4 Laparoscopy

Laparoscopy is not commonly necessary in patients with DSD, many of whom are diagnosed without direct visualisation of the internal genitalia. Congenital adrenal hyperplasia (CAH), for example, rarely needs laparoscopy as the internal genitalia are female (as confirmed on ultrasonography), and reconstruction of the external genitals is done via the perineum. There are, however, a number of clear situations where laparoscopy is indicated (Heloury and Plattner 1999; Hutson and Kimber 2005).

17.5 Indications for Laparoscopy

The following are the four main reasons for laparoscopy in patients with DSD:

1. Diagnosis of intra-abdominal anatomy when this is in doubt.
2. Biopsy or excision of dysplastic gonads containing Y chromosome.
3. Excision (or disconnection) of internal genital ducts as a single procedure or as part of an abdomino-perineal reconstruction.
4. The diagnosis of internal genital anatomy in girls (46,XX) with complex cloacal anomalies where there may be two separate uterine horns either or both of which may not be connected to a vagina. This can usually be undertaken during other operative procedures performed to manage the bowel obstruction or during closure of a colostomy.

17.5.1 Diagnosis of Internal Genital Anatomy

17.5.1.1 Androgen Insensitivity Syndrome

Androgen insensitivity, caused by an X-linked variant in the androgen receptor, makes the target tissues less sensitive to circulating androgens. It is the most common cause in which patients with 46,XY chromosomes and otherwise normal testes do not have a typical male phenotype. In the complete form of insensitivity (complete androgen insensitivity syndrome—CAIS) the androgen receptor is completely unresponsive to androgens, and the affected infant has phenotypically typical female external genitals and a vagina that may be slightly shorter. Both Müllerian and Wolffian ducts are absent, so there is no uterus or cervix. At puberty, secondary sex characteristics, including breast development, will occur as testosterone is converted in peripheral tissues into 17β-oestradiol. Development will be typically female apart from the absence or presence of only minimal pubic and axillary hair.

Patients with CAIS may present early in infancy or childhood as a female with an inguinal hernia (often containing a gonad) (see Chap. 13) or, more commonly, as adolescents with primary amenorrhoea (see Chap. 14).

A number of androgen insensitivity syndrome (AIS) patients have a variation in the androgen receptor, which allows a limited response to testosterone, leading to partial insensitivity (partial androgen insensitivity syndrome—PAIS) and atypical external genitalia because of partial virilisation. The Müllerian ducts are absent (as AMH is functioning normally), but only the proximal part of the Wolffian ducts are preserved (the epididymis and proximal vas deferens), where the concentration of hormone is sufficient to induce development, despite the limited receptor response.

Laparoscopy is not usually needed for the diagnosis of CAIS, as the testis is usually found within the inguinal hernia, and absence of the vas deferens confirms the diagnosis (Fig. 17.3). In female infants having laparoscopic herniotomy, the presence of testes but absence of the vasa deferentia, as well as absence of the uterus will suggest CAIS. Caution is required as phenotypic female infants with uterovaginal agenesis/MRKH have a higher rate of inguinal hernias than girls without this diagnosis and gonadal removal must not be undertaken, as these are normal functioning ovaries with ovum/follicles and offer the potential for fertility with surrogacy in the absence of the uterus (Oppelt et al. 2006, Kimberley et al. 2012). In the past where the diagnosis of CAIS has been made preoperatively (chromosome and/or testosterone analysis), a gonadectomy may have been performed at herniotomy. In contrast, today, where a testis is found unexpectedly in a hernial sac, biopsy of the gonads to confirm the diagnosis and establish the malignancy risk (Cools et al. 2017) would be undertaken prior to closing the hernial sac. It is now usual practice to delay gonadectomy until after puberty or not at all, as the malignancy risk is small (0.8%), and pubertal development can occur normally without hormone treatment. Gonadectomy in this setting can be undertaken laparoscopically with discussion and involvement of the adolescent or young adult.

In PAIS, laparoscopy may aid diagnosis, although the gonads usually are located in labioscrotal folds, and the status of the internal anatomy can sometimes (immediately after birth,

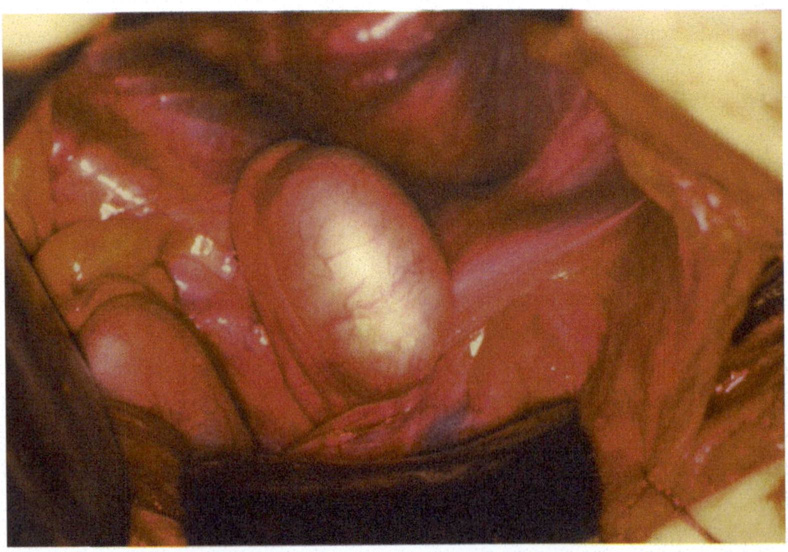

Fig. 17.3 Complete androgen insensitivity syndrome (CAIS) (shown here at a laparotomy), showing an intra-abdominal testis near the internal inguinal ring. Note the absence of Wolffian duct structures (epididymis and vas deferens), as well as Müllerian ducts behind the bladder

during maternal oestrogen impregnation) be confirmed by ultrasound scan or magnetic resonance imaging (MRI).

17.5.1.2 45,X/46,XY Mixed Gonadal Dysgenesis

In mixed gonadal dysgenesis (MGD), the karyotype is commonly 45,X/46,XY, but other patterns have been described. The mosaicism usually is expressed to a different extent in each urogenital ridge, leading to gonadal and genital duct asymmetry (see Chap. 8). In the commonest variant, one gonad is testicular (with an accompanying vas deferens), and the other gonad is an undifferentiated streak gonad (with an adjacent Müllerian duct structure).

Laparoscopy is useful in MGD to confirm the internal anatomy and to biopsy the gonads to establish the malignancy risk by undertaking appropriate tests for the immunohistochemical markers that suggest an increased malignancy risk (OCT3/4 and TSPY) (Looijenga et al. 2007). As these markers are elevated in immature gonads, interpretation of the results in light of the age of the young person is crucial to avoid false-positive interpretation of the results. Leaving genital structures, such as a Müllerian duct, which may be an entire uterine horn, is increasingly advocated in view of the evidence that uterine horns, even in the absence of a complete cervix, may have the potential to carry a pregnancy, and thus their removal would reduce options in the future (Deffarges et al. 2001; Kriplani et al. 2012).

17.5.1.3 Ovo-Testicular DSD

The external genitalia often are asymmetrical, and a number of chromosomal arrangements occur, although the commonest is 46,XX. In the latter situation, the peripheral blood is 46,XX, but, usually, there is clone of 46,XY cells in the urogenital ridge or gonads.

Laparoscopy will reveal the retained ovary or ovo-testis (Fig. 17.4.), allowing a management plan to be formed. One of the common varieties shows an intra-abdominal ovary (often on the left) and female genital tract (round ligament, hemi-uterus and tube and ovarian vessels). On the other side (often the right side), the vas deferens and gonadal vessels may disappear through the internal inguinal ring, connecting to a descended testis or ovo-testis.

17.5.1.4 Pure Gonadal Dysgenesis/46,XY Complete Gonadal Dysgenesis (Previously Called Swyer Syndrome)

These girls usually present in adolescence with failure of pubertal development, as the appearance at birth is unambiguously female regardless of the genetic make-up. Occasionally, these children are identified in childhood if a karyotype is done for other unrelated reasons, and increasingly neonates are identified in the setting of antenatal testing, revealing a karyotype not matching the birth phenotype (see Chaps. 11 and 21). The gonads are completely dysplastic and non-functioning—with no hormonal or fertility potential. Gonadectomy is recommended for prevention of malignancy, which approximates 30%, and puberty is induced by hormone treatment. The internal genitalia are feminine because of

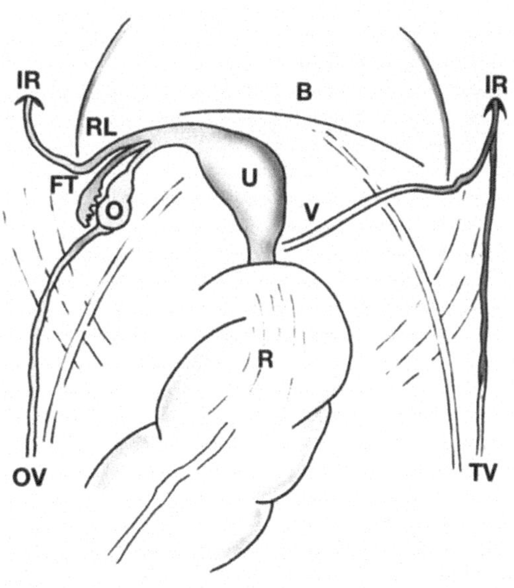

Fig. 17.4 Ovo-testicular DSD, showing one of the common varieties, with an intra-abdominal left ovary (O) and female genital tract (round ligament (RL); hemiuterus (U); fallopian tube (FT); ovarian vessels (OV). On the right side, the vas deferens (V) and testicular vessels (TV) disappear through the internal inguinal ring (IR) to reach a descended testis. The rectum (R) and bladder (B) and ureters (unlabelled) are shown

absence of testosterone and AMH, so carrying a pregnancy is potentially possible by *in vitro* fertilisation (IVF) using a donor egg (De Sutter 2001).

If laparoscopy is done during later childhood or adolescence (and prior to the commencement of oestrogen therapy), the uterine structure is likely to be very small. This structure can be missed by ultrasound if this is done at any time after the neonatal period when maternal oestrogens will be responsible for a more prominent uterus.

The ‘absent’ or rudimentary uterus on ultrasound and the very small uterus on laparoscopy have led to inexperienced surgeons and gynaecologists concluding that the uterus is absent. A vaginoscopy to confirm the presence of the cervix is usually adequate reassurance. In the presence of a 46,XY karyotype, streak gonads and absence of any virilisation or oestrogenisation, the diagnosis of pure or complete gonadal dysgenesis can be made. The small uterus will respond to oestrogens and achieve a normal size, menstruate and have the capacity to carry a pregnancy.

In view of the 3–5% rate of ectopic pregnancies in the context of *in vitro* fertilisation with embryo transfer, there is an argument for removal of the fallopian tubes at the time of gonadectomy (Marcus and Brinsden 2002).

17.5.1.5 Persistent Müllerian Duct Syndrome

This rare genital variation presents with completely male external genitalia with either impalpable testes or a hernia ipsilateral to an impalpable testis (*hernia uteri inguinalis*). Endoscopy provides the capacity to document the location of the gonads as well as identifying and/or removing the retained Müllerian ducts (uterus and Fallopian tubes), when they are complicated (recurrent urinary tract infections or epididymo-orchitis, inability to perform the orchidopexy). The lower part of the Müllerian remnant is usually left *in situ,* as the *vasa deferentia* drain into it.

17.5.1.6 Primary Amenorrhoea

Laparoscopy is only infrequently required in the assessment of teenagers presenting with primary amenorrhoea. Prior to undertaking this procedure, careful examination and simple investigations, including testosterone measurement if there is breast development but minimal pubic and axillary hair and an expert pelvic ultrasound will usually be adequate to clarify the diagnosis. Only occasionally, an MRI is required following appropriate hormonal tests and careful ultrasound, remembering that in the absence of secondary sexual characteristics, and thus low oestrogen, a pelvic ultrasound and even an MRI may fail to identify the prepubertal uterus.

Although laparoscopy is reported to be used in the context of diagnosing vaginal agenesis, the combination of primary amenorrhoea in the presence of normal secondary sexual characteristics, female reproductive hormones (follicle-stimulating hormone—FSH and oestrogens), karyotype and pelvic ultrasound with an absent uterus is more than adequate to make this diagnosis. The identification of non-cavitated uterine remnants is not important, as they are not responsible for any future problems. Fimbria and part of the fallopian tubes are often present either unilaterally or bilaterally.

17.5.1.7 Hypothalamic Hypogonadism

With this diagnosis, the adolescent girl will present with both primary amenorrhoea and pubertal delay. Hormonal investigations will reveal a very low FSH, luteinizing hormone (LH) and oestradiol. In this context, a pelvic ultrasound is likely to report an absent uterus or rudimentary uterus—when, in fact, it is a very small but completely formed uterus. At laparoscopy, the uterus may appear to be absent—to the inexperienced clinician, but fimbria, tubes, inactive ovaries and a small midline structure will be present. The uterus will respond to oestrogen and grow to a normal size, menstruate and will be able to carry a pregnancy.

17.5.2 Biopsy/Excision of Intra-Abdominal Gonads

This can be required in patients in whom chromosomal analysis shows the presence of a Y

Table 17.1 Y chromosome-containing conditions where laparoscopy may be useful

Condition	Karyotype	Pelvic anatomy
CAIS/PAIS	46,XY	Testes in pelvis/ inguinal hernia, absent vas deferens and uterus
MGD	45,X/46,XY	One testis (dysplastic) and vas, one streak gonad and uterine tube
Turner	45,X/46,XY	Turner phenotype but streak gonads contain some Y cells
Ovo-testicular DSD	46,XX/46,XY 46,XX	Testis + ovary Testis + ovo-testis Ovo-testis + ovo-testis Ovary + ovo-testis
Pure gonadal dysgenesis	46,XY	Streak gonads and female internal ducts
PMDS	46,XY	Testes plus both male and female ducts

chromosome, as seen in a range of (mostly rare) conditions (Table 17.1). This is because gonads containing the Y chromosome have: (1) a variable degree of testicular differentiation and (2) a propensity to undergo progressive dysplasia and thus a malignancy risk, related to the degree of dysplasia or differentiation and possibly the intra-abdominal temperature (37 °C).

Gonadal biopsy should be performed in any situation where the diagnosis remains uncertain, despite all other investigations. Where the gonad is heterogeneous, the possibility of ovo-testicular DSD or secondary tumour (gonadoblastoma, dysgerminoma or malignant seminoma) should be considered, and multiple biopsies with frozen section may be needed. In ovo-testicular DSD, the gonad may contain adjacent ovarian and testicular tissue forming an ovo-testis: the ovarian tissue may be at one or both poles with testicular tissue between. To avoid missing the diagnosis, a longitudinal wedge biopsy should be taken.

Gonadal biopsy also allows some further information to be gained regarding the malignancy risk of the gonad with the markers OCT3/4 and TSPY—although these markers are normally elevated in immature gonads (Looijenga et al. 2007). To differentiate between delayed maturation of a germ cell and preneoplasic state, staining with KIT Ligand (also known as Stem Cell Factor, SCF) is useful (Spoor et al. 2018).

Excision of streak gonads with presence of Y material is appropriate and should be undertaken as there is a significant risk of malignancy, and these gonads are non-functioning—from both an hormonal and fertility perspective.

Occasionally, prepubertal girls and adolescents may present with complex solid pelvic masses. The possibility of a dysgeminoma needs to be considered and an estimate of FSH is useful to rapidly identify an underlying gonadal dysgenesis, which can then be followed by FISH testing for Y genetic material. This then allows for surgery to remove not only the tumour mass but also the contralateral streak gonad.

Gonads that carry a lower malignancy risk or where there is some hormonal function require careful discussion and consideration before removal. Today, every attempt is made to do this at an age when the young person can be involved in the discussion.

The gonads of a person with CAIS are hormonally productive and have a low malignancy risk. These gonads should be left *in situ* and can be monitored. Some adults may choose to have them removed rather than have regular monitoring, particularly when this may be difficult and require annual MRI although for others an ultrasound is feasible, although its utility for diagnosis pre- or early malignant change is limited. On the other hand, if the testes are functioning with the production of testosterone, which is being converted to oestrogen peripherally, then avoiding gonadectomy allows the person to avoid taking exogenous hormones, usually in the form of oestrogens. There is no evidence that there is any fertility potential in the testes of people with CAIS.

For people with PAIS, the malignancy risk is such that biopsy is often undertaken to clarify the risk or identify premalignant changes. Newer data indicate that malignancy risk is however likely to be lower than previously estimated (see Chap. 7). In PAIS, although there is hormonal production and some receptor response, the fertility potential of the gonads is low (Cools et al. 2017).

The operative technique for removal of the gonads is determined by their size. Undifferentiated streak gonads are excised easily, as their blood supply is very meagre and can be diathermied. More substantial gonads or gonadal tumours need formal ligation of the gonadal vessels first.

17.5.3 Excision of Internal Genital Ducts

Laparoscopic excision of genital ducts may be considered in DSD where there are female internal ducts in a child being raised as a male (e.g. mixed gonadal dysgenesis and ovo-testicular DSD with unilateral Müllerian duct retention, and persisting Müllerian duct syndrome with bilateral duct retention). However, delay in excision is now recommended, if possible, until the gender identity of the individual is clear and consent by the individual can be given, unless the retained Müllerian duct is the source of complications (recurrent urinary tract infections—UTIs, epididymo-orchitis, stones). Also, there are some males with androgenic dysfunction where there is a remnant of the urogenital sinus (primitive lower vagina). In children being raised as females, laparoscopic removal of Wolffian duct remnants may be considered if symptomatic, as in some with ovo-testicular DSD.

17.5.4 Cloacal Anomalies

In the setting of anorectal anomalies, the presence of a structural Müllerian (uterine, cervical and/or vaginal) variation is reported to occur in 10% of girls (Levitt and Pena 2005) and up to 30% with the more complex cloacal anomalies (Levitt and Pena 2012). The Müllerian variations may range from utero-vaginal agenesis, vaginal agenesis with uterine structures present, uterine didelphys with a septate vagina, noncommunicating uterine horns unilaterally or bilaterally, cervical agenesis. Unlike many other scenarios, the Müllerian and renal variations may not be on the same side. As operative procedures will be involved to manage the urinary and bowel problems, it is appropriate to consider the involvement of a gynaecologist to ensure adequate inspection and documentation of the Müllerian tract at that time. Removal of apparently small uterine structures is no longer appropriate in view of the current knowledge regarding the potential to anastomose uterine horns without a cervix and thus at least attempt to preserve the possibility of future pregnancy (Deffarges et al. 2001; Kriplani et al. 2012). This anastomosis would be done in adolescence and can be deferred by suppressing menses until the young woman chooses to have the procedure.

Identification of uterine horns surgically is important, as visualisation with imaging in the setting of the bowel and urinary problems in the neonate can be challenging, and imaging later in childhood (with either ultrasound or MRI) is difficult due to the small size of these structures in the absence of oestrogens. Failure to clarify the presence or absence of the Müllerian structures can result in the presentation in adolescence of painful abdominal-pelvic masses associated with an obstructed uterus (Levitt et al. 1998; Warne et al. 2003). In the setting of a young person who has already undergone major surgery and likely to have experienced challenges with bladder and bowel, to have an unexpected painful surgical problem, is far from ideal.

17.6 Vaginoplasty

A range of techniques exist for the creation of a neovagina. In the majority of conditions where there is an absent vagina, the creation of a vagina is delayed until the girl reaches adolescence or early adulthood and can be involved in the decision-making process. The exception is in the setting of complex cloacal anomalies where correction of the urinary and bowel problems may necessitate mobilising and utilising some bowel segments—in which case creation of a neovagina with bowel at this time may be appropriate.

17.6.1 Mayer-Rokitansky-Küster-Hauser Syndrome and Complete Androgen Insensitivity Syndrome

Vaginal dilatation is primarily the technique that is utilised for creating a vagina (Cheikhelard et al. 2018). In both of these conditions, the vagina may already be a functional length which may not require any intervention for successful sexual activity.

A comprehensive review of the operative approaches and complications as well as sexual and functional outcomes of different techniques of vaginoplasty has been undertaken (McQuillan and Grover 2014a, b). Although the technique of bowel segment neovagina was previously popular in some countries, there has been a move away from this technique except in the difficult complex setting.

Surgical techniques all report a rate of bladder and bowel injuries. The laparoscopic techniques with the use of peritoneum (both the Davydov and the Luo techniques) appear to only require the daily dilatation, whereas the technique of creating a space and allowing epithelialisation (with both the Sheares' and the Vecchietti techniques) require the daily use of a vaginal mould, for 1–3 months (Qin et al. 2016).

Irrespective of technique to the approach of creating a neovagina, psychological support including peer support as well as physiotherapy are important.

17.6.2 Partial Müllerian Agenesis

There is increasing recognition that uterine horns, even those without a cervix, in girls with complex variations should be preserved due to the potential to surgically anastomose with a neovagina or even the vestibule, allowing the potential for future fertility.

Acknowledgement With acknowledgement to Chris Kimber who contributed to the first edition.

References

Alizai NK, Thomas DF, Lilford RJ, et al. Feminizing genitoplasty for congenital adrenal hyperplasia: what happens at puberty? J Urol. 1999;161(5):1588–91.

Bogdanska M, Morris A, Hutson JM, et al. Long-term urinary symptoms in adolescent and adult women with congenital adrenal hyperplasia. J Pediatr Urol. 2018;14(3):240.e241–5.

Bracka A. Buccal mucosa: good but not perfect. J Urol. 2011;185(3):777–8.

Callens N, van der Zwan YG, Drop SL, et al. Do surgical interventions influence psychosexual and cosmetic outcomes in women with disorders of sex development? ISRN Endocrinol. 2012;2012:276742.

Cheikhelard A, Bidet M, Baptiste A, et al. Surgery is not superior to dilatation for the management of vaginal agenesis in Mayer-Rokitansky-Küster-Hauser syndrome: a multicenter comparative obervational study in 131 patients. 2018.

Clausen NG, Kahler S, Hansen TG. Systematic review of the neurocognitive outcomes used in studies of paediatric anaesthesia neurotoxicity. Br J Anaesth. 2018;120(6):1255–73.

Cools M, Wolffenbuttel KP, Hersmus R, et al. Malignant testicular germ cell tumors in postpubertal individuals with androgen insensitivity: prevalence, pathology and relevance of single nucleotide polymorphism-based susceptibility profiling. Hum Reprod. 2017;32(12):2561–73.

Crawford JM, Warne G, Grover S, et al. Results from a pediatric surgical centre justify early intervention in disorders of sex development. J Pediatr Surg. 2009;44(2):413–6.

Creighton SM, Minto CL, Steele SJ. Objective cosmetic and anatomical outcomes at adolescence of feminising surgery for ambiguous genitalia done in childhood. Lancet. 2001;358(9276):124–5.

Creighton S, Alderson J, Brown S, et al. Medical photography: ethics, consent and the intersex patient. BJU Int. 2002;89(1):67–71; discussion 71–2.

De Sutter P. Gender reassignment and assisted reproduction: present and future reproductive options for transsexual people. Hum Reprod. 2001;16(4):612–4.

Deffarges JV, Haddad B, Musset R, et al. Utero-vaginal anastomosis in women with uterine cervix atresia: long-term follow-up and reproductive performance. A study of 18 cases. Hum Reprod. 2001;16(8):1722–5.

Farkas A, Chertin B. Feminizing genitoplasty in patients with 46XX congenital adrenal hyperplasia. J Pediatr Endocrinol Metab. 2001;14(6):713–22.

Grover SR, Loan D, Armstrong K, Henderson C, Hoan NT, Liem N, Warne G. Congenital adrenal hyperplasia in Vietnam: the issues confronting girls and their families and the surgical outcomes. World Congress Paed Adol Gynaecol Montpellier, 2010. p. 2.1–15.

Heloury Y, Plattner V. Laparoscopy and intersex. In: Bax NMA, Georgeson KE, Najaldin A, Valla J-S, editors.

Endoscopic surgery in children. New York: Springer-Verlag; 1999. p. 427–30.
Hendren WH. Surgical approach to intersex problems. Semin Pediatr Surg. 1998;7(1):8–18.
Hendren WH, Atala A. Use of bowel for vaginal reconstruction. J Urol. 1994;152(2 Pt 2):752–5; discussion 756–7.
Hester AG, Kogan SJ. The prostatic utricle: an under-recognized condition resulting in significant morbidity in boys with both hypospadias and normal external genitalia. J Pediatr Urol. 2017;13(5):492.e491–5.
Hrabovszky Z, Hutson JM. Surgical treatment of intersex abnormalities: a review. Surgery. 2002;131(1):92–104.
Hutson JM, Kimber C. Intersex. In: Najmaldin A, editor. Operative endoscopy and endoscopic surgery in infants and children. London: Hodder Arnold; 2005. p. 441–7.
Hutson J, Voigt R, Luthra M, et al. Girth-reduction clitoroplasty – a new technique: experience with 37 patients. Pediatr Surg Int. 1991;6:336–40.
Ing C, DiMaggio C, Whitehouse A, et al. Long-term differences in language and cognitive function after childhood exposure to anesthesia. Pediatrics. 2012;130(3):e476–85.
Jones BC, O'Brien M, Chase J, et al. Early hypospadias surgery may lead to a better long-term psychosexual outcome. J Urol. 2009;182(4 Suppl):1744–9.
Kimberley N, Hutson JM, Southwell BR, et al. Vaginal agenesis, the hymen, and associated anomalies. J Pediatr Adolesc Gynecol. 2012;25(1):54–8.
Kriplani A, Kachhawa G, Awasthi D, et al. Laparoscopic-assisted uterovaginal anastomosis in congenital atresia of uterine cervix: follow-up study. J Minim Invasive Gynecol. 2012;19(4):477–84.
Lean WL, Deshpande A, Hutson J, et al. Cosmetic and anatomic outcomes after feminizing surgery for ambiguous genitalia. J Pediatr Surg. 2005;40(12):1856–60.
Levitt MA, Pena A. Outcomes from the correction of anorectal malformations. Curr Opin Pediatr. 2005;17(3):394–401.
Levitt MA, Pena A. Anorectal malformations. In: Coran AG, Caldamone A, Adzick NS, editors. Pediatric surgery. Philadelphia: Saunders; 2012. p. 1289–310.
Levitt MA, Stein DM, Pena A. Gynecologic concerns in the treatment of teenagers with cloaca. J Pediatr Surg. 1998;33(2):188–93.
Looijenga LH, Hersmus R, Oosterhuis JW, et al. Tumor risk in disorders of sex development (DSD). Best Pract Res Clin Endocrinol Metab. 2007;21(3):480–95.
Manzoni G, Bracka A, Palminteri E, et al. Hypospadias surgery: when, what and by whom? BJU Int. 2004;94(8):1188–95.
Marcus SF, Brinsden PR. Analysis of the incidence and risk factors associated with ectopic pregnancy. Fertil Steril. 2002;78:918–31.
Marei MM, Fares AE, Abdelsattar AH, et al. Anatomical measurements of the urogenital sinus in virilized female children due to congenital adrenal hyperplasia. J Pediatr Urol. 2016;12(5):282.e281–8.
McQuillan SK, Grover SR. Systematic review of sexual function and satisfaction following the management of vaginal agenesis. Int Urogynecol J. 2014a;25(10):1313–20.
McQuillan SK, Grover SR. Dilation and surgical management in vaginal agenesis: a systematic review. Int Urogynecol J. 2014b;25(3):299–311.
Minto CL, Liao LM, Woodhouse CR, et al. The effect of clitoral surgery on sexual outcome in individuals who have intersex conditions with ambiguous genitalia: a cross-sectional study. Lancet. 2003;361(9365):1252–7.
Mostafa IA, Woodward MN, Shalaby MS. Cystoscopic-assisted laparoscopic excision of prostatic utricle. J Pediatr Urol. 2018;14(1):77–8.
Mureau MA, Slijper FM, van der Meulen JC, et al. Psychosexual adjustment of men who underwent hypospadias repair: a norm-related study. J Urol. 1995;154(4):1351–5.
Nordenskjold A, Holmdahl G, Frisen L, et al. Type of mutation and surgical procedure affect long-term quality of life for women with congenital adrenal hyperplasia. J Clin Endocrinol Metab. 2008;93(2):380–6.
Oppelt P, Renner SP, Kellermann A, et al. Clinical aspects of Mayer-Rokitansky-Kuester-Hauser syndrome: recommendations for clinical diagnosis and staging. Hum Reprod. 2006;21(3):792–7.
Passerini-Glazel G. A new 1-stage procedure for clitorovaginoplasty in severely masculinized female pseudohermaphrodites. J Urol. 1989;142(2 Pt 2):565–8; discussion 572.
Pena A, Hong A. The posterior sagittal trans-sphincteric and trans-rectal approaches. Tech Coloproctol. 2003;7(1):35–44.
Pena A, Filmer B, Bonilla E, et al. Transanorectal approach for the treatment of urogenital sinus: preliminary report. J Pediatr Surg. 1992;27(6):681–5.
Qin C, Luo G, Du M, et al. The clinical application of laparoscope-assisted peritoneal vaginoplasty for the treatment of congenital absence of vagina. Int J Gynaecol Obstet. 2016;133(3):320–4.
Riepe FG, Krone N, Viemann M, et al. Management of congenital adrenal hyperplasia: results of the ESPE questionnaire. Horm Res. 2002;58(4):196–205.
Roberts JP, Hutson JM. Reduction of scrotalized skin improves the cosmetic appearance of feminising genitoplasty. Pediatr Surg Int. 1997;12(2–3):228–9.
Schnitzer JJ, Donahoe PK. Surgical treatment of congenital adrenal hyperplasia. Endocrinol Metab Clin North Am. 2001;30(1):137–54.
Smith ED. Durham Smith repair of hypospadias. Urol Clin North Am. 1981;8(3):451–5.
Smith ED. Timing of surgery in hypospadias repair. Aust N Z J Surg. 1983;53(5):396–7.
Spoor JA, Oosterhuis JW, Hersmus R, et al. Histological assessment of gonads in DSD: relevance for clinical management. Sex Dev. 2018;12(1–3):106–22.
Warne SA, Wilcox DT, Creighton S, et al. Long-term gynecological outcome of patients with persistent cloaca. J Urol. 2003;170(4 Pt 2):1493–6.
Warne G, Grover S, Hutson J, et al. A long-term outcome study of intersex conditions. J Pediatr Endocrinol Metab. 2005;18(6):555–67.

Gynaecological Management

18

Sonia R. Grover

18.1 Introduction

The aim of gynaecological care of young women with a DSD is for the person to reach a healthy, happy state of well-being, with the capacity to have positive relationships, including the potential for enjoyable and fulfilling sexual relationships. The desire for fertility is a possibility that may be more difficult to fulfil with a DSD diagnosis, but this too requires consideration. These outcomes are dependent on a number of factors, apart from those directly relating to the features of the specific DSD or the direct medical and surgical care. Some of the other prerequisites include having a positive self-esteem and body image and the absence of depression. Thus, examining the gynaecological management issues and the outcomes cannot be done in isolation.

Although this chapter deals primarily with the management of adolescents and young women with DSDs, there are earlier events and medical experiences that may have a negative impact; therefore, there should be some effort to ensure that optimal parental information as well as the avoidance of potentially traumatic events in childhood are also part of the gynaecological input.

Some of the issues described here may be undertaken by clinicians and health professionals other than gynaecologists. The gynaecology team at The Royal Children's Hospital provides gynaecology care to the paediatric and adolescent age groups for a range of different problems and routinely explores psychosocial aspects of the young person's life as an integral part to the provision of this clinical service. The gynaecologists are therefore comfortable to provide some of the psychosocial discussions and to undertake basic sexual counselling. This has enabled us to identify those in greater need, or to identify when the young person is ready for further psychological input before a referral is made to the limited psychology services that are available within the public hospital setting. In other places, psychologists may be more readily available to explore the psychosocial adjustment in young people with DSDs; sexual counsellors may perform all of the discussions regarding sexual activity, or this may be shared between the psychologist and sexual counsellors. Another alternative is that a nurse practitioner linked to a DSD service may provide some of the primary psychotherapeutic support and be able to trigger the relevant referral to psychologist or sexual counsellors when indicated. The important issue is that the topics raised here are relevant for the long-term well-being of young women with DSDs, and someone needs to be comfortable in ensuring that these issues are explored.

S. R. Grover (✉)
Department of Gynaecology, The Royal Children's Hospital, Melbourne, VIC, Australia

Murdoch Children's Research Institute, Melbourne, VIC, Australia

Department of Paediatrics, University of Melbourne, Melbourne, VIC, Australia
e-mail: sonia.grover@rch.org.au

J. M. Hutson et al. (eds.), *Disorders|Differences of Sex Development*,
https://doi.org/10.1007/978-981-13-7864-5_18

18.2 Neonatal Period

18.2.1 Talking with Parents

Parents, when confronted with trying to understand the impact of a DSD on their baby, are trying to integrate a complex range of information which includes aspects regarding long-term outcomes. Although paediatricians and paediatric surgeons who care for the neonate are also likely to be involved in the care of young children and young adolescents, most do not have involvement in the reproductive health and sexual aspects of young or adult people with these diagnoses. Thus, the insights and perspectives regarding teenagers at school, their interaction with peers and responses to peer pressure around issues relating to menses and relationships, and for young people becoming sexually active may be outside their clinical experience. Parents often ask questions such as 'What will it be like for our baby (if she is raised female) when she grows up?', 'How will she feel when she does not have periods when her friends do?', 'How different will she be to her friends?', 'Will she fit in?', 'Will she be a normal girl?' and 'How will she cope?'

To be able to respond to these questions, careful answers are required that acknowledge the differences that are present in all children. Additionally, some discussion with parents regarding normal variations in behaviour of children and young people is essential. For some individuals with DSD, the likely behaviour patterns are a little more predictable, as children with congenital adrenal hyperplasia (CAH) are somewhat more likely to participate in 'tomboy' play activities (Berenbaum and Bailey 2003)—but we should remember that many girls can also be 'tomboys' without it signifying any underlying DSD.

Other behavioural aspects are more difficult to predict, as there is such a wide variation between individuals. Some groups of adolescents will talk about periods and others do not, so the question of whether their teenage adolescent will tell friends about 'not having periods' (if there is an absent uterus in the specific DSD diagnosis) is very dependent on specific teenage friendship groups.

Part of the parental concern, but not always voiced spontaneously, is regarding the future potential of their child to be able to undertake sexual activity as an adult. Clearly, any positive sexual activity is very dependent on finding the right partner, but for people with DSDs, the diagnosis itself does not preclude the possibility of having a successful sexual relationship. Part of this discussion is reminding parents that many factors can potentially influence sexual experiences and pleasure.

Speaking to parents from a context of having cared for adolescents and adult people with similar diagnoses to that of their baby offers some perspective and reassurance for the future.

18.2.2 Surgical Input

An additional role that a gynaecologist can play in the neonatal period is in supporting the paediatric surgeon. Although in theory gynaecologists could undertake the surgery in the infants, most gynaecologists have had no training in genital surgery in babies. In contrast, paediatric urologists and surgeons undertake surgery on babies with severe hypospadias and are thus familiar with the anatomy relating to the erectile tissue, nerve and vascular supply of the glans. Despite this, the gynaecologist can have an input in terms of 'fine-tuning' the genital surgery to ensure optimal functional outcomes. Additionally, it is beneficial for the gynaecologist to understand the surgical techniques used to assist in understanding the potential problems that may be present in adolescence and adulthood.

Aiming for the creation of labia minora in the infant with virilised genitalia has been incorporated into the genitoplasty by some paediatric surgeons since the 1980s (Kogan et al. 1983). The creation of a clitoral hood has not been mentioned in papers describing the operative technique of genitoplasty, yet this too can be readily achieved at the time of the feminising genitoplasty (see Chap. 17). Up to now, assessment of the presence of the clitoral hood has been omitted from the standardised genital assessment tools that have been developed to assess long-term outcomes of this surgery (Creighton et al. 2001; Nordenskjold et al. 2008).

18.2.3 Timing of Surgery

There is considerable debate regarding the timing of genital surgery. It is clear that there are arguments for and against this early surgery. As the gynaecologist in a team of clinicians caring for young people with DSD, one of the gynaecologist's responsibilities is to ensure that optimal surgical outcomes as measured by long-term outcomes are occurring in that centre.

In some countries, early surgery undertaken for virilised genitalia has not included the introitoplasty or vaginoplasty. Some have argued that the vaginoplasty should be omitted in early surgery due to the high rate of further surgery (Creighton 2004). Thus, rather than aiming for a one-stage procedure, acceptance that genital surgery will be two-stage, with the vaginal component delayed till adolescence (Creighton and Minto 2001), has been advocated.

When this has not been done for those girls with a uterus (most frequently those with CAH), medical concerns arise with the onset of puberty as to whether the menses will be able to adequately drain through the urogenital opening. Medical pressure then mounts to undertake surgery at 11–13 years of age. This is not the ideal age to undertake genital surgery. The 11–13-year-old teenager tends to be embarrassed and uneasy about their genitalia and is unlikely to be mature enough to fully understand why the surgery is required. An option is to suppress the menses, but this option then generates further medical consultations regarding menstrual suppression, intervention with medications (either progestagens, the continuous oral contraceptive pill, or the gonadotrophin-releasing hormone analogues) with the possibility of side effects from the medications and further medicalisation of the adolescent.

Research on individuals with hypospadias has indicated that surgery undertaken at an age when the child is able to remember the surgery is more likely to have a negative impact on body image, self-esteem and their psychosexual outcomes. These findings are independent of the actual anatomical and functional outcomes (Mureau et al. 1995; Jones et al. 2009). The potential psychological impact of delayed surgery has not been explored for individuals who undergo feminising genitoplasties, although Nordenskjold reported that 20 out of 29 women with CAH who had undergone clitoral surgery advocated early timing of surgery (Nordenskjold et al. 2008).

Data from the UK have revealed that when young people who had feminising genitoplasties were assessed, 89% were found to require further major surgery (Creighton and Minto 2001; Creighton et al. 2001). A similar study in Melbourne (Lean et al. 2005) and in Hanoi (Grover et al. 2010) revealed that although many would require dilatation, only a small number would require further surgery—most which were likely to be minor involving a revision introitoplasty. It is unclear whether this difference reflects the population studied or the initial surgery, the surgical technique and expertise of the original surgeon, or all of these factors. In both Hanoi and Melbourne, the provision of feminising genitoplasty surgery is at a single hospital in each city and the surgery is undertaken by a small number of experienced surgeons. In Hanoi, the study population was individuals (n = 40) attending for the annual CAH meeting day/clinic, whereas in Melbourne, young people >12 years (n = 32) who agreed to be examined in clinic made up 50% of all individuals who had had genitoplasties in the relevant time period, and these individuals were considered representative of the total population cared for at the Royal Children's Hospital, Melbourne. In contrast, the study population reported by Creighton et al. (2001) consisted of people from all over the UK recruited from the CAH support group or who had been seen in the London clinic, which is a specialised adolescent/adult clinic with referrals from all over the UK, thus representing quite a different cohort.

Thus, for some centres, where research has demonstrated poor long-term outcomes, it may be wise to advocate for delayed surgery. Alternatively, where the research outcomes demonstrate good results, then there is a place for supporting the early surgery.

18.2.4 Reproductive Prognosis

An additional role of the gynaecologist in the neonatal period exists in terms of offering information regarding the future fertility potential of reproductive tract structures present in the infant. In some babies with DSD, there may be a combination of typical male and typical female anatomical structures present. Previously, some of these structures were thought to be remnants or vestigial (Davies et al. 2004) and thus removed.

In the past, where a decision was made to raise a baby as a male, this would have led to the removal of any structures which were part of the typical female genital tract. Yet, these structures, in particular, a unicornuate uterus, are quite capable of successfully carrying a pregnancy. Thus, in a condition such as mixed gonadal dysgenesis, there may be a unicornuate uterus present on one side with an ipsilateral streak or non-functioning gonad, and on the contralateral side, a gonad producing testosterone, resulting in the external genitalia being partially virilised, although often with hypospadias present. For those babies where a decision is made to raise the child as a male, the question is whether the uterine structure should be removed. Although the majority of these infants if raised male are likely to identify as male when adult (Cohen-Kettenis 2005; Szarras-Czapnik et al. 2007), there are, nevertheless, some reports of dissatisfaction with gender of rearing. In these young people, preservation of the uterus would enable the possibility of carrying a pregnancy (with donor egg) should they choose to change their gender in adolescence. It may be appropriate to ligate the lower end of the vagina to prevent retrograde urine flow into the vagina, but removal of these Müllerian structure can be delayed till the gender identity of the individual has been clarified during adolescence.

18.3 Childhood

During childhood, there is very little need for significant medical or surgical input. Nevertheless, it is a time when gentle education may begin and encouraging this possibility with parents is appropriate. The opportunity to raise issues relating to diversity can be incorporated into responses. When families are having discussions about growing up, the fact that everyone is different can be incorporated into those discussions. During discussions about people having babies, the possibility that not everyone can have a baby, that some people need help to have babies, that other people chose to adopt and others decide not to have babies can all be raised in a non-threatening gentle manner.

During childhood, it is important to ensure that traumatic medical experiences are avoided. In the past, medical photographs were often taken with the young person standing naked for the picture. These experiences are often recounted by the young person when they are adults as unpleasant events. They have the potential of having a negative impact on self-esteem and body image.

Genital examinations are also often recalled as negative events subsequently impacting on future sexual experiences. These genital examinations often used to occur with several observers (junior doctors or medical students) present. In some settings, these genital examinations may also have included a vaginal examination. As no surgery to the genitalia should be required in childhood (after the possible genitoplasty undertaken as an infant), these examinations are unnecessary. Although it has been previously argued that a genital examination can give an indication of adequacy of hormone replacement in the setting of CAH, there are alternative means of assessing this (by blood tests, measuring blood pressure, looking for evidence of a cushingoid appearance or hirsutism and pigmentation) which are far less intrusive. Genital examination is therefore not indicated for this purpose.

As the long-term aim is for the young person to have a positive self-esteem and body image, the genital examination in a young person who does not understand why it is being done is usually not a positive contribution.

18.4 Adolescence

18.4.1 General Issues

An advantage of providing an adolescent gynaecology service is that it provides an ideal opportunity to begin to transition the care from one where the main communication is with the parent, to one where the focus of communication is with the patient herself. As this is the age when transition to autonomy begins to occur, it is opportune to work towards a consultation occurring without parents. Studies suggest that young people are not well informed about their diagnosis nor are they satisfied with their knowledge (Migeon et al. 2002; Nordenskjold et al. 2008), and an effort must be undertaken to ensure that the young person themself understands their diagnosis.

Psychotherapeutic groups for young people with DSD have led to the identification of a number of themes that are useful to explore (Grover and Loughlin 2002). Young people with DSD often report feeling different from their peers; relationships with peers and partners may be difficult due to concerns that their diagnosis should be a secret; the need for open disclosure; many report being informed of their diagnosis as a traumatic event, with features suggestive of a post-traumatic stress disorder; and fertility and infertility are issues that become more prominent as they become older adolescents. The psychotherapeutic groups are reported as positive experiences by many of the young women. Unfortunately, there is no work to clarify the respective benefit of meeting others face to face versus establishing contact via internet-based support groups or by email contact. The opportunity for the young women to be able to make contact or speak to others reduces the isolation and sense of being alone and different, unfortunately there is no comparative work that has been undertaken with adolescent males to know if the same applies to them.

Some of the anxiety relating to genital appearance may stem from the fact that for some young women, their genitalia were repeatedly examined in childhood. Over the past 15 years, a policy of not examining the genitalia in young children and adolescents until the young woman herself is interested in looking, with the aid of a hand-held mirror and consents to this being done, appears to have led to a decline in the anxiety about genital appearance in our patient population.

Hormonal treatment to allow the progression through pubertal changes and gain secondary sexual characteristics is required for a number of adolescent women with DSD.

Discussion around relationships, peer groups and establishing if the teenager is undertaking similar social activities to her peer groups is part of this assessment. Some exploration of what the young person understands about their diagnosis and what others have been told also gives some indication of how comfortable the young person is with their diagnosis. An adolescent in their mid-to-late teen years has usually formed close friendships, and disclosure to close friends of some of their diagnosis—whether it is that they have no periods or that having babies will be difficult—can usually be interpreted as a positive sign of adjustment to their diagnosis. The older adolescent who has not disclosed any information about their diagnosis to anyone suggests that for the young person, the diagnosis is such an enormous secret and so shameful that it cannot be shared. If referral for psychological support has not occurred prior to this point, then this signifies the need for such intervention.

Fertility and the issue of infertility are topics that are normally raised by gynaecologists. For some people with DSD, the presence of a uterus means that the potential to carry a pregnancy exists. For a person with a uterus but with a DSD diagnosis, the gonads are usually non-functioning; hence, a donor egg is required for a pregnancy to occur (e.g. XY or XX gonadal dysgenesis, mixed gonadal dysgenesis, ovotesticular DSD). For some diagnoses, in particular for those with Turner Syndrome, despite the presence of a uterus, there may be substantial risks associated with carrying a pregnancy (Bondy 2007), which need to be discussed with the young person. Another group of women who benefit from discussions regarding fertility are those with uterovaginal agenesis, where the young person has functioning ovaries but no uterus (and potentially, initially, no vagina). These women have the possibility of using a surrogate to carry their pregnancy. To date, a small number of successful uterine transplants (Brannstrom et al. 2018) have occurred followed by successful pregnancies.

18.4.2 Genital Appearance and Function

Where a feminising genitoplasty has been performed for those born with some virilisation of their external genitalia, clitoral, introital and labial surgery may have been undertaken.

Reports on the long-term outcomes of this surgery have often failed to describe the exact surgical technique that was used or the experience of the surgeon. The techniques used have changed over time ranging from clitoridectomy (or amputation), clitoral recession to girth-reduction procedures (Lean et al. 2007). Some studies reporting on the outcomes of surgery include data on the experience of the surgeon, in terms of the number of different surgeons who have operated on the patients in the cohort (Alizai et al. 1999; Lean et al. 2007; Nordenskjold et al. 2008), but the expertise of the surgeons is not mentioned by others (Kuhnle et al. 1995; Creighton et al. 2001; Minto et al. 2003a, b).

Reports on the outcomes of feminising genitoplasty are mixed, and it has only been in the past two decades that attempts to use a standardised approach to the assessment of the cosmetic and anatomical outcomes has occurred (Creighton et al. 2001; Nordenskjold et al. 2008). Analysis of anatomical and cosmetic outcomes has included assessment of clitoral size (see Table 18.1), introital size and labial appearance.

Creighton reported outcomes of 44 women as poor cosmetic outcomes in 41%, and with 89% requiring further major surgery to use tampons, or to have sexual intercourse (Creighton et al. 2001). In contrast, Lean et al. (2005) reported on 32 patients with 6% poor cosmetic outcomes. In this series, two-thirds of all the procedures were undertaken by one surgeon with a specialized interest in this area.

Table 18.1 Clitoral size in patients who had undergone clitoral surgery

	Normal	Absent	Small	Large	Very large
Alizai et al. (1999)	7/14	1/14	4/14	1/14	
Creighton et al. (2001)	26/44	3/44	3/44		9/44
Lean et al. (2005)	24/32	4/32	3/32	1/32	
Nordenskjold et al. (2008)	11/38	4/38		19/38	

Table 18.2 Clitoral size judged by women with CAH with and without surgery and controls (Nordenskjold et al. 2008)

Clitoral size according to the woman	Controls $n = 60$	Women with CAH, had clitoral surgery $n = 38$	Women with CAH, no clitoral surgery $n = 24$
Too large	0	8/38	13/24
Normal	60	19/38	11/24
Too small	0	6/38	0/24

Another critical perspective on surgical outcome, which has been omitted in many studies, is that of the patient self-report (see Table 18.2). It is important to note that without surgery there are concerns with satisfaction regarding clitoral size, despite the fact that much discussion in the literature has centred around the outcomes of surgery, ignoring the fact that the condition itself has resulted in a variation in the appearance of the genitalia, and the question should be whether the outcomes of surgery and postsurgical satisfaction are higher than amongst those who have not had surgery.

18.4.3 Vaginal Surgery

Vaginal surgery, in the setting of virilised genitalia, likewise has shown mixed results. Many report the need for repeat vaginal surgery in the setting of a planned one-stage feminising genitoplasty procedure (Alizai et al. 1999; Stikkelbroeck et al. 2003; Crouch et al. 2008). Despite the need for repeat surgery, some researchers have shown that this does not necessarily result in a negative long-term outcome (Stikkelbroeck et al. 2003).

Satisfaction with vaginal size (using a 5-point scale) in a cohort of women with CAH who had had surgery (n = 37), compared to a group who had not had surgery (n = 20) and compared to a control population (n = 60) has been reported by Nordenskjold et al. (2008). Of controls, only 51% were completely satisfied, although none were completely dissatisfied with their vagina. The completely satisfied rates for women with CAH who had had surgery and those who had not had surgery were 33% and 40%, respectively, with 30% of each of these groups being neither satisfied nor dissatisfied with their vaginas.

Women with vaginal agenesis also belong the diagnostic grouping of DSD, as their anatomy does not conform to the typical internal anatomy of females. The approach to the management of vaginal agenesis varies in different parts of the world. Dilators are generally used as the first-line approach to creating a vagina in the United Kingdom (Nadarajah et al. 2005), Australia (Kimberley et al. 2011) and increasingly in the USA (Gargollo et al. 2009; Oelschlager et al. 2016). This approach results in a >90% success rate. In some parts of Europe, the use of dilators is limited to the women who already have several centimetres of vagina (usually >4 cm). The alternative approach of using operative techniques, the Davydov (Davydov and Zhvitiashvili 1974), Vecchietti (Borruto 1992) and bowel segment vaginoplasties (Khen-Dunlop et al. 2007) are reported more often from Europe.

Although there has been a small study that demonstrated that the use of dilators did have a negative impact on self-esteem (Liao et al. 2006), the only study to compare women who had had surgical versus dilator therapy to create a vagina had only small numbers of surgical patients (Kimberley et al. 2011), with sexual function in this study similar in both groups. A further predictive factor for sexual function scores was better quality-of-life scores and greater time since diagnosis, underlying the fact that there are a number of factors that contribute to outcome apart from the technique of making a neovagina.

One of the challenges in the care of young women with vaginal agenesis is the timing and type of any intervention (Skinner and Quint 2017a, b; Committee on Adolescent Health Care 2018). In Tubingen, Germany, the decision to undertake surgery (a laparoscopic Vecchietti approach is used) is only made after completion of psychological assessment of the young woman (personal communication, Sara Brucker).

The approach to women with complete androgen insensitivity syndrome (CAIS) also varies from the use of dilators (Ismail-Pratt et al. 2007) to surgery. It is very hard to separate the negative impact that occurs when the information is given to the young person that 'their vagina is short', and the subsequent reporting by the young person that they feel as though their vagina is short. Minto reported that 77% of people with CAIS reported that they felt their vagina was small, yet clinical examination identified this in only 35% (Minto et al. 2003a, b).

Bladder exstrophy and cloacal exstrophy are now considered part of the DSD spectrum. In these conditions, variations of the vagina and uterus are common. In cloacal exstrophy, uterine didelphys is almost routinely present, although these structures may be associated with cervical agenesis and/or vaginal agenesis. A high level of suspicion is essential, as the exact internal reproductive tract anatomy has often not been adequately clarified in the neonatal period when the urinary and bowel anomalies are being corrected. These adolescents potentially then present at puberty acutely with obstructed systems with haematocolpos and/or haematometra. The young people with bladder exstrophy often have a lower vaginal stricture as a result of the corrective surgery to create a urethra and close the bladder. This will require correction either when they present with vaginal discharge or when they are ready to use tampons or commence sexual activity.

18.4.4 Genital Sensation and Sexual Function

A further aspect in establishing the long-term impact of genital surgery has been the assessment of sensation. Most of the studies that have been undertaken demonstrate a reduction in sensation following genital surgery (Crouch et al. 2008; Nordenskjold et al. 2008), but the relationship to altered sexual function is not as clear.

Quite a number of reports on sexual function and sexual quality of life in adults with DSD exist, although the quality of these reports varies (Kuhnle et al. 1995; Crouch et al. 2008; Warne 2008; Nordenstrom et al. 2010; Schonbucher et al. 2012). Although the results are inconsistent, overall, there is evidence suggesting that the sexual quality of life of individuals with DSD is reduced. The

Table 18.3 Reports on the ability to achieve orgasm in women with DSD—with and without genital surgery

	No clitoral surgery	Clitoral surgery
Minto et al. (2003a) All CAIS	39/59	
Minto et al. (2003b) DSD with ambiguous genitalia	6/19	7/18
Nordenstrom et al. (2010) All CAH	23/24	5/7 amputation10/10 recession8/11 reduction
Beerendonk (2010) mixed DSD population	8/13	11/18

impact of the medical and surgical care, as well as the psychosocial contributions, has not routinely been considered when assessment of sexuality and sexual function has been undertaken.

One approach to try to clarify this is to examine the studies that report on the ability of individuals identifying as female to achieve orgasm. When combining the studies that compare those individuals with DSD who have not had external genital surgery to those who have, there is no significant difference in the rate of orgasm ($Chi^2 = 1.08$, $p = 0.3$) (Table 18.3).

A study on the impact of body image and self-esteem on sexual function has shown that sexual function does not correlate with the severity of a carefully measured genital problem (genital prolapse) but rather with body image and distress scores (Lowenstein et al. 2009).

Ongoing involvement of clinicians, who are comfortable to explore issues relating to sexual function (e.g. sexual counsellors), and with the requisite knowledge regarding the potential problems that may occur as a result of the DSD, is critical.

The potential problems will differ for each of the DSD diagnoses. Individuals with CAH may choose to undergo further surgery or the use of dilators to achieve an adequate vagina for sexual activity and intercourse. Individuals with CAIS will mostly have an adequate vaginal length for intercourse, and exploration of other issues relating to sexual intercourse needs to occur prior to contemplating any surgical intervention, but this needs to explore the potential negative inputs relating to information given about vaginal length. Individuals with vaginal agenesis can most likely make their own vagina with the use of dilators, although some will require surgical intervention. Lubrication can be an ongoing issue for those with vaginal agenesis who were born without a hymen but use of a lubricant will assist.

18.5 Gonadal Surgery

For a number of the diagnoses encompassed by the expression DSD, there is no indication for any gonadal surgery. Conditions where there is typical ovarian function such as 46,XX bladder exstrophy, 46,XX cloacal exstrophy and vaginal agenesis ovarian function is completely normal. For women with CAH, ovarian function is also typical, although the negative impact of elevated androgens and potentially obesity may result in irregular menses.

For those conditions where there is an 46,XY karyotype and dysgenetic gonads (e.g. 46,XY complete gonadal dysgenesis, 45,X/46,XY mixed gonadal dysgenesis) the malignancy risk dictates a recommendation of removal of this non-functioning tissue.

In diagnoses such as CAIS, the question of gonadal removal is now openly discussed. For intra-abdominal testes, the risk of malignancy is marginally increased, and monitoring for any change in size with ultrasonography is an option. As these functional testes are producing testosterone which is being converted to oestrogens peripherally, they are serving a useful function. This is particularly the case, if performing a gonadectomy may result in difficulties accessing oestrogen replacement therapy, the cost of this replacement medication may be too high or where there may be issues with non-compliance. Thus, there is a clear argument for leaving the inguinal and labial testes *in situ*, as long as there is no associated inguinal hernia. Their location does carry the potential of pain or discomfort with sexual activity, and removal at that point may then be appropriate after careful discussions.

Gonadectomy for those with 46,XY conditions where virilisation has occurred at puberty (PAIS and 17β-HSD3) should be delayed until certainty regarding the gender identity of the young person has been adequately explored. Delay in undertaking the surgery, without any further virilisation, can be achieved with suppression of further hormones by the use of gonadotrophin-releasing-hormone antagonists.

18.6 Conclusion

The issues encompassed by the gynaecology input overlap with those of other members of the multidisciplinary team involved in the care of the young women with DSD. The exact role undertaken by each clinician is dependent on the clinicians themselves and their specific skills at each centre, but the range of issues that need to be explored are important and require the team to have discussions and good communication to ensure that these issues are covered.

A good understanding of the surgical techniques that may have been used in childhood, as well as having an understanding of surgical techniques that may be required to overcome complications, is necessary; it is therefore preferable for the clinician who will be undertaking the surgery to also be the one who is talking to the patient about potential problems. These problems may not become evident until the young person is trying to use tampons or is beginning to become sexually active and wishing to use their vagina. To clarify what the exact difficulties are requires close co-operation between the surgical members of the DSD team and good communication with counsellors if these clinicians are undertaking the sexual counselling. But most importantly, it requires open discussion and communication with the young person themself.

Timing the initiation of the discussions with the young person regarding adolescent issues, menses and sexual relationships is challenging. Having the opportunity to 'get to know' the young adolescent before this, to establish a trusting relationship, and one that is specifically with the young person (as distinct to the one with the parents) is part of this process. Gently exploring and tackling these issues before they have a negative impact on the adolescent's development and transition to adulthood is important.

References

Alizai NK, Thomas DF, Lilford RJ, et al. Feminizing genitoplasty for congenital adrenal hyperplasia: what happens at puberty? J Urol. 1999;161(5):1588–91.

Beerendonk C. Long term followup of women with disorders of sex development. Ano-rectal malformations, Nijmegen, The Netherlands. 2010.

Berenbaum SA, Bailey JM. Effects on gender identity of prenatal androgens and genital appearance: evidence from girls with congenital adrenal hyperplasia. J Clin Endocrinol Metab. 2003;88(3):1102–6.

Bondy CA. Care of girls and women with Turner syndrome: a guideline of the Turner syndrome study group. J Clin Endocrinol Metab. 2007;92(1):10–25.

Borruto F. Mayer-Rokitansky-Kuster syndrome: Vecchietti's personal series. Clin Exp Obstet Gynecol. 1992;19(4):273–4.

Brannstrom M. Current status and future direction of uterus transplantation. Curr Opin Organ Transplant. 2018;23(5):592–7.

Cohen-Kettenis PT. Gender change in 46,XY persons with 5alpha-reductase-2 deficiency and 17beta-hydroxysteroid dehydrogenase-3 deficiency. Arch Sex Behav. 2005;34(4):399–410.

Committee on Adolescent Health Care. ACOG Committee opinion no. 728: Müllerian agenesis: diagnosis, management, and treatment. Obstet Gynecol. 2018;131(1):e35–42.

Creighton SM. Long-term outcome of feminization surgery: the London experience. BJU Int. 2004;93(Suppl 3):44–6.

Creighton S, Minto CL. Managing intersex: most vaginal surgery in surgery should be deferred. BMJ. 2001;323:1264–5.

Creighton SM, Minto CL, Steele SJ. Objective cosmetic and anatomical outcomes at adolescence of feminising surgery for ambiguous genitalia done in childhood. Lancet. 2001;358(9276):124–5.

Crouch NS, Liao LM, Woodhouse CR, et al. Sexual function and genital sensitivity following feminizing genitoplasty for congenital adrenal hyperplasia. J Urol. 2008;179(2):634–8.

Davies MC, Creighton SM, Wilcox DT. Long-term outcomes of anorectal malformations. Pediatr Surg Int. 2004;20(8):567–72.

Davydov SN, Zhvitiashvili OD. Formation of vagina (colpopoiesis) from peritoneum of Douglas pouch. Acta Chir Plast. 1974;16(1):35–41.

Gargollo P, Cannon G, Diamond D, et al. Should progressive perineal dilatation be considered first line therapy for vaginal agenesis. J Urol. 2009;182(4 Suppl):1882–9.

Grover S, Loughlin E. Recurring themes from psychotherapeutic group work leading to the development of a clinical practice checklist for women with intersex and related conditions. IX European Congress in Paediatric and Adolescent Gynaecology. Florence. 2002.

Grover S, Loan D, Armstrong K, et al. Congenital adrenal hyperplasia in Vietnam: the issues confronting girls and their families and the surgical outcomes. FIGIJ Montpellier. 2010. P2.1–15.

Ismail-Pratt IS, Bikoo M, Liao LM, et al. Normalization of the vagina by dilator treatment alone in Complete Androgen Insensitivity Syndrome and Mayer-Rokitansky-Kuster-Hauser syndrome. Hum Reprod. 2007;22(7):2020–4.

Jones BC, O'Brien M, Chase J, et al. Early hypospadias surgery may lead to a better long-term psychosexual outcome. J Urol. 2009;182(4 Suppl):1744–9.

Khen-Dunlop N, Lortat-Jacob S, Thibaud E, et al. Rokitansky syndrome: clinical experience and results of sigmoid vaginoplasty in 23 young girls. J Urol. 2007;177(3):1107–11.

Kimberley N, Hutson JM, Southwell BR, et al. Well-being and sexual function outcomes in women with vaginal agenesis. Fertil Steril. 2011;95(1):238–41.

Kogan SJ, Smey P, Levitt SB. Subtunical total reduction clitoroplasty: a safe modification of existing techniques. J Urol. 1983;130(4):746–8.

Kuhnle U, Bullinger M, Schwarz HP. The quality of life in adult female patients with congenital adrenal hyperplasia: a comprehensive study of the impact of genital malformations and chronic disease on female patients life. Eur J Pediatr. 1995;154(9):708–16.

Lean WL, Deshpande A, Hutson J, et al. Cosmetic and anatomic outcomes after feminizing surgery for ambiguous genitalia. J Pediatr Surg. 2005;40(12):1856–60.

Lean WL, Hutson JM, Deshpande AV, et al. Clitoroplasty: past, present and future. Pediatr Surg Int. 2007;23(4):289–93.

Liao L, Doyle J, Crouch NS, et al. Dilation as treatment for vaginal agenesis and hypoplasia: a pilot exploration of benefits and barriers as perceived by patients. J Obstet Gynaecol. 2006;26(2):144–8.

Lowenstein L, Gamble T, Sanses TV, et al. Sexual function is related to body image perception in women with pelvic organ prolapse. J Sex Med. 2009;6(8):2286–91.

Migeon CJ, Wisniewski AB, Brown TR, et al. 46,XY intersex individuals: phenotypic and etiologic classification, knowledge of condition, and satisfaction with knowledge in adulthood. Pediatrics. 2002;110(3):e32.

Minto CL, Liao KL, Conway GS, et al. Sexual function in women with complete androgen insensitivity syndrome. Fertil Steril. 2003a;80(1):157–64.

Minto CL, Liao LM, Woodhouse CR, et al. The effect of clitoral surgery on sexual outcome in individuals who have intersex conditions with ambiguous genitalia: a cross-sectional study. Lancet. 2003b;361(9365):1252–7.

Mureau MA, Slijper FM, van der Meulen JC, et al. Psychosexual adjustment of men who underwent hypospadias repair: a norm-related study. J Urol. 1995;154(4):1351–5.

Nadarajah S, Quek J, Rose GL, et al. Sexual function in women treated with dilators for vaginal agenesis. J Pediatr Adolesc Gynecol. 2005;18(1):39–42.

Nordenskjold A, Holmdahl G, Frisen L, et al. Type of mutation and surgical procedure affect long-term quality of life for women with congenital adrenal hyperplasia. J Clin Endocrinol Metab. 2008;93(2):380–6.

Nordenstrom A, Frisen L, Falhammar H, et al. Sexual function and surgical outcome in women with congenital adrenal hyperplasia due to CYP21A2 deficiency: clinical perspective and the patients' perception. J Clin Endocrinol Metab. 2010;95(8):3633–40.

Oelschlager AM, Debiec K, Appelbaum H. Primary vaginal dilation for vaginal agenesis: strategies to anticipate challenges and optimize outcomes. Curr Opin Obstet Gynecol. 2016;28(5):345–9.

Schonbucher V, Schweizer K, Rustige L, et al. Sexual quality of life of individuals with 46,XY disorders of sex development. J Sex Med. 2012;9(12):3154–70.

Skinner B, Quint EH. Nonobstructive reproductive tract anomalies: a review of surgical management. J Minim Invasive Gynecol. 2017a;24(6):909–14.

Skinner B, Quint EH. Obstructive reproductive tract anomalies: a review of surgical management. J Minim Invasive Gynecol. 2017b;24(6):901–8.

Stikkelbroeck NM, Beerendonk CC, Willemsen WN, et al. The long term outcome of feminizing genital surgery for congenital adrenal hyperplasia: anatomical, functional and cosmetic outcomes, psychosexual development, and satisfaction in adult female patients. J Pediatr Adolesc Gynecol. 2003;16(5):289–96.

Szarras-Czapnik M, Lew-Starowicz Z, Zucker KJ. A psychosexual follow-up study of patients with mixed or partial gonadal dysgenesis. J Pediatr Adolesc Gynecol. 2007;20(6):333–8.

Warne GL. Long-term outcome of disorders of sex development. Sex Dev. 2008;2(4–5):268–77.

19 Psychosocial Support

Chloe A. Hanna

19.1 Psychosocial Support

The development of psychosocial support services and a focus on the long-term well-being of a person with a DSD has been identified as one of the key components in enhancing the medical care for families and individuals with DSD. At this time, there is not a shared or congruent ideology of what constitutes the best medical management by representatives from intersex advocacy groups and health professionals (Karkazis 2008; Garrett and Kirkman 2009). Some medical interventions offered to individuals with DSD, particularly, with respect to genital surgery and also some forms of hormonal management, have been challenged as infringing the human rights of the affected individual. As a consequence, should such interventions be deferred to a time where the individual can be involved in the decision-making process, psychosocial support may become the primary form of medical care for infants and children with DSDs and their families. Psychosocial support should provide assistance to families to adapt and accept the spectrum of physical presentations that result from these variations.

C. A. Hanna (✉)
Department of Gynaecology, The Royal Children's Hospital, Melbourne, VIC, Australia

Murdoch Children's Research Institute, Melbourne, VIC, Australia
e-mail: chloe.hanna@rch.org.au

19.2 Development of Psychosocial Systems and Sharing Information

The health management of individuals with DSD has evolved from controversial beginnings. Until relatively recently, full disclosure of information relating to their underlying DSD was not considered in the best interest of the person and family, as health providers deemed the knowledge to cause more psychological harm than good (Thomas 2003). The transition to full disclosure has occurred at different times in different parts of the world. Thus, the opportunities for individuals and their families to clearly understand their condition, provide informed consent for the types of management being offered and gain access to appropriate psychosocial supports has been limited. In turn, the well-being of individuals and their parents was compromised (Thomas 2003; Cull and Simmonds 2010; Hutson et al. 2012). This led to dissatisfaction with medical care and affected the long-term psychosocial development of the child (Karkazis 2008). In the 2006 Chicago consensus, it was determined that psychosocial supports played a critical role in the medical management of DSD (Lee et al. 2006). The consensus perspective emphasised the importance for clinical teams to disclose aetiology, review potential intervention options and the developmental outcomes expected at puberty with individuals and families as well as ongoing psychosocial supports. In Melbourne, Australia,

J. M. Hutson et al. (eds.), *Disorders|Differences of Sex Development*,
https://doi.org/10.1007/978-981-13-7864-5_19

The Royal Children's Hospital DSD patient care included key psychosocial elements such as full condition disclosure, a multidisciplinary team (MDT) approach and links to peer support from the 1980s (Warne 1992). The long-term goal of healthcare for people with DSD is considered a good quality of life, covering domains such as general health, self-esteem and body image, social life and relationships, ability to work, access to education, having a family and being an active member of the community (Nordenström 2015; Jones et al. 2016).

19.3 Psychosocial Implications of DSD

Psychosocial needs can loosely be defined as involving both psychological and social factors acknowledging the emotional, functional, mental, cultural and spiritual responses of a person (Johannsen et al. 2006). The psychosocial implications of having a DSD are broad and may differ greatly for each individual, each condition/diagnosis/aetiology and in different cultural/religious settings. Common psychosocial issues experienced by individuals with a DSD include issues relating to events at the time of diagnosis/disclosure, bodily integrity, self-esteem, gender identity, effect of medical intervention, general health, fertility and intimate relationships, as quality-of-life (QoL) outcomes are influenced by all these factors (Sutton et al. 2005; Hughes et al. 2006).

As families and specifically parents provide the principal care and psychosocial support to their children with a DSD, it is critical for the parents to receive family-centred support to promote overall quality of life (Rolston et al. 2015; Hanna 2013; Wolfe-Christensen et al. 2016). Parents of a child with a DSD may experience grief and loss, living with uncertainty, perceived stigma and stress regarding the diagnosis/disclosure, decision-making and medical management (Gomez-Lobo 2014; Rolston et al. 2015). Effective communication about clinical information delivered with sensitivity and compassion by members of the MDT results in better mental health of parents (Rolston et al. 2015; Pasterski et al. 2014; Crissman et al. 2011).

Both individuals with a DSD and their parents experience perceived social stigma regarding DSD that may challenge frequently encountered societal expectations of a binary sex and gender. The resulting stigma and secrecy regarding a person's health and body decreases their ability for psychosocial adaptation (Rolston et al. 2015).

Psychosocial support opportunities should be offered not only at specific junctures in the child's (and parent's) life but also on an ongoing basis throughout their medical care to adequately respond to individual care needs as they evolve and change over time (Hanna 2013; Pasterski et al. 2014).

19.4 What Is Psychosocial Support?

The term psychosocial support outlined in this book describes the current multidisciplinary team (MDT) approach to clinical care with the involvement of a DSD clinical coordinator. It includes but is not limited to:

- MDT care—team of health professionals from different disciplines (endocrinology, urology, gynaecology, allied health, clinical ethics) providing a shared-care approach for an individual/family;
- sharing of diagnosis information and medical interventions to individuals and families;
- informed decision-making;
- psychosocial counselling—face to face/telephone/online;
- counselling about interventions—including expected outcomes, the potential beneficial effects and possible side effects or negative outcomes of hormonal therapies or surgical interventions;
- access to up-to-date resources;
- continuity of care;
- provision of peer-support opportunities and referral to such agencies/groups; and,
- provision of summary information for the person to share with other health professionals when needed.

Definitive guidelines outlining specific psychosocial support are yet to be identified, although recognised as a key element of DSD management. Many components such as economic status, cultural beliefs and perception of DSD, resources and differences in educational levels influence the management of a person with DSD (Warne and Raza 2008). The majority of people with DSD seek and expect psychosocial support to be provided by their medical specialists, thus, psychological skills in all members of the MDT are essential (Hanna 2013; Jones et al. 2016). Even though a growing number of tertiary medical centres offer psychological support and links with peer-support groups, barriers still exist in accessing these forms of services (Leidolf et al. 2008; Mortimer 2017).

19.5 The Role of the Multidisciplinary Team

The MDT approach is recognised as best practice model of care for people with a DSD (Gomez-Lobo 2014; Hughes et al. 2006). The MDT is inclusive of clinicians from a range of medical specialities—endocrinology, gynaecology, urology, mental health, genetics, pathology, clinical coordinator (allied health) and clinical ethics. The team also involves external stakeholders when appropriate, such as peer-support groups, clinical researchers, general practitioners and community-service representatives. The role of the MDT is to provide holistic care by integrating each medical discipline into a unified clinical plan for each individual. This MDT approach enables specialists to work transparently with individuals while still providing continuity of care, streamline clinical pathways and identify gaps in care, in a patient-centred approach to care.

A team coordinator for an MDT is necessary for the varying disciplines to work as a unit (Sandberg and Mazur 2014). A dedicated role for DSD MDT clinical coordination enables a point of contact between the DSD MDT and families, as well as developing networks with peer support groups and other community organisations.

Each member of the MDT is responsible for providing psychosocial support or referral to a clinical coordinator or centralised team member such as a mental health clinician or social worker who has the knowledge base and appropriate skillset to provide support.

19.6 Multidisciplinary Team Clinical Meeting

The formation and the development of a structured DSD MDT meeting have been important steps in improving psychosocial care for individuals and families. These case conferences are confidential and enable the MDT to discuss patients' diagnosis and management decisions as well as examine human rights, ethics, recent research publications and new technologies. Cases are referred to the DSD MDT meeting to determine appropriate investigations, optimal management pathways and facilitate interdisciplinary communication (Sandberg and Mazur 2014). The meeting aims to discuss and achieve a consensus among clinicians in the role and timing of any further diagnostic investigations, options and reasons to consider any medical interventions, and relevant psychosocial supports. Consent from parent/caregiver is sought prior to their case being presented to the DSD MDT. This MDT care approach enables specialists to provide consistent holistic information and support to individuals/families. Recommendations are sent to relevant referring clinicians and added to the patient medical record. If a person presents with ongoing clinical complexity, it is usual for the case to be reviewed and discussed at further meetings.

19.7 Sharing Information About a DSD Diagnosis

The clinician's attitude and clinical practice in relation to disclosure of a DSD clearly influences the psychosocial development of an individual. Recommendations for informing an individual or parents about a diagnosis is necessary, taking into account the individual, the family and the cultural context (Sandberg et al. 2012). Intersex advocacy organisations have provided a space for affected individuals to voice their experiences and opinions of DSD management. This has stimulated further research into patient well-being and the development of DSD-management models (Karkazis 2008).

Over the past 30 years, clinicians supporting children and adolescents with DSD have developed skills and improved attitudes about the sharing of medical information with parents. A number of information booklets have been written to help with this, see Chap. 25 (Warne 1989). Doctors have an obligation to share what they have learned from medical observation and investigation about children in their care with parents and to their children, in a method that is appropriate for their age. Sharing of information about a diagnosis should take place with the individual and their family at regular intervals throughout their care to ensure ongoing improved understanding of their health and body (Cohen-Kettenis 2010).

It is important for the MDT to communicate information highlighting the different terminology associated with DSD. Although "DSD" is used in the medical community as an umbrella term, some Australian and international peer and advocacy groups use terms such as intersex or variation of sex characteristics. Many families prefer the specific condition name, which tends to be the practice of clinicians (Mortimer 2017). Australian peer-support groups encourage clinicians to share the spectrum of terms, normalising the range of expressions used, enabling families to access the range of information available on the internet.

Provision of both web-based resources and written information/hand outs are an essential form of psychosocial support for many people. Resources comprising accurate information, lived experiences and links to support services have been and continue to be developed for families to give them opportunities to access in their own time, and in a comfortable environment, and with the option of sharing this with other people if they want.

Bodily integrity is an important consideration for the clinical MDT when caring for individuals with DSDs. Individuals with DSDs are likely to have blood tests, physical examinations and other forms of medical interventions relating to their condition. It is within the role of health professionals to promote and educate families about bodily autonomy when sharing information about a DSD diagnosis (Box 19.1). Information for families about genital examination outlines the discussion and considerations health professionals can have when assisting their individuals (and family members) to make informed choices about having genital examinations (Box 19.2).

Box 19.1 Sharing Information About a Variation with a Child

Sharing Information with Young Children

It is important for parents to talk to their children about their condition; this should be completed in age-appropriate stages and supported by health professionals and counsellors. Use language that children are familiar with; consistent terminology should be used by both families and clinicians.

Key Discussion Points for Parents:

- Point about variations in everyone "*we are all different in many ways*". It is important for all children, not just those with DSD, to learn about the positive aspects of human diversity.
- Talk about the similarities between boys and girls—both physical attributes and social.
- Everyone is good at lots of things, but might need help with other things "that child there needs to wear glasses to help him see better".
- It is important to give your child an opportunity to talk about how they feel about taking medications and other medical interventions before and during. Talking to the doctor about what the side effects are can be useful.
- For some DSD diagnoses, fertility may be affected, so highlight that families can be made in different ways—adoption, IVF (with the help of someone else's egg/sperm), becoming a step parent, fostering, close friendships, or for some people having children is not a priority.
- Be clear and honest about why your child sees doctors at the hospital—"we

are going to the hospital for a check-up, our doctor will talk to us about how you are feeling, check how your body is working and growing—they might measure your height, your weight and sometimes ask you to have a blood test".

- Be open about what surgeries have occurred and why.
- Try to use correct terms for genitals—penis/phallus/clitoris; vulva/vagina/labia; scrotum; testes/gonads/ovaries.
- Providing opportunities for children and adolescents to talk about their bodily variation or previous genital surgeries could help normalize their body to them (Austin et al. 2011).
- If your child asks a question you do not know the answer to, be honest "I'm not sure of the answer, let's ask someone who may know, and learn about it together".

Box 19.2 Information for Families About Genital Examination

Parent and Patient Information About Physical Examinations.

Genital examinations are necessary when a baby or child presents with a DSD. This period can be very stressful for the family, especially if the baby has not yet been assigned a sex. An explanation of the different factors such as physical examination, hormone levels, genetic information and internal structures help inform the MDT to make the best decisions for a baby's health plan.

Why Are They Performed?

Newborns Physical Examinations for DSD

It is important for the clinical team to perform genital examinations to identify anatomy, this will help to understand how the baby gets rid of urine and faeces, this will also assess whether the baby was exposed to testosterone in the womb and where the gonads/testes/ovaries are located (this can be referred to as whether they are "palpable" in the pelvic region or not). A full explanation and option to opt out should be provided by clinicians to the parents/carers of the child.

For some children there will be an option for having surgery to change the genital anatomy. It is useful for the surgical team to have a medical professional photo of the area where surgery will be performed.

Parents are required to consent to this medical photography, this is voluntary, and parents can chose to opt not to have photos of the anatomy in their child/ren taken.

Paediatric and Adolescent Physical Examinations for DSD:

There are a few reasons for a child to require a physical examination, which are as follows:

- during the time of puberty, and if patient/child consents and would like information about their body;
- if there is pain or discomfort in the genital region;
- if there is a plan to do surgery;
- to assess puberty in boys;
- for the consideration of endocrine hormone therapies;
- post-surgery follow-up.

Although at times genital examinations are required for medical management, the clinician's approach to performing this type of examination should be completed with the cooperation from the child or adolescent wherever possible. If this consent is not supplied by the child it is worth considering not performing a genital examination (Quigley 2016).

Regular genital examinations in childhood and adolescence are likely to have negative impact to a person's mental health and their sense of self (Sandberg 2017).

Genital examinations that are completed in front of trainee groups can be experienced as very stigmatising events (Meyer-Bahlburg 2017).

A 2017 Victorian study found that many young people did not understand the reason for genital examinations, suggesting that clinicians could improve in communicating the reason for an examination (Tonkin-Hill 2018). Communication with the individuals and parents should sensitively explain the nature and reason for the physical examination, and to increase patient comfort and minimise stigma associated with bodily difference (Sandberg 2017).

19.8 Informing the Parents of Their Child's Condition/Variation

For parents, learning about their child's DSD diagnosis can be overwhelming, stressful and an isolating experience. Understanding complex medical information, uncertainty about sex of rearing (in some cases) and decisions about medical management including possible medical and/or surgical interventions that may be considered or recommended at different time points can take time, and concerns evolve and change as their child grows (Crissman et al. 2011). Educating parents about complex and unfamiliar matters that are potentially distressing requires the information to be presented in a form and manner that the parents can understand, according to their education and cultural background. Key time points for support and education are at the time of diagnosis (birth or later in life), prior to and during interventions, such as hormone therapies or surgery, pre-puberty, adolescence and transition to adult services.

19.9 Psychosocial Counselling Service for Families of an Infant with Uncertain Sex

The birth scenario is a varying experience that is not anticipated nor easily controlled. This may occur in the form of atypical genitalia at birth, or the phenotype of the newborn not matching the expected appearance on the basis of antenatal testing. Depending on the neonatal team's knowledge of DSD and timing of medical investigations, there may be a delay in the provision of clear information for parents. Parents themselves vary in their response to their infant's appearance depending on their personal capacities to cope with the unexpected and unknown, and also if they are vulnerable from significant prior losses and grief. With the assistance of the MDT, parents are involved in making informed decisions about the sex of their infant as well as participating in decisions about care pathways for their child, including the option of surgery and being comfortable with the outcomes of these decisions (Sanders et al. 2008). The decision is not made easily when, in many instances, there is no clearly defined optimal care pathway. In addition, there are differing views about infant surgery coming from sources such as adults with DSD, parent-support groups, varying outcomes reported in the medical literature, as well as, potentially, a range of perspectives within the family's MDT. Psychosocial support should be available during decision-making for medical interventions.

Psychosocial support for parents should include assistance to recover from the emotional stress at birth, to understand information and decision-making about DSD conditions and share information about the particular DSD.

A structured interview framework (Fig. 19.1) was developed by Elizabeth Loughlin in 2002 that sought to ensure a systematic assessment of psychosocial issues that may impact the family

Events surrounding the birth and ensuing days of investigations and decisions
1. Parents' response to ambiguous genitalia: adapted/ distressed/ traumatised/ not known (NK)
2. Mother's response shortly after birth: adapted/ distressed/ traumatised/ NK
3. Decision re gender at day 1 or 2: clear/dilemma/delayed/NK
4. Decision re gender by day: 0-2/3-7/8-14/15-30/>1/12/NK
5. Need to retell or delay gender to kin: yes/ no/ NK
6. Need to retell or delay gender to friends, community: yes/ no/ NK
7. Medical management (including clinical reports): clear/ unclear/ NK
8. Medical management (parents' perceptions): clear/ unclear/ NK
Infant
9. DOB Infant: .....
10. Birth: normal/ unexpected difficulties/ traumatic/ NK
11. Infant parallel serious health condition: yes/ no
12. Sex of baby decided: male/ female
13. Infant subsequently alive/deceased
Diagnosis
14. Diagnosis: CAH, CAIS, PAIS, MGD, ovotesticular DSD, Severe hypospadias, Klinefelter, other atypical genital appearance; other
15. Medical diagnosis at day: 0-2/3-7/8-14/15-13/>30/NK
Pre-existing issues
16. Pre-existing issues with infertility, miscarriage, neonatal loss or other loss that has impacted on self concept or parent relationship: yes/ no/ NK
17. Pre-existing mother or father with long-term problems in family of origin: yes/ no/ not
Cultural
18. Cultural background: English or Northern European/ Mediterranean/ Asian/ Muslim/ Indigenous & Islander
19. Residence: Victorian (Home state of hospital) metropolitan or rural city/ Victorian rural or small country town/ Interstate or interstate rural/ New Zealand and overseas
Emotional supports
20. Mother feels supported post-natally by partner, close family member: yes/ somewhat/ no/ NK
21. Maternal grandmother supportive and nearby: yes/ somewhat/ no/ NK

Fig. 19.1 The structured Interview

Parent–infant relationship
22. Mother, father observed attached to baby: yes/ developing/ no/ NK
23. Parental cultural preference or strong expectation for male or female: no preference/ boy/ girl/ acted on/ NK
Engagement
24. Parents engaged with psycho-social counselling, social work (2interviews 45- 90 minutes : yes/ somewhat/ no
25. Mother father engaged with medical investigations with discussion of options for surgery, and possibility of some uncertainty in DSD outcomes: yes / no/ NK
Follow up
26. Interested in psychosocial counsellor (outpatient or phone) (ie recognition that
they are experiencing huge adjustment, and infant will also): yes/ somewhat/ no/ NK
27. Willing to listen to existence of support groups and their style of support, even if do not want contact at present time: yes/ somewhat/ no/ NK
28. Acceptance that professional review – Medical specialist, Maternal Child Health nurse and other health personnel - is implicit in diagnosis
Service details
29. Referral day for psychosocial counselling: 0-2/3-5/6-15/16-90/3-6 months/1-2yr/>2-5yr
30. Referred by Surgeon/ Senior Endocrinologist/ Gynaecologist/ Endocrinologist 1/ 2/ 3/ Other
31. Date first seen by social worker......
32. Where first seen by social worker: ward /outpatients / maternity hospital/ telephone/ missing
33. Follow-up conducted: yes/ no
34. Date social work follow-up interview........
35. Where social work follow-up interview: ward/ outpatients/ maternity hospital/ telephone/ support group newsletter mailed/ letter/ missing
36. Social worker (SW): Endocrinology SW/ Neonate SW/ Neonate & Endo SW/ Other SW
37. Further extra follow-up clinically indicated: yes/ no
38. Individual SW comment about family: yes/ no Comments 1, 2, 3, 4 Individual family characteristics

Fig. 19.1 (continued)

as well as attachment between parents and infant/toddler was designed for use with parents of children aged 0–3 years with a DSD. This aimed:

- to prompt psychosocial support to cover all important issues and facts;
- to offer the parents emotional and social counselling around their experiences after the birth of their infant;
- to maintain a focus on the infant as the parents' new baby;
- to make a broad assessment of the family adaptation.

While the structured interview may not be appropriate in all scenarios, it is included here to highlight important considerations and themes that may impact families.

The following are some useful resources for caregivers and adolescent DSD families: The Royal Children's Hospital: https://www.rch.org.au/endo/differences-of-sex-development/.

19.10 Celebrating the Birth of a Baby with a DSD to Family and Friends

As the medical issues become clearer for parents, the dilemma of how to explain their infant's condition, and if necessary, how to delay or retell the sex to relatives and friends may become insistent and perplexing. Challenges surrounding the birth of an infant with different genital appearance relate to who and what to tell. Counselling points highlighted by the structured interview give an opportunity to assist parents to think about how to tell relatives and friends and yet preserve what they feel is right for their infant, their future child/adolescent's privacy and self-image. Parents want to rely on their own siblings and close friends for emotional support and yet want to keep the confidences about their baby—who cannot give permission—to a trusted few. Some families may choose to gather all the relatives to talk about the condition at the same time while others may decide to explain the details of the condition to only one set of grandparents. In small towns where families share local doctors, parents can be more cautious than city families about whom they tell. Published American guidelines for parents (www.dsd-guidelines.org) encourage straightforward explanation of their child's DSD to relatives and friends; support for this should be provided through the MDT.

Discussion with parents to devise their own strategies may include the following: (1) Decisions about who to tell and what to say to close family, to friends, to neighbours and to acquaintances. (2) Thoughts of what the future adolescent would wish parents to say. (3) Requests to doctors for full information about the condition so parents feel confident to speak to others on a variety of levels. For some parents and individuals, it is useful to have a prepared script of what type of information they will be sharing (and with whom), to assist with communicating with others about their child's condition. Support by the multidisciplinary team should be given to minimise percieved societal stigma surrounding variations that affect sex development, and reassurance for parents that these variations are normal occurrences.

19.11 Issues Faced by Families of Infants and Young Children with DSD

A clinical audit of the use of this structured interview was conducted with 70 families at our centre over a period of 5.5 years from July 2002 to January 2009.

There were 25 males and 45 females in the infant cohort, ($n = 70$). Parallel health issues were present in 23/70 families, and 21 had unexpected difficulties or trauma at delivery. There was a wide spread of referral day for psychosocial counselling, with 11 within 2 days of delivery and 11 more by 5 days. Fourteen were referred between 2 weeks and 6 months and 30 thereafter, the latter reflecting the number of families from interstate and overseas.

19.11.1 Adaptation

Parents in the cohort showed a range of adaptation, distress or trauma to the birth. Half the parents reported or were observed at the time of interview to be adapting to the unclear genital appearance, while 28 (40%) reported or were observed to express distress. Five families (7%) were still feeling traumatised, with 3% unknown. Mother's response shortly after birth showed more distress and trauma than parents together, with only 22 (31%) adapted.

19.11.2 Parent Pre-existing Issues

Issues surrounding infertility, miscarriage, neonatal loss or other loss were present in 11 families (16%), but in 25/70 (36%) it was not known.

19.11.3 Dealing with Uncertainties

The mother and/or father were observed to be engaged with medical investigations with discussion of options for surgery, and DSD outcomes in 59 families (84%). Many parents had the capacity to think about and tolerate some uncertainty in the future.

19.11.4 Family Issues

19.11.4.1 Decision Regarding the sex of rearing at Day 1 or 2

The decision regarding sex of rearing at day 1 or 2 was clear in 30 families (43%), but there were problems in 36 families (51%). Less than half the infants had a clear sex of rearing by the end of day 2. The following Tables 19.1 and 19.2 show a significant association between the parents' or the mother's response of adaptation to distress and trauma, and the decision about sex of rearing at day 1 or 2.

Table 19.1 Sex of rearing

Decision re sex of rearing at day 1 or day 2	No	Yes	Total
Clear	21	8	29
Dilemma/delayed	12	24	36
Total	33	32	65

$n = 65, p = 0.0006$ (Pearson Chi^2)

Table 19.2 Mother's response after birth

Decision re sex of rearing at day 1–2	Adapted	Distressed	Traumatised	Total
Clear	19	4	4	27
Dilemma/delayed	3	28	4	35
Total	22	32	8	62

$N + 62, p < 0.001$ (Pearson Chi^2)

Table 19.3 Sex of rearing

Need to retell or delay sex of rearing to kin	No	Yes	Total
Yes	9	18	27
No	22	12	34
Total	22	8	62

$N = 61, p = 0.015$ (Pearson Chi^2)

Table 19.4 Mother's response after birth

Need to retell or delay sex of rearing to kin	Adapted	Distressed	Traumatised	Total
Yes	2	23	2	27
No	20	7	5	32
Total	22	30	7	59

$N = 59, p < 0.001$

There was a need to retell or delay sex of rearing to relatives in 27 families (38.57%), and 21 families (30%) needed to retell or delay sex of rearing to friends and community. Overall, more than a third of parents had to retell or delay the sex of rearing to their relatives, and somewhat less than to friends and community (Table 19.3).

Cross-tabulation of parental distress and trauma and need to retell or delay sex of rearing to friends and community was not associated at a significant level. By contrast, the mother's response shortly after birth and the need to retell or delay sex of rearing to friends and community was highly significant (Table 19.4).

19.11.5 Other Selected Associations

Pre-existing issues of infertility, miscarriage or neonatal loss in the family were significantly associated with parental distress and trauma. Cultural background and residence were not significantly associated with parental distress and trauma. Whether the mother felt supported postnatally by father or close family was significantly associated with her response shortly after birth. However, whether the maternal grandmother was supportive and nearby was not associated with the mothers' response shortly after birth.

19.11.6 Discussion

This audit of the structured interview highlighted the parental characteristics to take into account during the psychosocial counselling interviews. The significant association of certain variables affirms family issues, namely the delay in deciding sex of rearing and need to retell or delay sex of rearing to relatives and friends as a stressor for parents. This indicates the need to address parent distress and psychosocial support for parent adaptation in these areas.

Certain pre-existing issues are associated with parental distress/trauma, as expected in families with a child with a serious health condition (Kazak et al. 2003). Other variables such as residence and cultural background were not associated with parental distress and trauma, as expected from clinical experience.

This audit highlights the importance of psychosocial counselling focusing on areas identified in this structured interview for parents of a newborn with a variation in sex development.

19.11.7 Issues for Families at Subsequent Counselling

Follow-up psychosocial support for parents and young persons self-referred, or re-referred by doctors for problems, reveals parents' preoccupations and family issues. Parents requested guidance about how to tell the young child aged 2–4 years about their DSD condition, or how to explain to the older child the unclear genital appearance of their sibling at birth. Parents worried about school-start for boys with hypospadias, and they also feared at the secondary school level, that the different appearance of the penis would affect their son's self-esteem and lead to teasing or bullying from other boys.

Some parents needed to go over the events post-birth again years later, which may reflect the depth of trauma they had experienced, even though their child was doing well. For girls with Turner syndrome, some families worried over their girls' self-concept, and ability to make friends, while their daughters wondered about future relationships and their infertility (Loughlin 2006).

The presence of the parents lessened when young women were referred to the paediatric and adolescent gynaecology clinic, which was available to people up to 24 years of age. In this clinic, issues raised in individual and group psychosocial counselling about the physical loss of their sexual and reproductive structures, infertility and beginning sexual relations; occasionally, the psychosocial counsellor saw parents for supportive counselling where the young woman were diagnosed later in adolescence. Questions of gender identity were rare but if present, were referred to the consultant psychiatrist.

19.11.8 What Does the Family Need from Psychosocial Services?

Families need to be given the ongoing opportunity for psychosocial counselling and resources in different formats (handouts/online/face-to-face) as soon as possible, ideally within a couple of days of hospital admission or referral to DSD MDT to cover all important family issues that are common, but with individualised counselling, particularly with regard to cultural responses to privacy in talking to others.

Follow-up counselling and opportunities for families to access a variety of psychosocial supports should be offered on an ongoing basis to both parents/family and individuals (Mortimer 2017; Tonkin-Hill 2018). Peer-support groups provide a valuable psychosocial service, benefitting a person's self-efficacy, empowerment and therapeutic qualities (Warne 2003; Hong et al. 2012). Internationally, peer-support organisations provide a spectrum of support, advocacy, education and resources. Opportunities to link in with these organisations should be provided regularly to individuals and families.

Discussion of pre-existing issues of prior infertility, assisted reproduction or pre- or neonatal loss may still be unresolved and will need extra counselling to address old trauma in order to adapt to their infant's DSD condition.

19.11.9 Sharing Information About a of Sex Development to a Child

Historically, the disclosure of a DSD to a child or adolescent presented an ethical dilemma for the DSD clinical team (Hutson et al. 2012). This was due to the health professional's fear of the psychological impact of knowing of such a diagnosis for an adolescent, which might lead to depression and suicide (Hutson et al. 2012). Misinformation and concealment provided by health professionals during this period has been consistently documented to encourage isolation, shame and stigma (Nordenström 2015). While learning of their diagnosis may trigger negative emotions and depression, positive implications of sharing a diagnosis using age-appropriate vocabulary with a child or adolescent have been recognised as best practice (Austin et al. 2011; Quigley 2009).

Knowing their own diagnosis allows a person to be able to participate with their healthcare, understand how it may affect them in other areas of life such as going through puberty, educational learning styles and reason for hormone effects (Tartaglia et al. 2008; Tonkin-Hill 2018). Access to psychosocial supports are essential through this period and should include opportunities for peer support to decrease any sense of isolation (Hanna 2013; Jones et al. 2016). Some of the key points needed for parents to help them talk to their children about their condition are listed in Box 19.1.

Acknowledgement With thanks and acknowledgement to the original author of this chapter—Elizabeth Loughlin.

References

Austin J, Tamar-Mattis A, Mazur T, et al. Disorders of sex development-when and how to tell the patient. Pediatr Endocrinol Rev. 2011;8(3):213–7; quiz 223.

Cohen-Kettenis PT. Psychosocial and psychosexual aspects of disorders of sex development. Best Pract Res Clin Endocrinol Metab. 2010;24(2):325–34.

Crissman HP, Warner L, Gardner M, et al. Children with disorders of sex development: a qualitative study of early parental experience. Int J Pediatr Endocrinol. 2011;2011(1):10.

Cull ML, Simmonds M. Importance of support groups for intersex (disorders of sex development) patients, families and the medical profession. Sex Dev. 2010;4(4–5):310–2.

Garrett CC, Kirkman M. Being an XY female: an analysis of accounts from the website of the androgen insensitivity syndrome support group. Health Care Women Int. 2009;30(5):428–46.

Gomez-Lobo V. Multidisciplinary care for individuals with disorders of sex development. Curr Opin Obstet Gynecol. 2014;26(5):366–71.

Hanna C. Exploring the psychosocial support services for women with differences of sex development. Master of genetic counselling. Melbourne, Victoria, Australia: University of Melbourne; 2013.

Hong Y, Peña-Purcell NC, Ory MG. Outcomes of online support and resources for cancer survivors: a systematic literature review. Patient Educ Couns. 2012;86(3):288–96.

Hughes IA, Houk C, Ahmed SF, et al. Consensus statement on management of intersex disorders. J Pediatr Urol. 2006;2:148–62.

Hutson J, Warne G, Grover SR (Eds). Disorders of sex development : an integrated approach to management. Heidelberg: Springer-Verlag Berlin Heidelberg; 2012.

Johannsen TH, Ripa CP, Mortensen EL, et al. Quality of life in 70 women with disorders of sex development. Eur J Endocrinol. 2006;155(6):877–85.

Jones T, Hart B, Carpenter M, et al. Intersex: stories and statistics from Australia. Cambridge, UK: Open Book Publishers; 2016.

Karkazis KA. Fixing sex : intersex, medical authority, and lived experience. Durham, NC: Duke University Press; 2008. p. 2008.

Kazak AE, Cant MC, Jensen MM, et al. Identifying psychosocial risk indicative of subsequent resource use in families of newly diagnosed pediatric oncology patients. J Clin Oncol. 2003;21(17):3220–5.

Lee PA, Houk CP, Ahmed SF, et al. Consensus statement on management of intersex disorders. International consensus conference on intersex. Pediatrics. 2006;118(2):e488–500.

Leidolf EM, Curran M, Scout, et al. Intersex mental health and social support options in pediatric endocrinology training programs. J Homosex. 2008;54(3):233–42.

Loughlin E. An unspoken presence in the lives of teens and young women with Turner syndrome. In: Balan R, Crawshaw M, editors. Sexuality and fertility issues in ill health and disability. London: Jessica Kingsley; 2006. p. 159–76.

Mortimer R. Supports for parents of children with differences of sex development. Faculty of Medicine, University of Melbourne. Melbourne, Australia: 2017.

Nordenström A. Psychosocial factors in disorders of sex development in a long-term perspective: what clinical opportunities are there to intervene? Horm Metab Res. 2015;47(5):351–6.

Pasterski V, Mastroyannopoulou K, Wright D, et al. Predictors of posttraumatic stress in parents of children diagnosed with a disorder of sex development. Arch Sex Behav. 2014;43(2):369–75.

Quigley C. Disorders of sex development: when to tell the patient. Baltimore, MD: Lawson Wilkins Pediatric Endocrine Society & Pediatric Academic Societies; 2009.

Rolston AM, Gardner M, Vilain E, et al. Parental reports of stigma associated with child's disorder of sex development. Int J Endocrinol. 2015;2015:980121.

Sandberg D, Mazur T. A noncategorical approach to the psychosocial care of persons with DSD and their families. 2014. https://doi.org/10.1007/978-1-4614-7441-8_5.

Sandberg DE, Gardner M, Cohen-Kettenis PT. Psychological aspects of the treatment of patients with disorders of sex development. Semin Reprod Med. 2012;30(5):443–52.

Sanders C, Carter B, Goodacre L. Parents' narratives about their experiences of their child's reconstructive genital surgeries for ambiguous genitalia. J Clin Nurs. 2008;17(23):3187–95.

Sutton EJ, McInerney-Leo A, Bondy CA, et al. Turner syndrome: four challenges across the lifespan. Am J Med Genet A. 2005;139a(2):57–66.

Tartaglia N, Howell S, Bornstein A. How to talk to your child about his or her diagnosis. In: KS&A families conference, Denver, CO. 2008.

Thomas B. A patient's view of ambiguous genitalia. Minerva Pediatr. 2003;55(5 Suppl 1):54–7.

Tonkin-Hill, G. Identifying the resource needs of adolescents with differences of sex development. Faculty of Medicine, University of Melbourne, Melbourne, Australia. 2018.

Warne GL. Your child with congenital adrenal hyperplasia. Melbourne, 1989: Department of Endocrinology and Diabetes, Royal Children's Hospital; 1989.

Warne G. The baby of uncertain sex. Pediatr Surg Int. 1992;7(4):244.

Warne G. Support groups for CAH and AIS. Great Britain: Williams & Wilkins; 2003.

Warne GL, Raza J. Disorders of sex development (DSDs), their presentation and management in different cultures (Report). Rev Endocr Metab Disord. 2008;9(3):227.

Wolfe-Christensen C, Wisniewski AB, Mullins AJ, et al. Changes in levels of parental distress after their child with atypical genitalia undergoes genitoplasty. J Pediatr Urol. 2016;13(1):32.e31–6.

20 Psychological Management in Adolescence and Beyond

Porpavai Kasiannan

The human story does not always unfold like a mathematical calculation on the principle that two and two makes four. Sometimes in life they make five or minus three; and sometimes the blackboard topples down in the middle of the sum and leaves the class in disorder and the pedagogue with a black eye.

Winston Churchill

20.1 Introduction

There has been growing interest in the study of infants, children, adolescents and adults with DSD since the 1990s, mainly stemming from the varied views of their medical and psychosocial management. It has long been acknowledged that psychological counselling and support should be an integral component of the multidisciplinary standard of care for children with such disorders. The Lawson Wilkins Paediatric Endocrine Society (LWPES) and the European Society for Paediatric Endocrinology (ESPE) produced the consensus statement on management of intersex disorders in 2006 (Hughes et al. 2006). The statement recommends that the evaluation and long-term management should be carried out at a centre with an experienced multi-disciplinary team that includes psychology/psychiatry (Hughes et al. 2006). Previously, the Hastings Centre group also recommended that families with children having intersex conditions require multidisciplinary care (Frader et al. 2004). More recent recommendations also support the need for psychological support during the various phases of assessment and treatment for DSD (Ahmed et al. 2016; Cools et al. 2018). Psychosocial support is essential to help families and individuals in relation to the choices and the daily context of life. These recommendations are based on the findings from various follow-up studies that highlight the psychosexual and psychosocial issues that many individuals with DSD face, as they develop from childhood to adolescents and adults. This chapter discusses these two aspects in DSD and their management.

P. Kasiannan (✉)
Pathways Foundation Kovai, Coimbatore, TN, India

20.2 Psychosocial and Psychosexual Issues in Adolescents and Adults with DSD

Human development is characterised by dynamic stages, which are influenced by internal and external factors from birth to death. Some stages may be characterised by stress and turmoil depending on the individual personality and the available social supports. Adolescence is the major transitional phase from childhood to adulthood, creating not only challenges and risks but also opportunities (Kleinemeier et al. 2010). Biological changes in adolescence include brain development leading to increased cognitive development and bodily changes with development of secondary sexual characters. Presence of a chronic physical illness is likely to be more

J. M. Hutson et al. (eds.), *Disorders|Differences of Sex Development*,
https://doi.org/10.1007/978-981-13-7864-5_20

stressful in an adolescent who even otherwise has a number of developmental tasks to negotiate. Psychosocial and psychosexual issues related to DSD influence one another and do not occur in isolation in general.

At the time of puberty, adolescents with DSD become aware of the difference in terms of pubertal development compared to peers, for example, amenorrhoea, lack of breast development and atypical appearance of genitalia. This could especially come as a shock in an adolescent who was either not diagnosed or not informed of the condition earlier. Atypical appearance of genitals and infertility may be of a lesser importance before puberty, but generally becomes a source of concern in adolescents (Cohen-Kettenis and Pfafflin 2003). Delayed or lack of puberty may lead to psychological difficulties at a stage where peer conformity is of prime importance. Cohen-Kettenis and Pfafflin (2003) describe low self-esteem and social insecurity because of physical differences, shyness in romantic and sexual relationships and fear and insecurity in talking about the condition with a potential partner.

20.3 Psychological Issues in DSD

20.3.1 Psychopathology

There have been only a handful of studies that have looked at the psychological outcomes in DSD. Research has looked at psychological functioning as an outcome of medical interventions and at psychosexual outcomes (gender dysphoria, sexual orientation and gender change) in follow-up studies. Research that focusses directly on psychosocial and psychosexual outcomes in children and youth, specific to diagnosis characteristics and treatment protocols, has been sparse. The reasons for this are that the conditions themselves are extremely rare, health care professionals having to be mindful of respecting people's privacy and lack of knowledge about the outcome for every patient (Roen and Pasterski 2013).

The main causes of psychological distress include shame or secrecy and taboo around the diagnoses. Psychological distress has been assessed directly only in some of these studies, which have been generally limited by small sample sizes, lack of standardised measures or selection bias (Schutzmann et al. 2009). Slijper et al. (1998) report increased risk for emotional problems in children and adolescents with DSD. Most studies on adolescents focus on physical development, especially the hormonal status and its changes during puberty. There are inconsistencies in these studies due to several problems including focussing only on one DSD condition, using different assessment methods, recruiting individuals without an accurate diagnosis, and lack of independence of care provider and researcher. Statistics are hampered by small sample sizes and lack of control groups. An observational study conducted by Kleinemeier et al. found no overall psychological impairments in adolescents with DSD but found special needs in the group, warranting support with shame, stigmatisation and coping with normative pressures. They observed that a need for hormonal treatment to induce puberty was a strong factor with regard to impaired well-being. The diagnostic groups that were under-represented in their study were the girls with no androgen effect and boys with DSD, the possible reasons that the girls being uninformed of their condition and denial associated with boys (Kleinemeier et al. 2010).

One long-term follow-up study of female individuals with congenital adrenal hyperplasia (CAH) found them to have negative body image and anxiety associated with sexuality (Kleinemeier et al. 2010). Studies of adolescents with CAH and urogenital abnormalities have not consistently found psychological impairment. In one study, female adolescents and adults with CAH were found to have higher scores on aggression scales than siblings and cousins. These findings are suggestive of prenatal androgen exposure, which is greater in the seriously affected salt-wasting type than in the simple virilising type (Cohen-Kettenis and Pfafflin 2003). Males with CAH had more psychiatric diagnoses, suicide and suicide attempts than their controls. Alcohol and substance misuse were increased, compared with controls, in both men and women (Falhammar et al. 2014). These difficulties were not found to be related to androgen effects and differences in genital development, some of which may be related to the glucocorticoid medication. It is important to make the correct comparisons, as results from one diagnostic group do not necessarily apply to the other groups (Nordenstrom 2015).

Few adult follow-up studies have been conducted on DSD populations. In Diamond and Watson's study population, 24 (62%) of those who had CAIS had considered suicide and 9 (23%) had attempted it. Among those who had PAIS, 11 (61%) had considered suicide and 3 (17%) had attempted it. The three who had attempted suicide did so before switching from their sex of rearing. Frequently, these considerations and attempts were associated with learning of their diagnosis or a problem with a specific amorous relationship (Diamond and Watson 2004). Another adult study (Warne et al. 2005), which fulfilled methodologically high standards on a group of heterogeneous adults found that the rates of psychological distress were similar to samples of persons with chronic somatic diseases. The group with DSD reported lower self-esteem, higher trait anxiety, higher extraversion and more interpersonal problems than one of the comparison groups (Warne et al. 2005). Schutzmann et al. (2009) conducted a pilot study on a diverse group of 37 adults with DSD using the Brief Symptom Inventory to assess self-reported psychological distress. Their results suggested that adults with DSD were markedly psychologically distressed with rates of suicidal tendencies and self-harming behaviour on a level comparable to that of non-DSD women with a history of physical or sexual abuse but concluded that their sample recruitment procedures did not permit a firm generalisation (Schutzmann et al. 2009).

According to Karkazis, there is a belief that if the child was not anatomically correct, this might lead to increased risk of suicide later in life. She reports that several adults whom she interviewed have considered suicide, and that their desperation did not result from diagnosis per se, but from how their family, physicians and society had perceived and treated them throughout their lives (Karkazis 2008). Schweizer et al. (2017) carried out a mixed-method study looking at coping and gender experiences in seven individuals with DSD living as women and concluded that psychological distress relates to the effects of medical treatment, and some of that relates to the experience of diverging from norms without having someone supportive to talk to about that. There are other losses that may result in the form of relationship breakdowns due to a partner's lack of understanding of the distress of an individual with a DSD or may be due to sexual incompatibilities.

An area worth considering is the long-term effects of surgery in infancy. Psychosocial adjustment is a complex phenomenon and is influenced by multifaceted inter-relationship between the child and family factors. Ludman summarises in her review that the period between 6 and 48 months was the most vulnerable developmental stage for developing adverse effects of hospitalisation. She reviewed studies exploring long-term effects of major paediatric surgery in congenital anomalies of the alimentary tract and concluded "despite inconsistencies, the evidence suggests that, irrespective of the presence of chronic health problems, children who require major paediatric surgery are at a two to three times greater risk for psychiatric disorder than healthy children" (Ludman 2006). This is an area that needs further attention in relation to the long-term effects of early surgery for DSD, as there are no methodologically sound studies that have evaluated this issue. Studies assessing the effect of deferred surgery on the domains of social acceptance, psychological well-being, parent–child bonding, body image and sexual functioning and comparing psychological outcomes with and without surgery are underway (Cools et al. 2018).

20.3.2 Quality of Life

Studies with results concerning quality of life in DSD have been scarce and inconsistent so far. Different results in different studies could be due to not only the use of different questionnaires, but also the size of the population studied and different cultural contexts. A Danish follow-up study of adult women (40 with 46,XX (CAH) and 30 with 46,XY DSD) reported impaired quality of life and affective stress compared to controls (Johannsen et al. 2006). Jurgensen et al. studied health-related quality of life (HRQoL) in 86 German children and found that it was lower regarding self-esteem, physical well-being and school functioning. This study also found poor parent–child agreement, with parents estimating their children's quality of life as higher in the above-mentioned parameters and lower in emotional well-being than the children themselves did. The number and timing of surgery and gender role behaviour did not correlate with HRQoL in the study. Out of 11 children who had gender dysphoria as assessed by gender identity interview, six (all with CAH) had significantly reduced HRQoL (Jurgensen et al. 2014). This finding is in contrast to earlier findings that 46,XX women with CAH do not have gender dysphoria.

There are other ways of assessing QoL as in this Norwegian study of 104 adult patients with CAH; disability benefits were received by 19% of the patients aged 18–27 years, as compared to 10% of the general population. They found that female patients were often single (53%), and the women had 21% of the expected number of children and significantly lower numbers among the salt-losing than simple virilising CAH individuals. The overall QoL scores were significantly impaired compared with normal population data (Nermoen et al. 2010).

In the Swedish registry study of CAH, 588 patients with a known severity in more than 80% of the cases and 100 controls per patient, matched for sex and year and place of birth, were compared for quality of life, such as an active life, being able to work, to form close relationships, and having children. Women with salt-wasting (SW) CAH had completed primary education less often with an odds ratio (OR) of 0.3, not explained by neonatal salt crisis or hypoglycaemia because the men did not differ from controls. Men and women in the less severe I172N genotype group were more likely to have an academic education (OR 1.8). Both men and women had more disability pensions (OR 1.5) and sick leave (OR 1.7). The men more often had long-lasting employment (OR 3.1) and were more often married (OR 1.6) and women were less often married (OR 0.7). Individuals had children less often (OR 0.3). The authors recommend identifying the mechanism behind the increased sick leave or disability pensions in future research, to improve medical and psychological care (Strandqvist et al. 2014).

Studies that look at psychological well-being also provide insight into QoL. In a German follow-up study of 110 adults, a worrying 30% of the patients scored below the cut-off for satisfaction with care. Women with CAH were more satisfied and women with XY-DSD conditions, androgen insensitivity and gonadal dysgenesis scored the lowest, indicating that individuals with more rare conditions have more difficulties finding appropriate care and that healthcare and psychological support are important factors for the outcome in these patient groups. The same study found the lowest satisfaction with care among those that stated that they had unmet needs for psychological support. An overwhelming 46% of individuals in an English study reported an ongoing need for psychological expertise. These findings may also suggest that psychological support to strengthen coping strategies and the ability to find access to care may coincide with a better sense of well-being (Nordenstrom 2015).

20.3.3 Sports and DSD

DSD came into public view when Caster Semenya, a South African athlete, won the 800-m sprint in the world championships in Berlin in 2009. As questions were raised by fellow athletes, the International Association of Athletes Federation (IAAF) required Semenya to undergo a full physical evaluation and gender verification testing including reports from a gynaecologist, an endocrinologist, a psychologist, a gender specialist and an internal medicine specialist. Subsequently, after a prolonged wait, Semenya was allowed to retain her title and was allowed to participate in sports. The results of the testing were not released for privacy reasons (O'Reilly 2010). There were a number of discussions in the media regarding gender, DSD and sports following this incident. This was not the first time DSD have taken centre stage in sports. There have been other reports of such incidents dating back to the 1930s.

Gender verification was mandatory until the 1996 Olympic Games in Atlanta, at which out of 3000 tests administered, eight showed up positive. Upon further examination, seven of those athletes were found to have AIS and the eight had an enzyme deficiency. All eight athletes were given the go-ahead to compete (O'Reilly 2010). Since discontinuing mandatory gender verification, the IOC has championed case-by-case evaluation of athletes with suspected gender disorders (Handley 2010). Following the Semenya case, a symposium of experts was held at Miami in January 2010 by the International Olympic Committee (IOC). Among the symposium's conclusions were recommendations that medical centres of excellence specialising in DSD be set-up around the world, that athletes have periodic pre-participation health exams, that athletes with a gender ambiguity be diagnosed and recommended treatment as quickly as possible and that rules of eligibility for competition for such athletes be established (Handley 2010) (O'Reilly 2010).

Against the backdrop of Semenya's case in May 2011, IOC and IAAF devised new policies based on the central assumption that atypically high levels of endogenous testosterone in women create an unfair advantage. Based on this, they set the upper limit of acceptable testosterone level to be 10 nmol/L in female athletes (Karkazis et al 2012). Karkazis et al. put forward arguments stating that scientific evidence did not support the notion that endogenous testosterone levels conferred athletic advantage in a straightforward or predictable way. They argued that athletic excellence was a product of complex entanglement of biological factors and material resources, which were not regulated by IAAF and IOC (Karkazis et al. 2012).

Variation in hormone levels even in typical females makes understanding baseline levels difficult. Robert Ritchie reports that there is no evidence that female athletes with DSD display sports-related physical attributes, which have not been seen in biologically normal female athletes (Ritchie et al. 2008). Ambiguity in gender can take many forms and can range from mild to pronounced. It is difficult to find the cut-off point where gender ambiguity becomes a genetic advantage and an unfair sporting advantage.

The story continues with new announcements from IAAF and IOC in 2018. IAAF is introducing a separate female classification for athletes with DSD. They will have to reduce the testosterone levels to no more than 5 nmol/L if they want to compete in events ranging from 400 m to a mile (Ingle 2018). IOC will also issue new guidelines to 55 sports from archery to wrestling, which will apply to the 2020 Tokyo Games capping the maximum level of testosterone to 5 nmol/L (Hellen 2018). These guidelines will affect transgender athletes as well. Sport is not the only arena where individuals with a DSD face issues. Other institutions, especially the armed forces, are another area where adults with DSD may face problems. Empirical research in this area is lacking. There is a general assumption that Western countries are more advanced than other nations regarding gender and sexuality. However, recognition of intersex and trans-sexual people is still rare in military and other higher offices even in the west.

20.4 Psychosexual Issues in DSD

20.4.1 Psychosexual Development

Psychosexual development is a species-centred conception of human development that includes sexual differentiation, sexual development, sexual behaviour, gender-typical social affiliation, pairing, reproduction and parental care. The concept of gender identity encompasses cognitive (understanding of being a boy or a girl) and affective (feelings of contentment with one's gender) components. The term gender identity is used to denote a person's sense of themselves being male, female or indeterminate. Gender role refers to behaviours, attitudes and personality traits that a society, in a given culture and historical period, designates as male or female social role (Cohen-Kettenis 2010). In adolescents and adults, gender role is measured using stereotypic masculine or feminine personality attributes or with regard to recreational and occupational interests and aspirations (Cohen-Kettenis 2010).

Psychosexual development is traditionally conceptualised as three components. Gender identity refers to a person's self-representation as male or female (with the caveat that some individuals may not identify exclusively with either). Gender role (sex-typical behaviours) describes the psychological characteristics that are sexually dimorphic within the general population, such as toy preferences, play and playmate preferences and physical aggression. Sexual orientation refers to the direction(s) of erotic interest (heterosexual, bisexual and homosexual) and includes behaviour, fantasies and attractions. Psychosexual development is influenced by multiple factors such as exposure to androgens, sex chromosome genes and brain structure, as well as social circumstances and family dynamics.

Theories have varied over the years regarding psychosexual development in children and adolescents. John Money reasoned that sex of rearing, if assigned early enough in childhood and if appropriately matched with external genitalia, is the most important determinant of gender identity. This theory dominated the rationale behind management of children with DSD during the major part of the 1990s (Karkazis 2008). Such neonatal interventions, although not affecting the children early on, do have implications for the adolescent and adult. Studies that followed did not support the concept that form and function and the appropriate environment alone were sufficient to determine future gender identity and gender role.

Gender identity is affected by neurobiological processes that interact with general and specific environmental influences (Reiner 2004). Gender identity reflects individual's understanding of themselves based on cultural norms of female and male. There are not many systematic studies that look at the typical psychosexual development in children. The focus on atypical gender behaviours in children ignores the broader and richer dimensions of human sexuality. Meyer–Bahlburg's review found very marked variations between syndromes in the prevalence of individuals who are not satisfied with their assigned gender and undergo gender change. He found gender change from female to male more frequent than from male to female and that gender identity problems were not prevalent even in female-raised individuals with a history of normal-male prenatal androgen exposure, and if they do develop, it may not occur before adolescence or even adulthood (Meyer-Bahlburg 2005). He concluded that there was no evidence to support a perspective of a specific biological factor overriding all others and determining gender identity.

20.4.2 Gender Dysphoria

Gender dysphoria denotes dissatisfaction with one's assigned gender. There is considerable evidence that individuals with a DSD experience gender incongruence or gender dysphoria and may wish to change from their assigned gender. Gender dysphoria generally is seen in 8.5–20% of individuals with DSD (Furtado et al. 2012). From a phenomenological perspective, DSD individuals with gender dysphoria have both similarities and differences to individuals with gender dysphoria with no known DSD. Developmental trajectories also have similarities and differences. The presence of a DSD is suggestive of a specific causal mechanism that may not be present in individuals without a diagnosable DSD. Gender dysphoria appears more frequently in the DSD population than in the general population, but it has been difficult to predict from karyotype, genital virilisation, prenatal androgen exposure and assigned gender (Cohen-Kettenis 2005; Zucker 1999).

The context in which gender problems occur in persons with DSD is sufficiently different from those without. Regarding gender dysphoria in non-DSD individuals, there is currently much speculation about genetic and/or hormonal, brain-specific mechanisms that underlie neuroanatomic changes and, thereby, induce a form of intersexuality that is limited to the central nervous system (Meyer-Bahlburg 2005). In the recent years, there has been an increasing societal acceptance of non-stereotypic gender presentations and non-binary gender identities marking an evolutionary change in our understanding and acceptance of gender variations. Despite growing recognition of gender identity being on a spectrum, most individuals with DSD identify with the gender assigned at birth.

20.4.3 Diagnosing Gender Dysphoria

The most recent version of the Diagnostic and Statistical Manual for Mental Disorders (DSM-5) has changed the diagnostic criteria for gender dysphoria to reflect the distinction between gender role behaviour/presentation from core gender identity. The new diagnostic criteria include the provision for a diagnosis in individuals with a DSD in contrast to the previous versions. The previous Diagnostic and Statistical Manual (DSM-IV-TR) of the American Psychiatric Association (2000) categorised individuals with intersexuality (DSD) and related conditions who experience gender identity problems as Gender Identity Disorder Not Otherwise Specified (GID-NOS).

DSM-5 Criteria for gender dysphoria in adolescents or adults require a marked incongruence between one's experienced/expressed gender and assigned gender, of at least 6 months' duration, as manifested by two or more indicators from six indicators of gender dysphoria. The indicators are a marked incongruence between one's experienced/expressed gender and primary and/or secondary sex characteristics (or, in young adolescents, the anticipated secondary sex characteristics), a strong desire to be rid of one's primary and/or secondary sex characteristics'(or, in young adolescents, a desire to prevent the development of the anticipated secondary sex characteristics) a strong desire for the primary and/or secondary sex characteristics of the other gender, a strong desire to be of the other gender (or some alternative gender different from one's assigned gender) a strong desire to be treated as the other gender (or some alternative gender different from one's assigned gender) and a strong conviction that one has the typical feelings and reactions of the other gender (or some alternative gender different from one's assigned gender).

The *International Classification of Diseases* (ICD 10) had different criteria for gender identity disorders in boys and girls and recommends the use of either Other Gender Identity Disorders or Gender Identity Disorder Unspecified category for those with intersexed conditions (WHO 1992). The updated version of *International Classification of Diseases* (ICD 11) includes gender incongruence that was previously classed as a mental disorder, under the new chapter "conditions related to sexual health". ICD 11 stresses that gender incongruence is "characterised by a marked and persistent incongruence between an individual's experienced gender and the assigned sex", and gender variant behaviour and preferences alone do not form the basis for diagnosis. The category is further divided into childhood and that of adolescence and adulthood, recognising that the presentation and needs and requirements of clinical approaches are different in the groups (WHO 2018).

The central aspect of medical decision-making early in life in DSD is assignment of gender. This has led to increased research into the different aspects of psychosexual development including assessment of gender identity, gender role and sexual orientation later in life. The best form of assessing gender identity is still good clinical evaluation by a trained mental health professional. Standards of care version 7 provides guidelines regarding competency requirements of mental health professionals and tasks related to assessment and referrals (Health 2011).

Various measurement tools are available to assess the psychosexual differentiation of individuals born with DSD (Zucker 2005). The main assumptions in the designing of these instruments were that the measures should be related to empirical evidence for normative gender differences, that some human behavioural sex differences have a parallel in non-human primates and that they should be consistent with or related to cultural definitions of masculinity and femininity (Zucker 2005). This again is based on the prevailing binary view of the world regarding gender differences. There are around 20 measures available for measuring gender identity in young children with equally distributed parents and child measures. Zucker discusses 11 measures to assess gender identity and four measures to assess sexual orientation. Measuring gender in a dichotomous fashion in adolescents and adults does not provide rich information a dimensional approach might provide. However, the psychometrics of such measures have not been studied in depth (Zucker 2005). Zucker's Gender identity questionnaire in adults attempts to measure gender identity and dysphoria in a dimensional manner and appears promising in studying adults with DSD. In adolescents, Utrecht gender dysphoria scale (UGDS) is useful in measuring adolescents' and adults' gender-related discomfort. This is a 12-item questionnaire that measures gender dysphoria in a dimensional way (Cohen-Kettenis and van Goozen 1997). Another scale Gender Identity/Gender Dysphoria questionnaire for adolescents and adults (GIDYQ-AA) (Deogracias et al. 2007) addresses subjective, somatic, social and socio-legal aspects. Studies conducted using these scales indicate that gender dysphoria can be reliably and validly measured. Body satisfaction can be measured using body image scale, which may be indicative of one's ability to adapt to one's body and of clinical expectations (Lindgren and Pauly 1975). This is particularly helpful in identifying individuals with low body dissatisfaction that extends beyond the sex characteristics and formulate appropriate psychological interventions.

20.4.4 Psychosexual Outcomes

Psychosexual development can be affected in DSD due to a number of factors, which include nature of the condition itself, medical interventions such as surgery or hormone replacement therapy, impact of delayed or precocious development, experience of stigmatisation or psychological trauma, societal expectations of gender role behaviour, dysphoria with assigned sex of rearing and comorbid mental health conditions (Kohler et al. 2014).

20.4.4.1 Congenital Adrenal Hyperplasia (CAH)

Prenatal androgen exposure is associated with certain aspects of psychosexual development, for example, cross-gender toy and play and playmate preference in CAH girls with severe mutation and marked genital virilisation. Reiner studied 84 individuals in a paediatric psychosexual development clinic and concluded that active prenatal androgen effects appeared to dramatically increase the likelihood of recognition of male sexual identity independent of sex of rearing (Reiner 2005). Other psychological characteristics like sexual orientation and maternal interest are also influenced by prenatal androgen exposure (Hughes et al. 2006). Some studies have reported male-typical behaviours and attributes, but not gender identity, in genetic females who were exposed to prenatal androgens from congenital adrenal hyperplasia. Several studies of girls with CAH from several different cultural settings also suggest that levels of androgen exposure early in development influence sex-typed play behaviour (Hines 2011). Hines notes that despite prenatal androgen exposure, virilised genitalia at birth and male-typical play behaviour girls with CAH assigned and raised as girls develop a female gender identity (Hines 2004). Dessens et al. reviewed the literature on gender identity, gender dysphoria and gender change in chromosomal females with CAH raised male or female. They found that 94.8% of individuals raised as female later developed gender identity as female but 5.2% had serious problems with gender identity. Among individuals raised as male, serious gender identity problems were reported in 12.1% of individuals (Dessens et al. 2005). Another review by de Vries et al. (2007) found that 10 of 217 (5%) of adolescents raised as female and adult women with CAH had some form of gender dysphoria. There is also some evidence that genetic girls with CAH reared as males can be content as men (Hines 2004). Hines, in her review, concluded that there was substantial evidence to associate CAH with reduced heterosexual orientation, reduced satisfaction with female sex of assignment and some evidence of increased tendency to physical aggression and reduced interest in infants and childcare. The majority of women with CAH are heterosexual, but the incidence of homosexuality compared to population norms is increased. Delayed psychosexual milestones, low interest in maternal role, lower than normal fertility and low sexual motivation are other findings (Cohen-Kettenis and Pfafflin 2003). When girls with CAH grow into adulthood, the majority identify as women but are about 600 times more likely than non-CAH women to express a desire to live as a man (Hines 2011).

20.4.4.2 Complete Androgen Insensitivity Syndrome (CAIS)

In CAIS childhood gender role behaviour, gender identity and sexual orientation in adulthood are the same as those in other females, which highlights the importance of sex hormones rather than sex chromosomes for psychological sex differentiation (Hines 2004; de Vries et al. 2007). Mazur reviewed all articles on CAIS, PAIS and micropenis published until 2004 and concluded that only 9.1% of individuals with PAIS changed gender and that gender dysphoria appeared to be a rare occurrence (Mazur 2005). This review acknowledged a number of limitations in the studies reviewed including varying degrees of accuracy in diagnoses, small sample sizes, lack of accurate descriptions of neonate's genitalia, sample from support groups, incomplete follow-up, lack of independent assessment of gender issues and lack of quality assessment methods. Due to these limitations, the results are unlikely to provide an accurate measure of gender identity outcome.

20.4.4.3 Partial Androgen Insensitivity Syndrome (PAIS)

Among individuals with PAIS, androgen biosynthetic defects, and incomplete gonadal dysgenesis, there is dissatisfaction with the sex of rearing in about 25% of individuals, whether raised male or female. In the review by De Vries et al., of 46 PAIS female-raised adolescent and adult individuals, five (11%) were gender dysphoric or changed gender and five among the 35 PAIS male-raised group were gender dysphoric or changed gender (de Vries et al. 2007). Available data support male rearing in all individuals with micropenis, taking into account equal satisfaction with assigned gender in those raised male or female, no need for surgery, and the potential for fertility in individuals reared male (Hughes et al. 2006).

20.4.4.4 Enzyme Deficiencies

In 1979, Imperato-McGinley reported that genetic males with 5-alpha-reductase deficiency (5α-RD) raised as females transitioned to male during puberty. Cohen-Kettenis reviewed studies on gender change in XY individuals more than 12 years of age raised as female who had 5α-RD, 17β-hydroxysteroid dehydrogenase deficiency (17β-HSD3) or previously known as 17-ketosteroid reductase deficiency (17-KRD). Gender role changes were reported in 56–63% of cases with 5α-RD and 39–64% of cases with 17β-HSD who were raised as girls. The changes were usually made in adolescence and early adulthood. In these two syndromes, the degree of external genital masculinisation at birth does not seem to be related to gender role changes in a systematic way. Cohen-Kettenis summarised that a masculine appearance in childhood, in association with masculine behaviour (perhaps both partially caused by prenatal exposure to androgens), make a gender role change likely after the pubertal changes, as they reinforce an already existing gender discomfort (Cohen-Kettenis 2005). Sobel and Imperato-McGinley in their review of XY intersexuality looked at the histories of individuals who have 5α-RD deficiency and 17β-HSD and concluded that gender identity was not merely a function of parental and societal influence. Even if raised as girls, these individuals were biologically driven to be male as a natural course of events (Sobel and Imperato-McGinley 2004), although this may not have been the case if the testes had been removed in early infancy. This is still an unresolved issue. In another review by de

Vries et al., 69 of 117 5α-RD-2 (59%), and 20 of 51 17β-HSD-3 (39%) persons reared as girls, and all older than 12 years, experienced gender dysphoria to the extent that they decided to live as boys/men (de Vries et al. 2007). Richter-Appelt et al. (2005) reported five persons with 5α-RD-2 and 17β-HSD-3 reared as girls, scored significantly lower on a "female gender identity scale" than a female comparison group and one of the five also had a significantly higher male gender identity score than the female comparison group on a "male gender identity scale".

Whether the proportion of those affected with 5α-RD-2 that ultimately change identity from female to male is relatively large or small, information on parental rearing styles, psychosexual development or more subtle signs of gender discomfort are essential for an understanding of the variability in gender identity outcome, and as of now, no reports provide such information (Sandberg et al. 2012).

20.4.4.5 Other DSD

Psychosexual development and sexual orientation have not been studied in depth in some DSD such as Turner syndrome. They have female gender identity with feminine interests and activities. One study suggested that they are more likely to show an undifferentiated psychosexual profile compared to other females (Hines 2004). Individuals with Klinefelter syndrome reported less sexual interest in girls and had a significantly later onset of masturbation (Diamond and Watson 2004). Gender expression in Klinefelter syndrome ranges from androgynous or feminine feelings to considering themselves as transgendered, intersex or trans-sexual (Diamond and Watson 2004). Despite such features, a large majority have masculine gender identities (Cohen-Kettenis and Pfafflin 2003).

There are considerable difficulties in evaluating individuals with rare disorders such as ovotesticular DSD and mixed gonadal dysgenesis. In males with 47,XYY DSD, gender identity was not a problem in general, other than few reports of gender identity problems and even trans-sexualism (Cohen-Kettenis and Pfafflin 2003). Grumbach's group noted that genetic males who had micropenis fared tolerably well even when reared female. Reiner found that males who were born with cloacal exstrophy, whether raised as male or castrated at birth and raised as female, demonstrate psychosocially and psychosexually dominant male-typical tendencies. He also noticed the ease of transition in many of the boys some of whom did not know their birth history. He concludes that prenatal androgen exposure and perhaps sex chromosome-specific neuronal properties influence gender role and, at least sometimes, creates male sexual identity, even if males are castrated at birth and reared female (Reiner 2004). Less systematic studies have been done in other rare DSD such as congenital penile agenesis, ovotesticular DSD, mixed gonadal dysgenesis, Leydig cell hypoplasia and vanishing testis syndrome, all of which are associated with genital malformation and ambiguity. For all DSD, it is important that investigators and authors conform to uniform nomenclature and definitions to ensure that data can be reliably analysed (Furtado et al. 2012).

20.5 Psychosocial Care in Adolescents and Adults

Caring for individuals with DSD involves the input of various disciplines. Although some DSD are primarily medical conditions that may require medical or surgical management, they also have significant impact on the individual's psychosocial and psychosexual life as discussed above. DSD may also impact the family and social life to varying degrees. There is emerging evidence that psychological support initially and on follow-up is an important component of a holistic approach to the individual's well-being. The consensus guidelines (Hughes et al. 2006) and Society for Endocrinology UK guidance (Ahmed et al. 2016) and the European consensus statement (Cools et al. 2018) acknowledge the significance of psychosocial care and the involvement of mental health staff with expertise in DSD. The importance of a psychologist, psychiatrist or similar professional in the management of DSD is not about pathologising DSD but rather is about the recognition of the exceptional personal and social issues a diagnosis of DSD presents (Brain et al. 2010). Psychological interventions vary between diagnoses and should be tailored to meet the individual needs. They include regular monitoring of psychological aspects, supporting ethical approval processes and regular validation of informed consent. According to Reiner, a child psychiatrist is an ideal candidate to be the "point player" on the treatment team (Reiner 2004).

Despite expert guidelines and consensus statements, not all individuals and families receive the psychosocial care that they need. A recent study has identified high need for psychological support for parents, especially in parents of children with XY-DSD with androgen effects other than hypospadias. The study also highlighted that out of the 40.4% of individuals who identified a need for psychological support, only 50% received the support adequately (Bennecke et al. 2015).

The important roles of the psychologist, psychiatrist or other mental health professional in DSD care are assessment and management of gender identity issues, information management including facilitating team decisions, addressing psychological aspects of surgery and management of issues of sexuality (Hughes et al. 2006; Brain et al. 2010; Cohen-Kettenis 2010; Ahmed et al. 2016). In adolescence, the individual may encounter learning and social problems, physical discrepancies compared to peers, precocious or delayed puberty, surgery, medication including hormones, nonsurgical genital treatment, for example, vaginal dilators and technical aids for sexual contact, infertility and sex reassignment. Individuals adapt and integrate aspects of their condition depending on the emotional and cognitive maturity, the amount of information received and the existing family and social support. Many of them, especially the ones with sex chromosomal DSD, may require speech and language therapy, assistance with learning, occupational therapy and medication for behaviour problems. All individuals diagnosed with DSD should be offered appropriate psychological assessment, emotional support, counselling and sometimes psychotherapy to enable them to lead a meaningful life despite vulnerabilities.

The mental health clinician in the multidisciplinary team should be knowledgeable in the various aspects of DSDs including current research. As basic requirements, they would need skills in acknowledging variety, complexity and individuality, be able to create an atmosphere of appreciation and acceptance and should be able to provide time, empowerment and encouragement (Cools et al. 2018).

20.5.1 Initial Diagnosis in Adolescents and Adults

Most cases of DSD are recognised in the neonatal period; later presentations in older children and young adults include previously unrecognised genital ambiguity; inguinal hernia in a girl; delayed or incomplete puberty; virilisation in a girl; primary amenorrhoea; breast development in a boy and gross and occasionally cyclical haematuria in a boy. Unless the family knows they carry X-linked CAIS, it is usually not diagnosed until abdominal testes herniate or menarche fails to occur. This can come as a huge shock to an adolescent who may react with feelings of rage and grief. They need appropriate support and treatment focussed on their feelings around body image, enhancing social skills and self-esteem and improving coping skills. They also will need help in coming to terms with the fact that their bodies will not change. Adolescents with DSD need appropriate psychosexual education tailored to their individual needs. The UK guidance (Ahmed et al. 2016) recommends that all adolescents with a newly diagnosed DSD or existing DSD requiring medical or surgical attention should be routinely offered clinical psychology input in addition to any support offered to their parents or wider family.

Rarely, the diagnosis of DSD comes as a surprise in adulthood. Occasionally, the first presentation may be to a psychologist or psychiatrist with gender dysphoria or more rarely due to gender verification tests done in athletes by sporting authorities. They require a thorough history and physical examination, karyotyping, consideration of the degree of brain masculinisation and psychiatric assessment. A thorough psychiatric assessment bearing all the dimensions of the bio-psycho-social model is warranted to make sense of the patient's gender, sexuality and general psychological well-being (Bostwick and Martin 2007). Potential psychiatric differential diagnoses include psychosis, somatic or religious delusions, body dysmorphic disorder, neurotic conflicts about sexual orientation and borderline or schizotypal personality disorders (Bostwick and Martin 2007).

20.5.2 Information Management

Information management in the DSD context involves disclosure of information both from clinicians to parents and child and from child and family to the wider environment (Cohen-Kettenis 2010). As initial emotions could be overwhelming for the individual and the family, explaining the condition as a natural variation in development would be much more helpful in helping them communicate with extended family and social network. In one study, parents reported post-traumatic stress disorder symptoms if they felt that they did not understand the information or perceived the information as confusing (Pasterski et al. 2014). There is a lot of confusion with regard to the use of the terms of "DSD" versus "intersex". Promoting a non-binary view on sex and gender in general could be helpful in focussing the discussion towards optimal care. Most individuals prefer to use the specific name of their condition rather than the broader DSD or intersex terms (Cools et al. 2018). Ongoing psychosocial support is necessary to help families process the diagnosis as well as for future decision-making.

When discussing treatment options for very young children, there is the potential conflict of interest between respect for the fundamental right of the child for physical and emotional integrity and self-determination and the right of the parents to serve as surrogate decision-makers and act in their child's best interests (Diamond et al. 2018). In a case study of three families whose children were recommended gonadectomy to eliminate tumour risk, parents valued a spectrum of options, transparency and team decision-making process (Diamond et al. 2018).

Being well informed about one's medical condition is associated with better psychological adjustment. Studies done in children with HIV suggest that children who know their HIV status have higher self-esteem than children who are unaware of their status. Parents who had disclosed the HIV status to their children experienced less depression than those who did not (AIDS 1999). Disclosures made to children and adolescents should consider not only their age but also the level of cognitive functioning, psycho-social maturity and the complexity of family dynamics. The mental health professional should be well informed in developmental issues and the impact of chronic illness on emotional well-being. As DSD have varied aetiology, presentation and long-term outcomes information provided will need to be appropriate to the clinical context. Transparent and complete information help individuals cope throughout their lives and set the stage for future discussions about risks and benefits of eventual interventions.

Young children with DSD would benefit from simple information regarding the nature of illness and about what they need to do to care for themselves. As children mature, they need to be fully informed about their condition and encouraged to actively participate in the treatment process. Appropriate resources in the form of children's books can be useful, a list of which are currently available in some support-group websites, (AISSG 2011). However, some parents may be reluctant to disclose to their children due to fear or perceived shame or to prevent negative emotional consequences. Parents also are likely to fear discrimination, stigmatisation or ostracism from other children and families. Such parents will need a lot of support and reassurance before information is disclosed to the children. Appropriate resources for parents should be provided whenever possible in the form of booklets, support groups and websites. Values regarding sexuality and gender vary between cultures, which can be another impediment to adequate disclosure. Despite the current trend in ethical practice being based on honesty and full disclosure, some physicians, especially in some cultures, may still be reluctant to disclose fully to the child or adolescent.

In adolescence, there is increasing awareness about their psychosexual development with focus on intimacy, sexual functioning, fertility and sharing information with peers. They may have a number of questions around these issues. The other issues that may be raised in adolescence include hormone replacement, need for regular medical follow-up, decisions about possible surgical interventions and issues around gender identity and sexuality. Discussing these issues may raise other difficult emotional issues. Issues around gender role behaviours and sexuality may give rise to significant anxiety if the condition is not fully understood, especially in the context of less than optimal cognitive processing, due to the emotional load. Repeated explanations tailored to the individual's developmental stage may be required. Apart from that, routine evaluation of psychosexual status will help the treating team in planning treatment, preventing problems and for providing guidance.

Disclosure is also paramount in obtaining informed consent for medical and surgical interventions in adolescents by enabling them to become well-informed participants in important health care decisions. Complete knowledge of their physical condition will also hopefully enable them to become resilient individuals with positive quality of life. It is important that young people with DSD know the whole truth about their condition, including their karyotype, anatomy and details of any previous interventions in childhood, if applicable. This is one area that may create a lot of discomfort for parents and clinicians. Information should be provided in a sensitive and thoughtful manner, focussing on the strengths of the individual with no ambiguity in the language used. Accurate written information in simple language should be provided at all stages of information provision. This gives the individual and the family opportunity to review the information in their own environment and to raise questions with the professional in the follow-up visits.

Families may also seek advice regarding disclosure to the wider social environment. Some parents may be reluctant to fully inform their children due to anxiety that the child might share the information with others and may become a target for bullying and ridicule. There are no clear guidelines regarding the consequences of sharing information with the wider environment. Clinicians generally base their advice on their own personal perspectives and intuition considering the individual family and social circumstances. Various aspects of this process need further study to improve clinicians' insight into how they time and share information with individuals and families. Studies comparing the development of children living in "informed" versus "uninformed" environments would be valuable (Cohen-Kettenis 2010).

Another area that requires appropriate disclosure is regarding potential gender identity issues in future. Evidence from the existing literature reveals that knowledge regarding predictability of gender identity problems in certain DSD is limited. It is important that individuals and parents are informed of this and appropriate psychological help offered to help understand the specific nature of problems. When full disclosure had been an issue, gaps in knowledge may persist into adolescence and adulthood. This can create a number of difficulties in the interpersonal relationships within the family system in adolescence. Even when there has been full disclosure, it is possible that some irreversible decisions have already been made, which may make the adolescent very angry. However, this situation is likely to be better resolved by further discussions than by a situation where the adolescent was not aware of their condition.

Child psychiatrists may be called to assess decisional capacity in complex cases for clinical decision-making and for legal requirements. Assessment of decisional capacity has three standard elements: (1) the ability to understand the nature of the medical problem; (2) the ability to appreciate the alternative medical responses to it (including the option of no treatment and the advantages and disadvantages of each option) and (3) the ability to express a choice. It is common to add a fourth element: the ability to apply reasonably stable personal values to the process of arriving at a considered preference (Kipnis 2004).

The nurturing of decisional capacity may be an important and realisable clinical goal in the multidisciplinary DSD team. Health care professionals need to assess decisional capacity in the individual patient and look for evidence of capacity in those who are between the ages of 7 and 14 years and for evidence of incapacity in those who are older than 14 years. A good framework to adopt would be that of Kipnis' "the work of the child and adolescent psychiatrist has to take into account the minor patient's present and future needs and interests and his/her emerging decisional capacity, the parents' responsibilities and aspirations for the child, and the state's interests in promoting sound child-rearing and protecting children from abuse and neglect" (Kipnis 2004).

20.5.3 Medical Trauma

A number of aspects of treatment in DSD include general concerns such as regular medication, frequent medical reviews including blood tests, surgery or other procedures and general physical well-being, which are similar to a chronic illness. These experiences can be stressful for both parents and children. Particular concerns in DSD are in relation to genital assessments. It is not appropriate for children or adolescents with DSD to be examined in grand rounds or educational sessions. However, their medical reviews may still involve whole-body examinations, genital exams and, sometimes, photographs and discussion with parents in the presence of the child or adolescent. Most interdisciplinary treatment teams are found in teaching institutions, where individuals may be examined by several individuals, in rooms crowded with other clinicians and trainees. Such experiences may be quite traumatic for some, leaving them vulnerable and feeling dehumanised (Tishelman et al. 2017). There is little research on the subjective perceptions and experiences of youth who have frequent medical and genetic exams (Tishelman et al. 2017). Recurrent genital examinations throughout life have the potential to increase feelings of embarrassment and anxiety, including psychological concerns about the appearance of external genitalia. One study found that impaired body satisfaction has resulted in adults with DSD apart from past negative experiences (Schweizer et al. 2017). As outlined elsewhere, genital examinations are no longer a routine part of an examination during outpatient review at our institution. They may, however be suggested if the clinical information an examination might provide cannot be acquired in another way. If this is the case, the reason for the examination must be clearly explained to the young person, along with the option to decline the examination if they prefer. Standard advice re presence of a support person or chaperone applies. If a genital examination is planned for a child, qualified members of the team can be involved in helping to reduce procedural anxiety by using distraction technique; the young person's privacy and dignity must also be respected at all times. Follow-up treatment and medication can sometimes have side effects and cause a lot of pain. This can be an important issue in adolescents who have vaginal surgery who may need dilation of the new vagina to prevent scarring.

The clinical guidelines for the management of DSD in childhood (Hughes et al. 2006) provide general recommendations for medical examination, which include suggestions for the clinician to remain calm, reassuring and open and to use the patient's preferred gender terminology. The guidelines also recommend minimising the number of healthcare professionals involved in caring for the child and the avoidance of repeated exams, particularly those that involve measurement. Trauma associated with medical care can be avoided by performing the genital exams and photographing only when absolutely necessary and, even when necessary, by taking time to explain the need for exams and photographs and by obtaining adequate informed consent and by meticulously observing confidentiality. Tishelman et al. (2017) reviewed the child sexual abuse and paediatric psychology literature and made specific recommendations in the context of medical examination of youth with DSD. They highlight the need for adequate information provided in a non-authoritative manner, open communication with children and care takers prior to the examination and for youth to have control of various aspects of the exam to the extent possible. They also recommend appropriate training for physicians in providing reassurance and full disclosure about findings. The recommendations also include assessing youth and family distress routinely, reducing possibility of stigma and shame and not forcing children to participate if acute distress is too high.

Psychological trauma was expressed by parents interviewed by Karkazis. They reported grieving not only for the loss of the son they thought they had but also for their imagined life in which they had pictured a perfect baby with no health concerns. Their concerns also extend in the longer term into fears that their child may have been assigned the wrong gender, anxieties about how the child will survive all the typical experiences of childhood, puberty and adulthood (Karkazis 2008).

20.5.4 Puberty and Sexuality

Puberty can prove very difficult for individuals with a DSD. This is generally the time when they consolidate their understanding of what having a DSD means in relation to their bodily and sexual development. For some, it may be the first time they learn about their DSD status. Sexuality and forming intimate relationships are important tasks of adolescence. Adolescents with DSD may have a number of anxieties in entering this phase, especially if they have a history of early medical trauma in the form of repeated genital examinations, medical photography or differential treatment by clinicians.

In general, sexual problems appear to occur more in DSD individuals than in non-DSD individuals. Some adolescents with DSD feel uncertain about sexual adequacy, sexual orientation or gender identity when they enter puberty. They may delay initiating intimate relationships due to their insecurities. Due to the nature of these difficulties, adolescents need adequate and timely medical and sexual education and also have the opportunity to discuss their concerns in private with a mental health clinician (Cohen-Kettenis 2010). The German clinical evaluation study found both adolescents and adults reported fewer experiences regarding love or sexual relationships than controls. Men with DSD and undervirilisation and women with DSD and androgen effects less often had a love relationship and adult women with DSD and androgen effects more frequently engaged in same-sex relationships than controls (Jurgensen et al. 2013). Around puberty, adolescents will need preparation for hormone therapy. They need accurate information regarding the need for hormones, forthcoming bodily changes, sexual thoughts and feelings. Sometimes, adolescents may rebel against their parents or their situation by non-compliance with treatment. They may need additional professional support at such crucial developmental stages. If vaginal dilation is required, success rates are good but are directly related to compliance. Support from a psychologist and supervision from a dedicated clinical nurse specialist are important. This usually provides an opportunity to explore worries about current and potential sexual relationships (Brain et al. 2010).

20.5.5 Gender Assignment and Reassignment

The most pertinent question that parents of children with DSD have is about gendered behaviour and sexual development. Neuropsychological research informs that gender-related behaviours likely develop as complex interactions of biological social and cognitive processes. Decisions on gender assignment can be made only after careful considerations of medical and psychosocial pros and cons, and it usually depends on the predicated optimal outcome. Unfortunately, adult gender identity cannot always be accurately predicted in some conditions. Gender assignment decision-making relies not only on the surgical possibilities, potential for fertility and need for hormone replacement but also on the potential for psychological and psychosexual functioning as male or female and the ability of parents to cope with uncertainties and complexities related to decision-making (Hughes et al. 2006; Cohen-Kettenis 2010). Sometimes, a correct diagnosis is made only after the child has been assigned to one gender, but the diagnosis may indicate appropriateness of assignment to the opposite gender. Moreover, in children with DSD, the process of gender development is likely to be different. The issue gets even more complex in an adolescent newly diagnosed with DSD. A degree of consensus exists for gender assignment for some diagnoses. In CAIS and CAH with moderate virilisation, the gender assignment as female is not disputed. However, there are no clear guidelines for other diagnoses like 5-alpha reductase deficiency and PAIS, to name a few.

It is clear from a number of follow-up studies discussed earlier the gender role behaviour may be inconsistent with assigned gender. This may be misconstrued as gender dysphoria by parents who may feel guilty for wrong decision-making. This anxiety can be avoided by regular follow-up by the treating team. Despite careful multidisciplinary assessment prior to gender assignment in DSD and regular reviews, there will be the occasional adolescent or adult who would later present with significant gender dysphoria. In such individuals, support for gender reassignment should be implemented with the help of the mental health clinician in the treating team. They may also need referral to a specialist gender assessment team for further management. Based on current literature, good clinical practice should include assessment of gender identity and gender role behaviour routinely by the multidisciplinary team not only at intake but also at periodic intervals as needed.

20.5.6 Gender Dysphoria and DSD

Gender dysphoria and gender change in individuals with DSD vary dramatically according to the type of DSD and gender assignment at birth (Meyer-Bahlburg 2005; de Vries et al. 2007). In cases of persistent gender dysphoria, the individual should be assessed by clinicians skilled in the assessment and management of gender dysphoria and gender change. The standards of care, version 7 of the World Professional Association for Transgender Health (WPATH), a professional organisation in the field of gender dysphoria, has a section dedicated to assessment and treatment of gender dysphoria in people with DSD (Health 2011). A thorough understanding of the gender variant behaviour against the broad background of functioning of the child and family is necessary. A number of instruments that are available to aid the assessment in gender-variant individuals are also useful in the cases of gender dysphoric children with DSD (Zucker 2005). Any decision regarding changing a person's birth-assigned sex or gender role should be taken only after a thorough assessment.

In adolescents with gender dysphoria, puberty-delaying hormones are generally initiated after Tanner stage 2 or 3. In contrast to gender dysphoric adolescents without DSD, agonadal adolescents with DSD do not need suppression of puberty. However, they may benefit from delaying hormone replacement therapy, which is likely to give them more time to reflect on their wish to change gender and to prepare psychologically and practically for gender change (Cohen-Kettenis 2010). Gender reassignment surgery is carried out only in adulthood and may be more complicated in individuals with DSD due to the effect of previous genital surgeries. WPATH recommends that certain criteria for treatment for gender dysphoria are usually not applicable to people with DSD, instead they are interpreted in light of the person's specific situation. Even genital surgery may be performed much earlier in individuals with DSD if the surgery is well justified by the diagnosis, by the evidence-based gender identity prognosis for the given syndrome and syndrome severity and by the individual's wishes (Health 2011).

20.5.7 Infertility

Sub- or infertility is a common consequence of DSD. Even in individuals where infertility is not a result of gonadal failure, it may still be an issue due to anatomical problems warranting intervention. Fertility outcome was investigated in the dsd-LIFE study, and the authors found that the fertility outcome was significantly reduced in all types of DSD (Slowikowska-Hilczer et al. 2017). In the total cohort of 1040 individuals, only 3.5% had been able to reproduce without assisted reproductive technology and 7% with it. They found that only 72% of the participants had received information on fertility, but 17% were not satisfied with the information. Advances in treatment of infertility and in preservation of sperm or ova for future use have increased the possibility of fertility options in some individuals with DSD. In many, infertility is untreatable. This in turn has a number of psychological implications, which need addressing from a young age, especially in adolescence so that they can make informed decisions about fertility choices. In rare cases where the diagnosis of DSD is made while being investigated for infertility, the psychological issues can be even more complex.

20.5.8 Role of Support Groups

The value of peer and parent support for many chronic medical conditions is widely accepted, and DSD, being lifelong conditions, which affect developmental tasks at many stages of life, are no exception. A number of support groups and organisations are available in different countries usually based on a particular condition like CAH or AIS. Support groups offer a safe place where individuals and families feel accepted without isolation or stigma and where very private concerns can be discussed with others who have experienced similar issues in life. They also provide ongoing support for the affected individual and parents to gather and explore information, promote autonomy and build knowledge and self-confidence regarding their condition and offer peer support to individuals and families. The UK guidance (Ahmed et al. 2016) recommends that contact details for national support groups and web resources should be supplied as routine as part of any written information.

While clinicians may appear focussed on gender and genital appearance as key outcomes, support groups' focus is on experiences associated with having a DSD.

Support groups complement the work of the health care team and, together, can help improve services and quality of life for individuals with DSD. Initiatives by support groups have led to improvements in management of DSD and research directed towards clinically relevant issues. Dialogue between health care professionals and support groups, and collaboration as partners is to be encouraged (Hughes et al. 2006).

20.6 Future Research Focus

The available data on the psychological and psychosexual outcomes of DSD are neither systematic nor comprehensive. Future follow-up studies on individuals should focus not only on the medical and surgical outcomes but also appropriately on psychological functioning, quality of life and psychosexual functioning and their outcomes. Research should also aim at developing measures and toolkits for identifying families that are at risk and made easily accessible (Cohen-Kettenis 2010). More rigorous research should be undertaken to formulate appropriate clinical guidelines for psychological assessment and management of the various types of DSDs and gender dysphoria in individuals with DSDs. Measures are already underway to address these issues.

The multidisciplinary providers of help for DSD are mainly based in paediatric services and should extend to include adult care. The study dsd-LIFE is a cross-sectional clinical outcome study of individuals with DSD, which aims to assess quality of life as a measure of psychosocial adaptation, psychosexual and mental health aspects as major outcomes. The data from the large sample from six European countries will provide a sufficient basis for evidence-based recommendations for improvement of clinical care (Rohle et al. 2017).

Studies should also be aimed at investigating the various aspects of information management including the timing, type and method of conveying information that is culturally sensitive. Qualitative and quantitative research in understanding the unique experiences of young people with DSD and their caregivers would lead to the development of evidence-based information management protocols. Evidence-based information/educational material regarding the various DSD conditions, their medical and psychological management should be developed for children, adolescents, families and professionals.

Although there is consensus regarding gender assignment at infancy, in some DSD conditions, there is no sound empirical basis in others. Gender assignment at birth to avoid future gender dysphoria or gender reassignment is one of the highly controversial issues in this field. DSDs are quite diverse and rare, which makes studying them systematically difficult. International collaborative efforts similar to the Euro-DSD project based at Cambridge University dsd-LIFE study are necessary for better understanding of DSD and implications for treatment. Long-term follow-up comparing psychosocial and psychosexual outcomes in individuals who had surgery as infants with those who did not is likely to help resolve the debate for and against surgery. Longitudinal studies on gender-normative and gender-variant development of children with DSD will help formulate appropriate gender care for people with DSD.

20.7 Summary

DSD affect not only anatomical and physiological development of the individual but also their thoughts, feelings, sense of self and relationships with immediate family and the extended social network. More individuals with a diagnosis of DSD survive and have longer lifespan with improved holistic care. The overall ultimate goal for treatment and care is good quality of life. Current knowledge about psychosocial outcomes and health-related quality-of-life data for individuals with different forms of DSD is limited. It is therefore paramount that DSD management always needs a multidisciplinary approach with a mental health professional, with expertise in DSD being an integral part of the team. Psychological support to the patient and the family should be an integral part of the treatment programme irrespective of age or the clinical condition. Psychological management should focus on providing accurate non-confusing information and preparing young adolescents to face the issues in life in general and sexual life in particular due to the consequences of the DSD and its treatment. Specific psychological interventions vary between different diagnoses and will need to be tailored to meet the individual needs including regular monitoring of general psychological well-being, assessment of gender identity where appropriate and regular validation of informed consent. Whilst certain aspects of the management of DSD clearly require input from a psychiatrist or psychologist, their actual role in the multidisciplinary team evolves with the team, and it is this dynamic integration of medical and psychological support that provides the best model of care. Understanding the psychological and psychosexual outcomes in individuals with DSD is a continuously evolving field. Not only the emerging evidence, but also the individual's lived experience, the family's predicament and the prevailing social construct need to be considered in depth when trying to formulate the best psychological care. There is strong need for identifying new and better ways to strengthen the individual's ability to cope with their condition. It is important to acknowledge that despite all the odds, many individuals with DSD are highly resilient, true to the words of Helen Keller "Although the world is full of suffering, it is also full of overcoming it".

References

Ahmed SF, Achermann JC, Arlt W, et al. Society for Endocrinology UK guidance on the initial evaluation of an infant or an adolescent with a suspected disorder of sex development (revised 2015). Clin Endocrinol. 2016;84(5):771–88.

AIDS C o P. Disclosure of illness status to children and adolescents with HIV infection. Pediatrics. 1999;103:164–6.

American Psychiatric Association. Diagnostic and statistical manual of mental disorders (4th ed., text revision). Washington, DC: American Psychiatric Association; 2000.

AISSG. 2011. http://www.aissg.org/#Books2.

Bennecke E, Werner-Rosen K, Thyen U, et al. Subjective need for psychological support (PsySupp) in parents of children and adolescents with disorders of sex development (dsd). Eur J Pediatr. 2015;174(10):1287–97.

Bostwick JM, Martin KA. A man's brain in an ambiguous body: a case of mistaken gender identity. Am J Psychiatry. 2007;164(10):1499–505.

Brain CE, Creighton SM, Mushtaq I, et al. Holistic management of DSD. Best Pract Res Clin Endocrinol Metab. 2010;24(2):335–54.

Cohen-Kettenis PT, Pfafflin P. Transgenderism and intersexuality in childhood and adolescence making choices. Thousand Oaks, CA: Sage Publications; 2003.

Cohen-Kettenis PT. Gender change in 46,XY persons with 5alpha-reductase-2 deficiency and 17beta-hydroxysteroid dehydrogenase-3 deficiency. Arch Sex Behav. 2005;34(4):399–410.

Cohen-Kettenis PT. Psychosocial and psychosexual aspects of disorders of sex development. Best Pract Res Clin Endocrinol Metab. 2010;24(2):325–34.

Cohen-Kettenis PT, van Goozen SH. Sex reassignment of adolescent transsexuals: a follow-up study. J Am Acad Child Adolesc Psychiatry. 1997;36(2):263–71.

Cools M, Nordenstrom A, Robeva R, et al. Caring for individuals with a difference of sex development (DSD): a consensus statement. Nat Rev Endocrinol. 2018;14(7):415–29.

Deogracias JJ, Johnson LL, Meyer-Bahlburg HF, et al. The gender identity/gender dysphoria questionnaire for adolescents and adults. J Sex Res. 2007;44(4):370–9.

Dessens AB, Slijper FME, Drop SLS. Gender dysphoria and gender change in chromosomal females with congenital adrenal hyperplasia. Arch Sex Behav. 2005;34(4):389–97.

Diamond M, Watson LA. Androgen insensitivity syndrome and Klinefelter's syndrome: sex and gender considerations. Child Adolesc Psychiatr Clin N Am. 2004;13(3):623–40, viii.

Diamond DA, Swartz J, Tishelman A, et al. Management of pediatric patients with DSD and ambiguous genitalia: balancing the child's moral claims to self-determination with parental values and preferences. J Pediatr Urol. 2018;14(5):416.e1–5.

Falhammar H, Frisen L, Norrby C, et al. Increased mortality in patients with congenital adrenal hyperplasia due to 21-hydroxylase deficiency. J Clin Endocrinol Metab. 2014;99(12):2715–21.

Frader J, Alderson P, Asch A, et al. Health care professionals and intersex conditions. Arch Pediatr Adolesc Med. 2004;158(5):426–8.

Furtado PS, Moraes F, Lago R, et al. Gender dysphoria associated with disorders of sex development. Nat Rev Urol. 2012;9(11):620–7.

Handley M. The IOC grapples with Olympic sex testing. Time Magazine. 2010.

Health WTWPAfT. Standards of care fot the health of transsexual, transgender and gender nonconforming people. 2011. http://www.wpath.org.

Hellen N. Transgender athletes face tougher Olympic rules. The Australian. 2018.

Hines M. Psychosexual development in individuals who have female pseudohermaphroditism. Child Adolesc Psychiatr Clin N Am. 2004;13(3):641–56, ix.

Hines M. Prenatal endocrine influences on sexual orientation and on sexually differentiated childhood behavior. Front Neuroendocrinol. 2011;32(2):170–82.

Hughes IA, Houk C, Ahmed SF, et al. Consensus statement on management of intersex disorders. Arch Dis Child. 2006;91(7):554–63.

Ingle S. IAAF doctor predicts intersex category in athletics within five to ten years. The Guardian. 2018.

Johannsen TH, Ripa CP, Mortensen EL, et al. Quality of life in 70 women with disorders of sex development. Eur J Endocrinol. 2006;155(6):877–85.

Jurgensen M, Kleinemeier E, Lux A, et al. Psychosexual development in adolescents and adults with disorders of sex development—results from the German Clinical Evaluation Study. J Sex Med. 2013;10(11):2703–14.

Jurgensen M, Lux A, Wien SB, et al. Health-related quality of life in children with disorders of sex development (DSD). Eur J Pediatr. 2014;173(7):893–903.

Karkazis K. Fixing sex: intersex, medical authority and lived experience. Durham and London: Duke University Press; 2008.

Karkazis K, Jordan-Young R, Davis G, Camporesi S. Out of bounds? A critique of the new policies on hyperandrogenism in elite female athletes. Am J Bioeth. 2012;12(7):3–16.

Kipnis K. Gender, sex, and professional ethics in child and adolescent psychiatry. Child Adolesc Psychiatr Clin N Am. 2004;13(3):695–708.

Kleinemeier E, Jurgensen M, Lux A, et al. Psychological adjustment and sexual development of adolescents with disorders of sex development. J Adolesc Health. 2010;47(5):463–71.

Kohler B, Jurgensen M, Kleinemeier E, et al. Psychosexual development in disorders of sex development. Boston: Springer; 2014.

Lindgren TW, Pauly IB. A body image scale for evaluating transsexuals. Arch Sex Behav. 1975;4(6):639–56.

Ludman L. Psychological aspects of pediatric surgery. In: Stringer MD, Oldham KT, Mouriquand PDE, editors. Pediatric surgery and urology: long term outcomes. Cambridge: Cambridge University Press; 2006.

Mazur T. Gender dysphoria and gender change in androgen insensitivity or micropenis. Arch Sex Behav. 2005;34(4):411–21.

Meyer-Bahlburg HF. Introduction: gender dysphoria and gender change in persons with intersexuality. Arch Sex Behav. 2005;34(4):371–3.

Nermoen I, Husebye ES, Svartberg J, et al. Subjective health status in men and women with congenital adrenal hyperplasia: a population-based survey in Norway. Eur J Endocrinol. 2010;163(3):453–9.

Nordenstrom A. Psychosocial factors in disorders of sex development in a long-term perspective: what clinical opportunities are there to intervene? Horm Metab Res. 2015;47(5):351–6.

O'Reilly. 2010. http://news.bbc.co.uk/go/pr/fr/-/02/hi/in_depth/8511176.stm.
Pasterski V, Mastroyannopoulou K, Wright D, et al. Predictors of posttraumatic stress in parents of children diagnosed with a disorder of sex development. Arch Sex Behav. 2014;43(2):369–75.
Reiner WG. Psychosexual development in genetic males assigned female: the cloacal exstrophy experience. Child Adolesc Psychiatr Clin N Am. 2004;13(3):657–74.
Reiner WG. Gender identity and sex-of-rearing in children with disorders of sexual differentiation. J Pediatr Endocrinol Metab. 2005;18(6):549–53.
Ritchie R, Reynard J, Lewis T. Intersex and the Olympic games. J R Soc Med. 2008;101(8):395–9.
Richter-Appelt H, Discher C, Gedrose B. Gender identity and recalled gender related childhood play-behaviour in adult individuals with different forms of intersexuality. Anthropol Anz. 2005;63(3):241–56.
Roen K, Pasterski V. Psychological research and intersex/DSD: recent developments and future directions. Psychol Sex. 2013; https://doi.org/10.1080/19419899.2013.831218.
Rohle R, Gehrmann K, Szarras-Czapnik M, et al. Participation of adults with disorders/differences of sex development (DSD) in the clinical study DSD-LIFE: design, methodology, recruitment, data quality and study population. BMC Endocr Disord. 2017;17(1):52.
Sandberg DE, Gardner M, Cohen-Kettenis PT. Psychological aspects of the treatment of patients with disorders of sex development. Semin Reprod Med. 2012;30(5):443–52.
Schutzmann K, Brinkmann L, Schacht M, et al. Psychological distress, self-harming behavior, and suicidal tendencies in adults with disorders of sex development. Arch Sex Behav. 2009;38(1):16–33.
Schweizer K, Brunner F, Gedrose B, et al. Coping with diverse sex development: treatment experiences and psychosocial support during childhood and adolescence and adult well-being. J Pediatr Psychol. 2017;42(5):504–19.
Slijper FM, Drop SL, Molenaar JC, et al. Long-term psychological evaluation of intersex children. Arch Sex Behav. 1998;27(2):125–44.
Slowikowska-Hilczer J, Hirschberg AL, Claasen-van der Grinten H. Fertility outcome and information on fertility issues in individuals with different forms of disorders of sex development: findings form the dsd-LIFE study. Fertil Steril. 2017;108(5):822–31.
Sobel V, Imperato-McGinley J. Gender identity in XY intersexuality. Child Adolesc Psychiatr Clin N Am. 2004;13(3):609–22, viii.
Strandqvist A, Falhammar H, Lichtenstein P, et al. Suboptimal psychosocial outcomes in patients with congenital adrenal hyperplasia: epidemiological studies in a nonbiased national cohort in Sweden. J Clin Endocrinol Metab. 2014;99(4):1425–32.
Tishelman AC, Shumer DE, Nahata L. Disorders of sex development: pediatric psychology and the genital exam. J Pediatr Psychol. 2017;42(5):530–43.
de Vries AL, Doreleijers TA, Cohen-Kettenis PT. Disorders of sex development and gender identity outcome in adolescence and adulthood: understanding gender identity development and its clinical implications. Pediatr Endocrinol Rev. 2007;4(4):343–51.
Warne G, Grover S, Hutson J, et al. A long-term outcome study of intersex conditions. J Pediatr Endocrinol Metab. 2005;18(6):555–67.
WHO. Multi axial version of ICD10: clinical description and diagnostic guidelines. Geneva: World Health Organisation; 1992.
WHO. Geneva: World Health Organisation; 2018.
Zucker KJ. Intersexuality and gender identity differentiation. Annu Rev Sex Res. 1999;10:1–69.
Zucker KJ. Measurement of psychosexual differentiation. Arch Sex Behav. 2005;34(4):375–88.

Genetic Counselling

21

David Amor

21.1 Introduction

DSD have a range of aetiologies, but for most DSD, genetic factors are prominent. As understanding of the genetic contributions increases, clinicians are increasingly faced with questions about why the DSD occurred and whether it will happen again. This chapter provides an overview of the process of genetic counselling, emphasizing the elements most relevant to genetic counselling for DSD, and then individual DSD, summarizing the specific aspects of genetic counselling for each condition.

21.2 Overview of Genetic Counselling

Genetic counselling is an important component of the management of people with DSD and their families and may take place in a variety of clinical settings. Genetic counselling for DSD frequently takes place within a multidisciplinary team, and it is typically carried out by clinical geneticists, genetic counsellors, or by other health professionals with specific expertise in genetic counselling.

Genetic counselling for DSD can take place at any stage of life but most commonly occurs in one of four clinical contexts:

1. a couple with personal or family history of DSD planning a pregnancy;
2. prenatal diagnosis of DSD;
3. following diagnosis of DSD in a neonate or young child; or,
4. an adolescent or young adult affected by DSD and seeking information about their own diagnosis.

Genetic counselling is a complex process that is difficult to encapsulate in a single definition; however, the content and process of genetic counselling typically includes, to varying degrees, six main elements (Harper 2010), which are summarized below.

21.2.1 Diagnostic and Clinical Aspects

Genetic counselling depends on accurate diagnosis, and it is essential that the diagnosis be made

D. Amor (✉)
Department of Neurodisability and Rehabilitation, The Royal Children's Hospital, Melbourne, VIC, Australia

Murdoch Children's Research Institute, Melbourne, VIC, Australia

Department of Paediatrics, University of Melbourne, Melbourne, VIC, Australia

Victorian Clinical Genetics Services, Melbourne, VIC, Australia
e-mail: david.amor@mcri.edu.au

J. M. Hutson et al. (eds.), *Disorders|Differences of Sex Development*,
https://doi.org/10.1007/978-981-13-7864-5_21

as firm as possible before risk[1] estimates are given. In addition to careful history and examination, additional data may be obtained from a variety of sources, such as interviewing multiple family members, seeking archived medical records, pathology reports and death certificates. In DSD, a careful endocrine, chromosome and molecular assessment is necessary before accurate genetic counselling can be given. Once a diagnosis is confirmed, it is important that the counsellor understands the natural history of the DSD and is able to communicate this to the individual and their family in a meaningful way.

21.2.2 Documentation of Family and Pedigree Information

The collection of family information is best achieved by drawing a family tree or pedigree. A clearly drawn pedigree provides a permanent record of genetic information in a particular family and conveys genetic information more clearly than other forms of family history documentation. Pedigrees drawn during the consultation also serve as a psychosocial tool, providing the opportunity to explore and better understand family dynamics and relationships. Careful inquiry may be required to elicit a family history of genital variation, information about which may not have been widely communicated within the family. Information about family history of stillbirth, neonatal death and consanguinity should also be sought.

Special care is required when drawing pedigrees in DSD families. Symbols used in constructing pedigrees include male (□), female (○) and sex unknown (◇); in DSD families, the symbols for male and female should be used to denote sexual identity rather than chromosomal sex. Where known, chromosome sex can be included as an annotation.

Although many DSD follow classical Mendelian inheritance, two points warrant emphasis. First, for X-linked recessive diagnoses that cause sex reversal (e.g. Androgen insensitivity syndrome—AIS), the pedigree at first glance may not suggest X-linked inheritance because affected individuals are phenotypically female rather than male. Second, there exist Mendelian DSD that are penetrant for only one chromosomal sex; for these diagnoses, the phenotype may skip one or more generations, and the risk of having an affected child is half of the genetic risk.

21.2.3 Recognition of Inheritance Patterns and Risk Estimation

Once all available information has been collated, it should be possible to make a risk estimation. In the setting of DSD, request for risk estimation usually takes one of three forms:

1. risk of having a second affected child;
2. risk of transmission from an affected parent to a child; or,
3. risk of having an affected child when a more distant relative is affected.

Risk figures in genetic counselling can be given either as odds (e.g. 'one in four') or as percentages (e.g. 25%), with the method of explanation tailored to the needs of the client. For Mendelian diagnoses, an exact risk can be given on the basis of the known inheritance pattern, typically ranging from 'negligible risk' to 50% risk. For chromosome variations and non-Mendelian diagnoses, risk estimation is usually empirical, based on observed data rather than theoretical predictions. The accuracy of empirical risk estimation depends on the quality of the available observed data and the degree to which it matches the client's personal situation. For very rare diagnoses, the only source of risk estimation might be from case reports of recurrence (or lack thereof).

[1] In this chapter, the term 'risk' is used in the context of the likelihood of a child of having a disorder/difference of sex development (DSD), but this term may not be appropriate in all clinical situations. In particular, when a particular DSD is viewed as a variation rather than a condition, terms such as 'chance' or 'likelihood' may be more appropriate. It is important to check in with parents to ensure they are comfortable with the language.

21.2.4 Communication

Genetic concepts are typically complex and need to be coupled with effective communication if genetic counselling is to be successful. Information about the psychological, psychosocial and practical impact of the diagnosis; genetic test results; natural history of the DSD; and available treatments should be conveyed in a way that is easily comprehended, taking into account the scientific literacy of the family. Genetic counselling must also be sensitive to the sexual identity of those affected, and care must be taken to avoid assuming that chromosomal sex will necessarily determine gender identity.

Most genetic counselling sessions are followed up by a letter in plain language to the client, summarizing the main points discussed and documenting any risk estimate. Finally, although generally distinct from psychotherapeutic counselling, genetic counselling frequently has a therapeutic element, arising from the willingness of the counsellor to listen to and acknowledge the client's experiences, the focus on the agenda of the client and the empathy shown during the consultation. Where possible sharing resources about these variations, including appropriate peer support contacts, should be included in this information.

21.2.5 Information on Available Options

Many genetic counselling sessions result in the client being presented with choices. In DSD genetic counselling, choices frequently centre on reproductive options, but they may also include decisions about whether to pursue further genetic testing, and whether to pass on information to other family members.

21.2.6 Support in Decision-Making and for Decisions Made

A key element underlying genetic counselling is non-directiveness; in practice, this means that a goal of genetic counselling is to provide clients with the appropriate information to enable them to make their own informed decisions, taking into account their attitudes, perceptions and beliefs. The genetic counsellor may facilitate and support the client's decision-making but should avoid advising the client on which choices to make. Finally, the genetic counsellor should assess the need for further counselling and follow-up.

21.3 Reproductive Options

For many DSD, there is a significant risk of recurrence for siblings or offspring; following diagnosis of these DSD, families are faced with difficult choices about future pregnancies. Reproductive choices are very personal, and not all options will be considered by all families. Where future pregnancies may have a DSD, there are six main reproductive options that may be available:

1. possibility of having another affected child;
2. deciding not to have further children;
3. prenatal diagnosis—some families may wish to know—to prepare themselves and their family or consider termination of pregnancy;
4. preimplantation genetic testing (PGT);
5. use of donor gametes or donor embryos; and,
6. adoption.

For some individuals with a DSD, reproduction using their own gametes will not be possible. For these people, conception using donor gametes may be possible, and provided the donor is not a genetic relative, the possibility of recurrence will be avoided.

21.4 Genetic Testing

Genetic testing is now a routine part of clinical practice and plays a key role in management of DSD, for which genetic testing falls into two categories: cytogenetic analysis and for single-gene disorders.

21.4.1 Cytogenetics

Cytogenetic analysis, and particularly information about the sex chromosomes, is a key part of the diagnostic process of DSD, and this is the only way to accurately diagnose chromosome DSD. Standard microscope karyotype should be performed in all cases, with at least 30 cells examined in order to exclude mosaicism. The presence of SRY is routinely tested using fluorescein *in situ* hybridization (FISH). Phenotypic sex determination involves a cascade of genes located on the autosomes and sex chromosome, and DSD have been associated with a number of autosomal deletions and duplications. Some of these include known DSD loci, such as SOX9, whereas others presumably harbour DSD genes that are yet to be discovered.

In recent years, traditional chromosome analysis has been replaced by chromosome microarray analysis, also known as molecular karyotyping. Chromosome microarray allows the determination of copy number at more than a million different loci across the genome, offering detection of small chromosome deletions and duplications at a resolution that is more than 100 times greater than microscopic karyotyping. Molecular karyotyping is a valuable diagnostic tool for detecting gene copy-number changes affecting known DSD genes and is also used for research to identify new DSD loci (Ledig et al. 2010). The diagnostic yield of molecular karyotyping is greatest in individuals with a DSD who have additional syndromal features, such as intellectual disability or associated birth defects. Despite the clear benefits of molecular karyotyping, microscopic karyotyping should still be performed in DSD cases due to its ability to detect balanced translocations and low-level mosaicism.

21.4.2 Gene Testing

Genetic testing for a number of DSD genes is now available on a clinical basis, including testing of SRY, androgen receptor (AR), DHH, NR5A1 (SF-1), SOX9, WT1 and CYP21A2. This number will undoubtedly increase as new genes are identified and linked to DSD. Detection of a specific gene variant can assist by confirming and refining a clinical diagnosis, clarifying the risk to other family members, and providing the opportunity for molecular prenatal diagnosis in future pregnancies. Families should be aware, however, that genetic testing does not provide clear answers in all cases. In some cases, a sequence variation of unknown significance may be identified. These are variations in DNA for which there is insufficient evidence to clearly classify the variant as being disease-causing. In other cases, no variant is identified, and there are several explanations for this finding. These include that a disease-causing variant is present in a gene that was not tested, or a gene that is yet to be discovered, or that there is a variant in the tested gene, but that it was not detected by the particular testing method used. In addition, failure to detect a causative pathogenic variant may be because the DSD is due to a non-genetic cause.

Testing for single genes is now mostly limited to cases where there is a strong suspicion of a pathogenic variant in a particular gene, based on clinical or biochemical phenotype. When multiple genetic aetiologies are being considered, a preferable approach is to use next-generation DNA sequencing (NGS), which enables large numbers of DSD genes to be simultaneously tested at relatively low cost, providing a new and valuable tool for the diagnosis of DSD. In the setting of 46,XY DSD, testing a 'panel' of 64 DSD genes has been shown to make a molecular diagnosis in about one-third of individuals tested (Baxter et al. 2015).

21.5 Genetic Counselling for Specific DSD

21.5.1 Sex Chromosome DSD

21.5.1.1 47,XXY

Klinefelter syndrome (47,XXY) is caused by the presence of an additional X chromosome in an otherwise male karyotype. Sibling recurrence risk for 47,XXY is low and probably not significantly increased compared to the background population risk, with only one documented occurrence of brothers with Klinefelter syndrome (Woods et al. 1997). There is a modest maternal age effect, resulting from approximately 30% of Klinefelter syndrome resulting from a maternal meiosis I error (Gardner and Amor 2018).

In the absence of medical intervention, men with Klinefelter syndrome are infertile. Instances of documented natural fertility are extremely rare (Laron et al. 1982; Terzoli et al. 1992; Juul et al. 2007) and may be accounted for by undetected XY/XXY mosaicism. In fact, testicular XY/XXY mosaicism appears to be relatively common, even in males with non-mosaic XXY on blood karyotype. Evidence from testicular biopsies of male with non-mosaic Klinefelter syndrome indicates that spermatogenesis, where present, originates not from XXY cells, but from foci of testicular tubules where the spermatogonia have a 46,XY karyotype, most likely representing clones of spermatogonia that have randomly lost one X chromosome.

Some men with Klinefelter syndrome are now able to become fathers with the assistance of testicular sperm extraction (TESE), which is able to obtain sperm in approximately 50% of XXY males (Fullerton et al. 2010). The chances of obtaining sperm might be improved if sampling and storage occur immediately after puberty; however, the benefits of this approach are yet to be proven (Gies et al. 2016). The few single sperms obtained by TESE are injected into the egg using intracytoplasmic sperm injection (ICSI). The first such child from a father with Klinefelter syndrome conceived using this technique was born in 1997 (Bourne et al. 1997), and since then more than 100 genetic children have been born to people with non-mosaic Klinefelter Syndrome (Fullerton et al. 2010).

These successes raise the question of whether there are genetic risks to the offspring. In terms of clinical outcome, results are reassuring, with only one documented instance of foetal XXY (Ron-El et al. 2000). Nonetheless, there is some evidence that sperm from XXY males have a higher incidence of aneuploidy compared to XY males, and that this aneuploidy affects autosomes as well as sex chromosomes (Levron et al. 2000; Rives et al. 2000). These aneuploidies are most likely the result of a compromised testicular environment rather than the presence of XXY cells per se, and the risk of variation is similar to that for azoospermic men with a 46,XY karyotype (Levron et al. 2000; Palermo et al. 2002). On the basis of this information, there may be a small increased risk for both sex chromosome and autosome aneuploidy in the offspring of XXY males, and preimplantation genetic diagnosis (PGD) or prenatal genetic diagnosis could be offered to these couples (Staessen et al. 2003).

For males with mosaicism XY/XXY in the blood, natural fertility may be possible, and a semen analysis in late adolescence can help predict the likelihood of natural pregnancy. In mosaic males with oligospermia or azoospermia, treatment with ICSI ± TESE may be beneficial, and XY/XXY mosaicism appears to be associated with a higher rate of sperm retrieval (Seo et al. 2004) and a lower rate of sperm aneuploidy (Ferlin et al. 2005) compared to non-mosaic XXY.

21.5.1.2 45,X

Turner syndrome (TS) is associated with partial or complete loss of one X chromosome (Nielsen and Wohlert 1991; Stochholm et al. 2006) and is characterized by ovarian insufficiency which occurs before puberty in most cases. Whilst infrequent at birth, 45,X karyotype is common at conception and is identified in approximately 10% of products of conception from spontaneous abortion (Kajii et al. 1980). There is no evidence of an increased risk of sibling recurrence.

Approximately 30% of women with TS have a mosaic karyotype in the peripheral blood, with a 45,X cell line detected in conjunction with one or more other cell line, for example, 45,X/46,XX, 45,X/47,XXX, and 45,X/46,XX/47,XXX, accounting for variability in phenotype and ovarian function (Hanson et al. 2001).

Spontaneous puberty occurs in 15–30% of girls with TS and 2–5% experience menarche (Pasquino et al. 1997). Oocytes are present in the ovaries of approximately a quarter of adolescents with TS, but spontaneous pregnancy is rare (Bernard et al. 2016), and for many women with TS, *in vitro* fertilization (IVF) with a donor egg is the most viable option. In a French study of 480 women with Turner syndrome, only 2/181 women (1.1%) with a non-mosaic 45,X karyotype achieved a spontaneous pregnancy (Bernard et al. 2016). In a woman with non-mosaic 45,X, any period of fertility is likely to be short-lived; in some centres, sampling and storage of oocytes in early adolescence, or ovarian cryopreservation in prepubertal girls, might offer a future possibility (Oktay et al. 2016).

Current evidence suggests that 45,X germ cells are unable to complete meiosis (Modi et al. 2003), suggesting that spontaneous pregnancy in women with 45,X TS relies on the presence of 46,XX germ cells in the ovaries, with the occasionally observed follicles originating from small numbers of 46,XX germ cells (Hall et al. 2006). Fertility is more likely to be retained in women with 45,X/46,XX mosaicism than standard monosomy (45,X), although premature ovarian insufficiency is common (Blair et al. 2001), and the risk of chromosomally atypical offspring in women with mosaic TS appears to be increased compared to the general population (Uehara et al. 1999; Sybert 2002; Bernard et al. 2016). Of note, a non-mosaic 45,X peripheral karyotype does not preclude the presence of 45,X/46,XX mosaicism in the ovary, and a peripheral blood karyotype is not a completely reliable predictor of ovarian status (Mortensen et al. 2010). In the study of Bernard et al. a pregnancy was achieved by 19/130 women with 45,X/46,XX mosaic Turner syndrome (Bernard et al. 2016).

A significant proportion of women with TS have a structural difference of the second X chromosome, resulting in partial X monosomy. Examples are deletion Xp, ring X and isochromosome Xq, and for these categories, mosaicism with 45,X or 46,XX cell lines is common. Many structural differences of the X chromosome are compatible with spontaneous menarche and pregnancy, and there are many examples of mother-daughter transmission (Lachlan et al. 2006). Risk to offspring is increased, and genetic counselling is recommended: male embryos that inherit the structurally atypical X will usually be non-viable, and female offspring are at risk of a more severe phenotype than the mother if X-inactivation does not completely favour the intact X.

Regardless of whether conception is spontaneous or assisted in TS, increased rates of miscarriage and foetal variation have been described (Bernard et al. 2016). In a review of the outcomes of 160 pregnancies in 74 women with TS, 29% resulted in miscarriage; 20% were associated with foetal anomalies, such as TS and Down syndrome; and 7% resulted in perinatal foetal death (Tarani et al. 1998). Intrauterine growth restriction and prematurity occur in approximately 50% (Bodri et al. 2006). In view of the high risk of foetal anomalies, antenatal diagnostic testing should be offered to all pregnant TS women, with the pregnancy managed as high risk from a foetal perspective. Miscarriages may be due to karyotypic variants such as TS or Trisomy 21, altered uterine environment related to developmental variation or poor endometrial receptivity due to hypo-oestrogenism (Abir et al. 2001; Doger et al. 2015; Bernard et al. 2016).

Pregnant women with TS require coordinated multidisciplinary tertiary medical and obstetric care, as they are at very high risk for complications during pregnancy, such as thyroid dysfunction, obesity, diabetes, hypertension, pre-eclampsia, deterioration of congenital heart disease, heart failure, aortic dissection and sudden death (Bernard et al. 2016).

21.5.1.3 45,X/46,XY

The karyotype 45,X/46,XY is associated with a broad range of clinical phenotypes from Turner syndrome to typical male. Presumably, these differences reflect the distribution of each cell line in different parts of the body, and particularly the presence of a Y-containing cell line in the gonad. Frequently, the Y chromosome is structurally atypical, with the structural variation presumably predisposing to loss during mitosis.

There is substantial difference in phenotype according to whether cases are ascertained prenatally or postnatally. Prenatally diagnosed cases are phenotypic male in 90% of cases but may be at later risk of infertility. The other 10% of prenatally ascertained cases exhibit phenotypic features of TS and/or genital variations (Telvi et al. 1999). Postnatally ascertained cases present with a broad range of phenotypes, including Turner syndrome, infertility in otherwise phenotypic males and genital variation. Although in theory Y chromosome instability might be familial, in practice, sporadic occurrence appears to be the rule. There is a risk of gonadoblastoma in dysgenetic gonads for individuals with a karyotype of 45,X/46,XY due to the Y chromosome component.

21.5.1.4 46,XX/46,XY

The 46,XX/46,XY karyotype usually results from the fusion of dizygotic twin XX and XY embryos (XX/XY chimerism), although several other mechanisms have been proposed. Associated phenotypes include ovotesticular DSD, genital ambiguity, phenotypic male and phenotypic female. Occurrence is always sporadic. 46,XX/46,XY is occasionally encountered at prenatal diagnosis; in this circumstance, both cell lines may be present in the foetus, or alternatively, the second cell line results from contamination of the sample by maternal cells, or from an undiagnosed 'vanished' twin (Amor et al. 1999).

21.5.2 46,XY DSD

21.5.2.1 46,XY Complete Gonadal Dysgenesis (Swyer Syndrome) and 46,XY Partial Gonadal Dysgenesis DSD

The category of 46,XY gonadal dysgenesis comprises two conditions that are phenotypically distinct but genitally overlapping.

1. 46,XY complete gonadal dysgenesis (CGD) is associated with a 46,XY karyotype, typical female external genitalia with typical Müllerian structures and underdeveloped gonads with no sperm production.
2. 46,XY DSD (partial gonadal dysgenesis) is characterized by ambiguous/atypical genitalia, dysgenic testes, reduced or absent sperm production and variable presence of Müllerian structures.

46,XY gonadal dysgenesis can be familial and is a unique example of a Mendelian condition that can be inherited as an X-linked recessive, Y-linked, autosomal dominant or autosomal recessive trait. When inheritance is autosomal, penetrance is typically limited to individuals with an XY karyotype.

About 15% of individuals have deletions or loss of function variants in the SRY gene that are detectable by FISH or gene sequencing. The contribution of other genes is unknown; however, duplication of the gene NR0B1 (DAX1) accounts for some X-linked 46,XY gonadal dysgenesis (Barbaro et al. 2007), homozygous (or compound heterozygous) variants in desert hedgehog (DHH) account from some autosomal recessive 46,XY gonadal dysgenesis (Canto et al. 2004), and autosomal dominant 46,XY gonadal dysgenesis can result from heterozygous variants in DHH, NR5A1 (SF1) (Philibert et al. 2010) and MAP3K1 (Pearlman et al. 2010).

Genetic testing is available and can be used to inform genetic counselling in familial and sporadic cases of non-syndromic 46,XY gonadal dysgenesis. Analysis of SRY and chromosome microarray analysis are the first-line genetic investigations, followed by genetic analysis of multiple genes via an NGS panel.

In familial cases of 46,XY gonadal dysgenesis and cases where a causative gene variant is identified, this information will inform genetic counselling. The identification of a gene variant allows carrier testing of family members and prenatal diagnosis in at-risk pregnancies.

Men with SRY variants are usually infertile; therefore, most variants arise *de novo* in the proband rather than being present in the father. Nonetheless, siblings of the proband might still be at low risk because of gonadal or somatic mosaicism in the father. Variants in SRY that result in partial loss of function can cause 46,XY DSD, and penetrance may be incomplete, complicating genetic counselling.

In cases where there is no family history and no identified genetic variant, the situation is less straightforward. No empiric sibling recurrence risk data exist, but risk is likely to be low. In the absence of molecular confirmation, prenatal diagnosis can be potentially offered by looking for the combination of an XY karyotype on chronic villus sampling (CVS), amniocentesis or non-invasive prenatal testing (NIPT) and female external genitalia on ultrasound scan.

Some individuals with 46,XY DSD may be able to reproduce with the aid of assisted reproduction technologies. For 46,XY women, assisted conception is possible if a uterus is present (Michala et al. 2008). Individuals with 46,XY may be able to reproduce using their own gametes and assisted reproduction technology. For variants affecting the SRY gene, the variants will be passed to all sons but not to daughters of the proband.

21.5.2.2 XY Ovarian DSD

The development of typical female anatomy and ovarian tissue (usually dysgenetic) in the presence of a 46,XY karyotype is very rare. There is a single case report of this presentation as an autosomal recessive entity caused by compound heterozygous variants in the gene CBX2 (Biason-Lauber et al. 2009).

21.5.2.3 Complete (CAIS) or Partial Androgen Insensitivity Syndrome (PAIS)

Androgen insensitivity syndrome is inherited as an X-linked recessive trait and is caused by variants in the androgen receptor (AR) at Xq11–12. The androgen receptor is the only gene known to be associated with AIS, and sequencing of the AR gene detects variants in >95% of individuals with CAIS. PAIS appears to be genetically heterogeneous and variants in the AR gene are found in <50% of individuals (Gottlieb and Trifiro 2017). Nearly 1000 different AR variants have been shown to cause AIS (http://androgendb.mcgill.ca/). The phenotype of CAIS is relatively consistent within families; however, the phenotypes of PAIS show intrafamilial variability (Deeb et al. 2005). *De novo* variants are relatively common, being observed in 27% of families with only one affected individual (Hiort et al. 1998); therefore, genetic testing is necessary to provide accurate genetic counselling. Gonadal mosaicism has also been reported for AIS (Boehmer et al. 1997); therefore, there is a small risk of recurrence even following an apparently *de novo* variant.

When an XX female is known to be heterozygous for an AR variant, for each offspring, there is a one in four chance of the offspring having a 46,XY karyotype and being affected by AIS, and a one in four chance of the offspring having a 46,XX karyotype and being a carrier of AIS. Prenatal diagnosis and preimplantation genetic testing (PGT) are available for AIS. Fertility may be preserved in some males with partial AIS, in which case all XX offspring will be carriers of AIS and all XY offspring will be unaffected males.

Note that AIS is allelic to Kennedy disease (Spinobulbar muscular atrophy), which is caused by expansion of a polyglutamine tract within the AR gene. People with Kennedy disease have mild AIS.

21.5.2.4 Hormone Biosynthetic Defects

Defects in androgen biosynthesis can lead to typical testis development but incomplete androgenization of male genitalia. Some conditions are accompanied by deficiencies of adrenal hormones. Examples are 17β-hydroxysteroid dehydrogenase deficiency, 3-beta-hydroxysteroid dehydrogenase deficiency, cholesterol desmolase deficiency and 17α-hydroxylase deficiency. Inheritance is autosomal recessive; therefore, there is a one in four risk of recurrence in each pregnancy; however, the genital phenotype is only expressed in individuals with a 46,XY karyotype.

Smith-Lemli-Opitz syndrome (SLOS) is a rare autosomal recessive multiple congenital anomaly syndrome caused by deficiency of the enzyme 7-dehydrocholesterol reductase. In XY individuals, there is incomplete androgenization of the male genitalia.

21.5.3 Rare Syndromes

21.5.3.1 Campomelic Dysplasia and SOX9

Campomelic dysplasia is a rare skeletal dysplasia characterized by long bone bowing (campomelia), cleft palate, club feet and distinctive facies. In XX individuals, typical female genital development occurs; however, most XY campomelic dysplasia individuals have either female or ambiguous/atypical external genitalia and variable internal genitalia. SOX9 is the only gene associated with campomelic dysplasia, and inheritance is autosomal dominant, although most cases result from *de novo* variants. About 5% of affected individuals have a chromosome translocation, visible in standard karyotype, disrupting the SOX9 locus at 17q24.3–25.1. Translocations are usually *de novo*, but parental karyotypes should, nonetheless, be checked, as translocations with breakpoints a long distance from SOX9 may have incomplete penetrance. The remaining 95% of individuals have a sequence change, or less commonly a large deletion, affecting SOX9. Germ line (Cameron et al. 1996) and somatic (Smyk et al. 2007) mosaicism for SOX9 variants has been reported. Notably, some individuals with SOX9 variants and ambiguous/atypical genitalia have typical skeletal development.

21.5.3.2 WT-1

Denys-Drash syndrome and Frasier syndromes are both caused by autosomal dominant variants in the gene WT-1 located at 11p13, with the majority of variants being *de novo*. Denys-Drash syndrome is characterized by early-onset nephropathy, increased risk of Wilms tumour and 46,XY DSD. In Frasier syndrome, nephropathy is later in onset, there is 46,XY complete gonadal dysgenesis, and tumour risk is primarily for gonadoblastoma. For both conditions, XX individuals usually have typical genital development.

21.5.4 Isolated Anomalies

21.5.4.1 Hypospadias

Hypospadias is a common variation where the urethra opens on the ventral side of the penis and is associated with a range of Mendelian syndromes, chromosome variations and DSD. For isolated hypospadias, the risk of recurrence in male siblings is around 1 in 20, and a similar risk applies for sons of an affected male. X-linked hypospadias has been reported in association with variants in the gene MAMLD1 (Fukami et al. 2006) and with variants in the androgen receptor (Allera et al. 1995).

21.5.4.2 Cryptorchidism

Cryptorchidism is a common presentation in males and is thought to result from a combination of genetic and environmental factors. The recurrence risk in male siblings of isolated cases is around 1 in 20 (Czeizel et al. 1981). Cryptorchidism is also associated with a range of Mendelian syndromes and chromosome variations.

21.5.5 46,XX DSD

21.5.5.1 XX Testicular DSD

Most males with XX testicular DSD arise as a result of the presence of SRY in an otherwise typical XX karyotype. The phenotype is similar to that of Klinefelter syndrome, with male external genitalia, small testes, azoospermia and, if untreated, signs of testosterone deficiency. In contrast to Klinefelter syndrome, males with XX testicular DSD do not have increased stature or learning difficulties (Ferguson-Smith et al. 1990). In most males with SRY+ XX testicular DSD, Yp material (including SRY) is present on the X chromosome as a result of atypical exchange during meiosis I during gametogenesis in the father. This is nearly always a sporadic event (Weil et al. 1994; Wang et al. 1995). Far less commonly, SRY has been translocated onto a terminal arm of an autosome (Dauwerse et al. 2006; Queralt et al. 2008), and in this circumstance, sex-limited autosomal dominant inheritance is observed. There is also on record a typically fertile XY individual in whom SRY was translocated onto the X chromosome (Abbas et al. 1993); in this circumstance, all XX offspring would have XX testicular DSD. Because of these rare familial occurrences, in order to prove sporadic occurrence, it is necessary to perform FISH to search for SRY in the father and confirm that SRY is located only on the Y chromosome. Men with SRY+ XX testicular DSD are infertile.

A minority of males with XX testicular DSD are SRY negative and presumably arise as a result from inappropriate activity of the gene cascade that is typically switched on only in response to SRY. Not surprisingly, atypical genitalia occur more commonly in these individuals. The cause of testicular development in these individuals is not well understood, but atypical dosage of genes in the sex-determining pathway is likely to play a part. One family has been reported with autosomal dominant sex-limited transmission of SRY-testicular DSD, resulting from a 178 kb duplication that is 600 kb upstream of SOX9 (Cox et al. 2011). In the absence of family history, risk of recurrence is likely to be low. XX testicular DSD has been diagnosed prenatally, following the detection of discordance between chromosomal and ultrasonographic sex (Trujillo-Tiebas et al. 2006).

21.5.5.2 46,XX Ovotesticular DSD

Individuals with 46,XX ovotesticular DSD have both testicular and ovarian tissue (containing spermatogonia or oocytes respectively either within the one gonad or in separate gonads). The karyotype on peripheral blood is 46,XX and SRY is absent. The likely explanation is localized activation of testicular development, for example, by cryptic mosaicism within the gonad for cells containing the SRY gene (Ortenberg et al. 2002; Queipo et al. 2002) or other mosaic variants that lead to testicular development. Most cases are sporadic, but the existence of rare familial cases (Ramos et al. 1996; Slaney et al. 1998) indicates the existence of X-linked or autosomal predisposition genes. Genomic rearrangements that increase the expression of SOX9 or SOX3 have been implicated in some cases (Grinspon and Rey 2016).

21.5.5.3 Congenital Adrenal Hyperplasia

Congenital adrenal hyperplasia (CAH) is a family of disorders characterized by impaired synthesis of cortisol from cholesterol in the adrenal cortex. At least eight forms exist, and all follow autosomal recessive inheritance. The most important type is 21-hydroxylase deficiency, which causes virilization in XX individuals and variable salt wasting in XX and XY individuals. Molecular testing of the gene *CYP21A2* detects variants in most cases and can be used for prenatal diagnosis. For families with familial CAH, genetic counselling is recommended to discuss future pregnancies and referral to an endocrinologist during a pregnancy to discuss the best management for the baby postnatally.

21.5.5.4 Rare Syndromes

Several rare syndromes exist in which male genital development occurs in the setting of an XX karyotype and other variations.

Variants in the R-Spondin1 gene cause a syndrome of XX testicular DSD, palmoplantar keratosis and squamous cell carcinoma of the skin (Parma et al. 2006). Inheritance is autosomal recessive, and in XY individuals, only PPK and SSC are present.

Microphthalmia with linear skin defects syndrome (MLS) is an X-linked male-lethal disorder associated with X-chromosome rearrangements that result in monosomy from Xpter to Xp22, including the gene HCCS. In some individuals, the chromosome rearrangement is an X;Y translocation, resulting in sex reversal due to translocation of SRY onto the X chromosome (Mucke et al. 1995).

Multiple congenital anomalies in association with 46,XX sex reversal have also been reported in an individual with a chromosome 22 duplication, 46,XX,dup(22)(q11.2q13). The person had male external genitalia and intrascrotal gonads (Seeherunvong et al. 2004).

21.5.5.5 Isolated Anomalies

Müllerian anomalies including uterine and vaginal agenesis, and duplication of the uterus and vagina, are relatively common, and undoubtedly underdiagnosed. Usually, individuals have typical ovarian function, and presentation is commonly at puberty with atypical menstruation or amenorrhea, or later with infertility or pregnancy complications. Although genetic factors are likely to contribute, most isolated Müllerian anomalies are sporadic, and risk of recurrence is low. There is a known association with renal and skeletal changes, which in its most severe form is known as Müllerian duct aplasia-unilateral renal aplasia-cervicothoracic somite dysplasia (MURCS) association (Duncan et al. 1979). MURCS association is usually sporadic, but familial forms exist, and autosomal dominant inheritance with incomplete penetrance has been suggested (Guerrier et al. 2006). Variations of female internal and external genitalia are also associated with a large number of rare genetic syndromes and a variety of chromosome anomalies.

References

Abbas N, McElreavey K, Leconiat M, et al. Familial case of 46,XX male and 46,XX true hermaphrodite associated with a paternal-derived SRY-bearing X chromosome. C R Acad Sci III. 1993;316(4):375–83.

Abir R, Fisch B, Nahum R, et al. Turner's syndrome and fertility: current status and possible putative prospects. Hum Reprod Update. 2001;7(6):603–10.

Allera A, Herbst MA, Griffin JE, et al. Mutations of the androgen receptor coding sequence are infrequent in patients with isolated hypospadias. J Clin Endocrinol Metab. 1995;80(9):2697–9.

Amor D, Delatycki MB, Susman M, et al. 46,XX/46,XY at amniocentesis in a fetus with true hermaphroditism. J Med Genet. 1999;36(11):866–9.

Barbaro M, Oscarson M, Schoumans J, et al. Isolated 46,XY gonadal dysgenesis in two sisters caused by a Xp21.2 interstitial duplication containing the DAX1 gene. J Clin Endocrinol Metab. 2007;92(8):3305–13.

Baxter RM, Arboleda VA, Lee H, et al. Exome sequencing for the diagnosis of 46,XY disorders of sex development. J Clin Endocrinol Metab. 2015;100(2):E333–44.

Bernard V, Donadille B, Zenaty D, et al. Spontaneous fertility and pregnancy outcomes amongst 480 women with Turner syndrome. Hum Reprod. 2016;31(4):782–8.

Biason-Lauber A, Konrad D, Meyer M, et al. Ovaries and female phenotype in a girl with 46,XY karyotype and mutations in the CBX2 gene. Am J Hum Genet. 2009;84(5):658–63.

Blair J, Tolmie J, Hollman AS, et al. Phenotype, ovarian function, and growth in patients with 45,X/47,XXX Turner mosaicism: implications for prenatal counseling and estrogen therapy at puberty. J Pediatr. 2001;139(5):724–8.

Bodri D, Vernaeve V, Figueras F, et al. Oocyte donation in patients with Turner's syndrome: a successful technique but with an accompanying high risk of hypertensive disorders during pregnancy. Hum Reprod. 2006;21(3):829–32.

Boehmer AL, Brinkmann AO, Niermeijer MF, et al. Germ-line and somatic mosaicism in the androgen insensitivity syndrome: implications for genetic counseling. Am J Hum Genet. 1997;60(4):1003–6.

Bourne H, Stern K, Clarke G, et al. Delivery of normal twins following the intracytoplasmic injection of spermatozoa from a patient with 47,XXY Klinefelter's syndrome. Hum Reprod. 1997;12(11):2447–50.

Cameron FJ, Hageman RM, Cooke-Yarborough C, et al. A novel germ line mutation in SOX9 causes familial campomelic dysplasia and sex reversal. Hum Mol Genet. 1996;5(10):1625–30.

Canto P, Soderlund D, Reyes E, et al. Mutations in the desert hedgehog (DHH) gene in patients with 46,XY complete pure gonadal dysgenesis. J Clin Endocrinol Metab. 2004;89(9):4480–3.

Cox JJ, Willatt L, Homfray T, et al. A SOX9 duplication and familial 46,XX developmental testicular disorder. N Engl J Med. 2011;364(1):91–3.

Czeizel A, Erodi E, Toth J. Genetics of undescended testis. J Urol. 1981;126(4):528–9.

Dauwerse JG, Hansson KB, Brouwers AA, et al. An XX male with the sex-determining region Y gene inserted in the long arm of chromosome 16. Fertil Steril. 2006;86(2):463.e461–5.

Deeb A, Mason C, Lee YS, et al. Correlation between genotype, phenotype and sex of rearing in 111 patients with partial androgen insensitivity syndrome. Clin Endocrinol. 2005;63(1):56–62.

Doger E, Cakiroglu Y, Ceylan Y, et al. Reproductive and obstetric outcomes in mosaic Turner's syndrome: a cross-sectional study and review of the literature. Reprod Biol Endocrinol. 2015;13:59.

Duncan PA, Shapiro LR, Stangel JJ, et al. The MURCS association: Müllerian duct aplasia, renal aplasia, and cervicothoracic somite dysplasia. J Pediatr. 1979;95(3):399–402.

Ferguson-Smith MA, Cooke A, Affara NA, et al. Genotype-phenotype correlations in XX males and their bearing on current theories of sex determination. Hum Genet. 1990;84(2):198–202.

Ferlin A, Garolla A, Foresta C. Chromosome abnormalities in sperm of individuals with constitutional sex chromosomal abnormalities. Cytogenet Genome Res. 2005;111(3–4):310–6.

Fukami M, Wada Y, Miyabayashi K, et al. CXorf6 is a causative gene for hypospadias. Nat Genet. 2006;38(12):1369–71.

Fullerton G, Hamilton M, Maheshwari A. Should non-mosaic Klinefelter syndrome men be labelled as infertile in 2009? Hum Reprod. 2010;25:588–97.

Gardner RJM, Amor DJ. Gardner and Sutherland's chromosome abnormalities and genetic counseling. New York: Oxford University Press; 2018.

Gies I, Oates R, De Schepper J, et al. Testicular biopsy and cryopreservation for fertility preservation of pre-

pubertal boys with Klinefelter syndrome: a pro/con debate. Fertil Steril. 2016;105(2):249–55.
Gottlieb B, Trifiro MA. Androgen insensitivity syndrome. GeneReviews®. 2017. doi: NBK1429 [book accession].
Grinspon RP, Rey RA. Disorders of sex development with testicular differentiation in SRY-negative 46,XX individuals: clinical and genetic aspects. Sex Dev. 2016;10(1):1–11.
Guerrier D, Mouchel T, Pasquier L, et al. The Mayer-Rokitansky-Kuster-Hauser syndrome (congenital absence of uterus and vagina)—phenotypic manifestations and genetic approaches. J Negat Results Biomed. 2006;5:1.
Hall H, Hunt P, Hassold T. Meiosis and sex chromosome aneuploidy: how meiotic errors cause aneuploidy; how aneuploidy causes meiotic errors. Curr Opin Genet Dev. 2006;16(3):323–9.
Hanson L, Bryman I, Barrenas ML, et al. Genetic analysis of mosaicism in 53 women with Turner syndrome. Hereditas. 2001;134(2):153–9.
Harper P. Practical genetic counselling. Oxford: Oxford University Press; 2010.
Hiort O, Sinnecker GH, Holterhus PM, et al. Inherited and de novo androgen receptor gene mutations: investigation of single-case families. J Pediatr. 1998;132(6):939–43.
Juul A, Aksglaede L, Lund AM, et al. Preserved fertility in a non-mosaic Klinefelter patient with a mutation in the fibroblast growth factor receptor 3 gene: case report. Hum Reprod. 2007;22(7):1907–11.
Kajii T, Ferrier A, Niikawa N, et al. Anatomic and chromosomal anomalies in 639 spontaneous abortuses. Hum Genet. 1980;55(1):87–98.
Lachlan KL, Youings S, Costa T, et al. A clinical and molecular study of 26 females with Xp deletions with special emphasis on inherited deletions. Hum Genet. 2006;118(5):640–51.
Laron Z, Dickerman Z, Zamir R, et al. Paternity in Klinefelter's syndrome—a case report. Arch Androl. 1982;8(2):149–51.
Ledig S, Hiort O, Scherer G, et al. Array-CGH analysis in patients with syndromic and non-syndromic XY gonadal dysgenesis: evaluation of array CGH as diagnostic tool and search for new candidate loci. Hum Reprod. 2010;25(10):2637–46.
Levron J, Aviram-Goldring A, Madgar I, et al. Sperm chromosome analysis and outcome of IVF in patients with non-mosaic Klinefelter's syndrome. Fertil Steril. 2000;74(5):925–9.
Michala L, Goswami D, Creighton SM, et al. Swyer syndrome: presentation and outcomes. BJOG. 2008;115(6):737–41.
Modi DN, Sane S, Bhartiya D. Accelerated germ cell apoptosis in sex chromosome aneuploid fetal human gonads. Mol Hum Reprod. 2003;9(4):219–25.
Mortensen KH, Rohde MD, Uldbjerg N, et al. Repeated spontaneous pregnancies in 45,X Turner syndrome. Obstet Gynecol. 2010;115(2 Pt 2):446–9.
Mucke J, Happle R, Theile H. MIDAS syndrome respectively MLS syndrome: a separate entity rather than a particular lyonization pattern of the gene causing Goltz syndrome. Am J Med Genet. 1995;57(1):117–8.
Nielsen J, Wohlert M. Chromosome abnormalities found among 34,910 newborn children: results from a 13-year incidence study in Arhus, Denmark. Hum Genet. 1991;87(1):81–3.
Oktay K, Bedoschi G, Berkowitz K, et al. Fertility preservation in women with Turner syndrome: a comprehensive review and practical guidelines. J Pediatr Adolesc Gynecol. 2016;29(5):409–16.
Ortenberg J, Oddoux C, Craver R, et al. SRY gene expression in the ovotestes of XX true hermaphrodites. J Urol. 2002;167(4):1828–31.
Palermo GD, Colombero LT, Hariprashad JJ, et al. Chromosome analysis of epididymal and testicular sperm in azoospermic patients undergoing ICSI. Hum Reprod. 2002;17(3):570–5.
Parma P, Radi O, Vidal V, et al. R-spondin1 is essential in sex determination, skin differentiation and malignancy. Nat Genet. 2006;38(11):1304–9.
Pasquino AM, Passeri F, Pucarelli I, et al. Spontaneous pubertal development in Turner's syndrome. Italian Study Group for Turner's Syndrome. J Clin Endocrinol Metab. 1997;82(6):1810–3.
Pearlman A, Loke J, Le Caignec C, et al. Mutations in MAP3K1 cause 46,XY disorders of sex development and implicate a common signal transduction pathway in human testis determination. Am J Hum Genet. 2010;87(6):898–904.
Philibert P, Leprieur E, Zenaty D, et al. Steroidogenic factor-1 (SF-1) gene mutation as a frequent cause of primary amenorrhea in 46,XY female adolescents with low testosterone concentration. Reprod Biol Endocrinol. 2010;8:28.
Queipo G, Zenteno JC, Pena R, et al. Molecular analysis in true hermaphroditism: demonstration of low-level hidden mosaicism for Y-derived sequences in 46,XX cases. Hum Genet. 2002;111(3):278–83.
Queralt R, Madrigal I, Vallecillos MA, et al. Atypical XX male with the SRY gene located at the long arm of chromosome 1 and a 1qter microdeletion. Am J Med Genet A. 2008;146A(10):1335–40.
Ramos ES, Moreira-Filho CA, Vicente YA, et al. SRY-negative true hermaphrodites and an XX male in two generations of the same family. Hum Genet. 1996;97(5):596–8.
Rives N, Joly G, Machy A, et al. Assessment of sex chromosome aneuploidy in sperm nuclei from 47,XXY and 46,XY/47,XXY males: comparison with fertile and infertile males with normal karyotype. Mol Hum Reprod. 2000;6(2):107–12.
Ron-El R, Strassburger D, Gelman-Kohan S, et al. A 47,XXY fetus conceived after ICSI of spermatozoa from a patient with non-mosaic Klinefelter's syndrome: case report. Hum Reprod. 2000;15(8):1804–6.
Seeherunvong T, Perera EM, Bao Y, et al. 46,XX sex reversal with partial duplication of chromosome arm 22q. Am J Med Genet A. 2004;127A(2):149–51.
Seo JT, Park YS, Lee JS. Successful testicular sperm extraction in Korean Klinefelter syndrome. Urology. 2004;64(6):1208–11.

Slaney SF, Chalmers IJ, Affara NA, et al. An autosomal or X linked mutation results in true hermaphrodites and 46,XX males in the same family. J Med Genet. 1998;35(1):17–22.

Smyk M, Obersztyn E, Nowakowska B, et al. Recurrent SOX9 deletion campomelic dysplasia due to somatic mosaicism in the father. Am J Med Genet A. 2007;143A(8):866–70.

Staessen C, Tournaye H, Van Assche E, et al. PGD in 47,XXY Klinefelter's syndrome patients. Hum Reprod Update. 2003;9(4):319–30.

Stochholm K, Juul S, Juel K, et al. Prevalence, incidence, diagnostic delay, and mortality in Turner syndrome. J Clin Endocrinol Metab. 2006;91(10):3897–902.

Sybert VP. Phenotypic effects of mosaicism for a 47,XXX cell line in Turner syndrome. J Med Genet. 2002;39(3):217–20.

Tarani L, Lampariello S, Raguso G, et al. Pregnancy in patients with Turner's syndrome: six new cases and review of literature. Gynecol Endocrinol. 1998;12(2):83–7.

Telvi L, Lebbar A, Del Pino O, et al. 45,X/46,XY mosaicism: report of 27 cases. Pediatrics. 1999;104(2 Pt 1): 304–8.

Terzoli G, Lalatta F, Lobbiani A, et al. Fertility in a 47,XXY patient: assessment of biological paternity by deoxyribonucleic acid fingerprinting. Fertil Steril. 1992;58(4):821–2.

Trujillo-Tiebas MJ, Gonzalez-Gonzalez C, Lorda-Sanchez I, et al. Prenatal diagnosis of 46,XX male fetus. J Assist Reprod Genet. 2006;23(5):253–4.

Uehara S, Yaegashi N, Maeda T, et al. Risk of recurrence of fetal chromosomal aberrations: analysis of trisomy 21, trisomy 18, trisomy 13, and 45,X in 1,076 Japanese mothers. J Obstet Gynaecol Res. 1999;25(6):373–9.

Wang I, Weil D, Levilliers J, et al. Prevalence and molecular analysis of two hot spots for ectopic recombination leading to XX maleness. Genomics. 1995;28(1): 52–8.

Weil D, Wang I, Dietrich A, et al. Highly homologous loci on the X and Y chromosomes are hot-spots for ectopic recombinations leading to XX maleness. Nat Genet. 1994;7(3):414–9.

Woods CG, Noble J, Falconer AR. A study of brothers with Klinefelter syndrome. J Med Genet. 1997;34(8): 702.

Cultural Differences in the Developing World

22

Tahmina Banu and Tanvir K. Chowdhury

Disorders/differences of sex development (DSD) are present in every country of the world with varied prevalence rates. Although knowledge about the aetiology and pathogenesis, investigation support, management and many other aspects has tremendously improved over the last 50 years, developing countries cannot yet take the full benefits of these. Poverty, lack of proper education, influence of culture and ethnic values, social stigma, misinterpretation of religion, fatalistic attitude, medical malpractice and lack of medical support are among the factors responsible for inadequate management of many DSD patients in the developing world. The consensus guideline for DSD advocates early and accurate diagnosis, multidisciplinary team involvement, an evidence-based process for decision-making, correct surgery by experts in a centre of excellence, adequate hormonal management and proper and long-term follow-up of patients (Warne and Raza 2008). However, controversies related to gender assignment, timing of surgery and disclosure of information have increased among patients, families and clinicians involved in the care. How have these factors and sociocultural impact touched the relationship among the persons involved in the care of DSD patients in the developing world? How are these countries dealing with their patients with DSD? This chapter will focus on the experience of managing DSD patients in a developing country and will discuss the cultural differences in developing countries with regard to different aspects of dealing with DSD patients.

T. Banu (✉) · T. K. Chowdhury
Chittagong Research Institute for Children Surgery (CRICS), Chittagong, Bangladesh

22.1 DSD Subtypes

In developed world, 46XX DSD is reported to be more commonly found. However, in most developing countries 46XY DSD is more common as reported by different studies. A 20-year study in South Africa showed that 57.5% of their DSD cohort was 46,XY DSD, 33% 46,XX and 9.5% had sex chromosomal DSD, although, due to absence of some specific hormonal assays, which is also similar in many other developing countries, 46,XY DSD could not be subcategorized (Ganie et al. 2016). An Egyptian study reported that 65.9% of their DSD patients were 46,XY DSD, with most of them having 5 α-reductase deficiencies (Mazen et al. 2008). In Sudan, the most common 46XY DSD was androgen insensitivity syndrome (Abdullah et al. 2012). In our centre, in Chittagong, Bangladesh, 64% cases were 46,XY DSD.

J. M. Hutson et al. (eds.), *Disorders|Differences of Sex Development*,
https://doi.org/10.1007/978-981-13-7864-5_22

Incidence of congenital adrenal hyperplasia (CAH) is relatively less in most developing countries. CAH was only 10% of all DSD cases in Durban which was the third most common diagnosis (Ganie et al. 2016). In our centre, 46,XX DSD comprised only 22%. The majority of CAH patients are non-salt wasting. On the contrary, in countries where newborn screening is available, salt-wasting CAH comprise 75% of babies diagnosed (Warne and Raza 2008). It can be assumed that many babies with salt-wasting CAH die undiagnosed in developing countries. In certain countries, there are also higher occurrences of certain other genetic forms. 5α-Reductase deficiency is more prevalent in Dominican Republic, Southern Lebanon and Papua New Guinea, and 17β-hydroxysteroid dehydrogenase deficiency is common in the Gaza Strip. 46,XX ovotesticular DSD is more common in South African blacks (Krstic et al. 2000; Warne and Raza 2008; Ganie et al. 2016).

22.2 Delayed Presentation

Delayed presentation is common in developing countries. Mean age at presentation in our centre was 8.7 years, 5 years ago. However, nowadays, we are starting to see more patients of younger age group and even neonates due to increasing awareness about management of DSD patients in our centre. In Durban, median age of presentation was 10 months with significant difference among aetiological groups. The majority (33%) of sex chromosome DSD patients presented after 10 years of age, two-thirds of whom had Turner syndrome. Diagnosis of Turner syndrome was missed by clinicians at infancy and childhood, and these patients presented at late childhood or adolescence with short stature and delayed puberty (Ganie et al. 2016). In a report from Nigeria, more than 80% had delayed presentation mostly due to delayed referral from primary and secondary-care centres (Ekenze et al. 2015). In male-dominant societies, it has been observed that parents seek medical advice for boys earlier than for girls. However, mean age of presentation of our DSD patients who were raised as girls was 6.8 years and that of boys was 9.7 years. Early virilization of girls noticed by parents may be the cause for earlier presentation for girls.

Delayed presentation has some particular negative influences in the diagnosis, medical management, surgical procedures and long-term outcome of patients. The window period of postnatal surge of gonadotrophins and sex steroids between 1 week and 3 months of age, which provides an important opportunity to investigate patients, is missed. Gonadotrophins and sex steroids including dehydroepiandrosterone sulfate, androstenedione, testosterone and dihydrotestosterone assay during mini-pubertal surge, before 6 months of age, help in the specific diagnosis of defects in testosterone synthesis or action in patients with 46XY DSD (Kuiri-Hanninen et al. 2014). Patients with CAH, who present late, remain exposed to ongoing virilization and develop male gender identity, and it is not uncommon to raise them as boys in developing countries. Gender-related problems have been found to be more in untreated DSD patients raised as girls who presented late than patients who received some treatment (Ediati et al. 2015). More cases of gender reassignment are reported from developing countries because of delayed presentation and wrong gender assignment in early childhood without appropriate medical evaluation. Delayed presentations of Turner syndrome had an impact on long-term outcome, because, if growth hormone therapy could be started in childhood, final height would have been improved (Davenport et al. 2007; Backeljauw 2008; Bolar et al. 2008).

Lack of adequate knowledge of health personnel regarding presentation of DSD is an important cause of delayed diagnosis and referral. In one-third of patients in Durban, who had earlier presented to hospital, diagnosis of DSD was missed, resulting in late presentations to endocrine or urologic clinics (Ganie et al. 2016). We also see many patients in whom the primary care physician missed the diagnosis. Very often, the primary physician advised the parents not to seek medical advice until puberty.

22.3 Investigations

Investigating DSD patients involves karyotyping, hormonal assays and imaging. Many centres in the developing countries do not have all the necessary facilities to completely evaluate a DSD patient. Even if the patients are referred to centres where the facilities are available, many cannot afford to go there due to financial constraints. The investigations are moderately expensive and many centres have to adopt ways of treating the patients applying clinical judgement, without the support of some important investigations. Often karyotyping is replaced by the Barr body test which makes it difficult to classify the patients according to the new consensus classification system. Proper genetic diagnosis is almost always impossible. Many centres do not have facilities to do laparoscopy or MRI. A report from Nigeria stated that they usually rely on mini pelvic laparotomy to assess the status of internal genitalia and gonads and do the Barr body estimation of buccal smear to determine genetic sex (Ekenze et al. 2015). We preferably do diagnostic laparoscopies rather than MRI, as MRI is costly and many cannot afford it. Laparoscopy is an important tool for us, and (Steven et al. 2012) showed that ultrasonography (USG) failed to identify Müllerian structures in 40% cases where laparoscopy allowed excellent visualization in complex DSD. Hormonal assays are also expensive. Parents of CAH patients do not always comply with repeated 17-OH progesterone level checks to monitor steroid therapy and come with complications of steroid treatment. The cost of most investigations has to be borne by the parents, and we have to plan investigations according to the financial capability of the family (Chowdhury et al. 2014b). If we advise an expensive investigation to a poor family, sometimes we have to miss the patient unless we arrange some funding for them to do the tests.

22.4 Treatment

Many patients are treated by inexpert doctors who do not have adequate knowledge of DSD. Hypospadias surgery is done not knowing the internal gonadal status. Proper counselling of the parents is not usually done due to lack of knowledge of the physician involved, and often misleading information is given making the management more complex. Parents' illiteracy often hinders proper counselling. The disease is not usually discussed with the patients due to lack of intellectual maturity of the children who are mostly dependent on their parents for many aspects of decision-making in their life, including even the decision to marry or choose a life partner. There is also involvement of relatives, local quack doctors, brokers and religious persons in the decision-making, who often guide them towards an unscientific way of treatment or no treatment. Many parents frequently change doctors and ultimately rely on the decision of quacks who show a cheaper way of managing things. All these factors lead to delay in the presentation to a proper centre and make treatment difficult. Even in the higher centres, multidisciplinary team involvement is not often practised, and usually, the surgeon and an adult endocrinologist are the persons involved in care. There is no paediatric endocrinologist, paediatric gynaecologist, professional genetic counsellor or paediatric psychologist in most hospitals. There is usually no patient-support group for DSD patients, and transition of adolescent patients to adult care is not methodically practised.

22.5 Sex Assignment

Societies are traditionally adherent to a binary system of gender which ensures reproductive success and continuation of species. Parents who bring their child with a DSD for medical advice usually want to raise the baby as a male or a female. The concept of third gender is not yet well accepted by the parents, although third gender is a legal right in Bangladesh, India and some other countries. This is usually confined to adult individuals who had decided to live as such. Many parents prefer male gender assignment because males enjoy social and economic independence in South Asian countries. A man can inherit his father's wealth, whereas a woman might inherit none or only half share depending on the culture. There is a lack of social security provisions such as pensions, which is why, when they are incapable of earning a livelihood, parents become totally dependent on their children for survival. In many cultures, the eldest son has special responsibilities for the welfare of the parents. In Hindu culture, the eldest son usually lights his parents' funeral pyre (Warne and Raza 2008). Most females are usually kept under the protection of their father, husband or son during different phases of their life. Many marriages are arranged by parents, and it is difficult to get an infertile girl married. Sometimes parents hide the fact and get the girl married, but often, this ends in divorce and the girl comes back to the parents' house to live with them. In cities, poor women usually manage to get a job in the garment or other manufacturing industries, or act as house maids, but in rural areas, where there is less chance of employment, they usually end up as a liability for the family.

The World Economic Forum has developed a grading system known as Global Gender Gap Index (GGGI) to characterize gender related variations among countries (World Economic Forum, 2017). This is based on economic participation and opportunity, educational attainment, health and survival and political empowerment (Meyer-Bahlburg 2017) (the 2017 GGGI ranked 144 countries from rank #1 [smallest gap between gender] to rank #144 [largest gap]). Scandinavian countries had the top ranks (#1 Iceland, #2 Norway, #3 Finland). Most developing countries had the largest gaps between genders, with men usually being in a better position. Among South Asian countries, Bangladesh ranked 47, Indonesia 84, India 108, Sri Lanka 109 and Pakistan 143. Most Middle East countries also had lowest ranks (Turkey #131, Egypt #134, Saudi Arabia #138, Iran #140, Syria #142 and Yemen #144) (World Economic Forum 2017, Table 3). This shows a striking gender bias towards males in most developing countries, which influences the decision-making during gender assignment for DSD patients.

For all the above reasons and many others, it is not uncommon in developing countries to raise DSD patients with some virilization as males (Sharma and Gupta 2012). There are reports of assignment of male gender regardless of karyotype, gonadal anatomy or fertility potentials from several countries such as Saudi Arabia, Turkey and Egypt because the male gender has a dominant role in the society. CAH girls who present late also develop a male gender identity, which plays an important role in the decision-making to raise her as a boy (Chowdhury et al. 2015). CAH patients, who had not been treated with steroid suppression, become progressively more virilized and during mid- to late childhood start to lead life as a boy. They develop a phallus, the size of which is usually more than the average size of normal boys for their age. The reared boy mixes well with other boys in the school and parents usually come to surgeons for the correction of hypospadias without having any understanding of the original defect or the status of gonads. Endeavour to raise him as a girl brings on catastrophe for the parents and the child, and they often refuse it. Many families and doctors prefer to raise him as an infertile male rather than a fertile woman. In Egypt, a 46,XX CAH patient first presented at 46 years as a man, with a male gender identity, complaining lack of erection. He denied any female behaviour and ultimately underwent hysterectomy (Mazen 2017). However, for CAH girls who present early, the general trend is to raise them as girls, do clitoral recession and feminizing genitoplasty and give steroid suppression. But many do not comply with steroid treatment well and come with complications of steroid overdose or under-treatment.

It is also not uncommon for 46,XY DSD babies with under-virilization to be raised as girls. This occurs due to inappropriate referral and lack of access to hormonal and genetic tests in some centres. Some of these patients develop gender atypical behaviour in later childhood which becomes noticeable by parents, and they seek further medical advice. Gender change is not always accepted easily by society and the family has to pass difficult times during the course of change, and, sometimes, they move out of the locality. Partial androgen insensitivity syndrome is another problematic condition for gender assignment. Children with a severe defect have almost female-looking genitalia and very mildly enlarged phallus. It is difficult to reconstruct them as males, but if they are raised as females, at some point they develop male gender identity, show aggression and become very upset and unsatisfied over the assigned sex. The situation becomes more complex if any feminizing genitoplasty had already been done on them. Many teenage patients with 5α-reductase deficiency reared as females also present with gender dysphoria (Joseph et al. 2017). In Egypt and Sudan, there is an increased rate of female circumcision, and about half of all women are circumcised. If 46,XY DSD patients raised as girls undergo circumcision, amputation of the phallus may occur and further genitoplasty becomes difficult (Mazen 2017).

However, we did not find much difficulty to convince a family to raise the baby as a female, especially when presented early, when the medical judgement led us to do so. To assign gender, due to lack of a paediatric psychologist, we rely on a gender identity questionnaire for children, child game participation questionnaire, parent report on child game participation questionnaire and sex-type toy play to aid in the decision-making of sex assignment. It has been shown that these have a good correlation with gender identity (Chowdhury et al. 2014a). The above tools help in the decision-making while we wait for appropriate sex assignment for these babies. Nonetheless, the consequences of gender reassignment are difficult for many patients to cope with, and they suffer from isolation and other forms of social and psychological difficulties which cannot often be addressed and taken care of. Gender identity confusion and cross-gender behaviour is more frequently observed in children with DSD raised as girls than as boys and most develop the wish to change gender during puberty or adulthood. In Indonesia, 21 (17 had 46,XY and 4 had 46,XX karyotype) of 118 DSD cases changed gender and all from female to male except one patient with cloacal anomaly (Ediati et al. 2015). The parents or the physician proposed the gender change in 8 patients, and 13 patients changed gender by themselves. The majority of the patients (76%) were late presenters. It has been shown that many adults with DSD in Indonesia experienced long-term gender problems, particularly those whose behaviour and interests were not in line with their assigned gender.

22.6 Socioeconomic and Cultural Influences

Different cultures treat DSD patients differently. The "serrer" of the Pokot tribe in Africa are banned from many social activities of their society (Hiort 2008). "Hijra" community in the Indian subcontinent is feared in some areas and respected in others (Joseph et al. 2017). In Vietnam, both the homosexuals and people born with genital anomaly are termed as "ai nam ai nu", which means "neither male nor female" which is often offensive for the DSD patients (Warne and Raza 2008).

Poverty is the most important setback for the adequate management of DSD patients in developing countries. Health budgets are largely consumed by public health priorities such as vaccination, antihelminthic program, tuberculosis and other infectious disease control and treatment of acute medical conditions (Warne and Raza 2008). Government healthcare systems cannot support many investigations or treatment modalities for DSD patients, and health insurance is in a preliminary stage and only affordable by higher economic societies. Community-based medical care cannot support patients of DSD. Telehealth is not practised in the hospitals and most private practices, and parents have to visit the doctor however minute the need might be. The economic consequences of multiple visits, admissions, investigations, surgeries and medication are often so large that families often search for alternate ways of managing the problem and usually find one, such as, alternative medicine or no treatment. Low levels of education makes the parents prone to superstition, social stigma and misinterpretation of religion, and all these factors hinder proper management of patients. Families are often large and there is always imbibition of different ideas from different family members and relatives which adds to the already prevailing confusion of the parents. In rural areas, the presence of large families and close interaction among neighbours make it almost impossible to hide the condition of the baby, and the child becomes a matter of gossip. In cities, parents often can keep the child isolated and travel to larger cities for treatment so that no one can know about the condition of the child. Parents of higher society often go abroad for treatment. The mother is sometimes blamed for giving birth to a malformed child. In India, two husbands sought divorce on this ground (Joseph et al. 2017). Marriage is an important phenomenon in the developing society, and whoever is not married is dealt with differently.

School support is not up to the mark most of the times, and children suffer bullying/abuse from peers, sometimes mocking from teachers. Hospitals are overcrowded and very little privacy is maintained most of the time. Very few healthcare providers appreciate the value of privacy, and children often have to endure the discomfort of examination in presence of many. In India, one gynaecologist, who delivered a child with DSD, declared the child to be hijra causing the mother both physical and mental trauma. On another occasion, hospital staff shared information of a DSD child and the baby became a matter of curiosity; some of the hospital staff looked at the genitalia and laughed at them (Joseph et al. 2017). These are actually very common scenarios in developing countries. All these factors make them vulnerable to depression, isolation, behavioural changes and psychologic disturbances. Moreover, these issues are not usually well diagnosed and not properly managed.

Some developing countries have higher levels of consanguinity. It has been suggested that it might be related to more DSD patients in these countries. In Western countries, the incidence of DSD has been estimated to be 1:5000, while Saudi Arabia and Egypt have an incidence of 1:2500 and 1:3000, respectively (Bashamboo and McElreavey 2014). Monogenic autosomal recessive disorders like 5α reductase-2 deficiency and CAH are the conditions which are associated with consanguinity. Two reports from Sudan observed parental consanguinity in 70% of cases (Abdullah et al. 2012; Ellaithi et al. 2011). Consanguinity rate in Egypt was 29–39% during the last 40 years, and there was 68.2% consanguinity rate among DSD patients (Mazen et al. 2008; Mazen 2017). Thirty percent of our DSD patients had consanguineous parents. However, none of the DSD patients in Durban had consanguineous parents, although 5% of them had positive family history (Ganie et al. 2016). There is clearly a need for further studies to address the relationship of consanguinity with DSD.

22.6.1 Hijra

In South Asia, the existence of the hijra community has a strong influence on the thinking process of parents when a DSD child is born. The word "hijra" originally stems from Urdu language, and hijras are commonly thought to be people who do not fit to binary categories of male or female either somatically or behaviourally, containing elements of both (Stenqvist 2015). They are also believed to be male-bodied feminine-identified people who have the spiritual power to bless or curse the newly wed and the newborn (Nanda 1999; Reddy 2005). They are legally treated as a third gender since 2014 in Bangladesh and India (Joseph et al. 2017). They are also referred to as hermaphrodites, eunuchs, transsexual, transvestite or intersex (Hossain 2012). Although they are commonly believed to be individuals who were born with an intersex condition, it has been found that they are a mixture of different individuals including people with DSD, boys who have been kidnapped and castrated or homosexual or transsexual individuals who join the group to earn their livelihood (Ammini et al. 2002). In India, their number has been estimated to be about half a million with Uttar Pradesh having the largest number (Nagarajan 2014). In Bangladesh it is about 30,000 to 150,000 (Firstpost 2013), with transgenders officially being a "third gender" in Bangladesh. Hijras live together in communes, dress as females with heavy makeup and adopt female behaviour with some exaggerations which are often inappropriate. They earn their living by collecting alms, extortions and performances at festivals, births and weddings. Hijras of Muslim, Christian and Hindu origins live in the same houses in Mumbai, Delhi, Chandigarh and Bengaluru, whereas in Gujarat and some other parts of India, they live apart (Nanda 1999). Hijras in Ayodhya in India are extremely respected because they are believed to be blessed by Ram for their devotion to his words (Nanda 1999). However, in Bangladesh, they are usually feared and cause discomfort because of their inappropriate behaviour, abusive speech and gestures and involvement with extortion. However, even if a transgender person wants to live a normal life, they are not well accepted in the society. One transgender man who used to work as a cleaner in a hospital was sacked from his job without paying his due salary and other service benefit when his identity was disclosed (Ahmed 2015). In certain regions, hijras take away children with DSD from their parents. This is one of the reasons that prevent some parents from seeking medical advice during infancy. However, awareness is gradually increasing among people to seek medical advice for DSD children and parents expect that with proper medical treatment, correct surgery, sex assignment and hormonal therapy their child will be able to lead a normal life.

22.6.2 Influence of Religion

Sex reassignment surgery for non-DSD transsexuals is legal in Iran and Egypt but banned in Indonesia (Mazen 2017; Meyer-Bahlburg 2017; Ediati et al. 2015). However, sex reassignment surgery for DSD patients is legal. Muslim laws in Malaysia, Saudi Arabia and Egypt give permission to do gender-assigning surgeries in cases of CAH and androgen insensitivity syndrome. These countries encourage involvement of a religious authority in the multidisciplinary team that manages the DSD patients. In Malaysia, it has been reported to be easier to convince Muslim families to assign female gender than to Chinese and Indian families residing there. The reason was thought that Malay Muslim women are entitled to inherit and control their own money, and a woman's fortune remains under her control even after divorce or when widowed, whereas within the ethnic Chinese and Indian communities, much more prestige is associated with the male role (Zainuddin and Mahdy 2017).

In Hindu religion, hijras have been linked to the action of various gods and believed to possess some divine power. The source of the power is believed to result from sexual abstinence which Hindu mythology associates with the powers of the ascetic (Nanda 1999). They are also believed to have the power to ruin by a curse.

22.7 Legal Issues

Birth registration is mandatory in Bangladesh, and it must be done before schooling and availing any social service. During registration, gender assignment has to be done. Parents usually assign a male or female gender according to the best fit. To change gender, a medical certificate from a qualified doctor explaining the reason and an affidavit from a lawyer is necessary. In Indonesia, a newborn must be assigned a female or male gender within 60 days for the birth certificate. Delayed registration or change in gender requires a legal procedure which seeks medical review (Ediati et al. 2015). Parents often face difficulties with birth registration of their child with DSD.

For infants and young children with DSD, ethical questions arise during gender assignment. The Fifth World Congress on Family Law and Children's Rights adopted a resolution to set ethical guidelines for managing DSD patients. The principles to guide the decision-making have been suggested to minimize physical and psychosocial risk to child, preserve potential for fertility, preserve or promote capacity to have satisfactory sexual relations, leave options open for the future and respect parents' wish and beliefs (Gillam et al. 2010). While ethical issues are under strict vigilance in the developed world, physicians in developing countries still enjoy some liberty in their approach to manage a DSD patient.

22.8 Problems with Compliance and Follow-Up

Adequate follow-up is a particular problem for developing countries. There are many dropouts, and people frequently change doctors since there is usually no well-organized referral system. Poor educational status makes it difficult to make them realize the importance of long-term follow-up in DSD patients. Poverty and many other factors, such as psychological stress of the baby from multiple examinations, multiple procedures, expensive investigations, lack of privacy, lack of support from medical staffs and long queues, make parents reluctant to visit doctors. There is also a lack of support groups to keep them motivated. A patient who underwent gonadectomy did not come for hormone replacement therapy and later presented to the gynaecology outpatient department with bone demineralization. Patients with gonadal tumours also do not maintain regular follow-up and are in danger of adverse outcome. However, patient counselling is not also always up to the mark.

Poor medical record management is another drawback in these countries. People have to carry their own medical records during visits to doctors or hospitals and sometimes the records are damaged by flood or fire, or lost. Hospital records are usually destroyed every few years due to scarcity of place for keeping records. There is also no digital record keeping in most hospitals. Doctors' interest is also low in dealing with DSD patients and doctors involved in their care are sometimes mocked by their peers. These are some of the reasons for lack of long-term outcome studies in DSD patients in developing countries.

22.9 Our Experience

What are the questions our parents of DSD patients frequently ask? Below is a list. We will end the discussion by sharing some stories of our patients.

Frequently asked questions by parents regarding DSD are as follows:

- Is the baby a boy or girl? (Confusion about gender)
- Will the patient survive?
- Why does it happen?
- Is it the mother's fault? (Blame on mother)
- Is it correctable?
- Should the patient be reared as boy or girl?
- Will they be able to lead their life as normal boy/girl?
- Is it ok for them to go to school?
- Will they be able to get married?
- Can the patient have children?
- Questions about the behavioural patterns.
- Why do they rub their vulva/perineum with pointed objects? (particularly in CAH, in clitoroplasty)
- Why couldn't it be prenatally diagnosed?
- Aasar of Jin/Pori? (Influence of invisible creatures)
- Ask for confidentiality—do not want other family members to know.

22.9.1 Some Stories

22.9.1.1 Story 1

MU, whose father is an expatriate, was born in a maternity hospital in the city where the baby's uncle used to work as a ward boy. The doctor announced her to be a girl and the baby was raised as a girl. The mother later delivered three other baby girls. This middle-class family always wished to have a boy. One day the mother noticed an erection of the penis over the clothes when the child was 14 years old, she became puzzled, discussed with her husband and they sought medical advice and was referred to us. The patient also noticed the anomaly at the same time and discussed with the mother about it. Karyotype showed 46,XY, and the patient was diagnosed as 46,XY DSD with scrotal hypospadias. Both testes were descended, there was no female internal genitalia on USG and cystoscopy showed a small vaginal remnant. The family became very happy to learn that he was a boy and they gave a feast in the community. The father believes that God has changed the gender of his child because he prayed to God during

"Hajj" to give him a boy. Many people came to see him and he got print and electronic media coverage. Orthoplasty was done, and he awaits hypospadias repair. The family gave him a male name, AM, and did all the necessary procedures to change name and gender in all certificates. He is a more than an average student and is in grade 10 now.

22.9.1.2 Story 2

In April 2016, SH, raised as a boy, was brought to CMCH with huge abdominal distension and was found severely ill, anaemic and anorexic. The patient also showed symptoms of failure to thrive. On further examination, the 13-year-old (46,XY) was found to have proximal hypospadias, enlarged breast and firm abdominal mass. The patient was diagnosed as having gonadoblastoma, mixed gonadal dysgenesis and horse shoe kidney. Family prioritized the other healthy children and overlooked this child because of financial and social issues. This patient was also sexually abused. In May 2016, laparotomy was done. A huge mass arising from left gonadal streak was removed with all the lymph nodes and seedlings, as many as possible. After the surgery, the patient did not come for follow-up. On 11 November 2017 (19 months later), the patient was brought again with weight loss, anaemia and recurrence. On 23 November 2017, the patient had been given one cycle of chemotherapy by bleomycin, etoposide and cisplatin and is on chemotherapy now.

22.9.1.3 Story 3

MM1, raised as a boy, came with the complaints of cyclical haematuria, pubic hair and axillary hair at the age of 7 years. He had a fully developed phallus of Prader 5. Laparoscopy showed streak gonad on the left with fallopian tube and left hemi-uterus, and an ovotestis on the right side. As the parents wanted to raise him as a boy, excision of vagina and left hemi-uterus with bilateral gonadectomy was done. He suffered from recurrent urinary tract infections and developed some behavioural changes. At last follow-up, he was found to be of short stature and had gynecomastia on and off. According to the advice of endocrinologist, he is on glucocorticoid/mineralocorticoid.

22.9.1.4 Story 4

MM2 was diagnosed as androgen insensitivity syndrome (46,XY DSD) 8 years ago and is now 19 years of age. During his regular testosterone injections, he developed persistent vomiting along with difficulty in micturition. He was also psychologically disturbed. He used to seek attention of doctors whenever he thought he was having some problem, whether it was insignificant or important. He had undergone fundoplication and orchidopexy. He also went to India for the purpose of treatment. He did not pursue school, and unsatisfied with the health system of Bangladesh or India he wants to consult new doctors.

22.9.1.5 Story 5

RR, raised as a boy, presented at 17 years with short stature (female facial features but behavioural attributes of a boy). After evaluation, the child was found to have 46,XX karyotype and had a Prader scale of 3. Ultrasound, laparoscopy and cystoscopic examination revealed presence of uterus and ovaries. The patient reported to have menstrual bleeding. The parents wanted to continue raising him as a boy which was also the desire of the child. The patient's father used to work in the Middle East, and he had three other daughters. The parents and the patient were informed that the patient would not be able to have any children in the future, but they persisted on converting the patient into a boy. So the female genital organs were removed and testosterone injections were advised regularly.

References

Abdullah MA, Saeed U, Abass A, et al. Disorders of sex development among Sudanese children: 5-year experience of a pediatric endocrinology clinic. J Pediatr Endocrinol Metab. 2012;25(11–12):1065–72.

Ammini AC, Gupta R, Kapoor A, et al. Etiology, clinical profile, gender identity and long-term follow up of patients with ambiguous genitalia in India. J Pediatr Endocrinol Metab. 2002;15(4):423–30.

Backeljauw P. Does growth hormone therapy before 4 years of age enhance the linear growth of girls with Turner's syndrome? Nat Clin Pract Endocrinol Metab. 2008;4(2):78–9.

Bashamboo A, McElreavey K. Consanguinity and disorders of sex development. Hum Hered. 2014;77(1–4):108–17.

Bolar K, Hoffman AR, Maneatis T, et al. Long-term safety of recombinant human growth hormone in turner syndrome. J Clin Endocrinol Metab. 2008;93(2): 344–51.

Chowdhury TK, Chowdhury MZ, Mili F, et al. Gender identity shows a high correlation with Prader score in patients with disorders of sex development (DSD) presenting in mid childhood. Pediatr Surg Int. 2014a;30(5):527–32.

Chowdhury TK, Kabir M, Chowdhury MZ, et al. The challenges in diagnosis and gender assignment in disorders of sex development presenting to a pediatric surgical unit in a developing country: the role of laparoscopy and simple tests for gender identity. J Pediatr Urol. 2014b;10(6):1255–60.

Chowdhury TK, Laila K, Hutson JM, et al. Male gender identity in children with 46,XX DSD with congenital adrenal hyperplasia after delayed presentation in mid-childhood. J Pediatr Surg. 2015;50(12):2060–2.

Davenport ML, Crowe BJ, Travers SH, et al. Growth hormone treatment of early growth failure in toddlers with Turner syndrome: a randomized, controlled, multicenter trial. J Clin Endocrinol Metab. 2007;92(9):3406–16.

Ediati A, Juniarto AZ, Birnie E, et al. Gender development in Indonesian children, adolescents, and adults with disorders of sex development. Arch Sex Behav. 2015;44(5):1339–61.

Ekenze SO, Nwangwu EI, Amah CC, et al. Disorders of sex development in a developing country: perspectives and outcome of surgical management of 39 cases. Pediatr Surg Int. 2015;31(1):93–9.

Ellaithi M, Kamel A, Saber O. Consanguinity and disorders of sexual developments in the Sudan. Sudan J Med Sci. 2011;6:267–70.

Ganie Y, Aldous C, Balakrishna Y. Disorders of sex development in children in KwaZulu-Natal Durban South Africa. J Pediatr Endocrinol Metab. 2016;30(1):11–8.

Gillam LH, Hewitt JK, Warne GL. Ethical principles for the management of infants with disorders of sex development. Horm Res Paediatr. 2010;74:412–8.

Hiort O. Alternative gender categories in different cultures: lessons to be learnt. Commentary on Lang and Kuhnle: intersexuality and alternative gender categories in non-Western cultures (Horm Res 2008;69:240–250). Horm Res. 2008;69(4):251–2.

Hossain A. Beyond emasculation: being Muslim and becoming Hijra in South Asia. Asian Stud Rev. 2012;36:495–513.

Joseph AA, Kulshreshtha B, Shabir I, et al. Gender issues and related social stigma affecting patients with a disorder of sex development in India. Arch Sex Behav. 2017;46(2):361–7.

Krstic ZD, Smoljanic Z, Vukanic D, et al. True hermaphroditism: 10 years' experience. Pediatr Surg Int. 2000;16(8):580–3.

Kuiri-Hanninen T, Sankilampi U, Dunkel L. Activation of the hypothalamic-pituitary-gonadal axis in infancy: minipuberty. Horm Res Paediatr. 2014;82(2):73–80.

Mazen IA. Clinical management of gender in Egypt: intersexuality and transsexualism. Arch Sex Behav. 2017;46(2):369–72.

Mazen I, Hiort O, Bassiouny R, et al. Differential diagnosis of disorders of sex development in Egypt. Horm Res. 2008;70(2):118–23.

Meyer-Bahlburg HF. Introduction to the special section on culture and variants of sex/gender: bias and stigma. Arch Sex Behav. 2017;46(2):337–9.

Nanda S. Neither man nor woman: the hijras of India. Belmont: Wadsworth Publishing Company; 1999.

Reddy G. With respect to sex: negotiating hijra identity in South India. Chicage: University of Chicago Press; 2005.

Sharma S, Gupta DK. Male genitoplasty for 46 XX congenital adrenal hyperplasia patients presenting late and reared as males. Indian J Endocrinol Metab. 2012;16(6):935–8.

Steven M, O'Toole S, Lam JP, et al. Laparoscopy versus ultrasonography for the evaluation of Mullerian structures in children with complex disorders of sex development. Pediatr Surg Int. 2012;28(12):1161–4.

Warne GL, Raza J. Disorders of sex development (DSDs), their presentation and management in different cultures. Rev Endocr Metab Disord. 2008;9(3):227–36.

Zainuddin AA, Mahdy ZA. The Islamic perspectives of gender-related issues in the management of patients with disorders of sex development. Arch Sex Behav. 2017;46(2):353–60.

Short, Medium and Long-Term Outcomes for DSD at The Royal Children's Hospital

23

John M. Hutson

23.1 Introduction

Although some children may present after the neonatal period, most babies are noted to have a DSD at birth when the genitalia are sufficiently atypical that immediate sex assignment by the midwife is difficult. This challenging situation needs a multidisciplinary team to manage the various psychological, psychosocial, hormonal and surgical issues (Houk et al. 2006).

Our hospital has been a tertiary centre specialising in DSD management for many years, and we continue to offer the option of surgical intervention to patients with DSD. Reasons in favour of early surgery include the maternal oestrogenic effect on the genitalia which appears to aid wound healing, benefits in terms of ease of post-operative care and satisfactory long-term results, which are described in this chapter (Lean et al. 2005; Warne et al. 2005; Crawford et al. 2009). Evidence from the outcomes of severe hypospadias repair has demonstrated that early surgery has a significant psychological benefit as the child has no long-term memory of their hospital experiences (Jones et al. 2009). While some centres have adopted a preference to defer feminising genital surgery until adolescence, published data from a cohort of women with CAH indicated the majority (20/29) stated a preference for early genital surgery (Nordenskjöld et al. 2008).

Currently, there remains a significant controversy surrounding early intervention in DSD. We continue to offer early surgical intervention for some children with DSD, as part of a multidisciplinary management strategy within a holistic treatment plan (see also Chap. 17). This chapter describes our short-term, medium-term and long-term outcomes.

23.2 Short-Term Results

Operative outcomes for infants with 46,XX congenital adrenal hyperplasia (CAH) have demonstrated that the complication rates are low. Of n = 72 identified from hospital databases (1974–2014), one had a significant operative complication (of bowel perforation). Approximately 50% had undergone surgery at <5 months of age, 10% between 6 and 12 months, 25% from 1 to 2 years of age and the remainder above this age (Bogdanska et al. 2018). (In recent years, the surgery is not being performed in babies <6 months of age.) Reoperation rates have been very low, with only two infants requiring repeat surgery (one associated with wound breakdown in an

J. M. Hutson (✉)
Department of Urology, The Royal Children's Hospital, Melbourne, VIC, Australia

Murdoch Children's Research Institute, Melbourne, VIC, Australia

Department of Paediatrics, University of Melbourne, Melbourne, VIC, Australia
e-mail: john.hutson@rch.org.au

J. M. Hutson et al. (eds.), *Disorders|Differences of Sex Development*,
https://doi.org/10.1007/978-981-13-7864-5_23

infant who was mobilising, and the other, for closure of the colostomy). Further surgery for revision of the feminising genitoplasty has consisted of only minor surgery (requiring only day stay or overnight admission), although dilators have been required by a few.

The records of children born between 1997 and 2003 (aged 5–10 years at the time of study) who had had their care at The Royal Children's Hospital (RCH) were reviewed after ethical approval (Crawford et al. 2009). The diagnosis, date of birth and dates of surgical intervention were recorded. After informed consent, the children were examined and the genitalia scored on a modified scale initially used by Creighton et al. (2001), and they also completed the paediatric quality-of-life (PedsQL) inventory (4.0) (Varni et al. 2001, 2002, 2003). In addition, parents also completed the parent-report version of the quality-of-life inventory, as well as the gender identity questionnaire for children (GIQC) (Johnson et al. 2004).

The physical examination included evaluation of gross anatomical and cosmetic factors using the following criteria: symmetry of the genitalia, clitoral size and position, number of perineal openings and size of the labia majora and minora. Males were evaluated for stretched penile length, testicular volume, symmetry of the genitalia, presence of chordee, position of the urethral meatus, scrotal position and degree of fusion, and location of the testes within the scrotum. An overall cosmetic score for the genitalia was given for both males and females from good, to satisfactory or poor. 'Good' was determined as the genitalia appeared normal with no abnormal features. 'Satisfactory' was described as up to two minor abnormalities but unlikely to be judged as abnormal by a non-medically trained person. 'Poor' was defined as the genitalia appeared abnormal, with three or more abnormal features.

The PedsQL Generic Score Scales (4.0), for both child and parent questionnaires, have been validated and contain 23 items divided into physical (eight items) and psychological (15 items) domains. Each question addresses whether or not an item has been a problem in the past month on a score from 0 (never a problem) to 4 (always a problem). The items are then scored in reverse and transformed into a scale of 100 so that higher scores indicate better quality of life.

The gender identity questionnaire for children (GIQC) is a validated parent-report questionnaire designed to screen for a gender identity disorder in paediatric populations (Johnson et al. 2004). The questionnaire contains 16 items addressing a range of sexual behaviours, and each one of these is scored on a 5-point Likert scale: higher scores indicate a same-gender behaviour, and lower scores indicate cross-gender behaviour.

Fifty-four children were identified from the medical records to be eligible for participation in the study. Ten patients were lost to follow-up, and three patients refused to participate. Sixteen girls had CAH, two had ovo-testicular DSD and one had XX virilisation. The diagnoses in the boys included five with 45,X/46,XY mixed gonadal dysgenesis, three partial androgen insensitivity syndrome (PAIS), three with ovo-testicular DSD and six with XY undervirilisation. There were five others with vanishing testis syndrome, Klinefelter syndrome, 5α-reductase-2 deficiency, 17β hydroxysteroid dehydrogenase (HSD) deficiency and placental insufficiency. The mean age at first surgical intervention was 13.2 months, and the mean age at follow-up was 7.5 ± 2.1 years.

Anatomical evaluation was undertaken on 13 of the 19 females, with 11 receiving a good cosmetic score and two receiving a satisfactory score. Twenty-one boys were examined, with 11 scored as good, 8 satisfactory and 2 poor (Fig. 23.1). The most commonly found atypical feature in the boys was short-stretched-penile length. In many cases, stretched penile length was reduced, with only 10 of 21 boys having a penile length within two standard deviations of the normal. Quality-of-life questionnaires showed that both children and parents rated their physical quality of life as being close to reported values for healthy children, with the only exception being the boys who rated their physical quality of life as lower (Crawford et al. 2009). For psychosocial quality of life, both children and their parents rated this lower than for healthy children, with boys scoring 67 and girls 76 (compared with normal values of 70 and 79, respectively) (Fig. 23.2a, b).

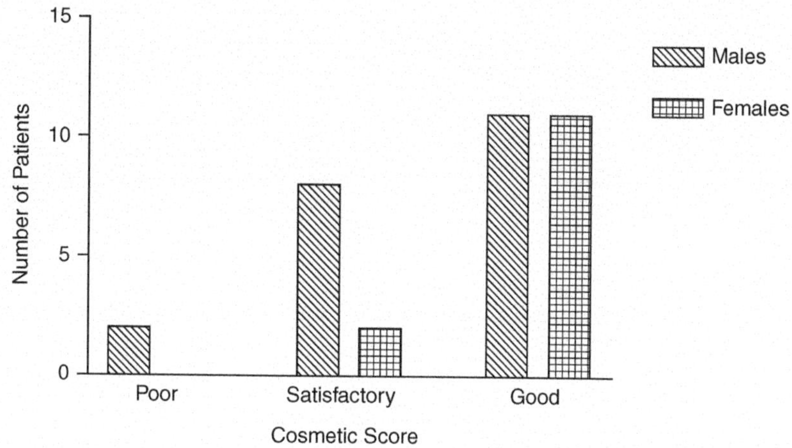

Fig. 23.1 Cosmetic results of early surgery by gender in 5–10-year-olds (Reproduced with permission from Crawford et al. 2009)

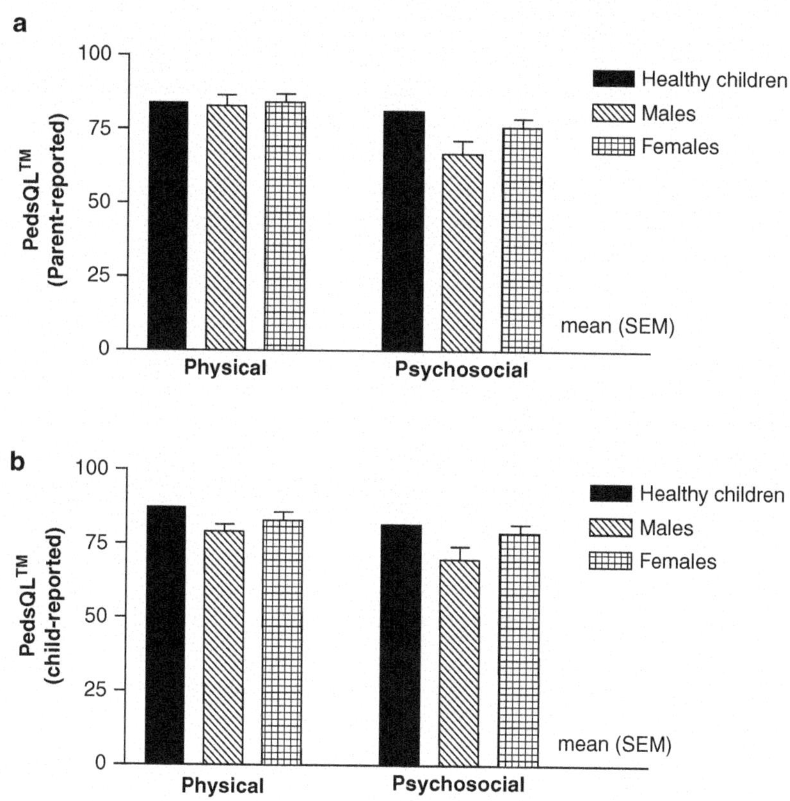

Fig. 23.2 (**a**) Parent-reported PedsQL™ scores: healthy children (Varni et al. 2003) (solid black bar), male DSD group (striped bar) and female DSD group (cross-hatched bar). (**b**) Child-reported PedsQL™ scores: healthy children (Varni et al. 2003) (solid black bar), male DSD group (striped bar) and female DSD group (cross-hatched bar) (Reproduced with permission from Crawford et al. 2009)

The mean scores for the gender identity questionnaire differed between females and males. The mean score for girls was 3.56, compared with 3.95 for boys. One male and three females (with CAH) had a score of 3 or less, which is in the range where there may be a risk of a gender identity disorder later in life (Fig. 23.3).

These short-term results showed that early genital surgery produced satisfactory cosmetic results for 100% of females and 90% of males. More importantly, when surgery was part of a holistic management plan, an early intervention strategy appeared to result in minimal impairment of quality of life or risk of gender dyspho-

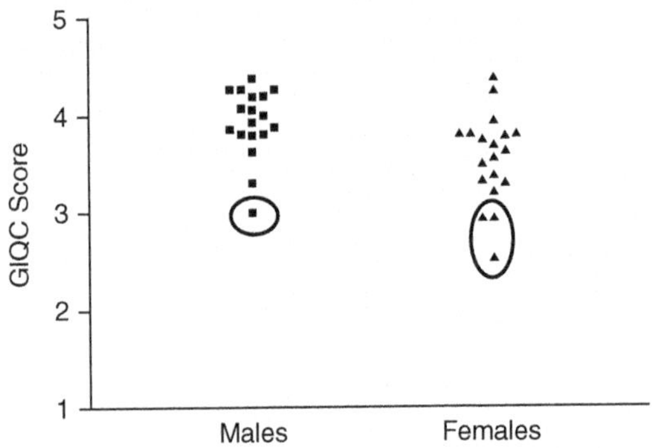

Fig. 23.3 Gender Identity Questionnaire for Children (GIQC) by gender. Data points within circles represent those children at risk of gender dysphoria or gender identity disorder. The three females with low scores had CAH, while the boy had PAIS (Reproduced with permission from Crawford et al. 2009)

ria. The finding that the majority of our younger patients had acceptable cosmetic results agrees with recent reports in the literature. Roll et al. (2006) found that 13 out of 19 patients had excellent results and 6 out of 19 had good cosmetic results on a 4-point scale.

The physical quality of life of these children, reported both by themselves and by their parents, was in the same range as that reported by normal children (5–7 years of age) except for males who had a lower physical quality of life. On the psychosocial scale, girls and their parents reported quality of life to be only slightly lower than that reported by normal children, while both boys and their parents had significantly lower psychosocial quality of life, which is probably related to the poorer cosmetic results related to the micropenis in the boys.

The gender questionnaire showed that these children had more cross-gender behaviour traits than children without a DSD. This is consistent with other studies of gender behaviour in boys with PAIS (Jurgensen et al. 2007) and in girls with CAH (Berenbaum and Bailey 2003). This behaviour is thought to be due to prenatal hormone exposure, which is well described in girls with CAH, although after puberty they did not experience higher levels of gender dysphoria (Zucker et al. 1996).

Although some patients were lost to follow-up, the records showed that these underwent fewer operations and were slightly older than those who were reviewed, suggesting that non-participants may actually have experienced better outcomes than those seen in the clinic. Many of these patients lost to follow-up were from interstate or overseas.

This review of short-term results did not reveal any significant concerns or problems arising as a consequence of early surgical intervention in DSD. When part of a holistic management plan, surgery produced good early cosmetic outcomes, achieved functional outcomes and minimal impairment of quality of life.

23.3 Medium-Term Results

We have also undertaken a medium-term follow-up of our female patients with DSD to examine the anatomical and cosmetic outcomes following early surgery with feminising genitoplasty (Lean et al. 2005). Patients were identified through the medical records who had undergone feminising genitoplasty between 1970 and 1991, with their age at time of review of 13–33 years. All girls and young women were reviewed in the paediatric and adolescent gynaecology clinic for follow-up. As part of their routine outpatient review, examination was undertaken with informed consent in those agreeing to genital examination. The patient held a hand mirror to enable herself to view the perineum while examination was being performed. A standard genital examination was carried out utilising a modified assessment from Creighton et al. (2001). This included scores for symmetry and overall genital proportions, clitoral position and size, appearance of vaginal introitus, and labial appearance and proportions (from normal to full fusion). Presence or absence of a clitoral hood was an addition to this standardised assessment. The quality of genital skin and the distribution of pubic hair was also assessed. Overall cosmetic outcomes were assigned into categories of ‘good’ (normal genital appearance unlikely to be judged abnormal by non-medical persons), ‘satisfactory’ (two or less minor anomalies unlikely to be judged abnormal by a non-medical person), or ‘poor’ outcome (genitalia abnormal, three or more abnormal features). Patients were divided into four groups

Table 23.1 Diagnoses and surgical procedures

Diagnosis	Number of patients (%)	Surgery	Number of patients
CAH	15 (45)	Clitoral reduction	23
MGD 45,X/46, XY	7 (17)	Clitoral recession	2
PAIS	5 (15)	Clitoral excision	3*
Ovotesticular DSD	0 (1)	Labial reconstruction	27
17β-HSD deficiency	3 (3)	V-Y vaginoplasty	29
Androgen exposure	1 (3)	Vaginal pull-through	5
Pan hypopituitarism	1(1)		

Reproduced with permission from Lean et al. 2005
*Two clitoral excisions were done elsewhere. One was done at RCH in the 1970's

depending on whether or not further treatment was required: no further treatment, dilatation, minor surgery or major surgery.

Eighty-two patients were identified from the medical records, and 21 of these had moved interstate or overseas and were lost to follow-up. A representative sample of 32 out of the remaining 61 patients were examined during the time course of the study, in the gynaecology clinic. Of those patients who were not examined, they had a similar range of diagnoses as those who were seen, and their surgical management was identical to those who were seen in the clinic.

The diagnoses of all patients and the 32 who were seen in the gynaecology clinic are listed in Table 23.1. Fifteen of these had CAH, while the remaining 17 had a range of other conditions. The mean age at examination was 18.4 years (range 12–32 years), with no significant difference between those patients with adrenal hyperplasia and other diagnoses.

Ten of the 32 patients had their first operation done elsewhere before being referred to The Royal Children's Hospital in Melbourne. The types of procedure are listed in Table 23.2. Half of the patients had a planned single-stage genital reconstruction, and 5 of these 16 needed vaginal dilatation in adolescence, and one patient had a repeat flap vaginoplasty at 9 years of age. One other adolescent girl had a further reduction of the bulk of the corpus spongiosum and corpora cavernosa and a vaginoplasty. Of the 16 having a planned single-stage procedure, 14 achieved a good cosmetic outcome. In 17 patients where more than one genital operation had been done, 10 (59%) had a good cosmetic outcome, and 5

Table 23.2 Anatomic outcomes of feminising genital surgery

	Normal	Abnormal
Clitoris	24	8 (1 large, 3 small, 4 absent)
Clitoral position	30	2
Vaginal introitus	20	12 (small)
Introital position	30	2
Labia majora	26	6 (1 small, 5 poor/ scrotal)
Labia minora	15	17 (4 small, 2 poor, 11 absent)

(29%) had satisfactory outcomes. Only two patients (12%) had poor cosmetic outcomes (Fig. 23.4).

Half the patients had had surgery before 2 years of age, and 12 of these had a good outcome, which was the same as those having surgery after 2 years of age.

Twenty-nine out of 32 patients had undergone clitoral reduction and vaginoplasty, and 27 had also had surgery to the labia. The majority of patients whose surgery was done by one of the dedicated surgeons in our team appeared to have a normal clitoris on examination. By contrast, those who had undergone reduction of the clitoris elsewhere by non-specialised surgeons showed the poorer outcomes, with the clitoris being either too small, too big or absent (Fig. 23.5).

Overall cosmetic outcome for the genitalia was graded as good in 23 out of 32 patients and was satisfactory in 7 with only 2 patients (6%) having an overall poor cosmetic appearance. Of the 22 patients who had been operated in our centre entirely, 19 had a good outcome and 3 had a

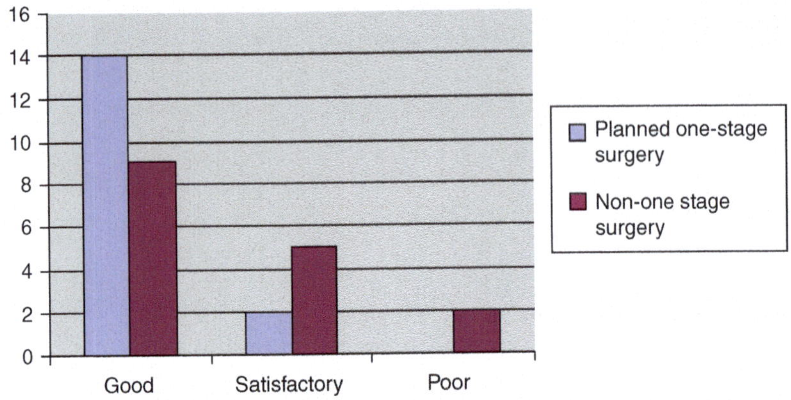

Fig. 23.4 Cosmetic outcomes in females of planned one-stage reconstruction (pale bar) versus multiple stages (dark bar) (Reproduced with permission from Lean et al. 2005)

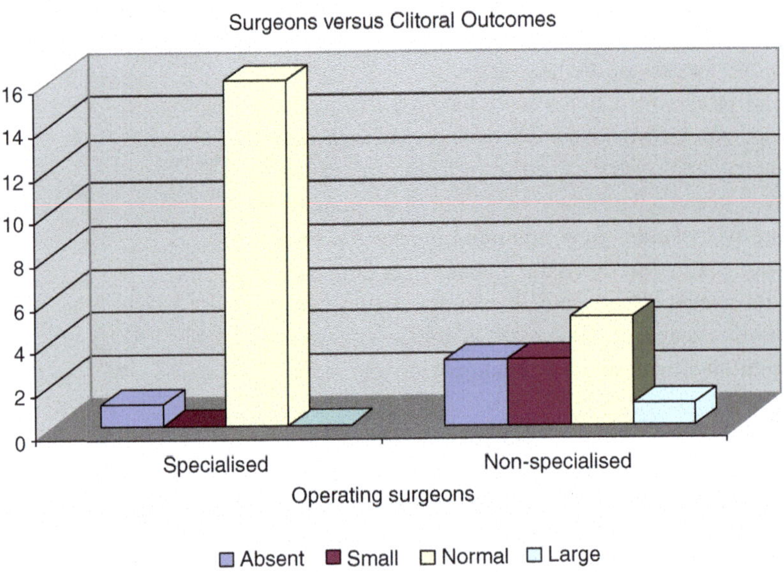

Fig. 23.5 Anatomic outcomes for clitoris versus experience of surgeon (dark grey bar; black bar, small; white bar, normal; light grey bar, large) (reproduced with permission of J Pediatr Surg)

satisfactory outcome. When overall and cosmetic outcomes were analysed on the basis of location of the initial surgery, it was found that those patients who had had their initial surgery at The Royal Children's Hospital had much better outcomes (18/22 compared with those who had had their initial surgery elsewhere 3/10).

This audit of medium- to long-term surgical results showed that planned one-stage surgery done in an institution with a dedicated team gave a better outcome than multistage surgery, which appeared to be associated with increased scarring and fibrosis.

These results support concentration of patients to a specialist referral centre. Sotiropoulos et al. (1976) reviewed 32 females between 5 and 22 years of age and reported good functional and cosmetic results following clitoral recession or resection. In their cohort, many girls who had vaginoplasty done before puberty required surgical revision in adolescence. Alizai et al. (1999) has also reported the need for repeat vaginoplasty in adolescence, with poor results correlating with surgeons' lack of expertise and experience. This correlation of surgical skill with outcome is consistent with our own results, where the poorest results were observed in surgery done by non-specialised surgeons. The different outcomes for vaginoplasty may relate to the different techniques used over 10–30 years. Other authors also reported satisfactory outcomes with single-stage infantile repair but have not provided a standardised assessment method (Azziz et al. 1986; Gonzalez and Fernandes 1990).

The results reported from centres in the UK, particularly those by Creighton et al. (2001), are in marked contrast to those reported here. Using similarly objective measures to those used in this study, they found that 41% of patients had poor cosmetic outcomes, and 98% required further treatment for cosmetic reasons. Moreover, of those women who had planned single-stage surgery in infancy or childhood, 89% required further major surgery. This is in stark contrast to our own studies where very few required further major surgery; in fact, only 2 out of 32 patients required further major surgery, 3 patients required minor vaginal surgery and 13 required dilatation. The reason for these very different results is probably related to the fact that the management of these patients in The Royal Children's Hospital has been centralised into a team of experts for many years, while the patients reported by Creighton et al. (2001) had been referred from various centres in the UK, and they were presumably biased to include those with poorer outcomes. Another difference between this review and the Creighton study is that our own patients were mostly examined in the outpatient clinic with the patient involved in the examination with a mirror, while in the series described by Creighton et al., many of the patients had their examination under anaesthesia. We found that examination under anaesthesia was infrequently required, and that examination in the clinic allowed the young woman to maintain some sense of self-control and autonomy.

Although our sample size was relatively small, and only half of those patients who were eligible were actually examined, the population seen was deemed to be representative of the total population of patients. One of the arguments in favour of early surgery is avoidance of long-term memory of the surgical procedure. This has not been studied often in patients having feminising genitoplasty but has been reviewed in our own clinic in patients raised as boys having hypospadias repair (Jones et al. 2009). When boys had surgery at an early age, which was completed prior to primary school, they demonstrated no serious psychological disturbance and no memory of the intervention at 13–15 years of age (Jones et al. 2009).

These results show that operations in early infancy done in a referral centre can produce satisfactory anatomical and cosmetic outcomes with a very low incidence of the need for major secondary surgery in adolescence. Although some adolescent girls needed dilatation of the vagina, this was done at the time that they were able to co-operate in the management, and it was perceived by them to be far superior to the need for further surgery. Single-stage surgery, if done by surgeons in an expert referral centre, can have a positive impact on anatomical and cosmetic outcome, obviating the need for major surgery in adolescence.

23.4 Long-Term Psychosocial and Psychosexual Outcomes in Young Adults

We have had a multidisciplinary team involved in the management of patients with DSD and have been pioneers in promoting full disclosure of the diagnosis to parents since 1984. Since 1992, the multidisciplinary team has met regularly to discuss and share experience about patients and their problems, with the addition of a clinic coordinator and expansion of the team meetings since 2016. This enabled us to develop a holistic, patient-centred model of care which has permitted us to provide parent support and encourage development of professional-parent discussion groups and counselling groups, as well as the production of educational material. Since 1996, we have aimed for full disclosure to patients as well as parents.

Although we felt we were doing well with their long-term management of psychological and psychosexual problems, outcomes in our young adult patients were unknown. We therefore decided to review our patients from 18 to 32 years of age to try and assess whether they were doing well enough on psychosocial and psychosexual issues (Warne et al. 2005).

Table 23.3 Diagnoses and identified gender of patients seen in long-term follow-up study

	Males	Females	Total
Mixed gonadal dysgenesis 45,X/46,XY (MGD)	1	1	2
Pure gonadal dysgenesis (PGD)		3	3
Congenital adrenal hyperplasia (CAH)	1	14	16
Complete androgen insensitivity syndrome (CAIS)		3	3
Partial androgen insensitivity syndrome (PAIS)	2	2	4
Vaginal agenesis		5	5
Severe hypospadias	11		11
17-β Hydroxysteroid dehydrogenase (17β-HSD) deficiency		1	2
5-α Reductase-2 deficiency	1		1
Post danazole therapy *in utero*		1	1
Cloacal anomaly		1	1
Bifid urethra and ectopic urethra	1		1
Total	17	31	50

Notes: (1) One person with CAH was assigned female and did not report identifying as male or female, and one person with 17β-HSD deficiency was assigned female now wishes to be identified as male, female, transgender and intersex. The two people (CAH and PAIS) who were assigned female and who now identify as male were included in the male column. (2) The phenotypic similarities of women with vaginal agenesis and CAIS result in similar long-term issues, thus the sample included participants with these diagnoses

The populations of this study included patients between 18 and 32 years of age who had been treated at The Royal Children's Hospital for a DSD. The sample, not surprisingly, comprised a range of conditions, the most common of which was CAH. We also included those boys with very severe penoscrotal hypospadias and children with AIS, gonadal dysgenesis as well as those girls with vaginal agenesis and other patients with rare conditions (Table 23.3). A total of 148 patients were identified on a search of the medical records, although 11 of these patients had died. From our initial list, we found that one patient had a congenital anomaly too minor to consider as part of the series and five patients had hypospadias that was not considered serious enough to be included in the DSD group. Thirty-one patients were lost to follow-up, three were excluded because they resided in remote locations and two were excluded because of intellectual disability. Of the 95 patients still potentially eligible to review, 27 declined to participate and 68 were sent study materials, and 50 of these returned completed questionnaires (Table 23.4). This gave us an overall participation rate of 53%.

To provide an adequate group of clinical control patients, we chose young people with Hirschsprung disease, which is a congenital anomaly affecting the bowel which typically requires surgery in infancy, as well as ongoing regular treatment and follow-up visits to the hospital. We found 51 patients with Hirschsprung disease in the database, and of those 27 completed a questionnaire, giving a participation rate of 53%. We also had a second control group of patients with insulin-dependent diabetes mellitus (IDDM). IDDM is a chronic illness usually diagnosed in childhood or adolescence, which requires regular visits to the endocrinologist for treatment and ongoing medical advice. There were 59 patients invited to participate, and 19 completed the questionnaires, with a participation rate of 32% (Table 23.5).

After approval by the human ethics committee, all potential participants were sent an invitation letter and consent form from the relevant medical specialist involved in their care. This was followed up by a telephone call to address any unresolved issues, and then, consenting participants were sent a questionnaire booklet, which was described as a quality-of-life and well-being survey, investigating the long-term outcomes of people who had been treated for conditions caused by variations in sexual development before birth. The patients with DSD were told that their responses would help provide an understanding of how medical management has affected different areas of their life. The

Table 23.4 Study measures

Construct	Measure	Scales	Scoring	Reliability
General health	Rand-36 Health Status Inventory (RAND-36 HSI)	Three composite scales labelled Physical Health, Mental Health and Global Health	Standardized scale T scores are calculated using item response theory and age-based normative weighting (mean = 50, SD = 10)	Cronbach's alpha coefficient estimates ranged from 0.73 to 0.95
Interpersonal problems	Inventory of Interpersonal Problems (IIP-32)	Eight subscales + a total score	Scores converted to standardized T scores (mean = 50, SD = 10)	Scale reliability coefficients ranged from 0.63 to 0.85
Personality	Eysenck Personality Questionnaire Revised (EPQR)	Three scales labelled Psychoticism, Neuroticism and Extraversion	Responses on a dichotomous scale (yes/no). Items are summed to compute scale scores	Scale reliability coefficients ranged from 0.61 to 0.88
Self-esteem	Coopersmith Self-esteem Inventory (SEI)	Total score	Items endorsed on a dichotomous scale ('like me' or 'unlike me') generating a total score	The reliability coefficient was 0.86
Anxiety	State-Trait Anxiety Inventory, Form Y (STAI)	Measures state anxiety—a level of emotional intensity at a given moment in time + trait anxiety—a stable personality characteristic of anxiety-proneness	Forty items are rated from 1 to 4 and summed to compute both a state and trait score, each having a range from 20 to 80	Reliability coefficients for the two scales were 0.93 and 0.94
Trauma symptoms	Impact of Event Scale—Revised (IES-R)	A 22-item questionnaire rates stressful events The three subscales closely follow the DSM-IV criteria for PTSD, measuring avoidance, intrusion (re-experiencing) and hyperarousal, together with a total score	Level of distress for each event is rated on a 5-point scale from 0 (not at all) to 4 (extremely). Subscale scores were computed by calculating the average score. A total scale score was computed by summing the three subscale scores	Reliability coefficients ranged from 0.84 to 0.94
Depression	Beck Depression Inventory, Short Form (BDI)	Total score	The 13 items are scored on a 4-point scale and summed to compute a total score	The reliability coefficient for the scale was 0.89
Gender identity	Personal Attributes Questionnaire (PAQ)	The questionnaire comprises a masculinity (or instrumental) scale, a femininity (or expressive) scale and a third masculinity-femininity scale consisting of items considered to be socially desirable for one sex, but not the other	Each item was scored from 0 to 4 and summed to compute scale scores. The feminine items on the masculinity-femininity scale are recoded so that high scores indicate masculinity	Reliability coefficients for the scales ranged from 0.57 to 0.72
	The Bem Sex Role Inventory (BSRI)	The inventory measures gender identity on the masculinity-femininity dimensional scale	Respondents rate 30 traits on a scale from 1 (never or almost never true) to 7 (always or almost always true). A difference score is then calculated, with T scores of 50 indicating a balance of masculinity and femininity	The reliability coefficient for the scale was 0.86
Body image	Body Parts Satisfaction Scale (BPSS)	A total score is used for the 24 body parts items. A separate single item measures 'overall body appearance'	The items are rated on a six point scale from 1 (extremely satisfied) to 6 (extremely dissatisfied), and are reverse-scored	The reliability coefficient for the scale was 0.91
Sexual awareness	The Sexual Awareness Questionnaire (SAQ)	The questionnaire comprises four scales labelled Sexual Consciousness, Sexual Monitoring, Sexual Assertiveness and Sex-Appeal Consciousness	The 36-items are rated on a 5-point scale from 0 (not at all characteristic of me) to 4 (very characteristic of me) and mean scale scores were calculated	Reliability coefficients for the scales ranged from 0.77 to 0.89
Sexual functioning and satisfaction	Individual items were borrowed and modified from various other inventories	Individual items measured sexual orientation and degree of arousal, desire and pain during sexual activity	The items are reported individually, and most were rated on a 5-point Likert scale	N/A

Reproduced with permission from Warne et al. (2005)

Table 23.5 Demographic characteristics of DSD and controls (Hirschsprung disease, HPD, insulin-dependent diabetes mellitus, IDDM)

		DSD	Control		
			HPD	IDDM	HPD + IDDM
		N = 50	*N* = 27	*N* = 19	*N* = 46
Age	*M* (SD)	25.1 (4.3)	25.3 (3.8)	26.4 (3.9)	25.7 (3.8)
Gender ("that you identify with")					
Male	*N* (%)	17 (35.4)	18 (66.7)*	11 (57.9)	29 (63.0)**
Female		31 (64.6)	9 (33.3)	8 (42.1)	17 (37.0)
Education					
Secondary School (year 12 or earlier)		21 (42.0)	11 (40.7)	6 (31.6)	17 (37.0)
Post-school qualification—university or TAFE		29 (58.0)	16 (59.3)	13 (68.4)	29 (63.0)
Marital status					
Married/de facto		12 (24.5)	9 (33.3)	5 (26.3)	14 (30.4)
Single/other		37 (75.5)	18 (66.7)	14 (73.7)	32 (69.6)
One or more children					
Yes		7 (14.6)	5 (18.5)	4 (21.1)	9 (19.6)
No		41 (85.4)	22 (81.5)	15 (78.9)	37 (80.4)
Socio-occupational status					
White-collar		26 (70.3)	16 (64.0)	14 (87.5)	30 (73.2)
Blue-collar		11 (29.7)	9 (36.0)	2 (12.5)	11 (26.8)

Note: The DSD group was treated as the base category for comparison with the control groups. *$p < 0.05$, **$p < 0.01$ (Reproduced with permission from Warne et al. 2005)

Hirschsprung disease and IDDM groups were informed that their responses could provide a useful comparison. Completion of the questionnaires was estimated to take 1–2 h.

For statistical analysis, composite scale scores were extrapolated if the person had responded to at least the majority of items. In those instances of missing data, an average score was computed from the items that were completed. Each variable was analysed in a separate analysis-of-variance for ordinal outcome variables, and logistic regression for dichotomous outcome variables; 95% confidence intervals were presented around the mean difference and an odds ratio was calculated.

At the time of data collection, the mean age of participants was 25 years (range 18–32 years). Although there were more females in the DSD group than in the control groups, there were no significant group differences in age, education or socio-demographic variables (Table 23.5).

There were no major differences in physical or mental health, depression, current anxiety, neuroticism, psychiatric or stressful life events (Table 23.6). The DSD participants were satisfied with their overall body appearance, although males with DSD were less satisfied than controls with the size and appearance of their external genitalia. The DSD patients were less likely to experience orgasm and tended to experience more pain during intercourse, and they also had more difficulties with penetration than the combined control groups. In addition, they were also more likely to have less frequent sexual activity than the control groups. However, DSD patients did not differ from the control groups in the level of sexual desire or enjoyment of sexual activities (Table 23.7). These results show that patients with DSD have positive psychosocial and psychosexual outcomes, even when treatment was begun more than 40 years ago, although some problems persist with sexual activity.

This detailed review of long-term psychosocial and psychosexual outcomes showed that young adults with DSD who were treated at The Royal Children's Hospital had relatively good outcomes. They did not differ from young adults with Hirschsprung disease or diabetes on such measures as general physical and mental health or post-traumatic stress disorder symptoms. More importantly, the DSD patients showed mean scores on most of these measures that were

Table 23.6 General health and psychosocial functioning

	DSD		Control						Total
			HPD		IDDM		HPD + IDDM		
	Mean	SD	Mean	SD	Mean	SD	Mean	SD	*N*
RAND-36 HSI: Physical health composite	46.5	(10.7)	48.8	(12.1)	46.1	(12.9)	47.7	(12.4)	94
RAND-36 HSI: Mental health composite	47.9	(11.7)	48.6	(12.9)	47.8	(12.8)	48.3	(12.7)	93
RAND-36 HSI: Global health composite	47.2	(10.9)	48.1	(13.1)	46.4	(13.5)	47.4	(13.1)	91
Beck Depression Inventory	4.5	(5.1)	3.7	(4.6)	5.6	(6.0)	4.5	(5.2)	95
Coopersmith Self-esteem Inventory	62.8	(19.6)	77.0**	(20.5)	62.7	(23.9)	71.1	(22.8)	96
STAI: State anxiety	38.4	(11.6)	34.0	(12.7)	40.0	(14.9)	36.5	(13.8)	96
STAI: Trait anxiety	41.3	(11.1)	35.5*	(12.5)	41.6	(14.2)	38.0	(13.4)	96
EPQ-R short version: Psychoticism	3.2	(2.1)	3.2	(2.4)	2.5	(2.0)	2.9	(2.3)	95
EPQ-R short version: Extraversion	8.2	(3.4)	9.5	(2.6)	5.3**	(3.8)	7.8	(3.7)	95
EPQ-R short version: Neuroticism	6.4	(3.4)	5.3	(3.5)	6.1	(3.1)	5.6	(3.3)	95
Inventory of Interpersonal Problems: Total score	55.4	(10.3)	49.3*	(8.0)	55.9	(10.2)	52.1	(9.5)	95
Impact of Event Scale Revised: Total score	4.6	(2.7)	3.6	(2.1)	3.7	(2.8)	3.6	(2.4)	94

Note: The DSD group was treated as the base category for comparison with the control groups. $^{*}p < 0.05$, $^{**}p < 0.01$ (Reproduced with permission from Warne et al. 2005)

not indicative of any clinically significant problem likely to impede general life functioning. The DSD patients reported lower self-esteem and higher anxiety traits than the Hirschsprung patients, indicating that they tended to be more self-disapproving and perceived stressful situations as more threatening. However, they scored no more severely than those with other chronic illnesses such as diabetes. Overall, these findings were consistent with earlier reports of positive psychosexual and general health outcomes in women with CAH and other forms of DSD.

The males tended to report lower levels of satisfaction with their genitalia than control groups, which is probably related to genital size similar to that reported by Gupta et al. (2010). In addition, compared to other groups, the DSD patients reported more problems during sexual intercourse. Despite this, DSD patients did not differ from the control groups on self-reported enjoyment of sexual activity or level of sexual desire.

One of the weaknesses of a longitudinal study such as this is the concern that non-participants may have had a poorer outcome. However, in this study, participation over 53% is comparable with many other studies in the literature. Also, the similar or lower rates of participation in the two control groups suggest that participation was a function of the method of contact rather than the underlying disorder.

Despite some of these limitations, this long-term review indicated a generally positive psychosocial and psychosexual outcome, which is in contrast to many other studies reported in the literature (Creighton et al. 2001; Schober 2001; Minto et al. 2003; Reiner and Gearhart 2004). This supports a holistic approach by a multidisciplinary specialised team, which we feel strongly should include mental health and social work, working in close liaison with support groups. The readiness of clinicians in our group to disclose and openly discuss the diagnosis and broader issues, such as sexuality, is likely to be important in the long-term outcome. As all the participants in this follow-up study had genital reconstructive surgery in infancy or early childhood, the results did not support a change in this practice.

Table 23.7 Psychosexual measures

		DSD		Control						Total
				HPD		IDDM		HPD + IDDM		*N*
BPSS: Satisfaction with size of sex organs	M(SD)	3.8	(1.6)	4.6*	(0.9)	4.3	(1.4)	4.5*	(1.1)	90
BPSS: Satisfaction with appearance of sex organs	M(SD)	3.8	((1.6)	4.7*	(0.8)	4.2	(1.5)	4.5*	(1.1)	90
BPSS: Satisfaction with overall body appearance	M(SD)	4.0	(1.3)	4.6*	(0.8)	3.9	(1.3)	4.3	(1.1)	92
BPSS: Total score (for all 24 body part items)	M(SD)	105.9	(16.4)	110.0	(12.3)	104.4	(17.2)	107.7	(14.6)	93
SAQ: sexual-consciousness subscale	M(SD)	2.6	(0.9)	3.1*	(0.7)	2.5	(0.7)	2.9	(0.7)	92
SAQ: sexual-monitoring subscale	M(SD)	2.1	(0.8)	2.1	(0.7)	2.1	(0.9)	2.1	(0.8)	92
SAQ: sexual-assertiveness subscale	M(SD)	1.7	(0.8)	2.0	(1.0)	1.4	(0.9)	1.7	(1.0)	92
SAQ: sex-appeal-consciousness subscale	M(SD)	1.4	(1.2)	1.7	(1.0)	0.9	(1.2)	1.4	(1.1)	93
Males: PAQ Masculinity (or instrumental) scale	M(SD)	21.3	(5.3)	21.7	(5.3)	18.1	(4.9)	20.3	(5.4)	45
Females: PAQ Masculinity (or instrumental) scale	M(SD)	21.1	(4.1)	22.6	(3.8)	19.6	(4.2)	21.2	(4.2)	48
Males: PAQ Femininity (or expressive) scale	M(SD)	21.8	(4.1)	22.9	(4.5)	21.7	(3.4)	22.4	(4.1)	45
Females: PAQ Femininity (or expressive) scale	M(SD)	22.3	(4.4)	25.0	(2.6)	25.0	(3.7)	25.0*	(3.1)	48
Males: PAQ Masculinity-Femininity scale	M(SD)	14.7	(3.6)	15.8	(5.3)	13.9	(4.5)	15.1	(5.0)	45
Females: PAQ Masculinity-Femininity scale	M(SD)	14.8	(3.7)	15.7	(4.2)	13.0	(5.8)	14.4	(5.1)	48
Males: BSRI Difference score (femininity-masculinity)	M(SD)	49.7	(10.5)	49.7	(12.2)	54.1	(11.8)	51.4	(12.1)	45
Females: BSRI Difference score (femininity-masculinity)	M(SD)	49.8	(9.8)	55.9	(6.3)	53.4	(12.4)	54.7	(9.4)	49
Males: Difficulties achieving erection										45
More than half the time	%	6.3		5.6				3.4		
Sometimes (about half the time)	%	6.3		11.1				6.9		
Less than half the time	%	87.5		83.3		100.0		89.7		
Females: Become lubricated ("wet") during sexual activity										46

Table 23.7 (continued)

		DSD		Control						Total
				HPD		IDDM		HPD + IDDM		*N*
More than half the time	%	77.4		85.7		87.5		86.7		
Sometimes (about half the time)	%	9.7				12.5		6.7		
Less than half the time	%	12.9		14.3				6.7		
Experience orgasm (climax) during sexual activity	M(SD)	3.9	(1.1)	4.3	(1.0)	4.4	(0.9)	4.3*	(0.9)	87
Experience any pain during intercourse	M(SD)	1.9	(1.1)	1.6	(0.9)	1.4	(0.6)	1.5	(0.8)	85
Experience any difficulty with penetration	M(SD)	2.2	(1.5)	1.6	(0.9)	1.4*	(0.6)	1.5**	(0.8)	86
How many times during the last month you have had sexual activity										93
Less than several times a week	%	50.0		23.1*		26.3		24.4*		
Several times a week or more	%	50.0		76.9		73.7		75.6		
Sexual preference										91
Heterosexual	%	84.8		92.3		94.7		93.3		
Bisexual	%	8.7		3.8				2.2		
Lesbian/gay	%	6.5		3.8		5.3		4.4		
How enjoyable are sexual activities for you?	M(SD)	3.9	(1.0)	4.3	(0.9)	4.0	(0.7)	4.2	(0.9)	89
Level of sexual desire										92
High or very high	%	62.5		68.0		68.4		68.2		
Moderate	%	29.2		32.0		15.8		25.0		
Low, very low or none at all	%	8.3				15.8		6.8		

Note: The DSD group was treated as the base category for comparison with the control groups. *$p < 0.05$, **$p < 0.01$ (Reproduced with permission from Warne et al. 2005)

References

Alizai NK, Thomas DF, Lilford RJ, et al. Feminizing genitoplasty for congenital adrenal hyperplasia: what happens at puberty? J Urol. 1999;161(5):1588–91.

Azziz R, Mulaikal RM, Migeon CJ, et al. Congenital adrenal hyperplasia: long-term results following vaginal reconstruction. Fertil Steril. 1986;46(6):1011–4.

Berenbaum SA, Bailey JM. Effects on gender identity of prenatal androgens and genital appearance: evidence from girls with congenital adrenal hyperplasia. J Clin Endocrinol Metab. 2003;88(3):1102–6.

Bogdanska M, Morris A, Hutson JM, et al. Long-term urinary symptoms in adolescent and adult women with congenital adrenal hyperplasia. J Pediatr Urol. 2018;14(3):240.e241–5.

Crawford JM, Warne G, Grover S, et al. Results from a pediatric surgical centre justify early intervention in disorders of sex development. J Pediatr Surg. 2009;44(2):413–6.

Creighton SM, Minto CL, Steele SJ. Objective cosmetic and anatomical outcomes at adolescence of feminising surgery for ambiguous genitalia done in childhood. Lancet. 2001;358(9276):124–5.

Gonzalez R, Fernandes ET. Single-stage feminization genitoplasty. J Urol. 1990;143(4):776–8.

Gupta D, Bhardwaj M, Sharma S, et al. Long-term psychological adjustments, satisfaction related to gender and the family equations in disorders of sexual differentiation with male sex assignment. Pediatr Surg Int. 2010;26(10):958.

Houk CP, Hughes IA, Ahmed SF, et al. Summary of consensus statement on intersex disorders and their management. International Intersex Consensus Conference. Pediatrics. 2006;118(2):753–7.

Johnson LL, Bradley SJ, Birkenfeld-Adams AS, et al. A parent-report gender identity questionnaire for children. Arch Sex Behav. 2004;33(2):105–16.

Jones BC, O'Brien M, Chase J, et al. Early hypospadias surgery may lead to a better long-term psychosexual outcome. J Urol. 2009;182(4 Suppl):1744–9.

Jurgensen M, Hiort O, Holterhus PM, et al. Gender role behavior in children with XY karyotype and disorders of sex development. Horm Behav. 2007;51(3):443–53.

Lean WL, Deshpande A, Hutson J, et al. Cosmetic and anatomic outcomes after feminizing surgery for ambiguous genitalia. J Pediatr Surg. 2005;40(12):1856–60.

Minto CL, Liao LM, Woodhouse CR, et al. The effect of clitoral surgery on sexual outcome in individuals who have intersex conditions with ambiguous genitalia: a cross-sectional study. Lancet. 2003;361(9365):1252–7.

Nordenskjöld A, Holmdahl G, Frisén L, Falhammar H, Filipsson H, Thorén M, Janson PO, Hagenfeldt K. Type of mutation and surgical procedure affect long-term quality of life for women with congenital adrenal hyperplasia. J Clin Endocrinol Metab. 2008;93(2):380–6. Epub 2007 Nov 20.

Nordenström A. Psychosocial factors in disorders of sex development in a long-term perspective: what clinical opportunities are there to intervene? Horm Metab Res. 2015;47(5):351–6.

Reiner WG, Gearhart JP. Discordant sexual identity in some genetic males with cloacal exstrophy assigned to female sex at birth. N Engl J Med. 2004;350(4):333–41.

Roll MF, Kneppo C, Roth H, et al. Feminising genitoplasty: one-stage genital reconstruction in congenital adrenal hyperplasia: 30 years' experience. Eur J Pediatr Surg. 2006;16(5):329–33.

Schober JM. Sexual behaviors, sexual orientation and gender identity in adult intersexuals: a pilot study. J Urol. 2001;165(6 Pt 2):2350–3.

Sotiropoulos A, Morishima A, Homsy Y, et al. Long-term assessment of genital reconstruction in female pseudohermaphrodites. J Urol. 1976;115(5):599–601.

Varni JW, Seid M, Kurtin PS. PedsQL 4.0: reliability and validity of the Pediatric Quality of Life Inventory version 4.0 generic core scales in healthy and patient populations. Med Care. 2001;39(8):800–12.

Varni JW, Seid M, Knight TS, et al. The PedsQL 4.0 Generic Core Scales: sensitivity, responsiveness, and impact on clinical decision-making. J Behav Med. 2002;25(2):175–93.

Varni JW, Burwinkle TM, Seid M, et al. The PedsQL 4.0 as a pediatric population health measure: feasibility, reliability, and validity. Ambul Pediatr. 2003;3(6):329–41.

Warne G, Grover S, Hutson J, et al. A long-term outcome study of intersex conditions. J Pediatr Endocrinol Metab. 2005;18(6):555–67.

Zucker KJ, Bradley SJ, Oliver G, et al. Psychosexual development of women with congenital adrenal hyperplasia. Horm Behav. 1996;30(4):300–18.

Outcomes of Individuals with DSD: A World View

24

Aurore Bouty, Sonia R. Grover, and John M. Hutson

24.1 Introduction

DSD consist of a wide range of diagnoses, with different aetiologies, and term outcomes are different between subgroups. Outcomes in the past used restricted and often non-standardised approaches to assessment. They never had any input from individuals with the diagnosis themselves. Today, most studies endeavour to use standardised, validated questionnaires and assessment and would also endeavour to have input from DSD-affected individuals, in their study design and development, to ensure that the outcomes being measured are relevant to the individuals themselves.

Clinical management is subject to multiple controversies, such as decisions regarding the sex of rearing (often referred to as 'gender assignment'), appropriateness and timing of genital surgery and disclosure (Adam and Vilain 2017). There have been major changes in the field in the past few decades, partly due to better understanding and knowledge from healthcare providers of the different aetiologies, implications and specific risks of each subtype (Ahmed et al. 2013). However, many of the changes are due to the work of patients' advocacy groups and families (Tamar-Mattis 2014), leading to debate as well as involvement of politicians (https://rm.coe.int/human-rights-and-intersex-people-issue-paper-published-by-the-council-/16806da5d4) (Cools et al. 2016). Thus, given that outcome studies are attempts to measure the effects of management undertaken in the past, by their very nature, they will be measuring management of the past, rather than outcomes of current practice. In a setting where there have been substantial changes in attitude, knowledge and management, these outcome studies will often not reflect current attitudes, knowledge and management.

In this chapter, some discussion regarding the factors that are important to consider when reading outcome studies is explored first as well as the potential indices that can be assessed or

A. Bouty
Department of Urology, The Royal Children's Hospital, Melbourne, VIC, Australia

Murdoch Children's Research Institute, Melbourne, VIC, Australia
e-mail: aurore.bouty@rch.org.au

S. R. Grover
Department of Gynaecology, The Royal Children's Hospital, Melbourne, VIC, Australia

Murdoch Children's Research Institute, Melbourne, VIC, Australia

Department of Paediatrics, University of Melbourne, Melbourne, VIC, Australia
e-mail: sonia.grover@rch.org.au

J. M. Hutson (✉)
Department of Urology, The Royal Children's Hospital, Melbourne, VIC, Australia

Murdoch Children's Research Institute, Melbourne, VIC, Australia

Department of Paediatrics, University of Melbourne, Melbourne, VIC, Australia
e-mail: john.hutson@rch.org.au

J. M. Hutson et al. (eds.), *Disorders|Differences of Sex Development*,
https://doi.org/10.1007/978-981-13-7864-5_24

should be considered before a review of some of the main long-term outcomes by DSD subtype.

24.2 Understanding Outcome Studies: Factors Influencing Interpretation

24.2.1 Recruitment

Most studies experience difficulties in recruitment to long-term follow-up studies. Participation rates are usually low amongst the specified or identified cohorts (which may be from a hospital database, from a cluster of clinic patients seen over a specified interval, from a national database or from support groups or a mixture of these). Most will have a high 'lost to follow-up' rate. This creates major difficulties in knowing whether it is appropriate to extrapolate the study results to those patients who did not answer and whether the non-participants were satisfied or not. In studies reported in the literature only a decade ago, the size of the potential cohort was often not reported, so it was even harder to know the participation rate, let alone how representative the study population was from the original potential cohort.

Many hospitals even today do not have database systems for ensuring that individuals with DSD are recorded; this particularly applies if these specialised services are not centralised.

Locating potential participants with the relevant inclusion criteria for a study does not guarantee recruitment and participation with completion of the study questionnaires or assessments. With a large range of possible outcomes to be measured in potentially a quite varied population, most studies opt to limit the range of issues to be explored in a specific study—for the sake of the individuals participating in the study and in the hope that those approached to participate will not be 'put off' by the large number of study questions and the time involved in undertaking this.

24.2.2 Cohort Participant's Profile

Study cohorts vary—from studies recruiting within a single hospital (Warne et al. 2005; Lean et al. 2007) to those recruiting within one hospital but who receive selected potentially complex referrals from wider sources; to cohorts recruited from hospital databases from a few specialised centres within a country (Nordenskjold et al. 2008) or recruited nationwide from a range of hospitals as well as other sources (Schweizer et al. 2017) where the individuals may thus have potentially experienced very different managements in different hospitals and a range of clinicians; to those recruited from support groups. Cohorts may also represent a mixed population of DSD, for example, where all those born with 'ambiguous genitalia' are recruited (Creighton 2001), but where there are a range of diagnostic groups, or people born without a uterus, where both women with CAIS and those with MRKH are participants, yet one group has fertility potential through surrogacy or uterine transplant and the other does not.

24.2.3 Health Resources

Outcome studies will also be influenced by the resources and health care available in a country. Delay in diagnosis, due to limited health education and resources may be in the form of delayed diagnosis at birth—which can have fatal consequences for those born with CAH (Zainuddin et al. 2013). Alongside these life-threatening risks linked to reduced access to health services are those relating to compromised, potentially risky suboptimal steroid replacement, which may then result in virilisation with flow-on impacts on outcomes (Armstrong et al. 2006).

A number of issues, as well as those relating to health resources, are demonstrated and apparent in the comprehensive review of the long-term outcomes in individuals with 5α-reductase-2 deficiency and 17β-hydroxysteroid dehydrogenase-3 deficiency (Cohen-Kettenis 2005). In this review, over 50% of cases came from resource-limited countries, half were cases reported before 1990 and despite several of the individuals having atypical genitalia at birth, almost all were raised female. This review reported a significant rate of gender change amongst individuals when they reached adolescence. Concerns regarding the applicability of this study today include the late diagnosis in many cases likely to be related to limited health resources in those countries, the differences in management of the child with atypical genitalia today compared to those in 1970 or 1990 and the potential of cultural influences on some of the decision-making.

Thus, the outcomes are already potentially very different for a range of reasons other than the type of DSD being reviewed.

The capacity to access care due to cost and distance will all contribute. Reports from Vietnam and Malaysia have both noted the considerable cost to families to access care, and in Malaysia, some differences in outcome may be due to these factors. To travel to the centre offering care may require an entire family to undertake 2–4 days for the return trip, with loss of income for both parents and missed schooling for the individual and their siblings.

24.2.4 Regional Cultural Preferences

The impact of cultural preference for one gender or another may have a range of reasons. These factors may impact on parental decision-making or decisions by a young adult when recognition of the DSD occurs including marriage-ability, employment, inheritance, acceptance of same-sex partners (in countries where this is illegal, the option of 'becoming' the other gender may make this more 'acceptable'), (see Chap. 22).

24.2.5 Cohort: Medical Care and Expertise of Their Carers

The availability of specialised medical care as well as access to clinical investigations will impact on outcome measures.

The spectrum of available testing may range from only limited availability of hormonal or karyotype testing, through to some centres having specific DSD panels to explore potential gene variations. In the past, any undervirilised male was classified as having PAIS, whereas now, far more specific diagnoses are possible, encompassing a range of conditions with now recognised, quite varied outcomes.

The availability of genetic testing also impacts on the timing of diagnosis. With increasing availability of antenatal testing (see Chap. 11; ultrasound, amniocentesis, chorionic villous sampling and now non-invasive prenatal testing), diagnosis of discordance between expected phenotypes of a neonate or even a precise diagnosis may be possible antenatally. Thus, a girl with complete gonadal dysgenesis diagnosed this early now has the possibility of having their infertility issues and options introduced gradually through childhood by informed and supported parents, rather than learning of the problem in her mid-teens.

A further example of this is the specific genotype testing for CAH that is available in Sweden (Nordenskjold et al. 2008), which has allowed a correlation between genotypes and a range of specific outcomes. In contrast, in Melbourne, where despite the availability of DSD genome panels, outcome studies of cohorts of individuals with CAH do not include CAH genotyping due to lack of availability of this testing, which is expensive, and where the benefit to date of genotyping has not been acknowledged. Thus, any difference in the availability of testing limits some of the detail and value that could otherwise be achieved and limits the capacity to directly compare results and outcomes.

Outcomes reported by clinicians (e.g. cosmetic outcomes) will not be the same as the outcomes reported by the affected individuals.

As mentioned in the surgical chapter (Chap. 17), the question of surgical technique and the experience of the surgeon are also relevant, yet usually not reported.

Other clinical issues that may impact on an individual's well-being, their body image and self-esteem and, thus, their long-term quality of life include medical photographs and repeated genital examinations, yet they are usually not mentioned or acknowledged (Creighton et al. 2002).

The expertise of the clinicians involved in the care of individuals may vary substantially. This issue has already been mentioned in the context of the experience of the surgeon and will be discussed further later in this chapter.

24.2.6 Cohort Age—Changes in Care over Time

A substantial problem with outcome studies is that time needs to have passed before the outcome can be measured. In that time, there may have been further advances in science, allowing far more specific management approaches. Genetic testing now allows for more accurate diagnosis of DSD, and knowledge regarding malignancy risk for specific diagnoses with the added tool of markers to help predict the gonads at risk of malignant change, allows for care to be specific to the individual.

Surgical techniques have also changed in many places over time, although the largely unchanged surgical technique of genitoplasty for over 40 years at RCH may be an exception to this (see Chap. 17).

24.3 Measuring Outcomes

The measurement tools for assessing outcomes have changed over time. A clear example of this is the reporting in the past on sexual function following surgery to create a vagina, which consisted of surgeons asking whether the individual was sexually active and whether she was sexually satisfied, with response options being either yes or no or by asking her current partner if they were sexually satisfied (McQuillan and Grover 2014). Since then, standardised measures have been introduced with increased recognition that a range of factors will impact on outcome, but some of the key factors that need consideration will be described (see Chaps. 20 and 23).

24.3.1 Quality of Life, Well-Being Measures

Earlier studies often omitted measures relating to quality of life, body image and self-esteem. Studies undertaken to assess satisfaction with outcomes that fail to acknowledge the impact of this range of measures may well conclude that there has been a negative outcome, but in the absence of these assessments, it will be difficult to know whether this is an association or causative factor. The more information that is known, the more complete is the outcome information.

A prime example of this is reporting on sexual function when body image and self-esteem have not been studied. A conclusion drawn from this information provides a very limited result, which will be very difficult to interpret. The relationship between these issues has been well described and assessed in an unrelated clinical problem of pelvic floor prolapse, which occurs in women (Lowenstein et al. 2009). Here, there is a clear association between body image and sexual function, rather than the anatomical finding relating to the severity of the prolapse. Parallel to this is the need to know whether individuals with a DSD have any altered body image, depression, general well-being assessments compared to controls and then how this relates to their satisfaction with genital appearance.

24.3.2 Gender Outcomes

In the largest international DSD cohort to date, gender change was reported by 5% of the participants, including identifying outside of the binary male/female genders (Kreukels et al. 2018). The rate of gender change varies depending on which condition is being considered (see Chaps. 6–8 for details regarding specific diagnoses) and also the era, location including cultural influences and health resources when the study was undertaken (see above).

Gender behaviour has been explored amongst individuals with 46,XX CAH, within four specific genotypes, with a clear correlation demonstrating increased gender-atypical occupations and behaviour, which likely reflected higher exposure to prenatal androgens (Frisen et al. 2009). This study also identified that the impact of the disease on upbringing and interpersonal relationships did not correlate with disease severity, suggesting that other factors including coping strategies play an important role in psychosocial adaptation. Although specific issues vary among individuals from different groups of DSD, a number of individuals with DSD do exhibit altered body image and self-esteem, and this needs to be addressed in the setting of holistic care (van de Grift et al. 2018) (see Chaps. 20 and 23).

24.3.3 Risk of Malignancy

Malignancy risk varies substantially depending on the condition: from those that have no increased risk of malignancy—with normal ovaries or testes (e.g. the non-hormonal DSD), through to conditions where dysgenetic gonads may carry a risk of 30%. Knowledge regarding the relative risks of malignancy has changed dramatically over the last few decades. Additionally, specific genetic markers are now known and can assist in prediction of malignancy risk in some conditions. Comparing management decisions and outcomes regarding gonadectomy needs to be carefully placed in the era in which the study was reported due to these advances in understanding (see Chaps. 7, 11 and 21).

24.3.4 Fertility Potential

Fertility potential relates to the presence of functioning gonads with gametes (either sperm or ova). The capacity to carry a pregnancy is dependent on the presence of a uterine body (with a unicornuate uterus capable of achieving this, as well as a uterine body with some degree of cervical dysgenesis). However, uterine transplants have now been successfully undertaken and offer some hope for those born without a uterus (see Chap. 18). The use of a donor egg allows an individual who does not have functioning ovaries to carry a pregnancy, although the offspring will have different genetic makeup. These options will be very dependent on the country where a study is occurring. Hence, in Sweden, where surrogacy is illegal, uterine transplant has been studied and progressed. In contrast, in countries where surrogacy is legal (and at least potentially affordable) (e.g. Australia), this option is the current option that may be taken up instead. *In vitro* fertilisation is not allowed for religious reasons in a number of countries; hence, reports on fertility outcomes for individuals with DSD will be influenced by factors other than the underlying diagnosis.

The capacity to achieve a pregnancy without assistance also requires the capacity for the ejaculate to pass from an erectile penis. Immature sperm extraction from a testicular biopsy and storage is another area of growing interest, which, albeit with no clear techniques yet available for maturation, is developing.

24.3.5 Measuring Surgical Outcomes

Surgery in the setting of DSD has been the topic of considerable debate and discussion over the last decade. This debate is complicated by the 'lumping' of all surgeries together. The argument against genital surgery in infancy relates to reports of poor outcomes, the need for repeat surgery, poor sexual function, altered/loss of sensation, lack of input by the individual in the decision-making (making this a Human Rights issue) and regret regarding surgery due to loss of function and reduced sensation, or the undertaking of the wrong surgery (i.e. feminising, rather than masculinising) (Gorduza et al. 2018).

It is important to recognise that surgery in the setting of DSD is highly variable.

Some conditions such as cloaca and bladder exstrophy can be associated with problems such as exposed bladder or imperforate anus—such that the surgery is absolutely essential.

For gonadal surgery, with increased knowledge, undertaking gonadectomies in infancy is now limited to settings where the malignancy risk has been defined and is deemed to be significantly increased (potentially as high as 30–50%) and after appropriate discussion; only then, would surgery be undertaken. This would be done with parental consent after discussion with a multidisciplinary team, if there is a gonadal cancer risk, and in these settings, the gonads are usually non-functioning from both a fertility potential and a hormone production perspective. Referral for further discussion at an ethics committee would be undertaken if the decision-making was more complicated or conflicted.

The debate lies with those conditions where delay in undertaking surgery could be done so that the young person can be involved in the decision-making.

In the past, there were a number of conditions where the sex of rearing was female, yet current understanding and capacity to accurately make a diagnosis means that the long-term gender identity outcomes, albeit recognising the limitations of outcome studies, is better known and understood.

Feminising genitoplasty is one of the most controversial topics in contemporaneous Paediatric Urology. This is because reports on long-term results of this procedure are conflicting and mainly of low quality (Jesus 2018). The major issues with these reports are those mentioned earlier in this chapter, but additionally, studies often do not include non-operated controls, often have missing information regarding pre-surgical degree of virilisation and quality of post-operative hormonal treatment. More importantly, there are no uniform criteria to evaluate clitoral size; few studies on genital sensitivity using very mixed techniques and reports often include surgical techniques that have since been abandoned. Exact techniques used are often not described. The experience at RCH where the same operative technique has been utilised for over 40 years is probably the exception to this, and thus, the long-term outcomes remain useful for current practice (see Chap. 23).

For infants with 46,XX CAH, born with atypical virilised genitalia, who are raised in a country, or part of a country, where access to medical care is limited or where a late diagnosis of CAH has occurred, undertaking feminising genitoplasty may be the wrong decision, as the socioeconomic setting may predispose to ongoing virilisation (and the risks associated with under-replacement of steroids including fatality) and thus an increased likelihood that the individual will identify as male during adolescence. Nevertheless, there are reports of serious sepsis in the setting of haematocolpos due to inadequate drainage of menstrual fluid.

In contrast, for infants with 46,XX CAH, born with atypical virilised genitalia, who are raised in a country where there is access to good medical care, it is almost certain that the individual will identify as female. With good control of CAH, it is likely that she will menstruate and thus will need an adequate outflow tract for menstrual fluid (for which she may choose to use tampons). Furthermore, most individuals in this setting, whatever their sexual orientation, are likely to undertake sexual activities that may encompass penetration into their vagina. Thus, she is likely to want and need a vagina. The question then remains as to what is the best surgical technique to use and when is the best time to undertake the surgery. In the past few decades, this was undertaken routinely in infancy. More recently, this has been challenged as unnecessary to be done at this age, usually requires significant further surgery, has poor cosmetic and anatomical outcomes (Creighton et al. 2001) and is an infringement of the human rights of the child.

These are valid concerns, but there remains room for uncertainty and questions. First, there are reports that women with CAH are unhappy with their genital appearance whether or not they have had surgery (Nordenskjold et al. 2008) and the outcomes were influenced by the type of surgery that had been undertaken (Nordenskjold et al. 2008). Reports on outcomes are quite mixed, with not all reporting poor outcomes (Stikkelbroeck et al. 2003; Lean et al. 2005), and thus, the poor outcome report almost certainly reflects a selected cohort of women with poor outcomes whose subsequent care has been aggregated at a specified centre. Although uncommon, there are some reports of complications arising from relative urinary obstruction or urinary pooling, likewise with sepsis arising from menstrual or vaginal secretion obstruction. If the presumption can be made that introital surgery will eventually be required (which, in CAH, in a country with good health resources is likely to be the case) and that in experienced hands, the outcomes can be satisfactory/good from both a cosmetic and an anatomic perspective, then, this surgery may be a reasonable consideration. Added to this is the evidence that women who have undergone this surgery in childhood do not report a wish that it had not been done. Then in this selected population, where a centre has its own outcome studies demonstrating these outcomes, undertaking surgery by competent experienced surgeons during infancy is not so unreasonable.

In contrast, there are no data on the outcomes of individuals with 46,XX raised female who have delayed surgery—their body image, self-esteem, sexual function and urinary function, let alone the cosmetic and anatomic surgical outcomes. There is evidence from males that suggests that undertaking genital surgery prior to 3 years of age does not leave a negative impact on self-esteem and body image as compared to genital surgery after this age (Mureau et al. 1995; Jones et al. 2009). (Timing of this surgery is challenging—as genital surgery in young adolescents (perimenarchal) is not optimal due to the typical self-consciousness and embarrassment that are commonly seen in this age group.) Leaving surgery to mid-teens (presuming that menstrual outflow has not been obstructed and required more urgent intervention), then leaves the teenager unable to undertake sexual activity at a time when her peers may be doing this. It is unknown whether this would have any negative psychological consequences.

One further risk that has not been discussed is the potential lack of surgical expertise if there is to be 15 years of absolutely no surgery (if a complete moratorium for genital surgery was introduced as has occurred in Malta). Will there be the expertise to undertake the surgery when these women request surgery for tampon use and penetrative sexual activities, or even if there are acute septic complications? Thus, there are many unknown reasons associated with delaying all genital surgeries, and this must be set against the information from some centres, which report that the majority of those raised female with CAH are actually satisfied with their outcome and timing of surgery.

As alluded to earlier, there are other DSD diagnoses where the outcome of gender identity clearly leans the decision-making away from undertaking early surgery where it can be avoided—to allow the individual both to be part of the decision-making and to maximise the options available for that individual.

24.4 Outcomes by DSD Classification

DSD were reclassified in 2005 (Hughes 2008). Although most stakeholders would recognise the imperfection of this classification system, it is the current reference and will be used in this review to structure the exploration of outcomes.

Each DSD outcome will be examined from the perspective of issues relating to the diagnosis itself, those relating to medical care and those relating to surgery (if required).

24.4.1 46,XX DSD

Overall morbidity in 46,XX males is increased compared to age-matched male controls but mortality is not. Education and income are lower than those in the general population, as well as fatherhood rate (Berglund et al. 2017).

24.4.1.1 Congenital Adrenal Hyperplasia (21-Hydroxylase Deficiency) (CAH)

CAH is a lifelong life-threatening condition that poses multiple challenges to affected individuals and their families. In addition to physiological concerns of optimal hormone replacement therapy and treatment monitoring, parents and later individuals themselves face psychological and behavioural aspects of chronic illness (Speiser et al. 2010).

Individuals with CAH are steroid dependent for life in order to replace deficient levels of cortisol and/or aldosterone and minimise androgen excess. The ultimate goal is to prevent virilisation in females, optimise growth and protect fertility. However, excess of hydrocortisone can have adverse effects, such as growth suppression and obesity, while insufficient replacement places the patient at risk of precocious puberty and adrenal crisis (Merke and Bornstein 2005).

In a retrospective cross-sectional study, Mendes-Dos-Santos et al. (2011) demonstrated that children with treated CAH had similar heights to controls of the same age, but that they had higher body fat. Similarly, Moreira et al. (2013) found a higher prevalence of obesity and metabolic syndrome in these children. However, the authors also commented that familial predisposition was a significant determining factor in CAH patients.

Bone mineral density has not been shown to be influenced by treatment with glucocorticoids. However, bone ages of poorly controlled or later diagnosed children were higher than those in tightly controlled, early-diagnosed groups (Cetinkaya and Kara 2011).

Although female sex of rearing is most common for babies born with CAH in Western countries and those with good access to health care, an important proportion of them are raised as boys in many developing countries. For instance, a retrospective study in Turkey identified surgical complications and emotional difficulties for the family when the change to female gender and surgery occurred after 2.5 years of age. The authors acknowledge that traditional, cultural and economic factors certainly play an important role in these difficulties (Ozbey et al. 2004). Likewise, in Jordan, 15% of 46,XX CAH patients were reconstructed (including gonadectomy and hysterectomy) and raised as male (Al-Maghribi 2007). In resource-limited countries, health education and literacy, access to medical care (due to cost and travel time, hence loss of income) as well as access to medications (due to cost and availability) results in suboptimal management of CAH, ongoing elevated androgens and virilisation of individuals with 46,XX CAH (Armstrong et al. 2006; Zainuddin et al. 2014) (see Chap. 22).

Many studies have looked at the impact of high concentrations of androgens on developing brain, in particular *in utero*, on both sexual orientation and gender identity. During childhood, many studies focus on toy preferences. Studies from Europe have shown that girls with CAH were more interested in masculine toys, such as cars or construction toys, than controls (Nordenstrom et al. 2002; Servin et al. 2003; Wong et al. 2013). Additionally, two-thirds of the more virilised girls reported a boy as their best friend compared to none of the controls and very few of those with milder forms. It has also been recently suggested that prenatal androgen exposure increased cross-gender identification (Pasterski et al. 2015). Gender identity is one's internal sense of being male or female, independently of gonadal sex. The vast majority (95%) of patients raised as female are satisfied and non-dysphoric in adulthood (Dessens et al. 2005). Gender dysphoria is a rare finding in CAH, although hormonal control, social, familial and religious beliefs have an important impact on gender identity in these patients (Razzaghy-Azar et al. 2017). Results from a study in Bangladesh also suggested that delayed treatment for CAH may favour male gender identity (Chowdhury et al. 2015), and results from Malaysia suggest that limited access to care (due to greater distance to care, rural and lower income) all contributed to dissatisfaction with female identity (Zainuddin et al. 2014). Results are more contrasted for the most virilised cases raised as male (Lee et al. 2010). Results on gender identity do not correlate with the severity of CAH nor with the degree of genital virilisation, demonstrating that genital appearance at birth is not the best predictor of gender outcomes in 46,XX CAH and that one has yet to understand the determinants of gender identity in CAH and in the general population (Berenbaum and Bailey 2003). With regards to sexual orientation, it has been shown that non-heterosexual behaviours are increased in women with CAH, with 20–30% of women reporting bisexual/homosexual fantasies and 3–6% having non-heterosexual partners (Zucker et al. 1996; Gastaud et al. 2007). As opposed to results with gender identity, the level of non-heterosexual tendencies increased with the severity and the form of the condition: 47% for the salt-wasting form, 33% for the simple virilising form and 24% for the non-classical form, respectively (Meyer-Bahlburg 2008). This aligns with the work undertaken where CAH CYP21A2 genotyping has been performed, and of those with the null genotype, 50% are reported to have a non-heterosexual orientation (Frisen et al. 2009). Taken together, it appears that *in utero* androgen exposure on an XX background affects sexual fantasies in women with CAH.

Cognitive differences are also present between men and women and have been largely studied in patients with DSD to evaluate the action of androgens on the brain. In particular, spatial awareness and mental rotation ability demonstrate a striking difference, with males outperforming females (Geiser et al. 2008). On average, 46,XX females with CAH outperform their matched controls on those tests, and the results correlate with the severity of the disease (Hampson and Rovet 2015). On the other hand,

46,XY males with CAH perform worse than their unaffected matched controls (Berenbaum et al. 2012). Therefore, there might be both an optimal time and level of androgen exposure during development (Bramble et al. 2017).

In the Swedish registry of individuals with CAH, 588 patients with a known severity in more than 80% of the cases were compared for education and quality of life, being able to work as well as a range of other factors to 100 controls per patient, matched for sex, year and place of birth. Women with salt-wasting (SW) CAH had completed primary education less often with an odds ratio (OR) of 0.3, with this difference not explained by neonatal salt crisis or hypoglycaemia because the men did not differ from controls. Men and women with less severe CAH genotype were more likely to have an academic education (OR 1.8). Both men and women had more disability pension (OR 1.5) and sick leave (OR 1.7), although the men were more often in long-lasting employment (OR 3.1) (Strandqvist et al. 2014). These findings were supported by a Norwegian study of adults with CAH (Nermoen et al. 2010) and likewise, a study from Malaysia on individuals with 46,XX CAH found higher rates of learning difficulties (Zainuddin et al. 2014), although in this population, the impact of adrenal crises may be an added factor.

A range of potential factors are thought to influence education and employment outcomes, rather than the underlying condition, and research to identify the underlying mechanisms would be valuable to thus improve medical and psychological care (Strandqvist et al. 2014).

Early surgical management of CAH has been driven partly by the risk of urinary tract infections (UTI). However, recent reports state that the incidence of UTI in these children is similar to that of the general population and that this should not be a reason to undertake genital surgery (Nabhan et al. 2006).

Regarding clitoroplasty, most patients report good subjective post-operative clitoral sensation, while poor clitoral sensation is directly correlated to multiple clitoral surgeries (Frost-Arner et al. 2003; Fagerholm et al. 2011), clitoral amputation or non-preservation of the neuro-vascular bundles (Zhen et al. 2016). Researchers have tried to objectively measure genital sensitivity using traditional devices for neurological evaluation (Frost-Arner et al. 2003; Yang et al. 2008; Nordenstrom et al. 2010). Studies utilising an instrument specifically designed to quantify genital sensitivity (Genito Sensory Analyser, GSA) were, nevertheless, limited by selection biases and recruitment limited to 30% of patients and 50% of controls (Crouch et al. 2004, 2008; Lesma et al. 2014; Zhen et al. 2016). Furthermore, sensitivity test results may not correspond to 'real' sensation during sexual activity, as despite abnormal responses on instrumental analyses, most patients report a sexual life comparable to unaffected women (Lesma et al. 2014). The sensitivity is related to the type of clitoroplasty performed, with nerve-sparing ventral clitoroplasty showing better sensitivity (Salle et al. 2012). Finally, it has also been shown a correlation between outcomes and genotype (Nordenstrom et al. 2010).

With respect to the cosmetic outcome of feminising genitoplasty, it is striking that evaluations on external appearance from patients do not correlate with assessments by clinicians (Stikkelbroeck et al. 2003; Nordenstrom et al. 2010). Moreover, there were inter-observer variations between clinicians.

The paper that drew most of the attention on long-term outcomes of feminising genitoplasty reported high rates of vaginal stenosis, and over two-thirds requiring major surgery (Creighton 2001). However, no details about the diagnosis or previous surgical technique were provided, nor expertise of the original surgeons. Other authors also report a high incidence of vaginal stenosis but with much fewer major surgeries required. In the vast majority of cases, self-dilatations or introitoplasty is sufficient (Fagerholm et al. 2011; Stikkelbroeck et al. 2003). Genital pain during intercourse is more frequent than that among controls (Fagerholm et al. 2011). Although the absence of perineal body and posterior fourchette has obstetrical consequences and favour dyspareunia, they are directly related to flap or cutback vaginoplasties (Fagerholm et al. 2011) and are probably uncommon after urogenital sinus mobilisation; however, long-term results are lacking.

Adult females with CAH report less frequent sexual activity with a partner (Creighton 2001; Fagerholm et al. 2011) and lower frequency of orgasms (Lesma et al. 2014). Interestingly, those results were not seen among patients with AIS and feminising genitoplasty, raising the possibility of these outcomes to be related partly to the disease itself and not the surgery (Fagerholm et al. 2011). Additionally, sexual function and avoidance do not differ between individuals with CAH whether or not they have had a feminising genitoplasty, with both groups reporting infrequent intercourse, avoidance, anorgasmia and penetration difficulties (Crouch et al. 2008).

In two papers that evaluated the opinion of the patients on the timing of their surgery, 71% of them thought it was correct (median age at first operation 2.1 years). No patient with CAH believed they should not have been operated at all (Stikkelbroeck et al. 2003). In contrast, a study exploring the long-term outcomes of 46,XX individuals with CAH in Malaysia included 59 of 61 identified individuals. The majority were pleased with surgery being performed in infancy, but there were three individuals who would have preferred surgery to have been undertaken in adulthood. It is worth noting that these individuals also had delayed diagnosis, were undertreated due to challenges in accessing medications and care and had gender dysphoria (Zainuddin et al. 2014). Less clear, however, are the opinions regarding the timing of secondary vaginoplasties (Stikkelbroeck et al. 2003).

Urinary outcome following feminising genitoplasty are generally good with similar lower urinary tract symptoms reported in a cohort of patients and in controls (Fagerholm et al. 2013). Urogenital sinus mobilisation, the most commonly used technique during genitoplasty currently, is still at its early days, but most reports are favourable (Palmer et al. 2012; Ludwikowski and Gonzalez 2013), despite one study reporting a high rate of incontinence (Stites et al. 2017).

Short-term operative outcomes are infrequently reported, but the RCH experience consisted of 72 individuals with 46,XX CAH identified from hospital databases (1974–2014), with only one who had a significant operative complication (of bowel perforation). Approximately 50% had undergone surgery at <5 months of age, 10% between 6 and 12 months, 25% from 1 to 2 years of age and the remainder, above this age (Bogdanska et al. 2018). (In recent years, surgery is not being performed in babies <6 months of age.) Re-operation rates have been very low, with only two infants requiring repeat surgery (one associated with wound breakdown in an infant who was mobilising and the other for reversal of the colostomy). Further surgery for revision of the feminising genitoplasty has consisted of only minor surgery (requiring only day stay or overnight admission), although dilators have been required by some.

The outcomes at 5–10 years of age of a cohort of predominantly girls with CAH (16 of 18 participants) who had genital assessment ($n = 13$) as well as quality of life assessment, and parent report version of the quality of life inventory and gender identity questionnaire demonstrated a 'good' cosmetic score in 11/13 and satisfactory in two (using a standardised assessment based on the Creighton study) (Creighton et al. 2001). Quality of life scores for both the child and the parental version were within the normal range (Crawford et al. 2009).

24.4.1.2 46,XX Ovo-Testicular DSD

In 60–82% of cases, the karyotype in human ovo-testicular DSD is 46,XX (Wiersma 2004; Verkauskas et al. 2007). Others may be 46,XY, 46,XX/46,XY chimeras or have other karyotypes. The genital appearance ranges from complete male to complete female, but many have ambiguous genitalia. Both ovarian and testicular tissues coexist in the person, with the distribution of one versus the other varying considerably between individuals (van Niekerk and Retief 1981). This wide spectrum of presentation and genetic complement makes sex of rearing a case-by-case decision (Diamond et al. 2018). The proportion of gender dysphoria is difficult to adequately evaluate, as the diagnosis is rare (Furtado et al. 2012). While an ovo-testis may have two distinct poles, an even distribution throughout the length of the gonad is commonly seen. An ovary containing fertile oocytes is possible on one side (most commonly the left) with an ovo-testis or dysplastic gonad on the other, but the testicular element degenerates faster than the ovary, and male fertility is rarely if ever possible.

Testosterone production, however, may be adequate, with report of spontaneous puberty (Matsui et al. 2011). The risk of gonadal malignancy is low unless a Y chromosome is present in the gonad (Looijenga et al. 2007). Female sex of rearing, which preserves the chance of fertility, has been the preferred option in many cases, and in these, the testicular component can be removed to prevent unwanted testosterone secretion and reduce the risk of malignancy (Damiani et al. 1997, 2005; Krstic et al. 2000; Verkauskas et al. 2007; Diamond et al. 2018).

24.4.1.3 46,XX Testicular DSD

In this condition (formerly known as XX male syndrome), similarities to Klinefelter syndrome are very strong, although men with 46,XX DSD are shorter than men with Klinefelter syndrome and men in the general population (Vorona et al. 2007). The gonads are dysgenetic and infertility is the rule. The *SRY* gene is expressed in some but not in all, affected individuals (Abusheikha et al. 2001; Chiang et al. 2013; Eggers et al. 2016).

24.4.1.4 46,XX Müllerian Agenesis Syndrome

While not associated with sexual ambiguity, the Mayer–Rokitansky–Küster–Hauser syndrome (Morcel et al. 2007) is in the spectrum of DSD, with an incidence of 1 in 4500. Typically, the uterus and vagina are absent, but there is some variation in anatomy such as partial/incomplete Műllerian duct fusion and unilateral renal agenesis. The ovaries may be ectopic, either higher in the pelvis or in the inguinal canal (Demirel et al. 2012) where they may be associated with inguinal hernias, which occur more often in these girls (Oppelt et al. 2006; Kimberley et al. 2012). Treatment of the vaginal hypoplasia does not always require surgery, as the vagina is able to lengthen in response to stretching over time, as in regular and frequent sexual intercourse (Cheikhelard et al. 2018). While isolated cases of ovarian cancer have been reported, it is unclear if the overall risk is increased (Huepenbecker et al. 2017; Juusela and Gimovsky 2017). Although reported, cancer in Müllerian duct remnants does not appear to be increased. Women with the condition may have a range of emotional difficulties related to absence of a womb and benefit from professional counselling and involvement in peer support groups.

Surrogacy can be used to achieve genetic children, as individuals with uterine agenesis have normal functioning ovaries. This option is not available in many countries. Uterine transplant has now been undertaken successfully on a number of occasions with successful pregnancy outcomes (Brannstrom 2018) mostly using live donors, although there are some recent reports on deceased donors.

24.4.2 46,XY DSD

Overall morbidity in 46,XY females was increased compared to age-matched controls from male and female general populations, but mortality was not. Individuals performed well from education and income perspectives, although their DSD seemed to impact on the prospects of family life, with lower cohabitation and motherhood rates (Berglund et al. 2018).

24.4.2.1 Complete Androgen Insensitivity Syndrome (CAIS)

The experience of women with CAIS has been documented very eloquently by an international patient-advocacy group (http://www.aissg.org/). In the past, the genetic details of the condition to individuals and their parents were often not disclosed. Full disclosure has been advocated and practised now for over 20 years in many places within a more holistic, multidisciplinary context (Warne 1989; Lee and Money 2004). Gender identity is typically female (Hines et al. 2003), and both breast size and body shape are typically within the population standard ranges. Pubic and axillary hair is scanty or absent. Women with CAIS have no uterus, and the loss of fertility potential may impact body image and self-esteem (Wisniewski et al. 2000; Wisniewski and Migeon 2002; Minto et al. 2003; Fliegner et al. 2014). The vaginal length is usually adequate, although the attitude towards this and the recommendations for dilatation or surgery varies substantially around the world. Surgery is not usually required; sexual intercourse or use of dilators can effectively lengthen the vagina if there is any concern. There are a number of surgical procedures that have been used, although the use of dilators has the fewest complications (McQuillan and Grover 2014). The gonads are often in a superficial inguinal position and may be the source of pain during sexual intercourse. This in theory may become a reason for choosing to have them removed. There is a slightly increased risk of *pre-* or *in situ* germ cell neoplasia (10–15%) but those rarely become invasive (Cools et al. 2017; Skakkebaek 1979; Handa et al. 1995; Sakai et al. 2000; Nojima et al. 2004; Hannema et al. 2006; Looijenga et al. 2007; Robboy and Jaubert 2007). Current recommendations are to leave the gonads *in situ* until after puberty has been completed, and at that age, the patient can then decide whether they prefer to retain them with ongoing monitoring or have a prophylactic gonadectomy (Cools and Looijenga 2017).

Women with CAIS have an increased risk of osteoporosis whether or not they have their gonads (Soule et al. 1995; Bertelloni et al. 1998; Mizunuma et al. 1998; Sobel et al. 2006; Danilovic et al. 2007). Although adult circulating testosterone levels are sometimes high (about 50 nmol/l) if the gonads have not been removed, as the skeleton is unresponsive to testosterone, bone mineral density will reflect the rate of conversion of testosterone to oestrogen. Oestrogen levels in individuals with CAIS are higher than those in men, but lower than those in women with ovaries. Therefore, it is possible that women with CAIS who have their gonads may benefit from having their bone density monitored to ensure identification of individuals who might warrant treatment with additional oestrogen to prevent osteoporosis (Warne et al. 2005).

There has been some discussion amongst women with CAIS who had their testes removed (prior to current practices), advocating for the use of testosterone replacement therapy rather than oestrogens. As the testosterone must be converted to oestrogens to have any effect, the benefit of this approach has yet to be established.

Women with CAIS, being XY, are candidates for red–green colour blindness, a condition otherwise confined to males, and they are on average slightly taller than average women. Being an X-linked trait, CAIS may affect sisters, maternal aunts and other female relatives on the maternal side. The mother who carries the gene often has a reduced amount of pubic and axillary hair.

24.4.2.2 Partial Androgen Insensitivity Syndrome (PAIS)

PAIS is associated with great phenotypic diversity, and the phenotype is poorly predicted from the genotype (Deeb et al. 2005). Within a single family (the condition is inherited as an X-linked trait), it is possible for some individuals to have atypical genitalia and for others to have a micropenis (without hypospadias) and gynaecomastia.

One study reported that nearly 25% of subjects with PAIS were dissatisfied with their adult gender identity, regardless of whether they had been reared male or female (Migeon et al. 2002). It should be noted, however, that in the majority, gender identity followed the sex of rearing (Gangaher et al. 2016). The policy regarding genital surgery in babies and children with PAIS has changed substantially, with a male sex of rearing in the vast majority of cases of PAIS because it preserves choice. High-dose testosterone therapy (Grino et al. 1989) has potential for enlarging the penis. An important part of the problem, however, is making an accurate diagnosis. The recent progress in genetic testing now allows more individuals to have an accurate diagnosis, in contrast to the past where androgen insensitivity syndrome had been used as an expression to cover all undervirilised males (see Chap. 21).

The risk of testicular cancer was considered high (55%) in intra-abdominal testes of males with PAIS (Hughes et al. 2006). However, recent data suggest that this risk is not higher in PAIS compared to CAIS. Therefore, decision on the management strategy to adopt is essential (Cools and Looijenga 2017). For scrotal testes, it would involve 6-monthly palpation and a biopsy looking for germ cell neoplasia *in situ* (GNCIS) (Faure et al. 2016). Retention of testes can be associated with the development of adolescent gynaecomastia, which may require bilateral mastectomies.

24.4.2.3 5α-Reductase-2 Deficiency

As first described (Imperato-McGinley et al. 1979), in those raised female, 5α-reductase-2 deficiency causes a gradual gender identity change from female to male at puberty in a significant number of individuals, if the testes have been retained (Cohen-Kettenis 2005). This has made it difficult to define a policy suitable for all environments (Houk et al. 2005). Gynaecomastia does not develop. The adult penis is typically small. Dihydrotestosterone treatment has been given with encouraging results in children (Charmandari et al. 2001). The risk of testicular cancer appears to be relatively low. The pattern of inheritance is autosomal recessive. Some individuals, not recognised as having this condition, and raised females may be able to decide as an adolescent whether to change gender.

24.4.2.4 17β-Hydroxysteroid Dehydrogenase (17β-HSD) Deficiency

17β-Hydroxysteroid dehydrogenase deficiency, like 5α-reductase-2 deficiency, may cause a transition in gender identity from female to male in some individuals (Rosler 2006), with response to produced testosterone being greater. For the individual who was not identified at birth, and reaches adolescence, discussion and any decision need to be carefully made with the young person themselves. The phenotype is seen only in genotypic males; affected females have no symptoms. The pattern of inheritance is autosomal recessive.

24.4.2.5 46,XY Lipoid Adrenal Hyperplasia and 46,XY, 17β-Hydroxylase Deficiency

These two forms of CAH are both extremely rare. Lipoid adrenal hyperplasia, caused by a deficiency of the steroid acute regulatory protein (StAR), is associated with a complete block in steroid hormone secretion by both the adrenals and the testes, so that all subjects, whether XX or XY, have a female phenotype (Miller 2007). The prognosis is good, once the diagnosis has been made and treatment started with both a glucocorticoid and a mineralocorticoid. Oestrogen replacement is needed to induce puberty and is continued life-long.

17β-Hydroxylase deficiency (Kater and Biglieri 1994) also results in a female phenotype in genotypic males, and there is no uterus; but, unlike lipoid adrenal hyperplasia, it is associated with glucocorticoid-suppressible hypertension due to the accumulation of mineralocorticoid precursors.

24.4.2.6 46,XY Complete Gonadal Dysgenesis

Women with 46,XY complete gonadal dysgenesis differ from women with CAIS in that spontaneous breast development at adolescence does not occur. Serum FSH and LH levels are high due to primary gonadal failure. Hormone replacement therapy is able to induce secondary sex characteristics including menses because women with this condition have a uterus. It is possible for them to carry a pregnancy if an embryo is implanted into the uterus and appropriate hormonal support is administered. Streak gonads should be excised at diagnosis, as they have no hormonal function, no fertility potential and carry a high risk of malignancy (Huang et al. 2017). Gender identity is female (McCarty et al. 2006).

24.4.2.7 46,XY Partial Gonadal Dysgenesis (GD)

The 46,XY form of partial GD is quite rare, but it is the subject of considerable interest to basic researchers into the genetic regulation of gonadal differentiation, who are now applying new gene discovery strategies (Croft et al. 2016; Eggers et al. 2016). More commonly, partial gonadal dysgenesis is associated with a 45,X/46,XY mosaic karyotype and discussion about long-term outcome will be found later in this chapter.

24.4.2.8 Persistent Müllerian Duct Syndrome

There are no long-term outcome studies on this very rare condition, which is due to mutations in either the gene for *AMH* or the AMH receptor gene. The usual anatomy is that the two vasa deferentia are enclosed within the lateral walls of the Müllerian remnant. Testes are often undescended, and the risk of malignant transformation is reported to be as high as 30%, whereas the risk of malignancy of the Müllerian remnant is less (Picard et al. 2017). Conservation of the Müllerian structures is now preferred to ensure that future options are available for the individual, although there are no reports of gender change in the literature.

24.5 Cloacal Exstrophy

Genetic males with cloacal exstrophy have normal testes, but the penis is severely hypoplastic and bifid. A generation ago, these babies would have had their testes removed and female genitalia constructed, then raised female. The long-term outcome was disastrous; most of those treated in this way grew up with an unequivocally male gender identity (Reiner and Gearhart 2004). This practice has now stopped, and patients would be raised as male. However, one must acknowledge that cloacal exstrophy remains one of the most challenging congenital anomalies, with persistent poor long-term outcomes from a urological, gastro-intestinal, sexual and psychological point of view (Vliet et al. 2015).

Genetic females with cloacal exstrophy will have normal ovaries, but their Müllerian tract will be variably affected. It is possible to have two separate uterine horns, with or without cervices and no vagina. It is crucial that consideration be given to the potential for the uterine horns to be anastomosed in the future to the vestibule, vagina or neovagina and thus potentially offer a fertility option.

24.6 Sex Chromosome DSD

24.6.1 45,X/46,XY Mixed Gonadal Dysgenesis

The phenotype varies widely from completely typical male or female to neonates with ambiguous genitalia (Muller et al. 1999). The mosaicism ratio, which varies between tissues, may explain the phenotype and may vary between tissues (Hatano et al. 2018). Similar to cases of ovo-testicular DSD, the decision regarding sex of rearing is difficult and a multidisciplinary approach is paramount (Diamond et al. 2018). The rate of gender dysphoria is difficult to evaluate in this population due to very small numbers (Furtado et al. 2012). However, this highlights the importance of not performing early irreversible surgery that would restrict options in the future, especially when the child is asymptomatic (Öcal et al. 2009). The exact risk of malignancy remains unclear and may vary according to phenotype. However, it is overall considered to be moderately elevated, and strategies have been proposed depending on the position and histologic features of the gonads (Wolffenbuttel et al. 2016).

24.6.2 47,XXY Klinefelter Syndrome with Atypical Genitalia

Although genital ambiguity is not usually a feature of Klinefelter syndrome, it does occur (Lee et al. 2007) and can be associated with gender dysphoria. It is important that Klinefelter syndrome is recognised, as it carries risks of malignancy (De Sanctis et al. 2013) and decreased fertility, which needs to be specifically addressed (Rives et al. 2018). Boys with Klinefelter syndrome can present with neurocognitive and endocrine symptoms and benefit from multidisciplinary management (Gravholt et al. 2018).

24.7 Discussion and Conclusion

Scientific studies that have been conducted have tried to measure outcomes utilising standardised validated assessment tools for body image, satisfaction with the body and the genitalia, sexual feelings and sexual activity, general health, urinary problems, mental health and, broadly, quality of life. They reveal that the quality of life for many people with DSD is mixed.

Little information is available about how to help people born with DSD and atypical genitalia to build the self-esteem needed to establish healthy intimate and sexual relationships. Efforts to understand the resource needs (Mortimer 2017; Tonkin-Hill 2018) and to increase the support to these individuals and their families have been made, with the establishment of multidisciplinary teams and DSD coordinators.

DSD present many challenges for people living with the conditions, their parents and the health professionals who care for them (Slijper et al. 1998; Thyen et al. 2005). It is an advance that so many centres are now reporting long-term outcome data and the fact that these reports are not only from centres able to devote a high level of human and technical resources but importantly also from very poor countries with very different cultural beliefs and traditions (see Chap. 22) (Ammini et al. 2002; Warne and Raza 2008; Zainuddin et al. 2014).

The management of DSD requires a MDT approach, properly funded and working from a strong evidence base. Ideally, patient advocacy groups should be involved, and where relationships between local practitioners and local support groups have become frayed, mediation to achieve compromise and positive engagement would be helpful. More research into basic mechanisms of sex differentiation, the determinants of gender identity and epidemiology is needed. Highly specialised diagnostic facilities should be centralised within countries and even regions. International collaborations to generate sufficient numbers for the study of very rare disorders are being established and should provide better information on which to base new management protocols.

Acknowledgement With thanks and acknowledgement to Professor Garry L. Warne AM who wrote the original version of this chapter.

References

Abusheikha N, Lass A, Brinsden P. XX males without SRY gene and with infertility. Hum Reprod. 2001;16(4):717–8.

Adam MP, Vilain E. Emerging issues in disorders/differences of sex development (DSD). Am J Med Genet C Semin Med Genet. 2017;175(2):249–52.

Ahmed SF, Bashamboo A, Lucas-Herald A, et al. Understanding the genetic aetiology in patients with XY DSD. Br Med Bull. 2013;106:67–89.

Al-Maghribi H. Congenital adrenal hyperplasia: problems with developmental anomalies of the external genitalia and sex assignment. Saudi J Kidney Dis Transpl. 2007;18(3):405–13.

Ammini AC, Gupta R, Kapoor A, et al. Etiology, clinical profile, gender identity and long-term follow up of patients with ambiguous genitalia in India. J Pediatr Endocrinol Metab. 2002;15(4):423–30.

Armstrong KL, Henderson C, Hoan NT, et al. Living with congenital adrenal hyperplasia in Vietnam: a survey of parents. J Pediatr Endocrinol Metab. 2006;19(10):1207–23.

Berenbaum SA, Bailey JM. Effects on gender identity of prenatal androgens and genital appearance: evidence from girls with congenital adrenal hyperplasia. J Clin Endocrinol Metab. 2003;88(3):1102–6.

Berenbaum SA, Bryk KL, Beltz AM. Early androgen effects on spatial and mechanical abilities: evidence from congenital adrenal hyperplasia. Behav Neurosci. 2012;126(1):86–96.

Berglund A, Johannsen TH, Stochholm K, Aksglaede L, Fedder J, Viuff MH, Main KM, Gravholt CH. Incidence, prevalence, diagnostic delay, morbidity, mortality and socioeconomic status in males with 46,XX disorders of sex development: a nationwide study. Hum Reprod. 2017;32(8):1751–60. https://doi.org/10.1093/humrep/dex210.

Berglund A, Johannsen TH, Stochholm K, et al. Morbidity, mortality, and socioeconomics in females with 46,XY disorders of sex development: a nationwide study. J Clin Endocrinol Metab. 2018; 103(4):1418–28.

Bertelloni S, Baroncelli GI, Federico G, et al. Altered bone mineral density in patients with complete androgen insensitivity syndrome. Horm Res. 1998;50(6):309–14.

Bogdanska M, Morris A, Hutson JM, et al. Long-term urinary symptoms in adolescent and adult women with congenital adrenal hyperplasia. J Pediatr Urol. 2018;14(3):240.e241–5.

Bramble MS, Lipson A, Vashist N, et al. Effects of chromosomal sex and hormonal influences on shaping sex differences in brain and behavior: lessons from cases of disorders of sex development. J Neurosci Res. 2017;95(1–2):65–74.

Brannstrom M. Current status and future direction of uterus transplantation. Curr Opin Organ Transplant. 2018;23(5):592–7.

Cetinkaya S, Kara C. The effect of glucocorticoid replacement therapy on bone mineral density in children with congenital adrenal hyperplasia. J Pediatr Endocrinol Metab. 2011;24(5–6):265–9.

Charmandari E, Dattani MT, Perry LA, et al. Kinetics and effect of percutaneous administration of dihydrotestosterone in children. Horm Res. 2001;56(5–6):177–81.

Cheikhelard A, Bidet M, Baptiste A, et al. Surgery is not superior to dilation for the management of vaginal agenesis in Mayer-Rokitansky-Kuster-Hauser syndrome: a multicenter comparative observational study in 131 patients. Am J Obstet Gynecol. 2018;219(3):281.e281–9.

Chiang HS, Wu YN, Wu CC, et al. Cytogenic and molecular analyses of 46,XX male syndrome with clinical comparison to other groups with testicular azoospermia of genetic origin. J Formos Med Assoc. 2013;112(2):72–8.

Chowdhury TK, Laila K, Hutson JM, et al. Male gender identity in children with 46,XX DSD with congenital adrenal hyperplasia after delayed presentation in mid-childhood. J Pediatr Surg. 2015;50(12):2060–2.

Cohen-Kettenis PT. Gender change in 46,XY persons with 5alpha-reductase-2 deficiency and 17beta-hydroxysteroid dehydrogenase-3 deficiency. Arch Sex Behav. 2005;34(4):399–410.

Cools M, Looijenga L. Update on the pathophysiology and risk factors for the development of malignant testicular germ cell tumors in complete androgen insensitivity syndrome. Sex Dev. 2017;11(4):175–81.

Cools M, Wolffenbuttel KP, Hersmus R, et al. Malignant testicular germ cell tumors in postpubertal individuals with androgen insensitivity: prevalence, pathology and relevance of single nucleotide polymorphism-based susceptibility profiling. Hum Reprod. 2017;32(12):2561–73. https://doi.org/10.1093/humrep/dex300.

Cools M, Simmonds M, Elford S, et al. Response to the Council of Europe Human Rights Commissioner's issue paper on human rights and intersex people. Eur Urol. 2016;70(3):407–9.

Crawford JM, Warne G, Grover S, et al. Results from a pediatric surgical centre justify early intervention in disorders of sex development. J Pediatr Surg. 2009;44(2):413–6.

Creighton S. Surgery for intersex. J R Soc Med. 2001;94(5):218–20.

Creighton SM, Minto CL, Steele SJ. Objective cosmetic and anatomical outcomes at adolescence of feminising surgery for ambiguous genitalia done in childhood. Lancet. 2001;358(9276):124–5.

Creighton S, Alderson J, Brown S, et al. Medical photography: ethics, consent and the intersex patient. BJU Int. 2002;89(1):67–71. discussion 71-62

Croft B, Ayers K, Sinclair A, et al. Review disorders of sex development: the evolving role of genomics in diagnosis and gene discovery. Birth Defects Res C Embryo Today. 2016;108(4):337–50.

Crouch NS, Minto CL, Laio LM, et al. Genital sensation after feminizing genitoplasty for congenital adrenal hyperplasia: a pilot study. BJU Int. 2004;93(1):135–8.

Crouch NS, Liao LM, Woodhouse CR, et al. Sexual function and genital sensitivity following feminizing genitoplasty for congenital adrenal hyperplasia. J Urol. 2008;179(2):634–8.

Damiani D, Fellous M, McElreavey K, et al. True hermaphroditism: clinical aspects and molecular studies in 16 cases. Eur J Endocrinol. 1997;136(2):201–4.

Damiani D, Guedes DR, Damiani D, et al. True hermaphroditism: experience with 36 patients. Arq Bras Endocrinol Metabol. 2005;49(1):71–8.

Danilovic DL, Correa PH, Costa EM, et al. Height and bone mineral density in androgen insensitivity syndrome with mutations in the androgen receptor gene. Osteoporos Int. 2007;18(3):369–74.

De Sanctis V, Fiscina B, Soliman A, et al. Klinefelter syndrome and cancer: from childhood to adulthood. Pediatr Endocrinol Rev. 2013;11(1):44–50.

Deeb A, Mason C, Lee YS, et al. Correlation between genotype, phenotype and sex of rearing in 111 patients with partial androgen insensitivity syndrome. Clin Endocrinol. 2005;63(1):56–62.

Demirel F, Kara O, Esen I. Inguinal ovary as a rare diagnostic sign of Mayer-Rokitansky-Kuster-Hauser syndrome. J Pediatr Endocrinol Metab. 2012;25(3–4):383–6.

Dessens AB, Slijper FME, Drop SLS. Gender dysphoria and gender change in chromosomal females with congenital adrenal hyperplasia. Arch Sex Behav. 2005;34(4):389–97.

Diamond DA, Swartz J, Tishelman A, et al. Management of pediatric patients with DSD and ambiguous genitalia: balancing the child's moral claims to self-determination with parental values and preferences. J Pediatr Urol. 2018;14(5):416.e1–5.

Eggers S, Sadedin S, van den Bergen JA, et al. Disorders of sex development: insights from targeted gene sequencing of a large international patient cohort. Genome Biol. 2016;17(1):243.

Fagerholm R, Santtila P, Miettinen PJ, et al. Sexual function and attitudes toward surgery after feminizing genitoplasty. J Urol. 2011;185(5):1900–4.

Fagerholm R, Rintala R, Taskinen S. Lower urinary tract symptoms after feminizing genitoplasty. J Pediatr Urol. 2013;9(1):23–6.

Faure A, Bouty A, O'Brien M, et al. Testicular biopsy in prepubertal boys: a worthwhile minor surgical procedure? Nat Rev Urol. 2016;13(3):141–50.

Fliegner M, Krupp K, Brunner F, et al. Sexual life and sexual wellness in individuals with complete androgen insensitivity syndrome (CAIS) and Mayer-Rokitansky-Kuster-Hauser Syndrome (MRKHS). J Sex Med. 2014;11(3):729–42.

Frisen L, Nordenstrom A, Falhammar H, et al. Gender role behavior, sexuality, and psychosocial adaptation in women with congenital adrenal hyperplasia due to CYP21A2 deficiency. J Clin Endocrinol Metab. 2009;94(9):3432–9.

Frost-Arner L, Aberg M, Jacobsson S. Clitoral sensitivity after surgical correction in women with adrenogenital syndrome: a long term follow-up. Scand J Plast Reconstr Surg Hand Surg. 2003;37(6):356–9.

Furtado PS, Moraes F, Lago R, et al. Gender dysphoria associated with disorders of sex development. Nat Rev Urol. 2012;9(11):620–7.

Gangaher A, Chauhan V, Jyotsna VP, et al. Gender identity and gender of rearing in 46 XY disorders of sexual development. Indian J Endocrinol Metab. 2016;20(4):536–41.

Gastaud F, Bouvattier C, Duranteau L, et al. Impaired sexual and reproductive outcomes in women with classical forms of congenital adrenal hyperplasia. J Clin Endocrinol Metab. 2007;92(4):1391–6.

Geiser C, Lehmann W, Eid M. A note on sex differences in mental rotation in different age groups. Intelligence. 2008;36(6):556–63.

Gorduza DB, Quigley CA, Caldamone AA, et al. Surgery of anomalies of gonadal and genital development in the "post-truth era". Urol Clin North Am. 2018;45(4):659–69.

Gravholt CH, Chang S, Wallentin M, et al. Klinefelter syndrome: integrating genetics, neuropsychology, and endocrinology. Endocr Rev. 2018;39(4):389–423.

Grino PB, Isidro-Gutierrez RF, Griffin JE, et al. Androgen resistance associated with a qualitative abnormality of the androgen receptor and responsive to high dose androgen therapy. J Clin Endocrinol Metab. 1989;68(3):578–84.

Handa N, Nagasaki A, Tsunoda M, et al. Yolk sac tumor in a case of testicular feminization syndrome. J Pediatr Surg. 1995;30(9):1366–7; discussion 1367–8

Hannema SE, Scott IS, Rajpert-De Meyts E, et al. Testicular development in the complete androgen insensitivity syndrome. J Pathol. 2006;208(4):518–27.

Hampson E, Rovet JF. Spatial function in adolescents and young adults with congenital adrenal hyperplasia: clinical phenotype and implications for the androgen hypothesis. Psychoneuroendocrinology. 2015;54:60–70. https://doi.org/10.1016/j.psyneuen.2015.01.022. Epub 2015 Feb 2.

Hatano M, Fukuzawa R, Hasegawa Y. The mosaicism ratio of 45,X may explain the phenotype in a case of mixed gonadal dysgenesis. Sex Dev. 2018;12(4):175–9.

Hines M, Ahmed SF, Hughes IA. Psychological outcomes and gender-related development in complete androgen insensitivity syndrome. Arch Sex Behav. 2003;32(2):93–101.

Houk CP, Damiani D, Lee PA. Choice of gender in 5alpha-reductase deficiency: a moving target. J Pediatr Endocrinol Metab. 2005;18(4):339–45.

Huang H, Wang C, Tian Q. Gonadal tumour risk in 292 phenotypic female patients with disorders of sex development containing Y chromosome or Y-derived sequence. Clin Endocrinol. 2017;86(4):621–7.

Huepenbecker SP, Divine L, Chu CS, et al. Two sisters with Mayer-Rokitansky-Kuster-Hauser syndrome and serous adenocarcinoma of the ovary. Gynecol Oncol Rep. 2017;22:13–5.

Hughes IA. Disorders of sex development: a new definition and classification. Best Pract Res Clin Endocrinol Metab. 2008;22(1):119–34.

Hughes IA, Houk C, Ahmed SF, et al. Consensus statement on management of intersex disorders. Arch Dis Child. 2006;91(7):554–63.

Imperato-McGinley J, Peterson RE, Gautier T, et al. Androgens and the evolution of male-gender identity among male pseudohermaphrodites with 5alpha-reductase deficiency. N Engl J Med. 1979;300(22):1233–7.

Jesus LE. Feminizing genitoplasties: Where are we now? J Pediatr Urol. 2018;14(5):407–15. https://doi.org/10.1016/j.jpurol.2018.03.020. Epub 2018 Apr 26.

Jones BC, O'Brien M, Chase J, et al. Early hypospadias surgery may lead to a better long-term psychosexual outcome. J Urol. 2009;182(4 Suppl):1744–9.

Juusela AL, Gimovsky ML. Intraoperative hemorrhage requiring emergent hysterectomy: failed conservative management of a cervical placenta accreta. J Gynecol Surg. 2017;33(5):215–8.

Kater CE, Biglieri EG. Disorders of steroid 17 alpha-hydroxylase deficiency. Endocrinol Metab Clin North Am. 1994;23(2):341–57.

Kimberley N, Hutson JM, Southwell BR, et al. Vaginal agenesis, the hymen, and associated anomalies. J Pediatr Adolesc Gynecol. 2012;25(1):54–8.

Kreukels BPC, Kohler B, Nordenstrom A, et al. Gender dysphoria and gender change in disorders of sex development/intersex conditions: results from the dsd-LIFE study. J Sex Med. 2018;15(5):777–85.

Krstic ZD, Smoljanic Z, Vukanic D, et al. True hermaphroditism: 10 years' experience. Pediatr Surg Int. 2000;16(8):580–3.

Lean WL, Deshpande A, Hutson J, et al. Cosmetic and anatomic outcomes after feminizing surgery for ambiguous genitalia. J Pediatr Surg. 2005;40(12):1856–60.

Lean WL, Hutson JM, Deshpande AV, et al. Clitoroplasty: past, present and future. Pediatr Surg Int. 2007;23(4):289–93.

Lee PA, Money J. Communicating with parents of the newborn with intersex: transcript of an interview. J Pediatr Endocrinol Metab. 2004;17(7):925–30.

Lee YS, Cheng AW, Ahmed SF, et al. Genital anomalies in Klinefelter's syndrome. Horm Res. 2007;68(3):150–5.

Lee PA, Houk CP, Husmann DA. Should male gender assignment be considered in the markedly virilized patient with 46,XX and congenital adrenal hyperplasia? J Urol. 2010;184(4 Suppl):1786–92.

Lesma A, Bocciardi A, Corti S, et al. Sexual function in adult life following Passerini-Glazel feminizing genitoplasty in patients with congenital adrenal hyperplasia. J Urol. 2014;191(1):206–11.

Looijenga LH, Hersmus R, Oosterhuis JW, et al. Tumor risk in disorders of sex development (DSD). Best Pract Res Clin Endocrinol Metab. 2007;21(3):480–95.

Lowenstein L, Gamble T, Sanses TV, et al. Sexual function is related to body image perception in women with pelvic organ prolapse. J Sex Med. 2009;6(8):2286–91.

Ludwikowski BM, Gonzalez R. The surgical correction of urogenital sinus in patients with DSD: 15 years after description of total urogenital mobilization in children. Front Pediatr. 2013;1:41.

Matsui F, Shimada K, Matsumoto F, et al. Long-term outcome of ovotesticular disorder of sex development: a single center experience. Int J Urol. 2011;18(3):231–6.

McCarty BM, Migeon CJ, Meyer-Bahlburg HF, et al. Medical and psychosexual outcome in women affected by complete gonadal dysgenesis. J Pediatr Endocrinol Metab. 2006;19(7):873–7.

McQuillan SK, Grover SR. Systematic review of sexual function and satisfaction following the management of vaginal agenesis. Int Urogynecol J. 2014;25(10):1313–20.

Mendes-Dos-Santos CT, Lemos-Marini SH, Baptista MT, et al. Normalization of height and excess body fat in children with salt-wasting 21-hydroxylase deficiency. J Pediatr. 2011;87(3):263–8.

Merke DP, Bornstein SR. Congenital adrenal hyperplasia. Lancet. 2005;365(9477):2125–36.

Meyer-Bahlburg HFL. Treatment guidelines for children with disorders of sex development. Neuropsychiatr Enfance Adolesc. 2008;56:345–9.

Migeon CJ, Wisniewski AB, Brown TR, et al. 46,XY intersex individuals: phenotypic and etiologic classification, knowledge of condition, and satisfaction with knowledge in adulthood. Pediatrics. 2002;110(3):e32.

Miller WL. Steroidogenic acute regulatory protein (StAR), a novel mitochondrial cholesterol transporter. Biochim Biophys Acta. 2007;1771(6):663–76.

Minto CL, Liao KL, Conway GS, et al. Sexual function in women with complete androgen insensitivity syndrome. Fertil Steril. 2003;80(1):157–64.

Mizunuma H, Soda M, Okano H, et al. Changes in bone mineral density after orchidectomy and hormone replacement therapy in individuals with androgen insensitivity syndrome. Hum Reprod. 1998;13(1O):2816–8.

Morcel K, Camborieux L, Guerrier D. Mayer-Rokitansky-Kuster-Hauser (MRKH) syndrome. Orphanet J Rare Dis. 2007;2:13.

Moreira RP, Villares SM, Madureira G, et al. Obesity and familial predisposition are significant determining factors of an adverse metabolic profile in young patients with congenital adrenal hyperplasia. Horm Res Paediatr. 2013;80(2):111–8.

Mortimer R. Supports for parents of children with differences of sex development. MDRP thesis, University of Melbourne. 2017.

Muller J, Ritzen EM, Ivarsson SA, et al. Management of males with 45,X/46,XY gonadal dysgenesis. Horm Res. 1999;52(1):11–4.

Mureau MA, Slijper FM, van der Meulen JC, et al. Psychosexual adjustment of men who underwent hypospadias repair: a norm-related study. J Urol. 1995;154(4):1351–5.

Nabhan ZM, Rink RC, Eugster EA. Urinary tract infections in children with congenital adrenal hyperplasia. J Pediatr Endocrinol Metab. 2006;19(6):815–20.

Nermoen I, Husebye ES, Svartberg J, et al. Subjective health status in men and women with congenital adrenal hyperplasia: a population-based survey in Norway. Eur J Endocrinol. 2010;163(3):453–9.

van Niekerk WA, Retief AE. The gonads of human true hermaphrodites. Hum Genet. 1981;58(1):117–22.

Nojima M, Taguchi T, Ando Y, et al. Huge seminoma developed in a patient with testicular feminization. J Obstet Gynaecol Res. 2004;30(2):109–12.

Nordenskjold A, Holmdahl G, Frisen L, et al. Type of mutation and surgical procedure affect long-term quality of life for women with congenital adrenal hyperplasia. J Clin Endocrinol Metab. 2008;93(2):380–6.

Nordenstrom A, Servin A, Bohlin G, et al. Sex-typed toy play behavior correlates with the degree of prenatal androgen exposure assessed by CYP21 genotype in girls with congenital adrenal hyperplasia. J Clin Endocrinol Metab. 2002;87(11):5119–24.

Nordenstrom A, Frisen L, Falhammar H, et al. Sexual function and surgical outcome in women with congenital adrenal hyperplasia due to CYP21A2 deficiency: clinical perspective and the patients' perception. J Clin Endocrinol Metab. 2010;95(8):3633–40.

Ocal G, Berberoğlu M, Siklar Z, Bilir P. Gender dysphoria and gender change in an adolescent with 45,X/46,XY mixed gonadal dysgenesis. Exp Clin Endocrinol Diabetes. 2009;117(6):301–4. https://doi.org/10.1055/s-0028-1085999. Epub 2008 Oct 1.

Oppelt P, Renner SP, Kellermann A, et al. Clinical aspects of Mayer-Rokitansky-Kuester-Hauser syndrome: recommendations for clinical diagnosis and staging. Hum Reprod. 2006;21(3):792–7.

Ozbey H, Darendeliler F, Kayserili H, et al. Gender assignment in female congenital adrenal hyperplasia: a difficult experience. BJU Int. 2004;94(3):388–91.

Palmer BW, Wisniewski AB, Schaeffer TL, et al. A model of delivering multi-disciplinary care to people with 46 XY DSD. J Pediatr Urol. 2012;8(1):7–16.

Pasterski V, Zucker KJ, Hindmarsh PC, "Hughes IA, Acerini C, Spencer D, Neufeld S, Hines M. Increased cross-gender identification independent of gender role behavior in girls with congenital adrenal hyperplasia: results from a standardized assessment of 4- to 11-year-old children. Arch Sex Behav. 2015;44(5):1363–75. doi: https://doi.org/10.1007/s10508-014-0385-0. Epub 2014 Sep 20.

Picard JY, Cate RL, Racine C, et al. The persistent Mullerian Duct syndrome: an update based upon a personal experience of 157 cases. Sex Dev. 2017;11(3):109–25.

Razzaghy-Azar M, Karimi S, Shirazi E. Gender identity in patients with congenital adrenal hyperplasia. Int J Endocrinol Metab. 2017;15(3):e12537.

Reiner WG, Gearhart JP. Discordant sexual identity in some genetic males with cloacal exstrophy assigned to female sex at birth. N Engl J Med. 2004;350(4):333–41.

Rives N, Rives A, Rondanino C, et al. Fertility preservation in Klinefelter syndrome patients during the transition period. Endocr Dev. 2018;33:149–57.

Robboy SJ, Jaubert F. Neoplasms and pathology of sexual developmental disorders (intersex). Pathology. 2007;39(1):147–63.

Rosler A. 17 Beta-hydroxysteroid dehydrogenase 3 deficiency in the Mediterranean population. Pediatr Endocrinol Rev. 2006;3(Suppl 3):455–61.

Sakai N, Yamada T, Asao T, et al. Bilateral testicular tumors in androgen insensitivity syndrome. Int J Urol. 2000;7(10):390–2.

Salle JL, Lorenzo AJ, Jesus LE, et al. Surgical treatment of high urogenital sinuses using the anterior sagittal transrectal approach: a useful strategy to optimize exposure and outcomes. J Urol. 2012;187(3):1024–31.

Schweizer K, Brunner F, Gedrose B, et al. Coping with diverse sex development: treatment experiences and psychosocial support during childhood and adolescence and adult well-being. J Pediatr Psychol. 2017;42(5):504–19.
Servin A, Nordenstrom A, Larsson A, et al. Prenatal androgens and gender-typed behavior: a study of girls with mild and severe forms of congenital adrenal hyperplasia. Dev Psychol. 2003;39(3):440–50.
Skakkebaek NE. Carcinoma-in-situ of testis in testicular feminization syndrome. Acta Pathol Microbiol Scand A. 1979;87(1):87–9.
Slijper FM, Drop SL, Molenaar JC, et al. Long-term psychological evaluation of intersex children. Arch Sex Behav. 1998;27(2):125–44.
Sobel V, Schwartz B, Zhu YS, et al. Bone mineral density in the complete androgen insensitivity and 5alpha-reductase-2 deficiency syndromes. J Clin Endocrinol Metab. 2006;91(8):3017–23.
Soule SG, Conway G, Prelevic GM, et al. Osteopenia as a feature of the androgen insensitivity syndrome. Clin Endocrinol. 1995;43(6):671–5.
Speiser PW, Azziz R, Baskin LS, et al. Congenital adrenal hyperplasia due to steroid 21-hydroxylase deficiency: an Endocrine Society clinical practice guideline. J Clin Endocrinol Metab. 2010;95(9):4133–60.
Stikkelbroeck NM, Beerendonk CC, Willemsen WN, et al. The long term outcome of feminizing genital surgery for congenital adrenal hyperplasia: anatomical, functional and cosmetic outcomes, psychosexual development, and satisfaction in adult female patients. J Pediatr Adolesc Gynecol. 2003;16(5):289–96.
Stites J, Bernabe KJ, Galan D, et al. Urinary continence outcomes following vaginoplasty in patients with congenital adrenal hyperplasia. J Pediatr Urol. 2017;13(1):38.e31–7.
Strandqvist A, Falhammar H, Lichtenstein P, et al. Suboptimal psychosocial outcomes in patients with congenital adrenal hyperplasia: epidemiological studies in a nonbiased national cohort in Sweden. J Clin Endocrinol Metab. 2014;99(4):1425–32.
Tamar-Mattis A. Patient advocate responds to DSD surgery debate. J Pediatr Urol. 2014;10(4):788–9.
Thyen U, Richter-Appelt H, Wiesemann C, et al. Deciding on gender in children with intersex conditions: considerations and controversies. Treat Endocrinol. 2005;4(1):1–8.
Tonkin-Hill G. Identifying the resource needs of adolescents with differences of sex development. Medicine. Melbourne, Australia: University of Melbourne; 2018.
van de Grift TC, Cohen-Kettenis PT, de Vries ALC, BPC K, (on behalf of dsd-LIFE). Body image and self-esteem in disorders of sex development: a European multicenter study. Health Psychol. 2018;37(4):334–43. https://doi.org/10.1037/hea0000600.
Verkauskas G, Jaubert F, Lortat-Jacob S, et al. The long-term followup of 33 cases of true hermaphroditism: a 40-year experience with conservative gonadal surgery. J Urol. 2007;177(2):726–31; discussion 731.
Vliet R, Roelofs LA, Rassouli-Kirchmeier R, et al. Clinical outcome of cloacal exstrophy, current status, and a change in surgical management. Eur J Pediatr Surg. 2015;25(1):87–93.
Vorona E, Zitzmann M, Gromoll J, et al. Clinical, endocrinological, and epigenetic features of the 46,XX male syndrome, compared with 47,XXY Klinefelter patients. J Clin Endocrinol Metab. 2007;92(9):3458–65.
Warne GL. Your child with congenital adrenal hyperplasia. Australia: Department of Endcrinology and Diabetes, Royal Children's Hospital; 1989.
Warne GL, Raza J. Disorders of sex development (DSD), their presentation and management in different cultures. Rev Endocr Metab Disord. 2008;9(3):227–36.
Warne G, Grover S, Hutson J, et al. A long-term outcome study of intersex conditions. J Pediatr Endocrinol Metab. 2005;18(6):555–67.
Wiersma R. True hermaphroditism in southern Africa: the clinical picture. Pediatr Surg Int. 2004;20(5):363–8.
Wisniewski AB, Migeon CJ. Long-term perspectives for 46,XY patients affected by complete androgen insensitivity syndrome or congenital micropenis. Semin Reprod Med. 2002;20(3):297–304.
Wisniewski AB, Migeon CJ, Meyer-Bahlburg HF, et al. Complete androgen insensitivity syndrome: long-term medical, surgical, and psychosexual outcome. J Clin Endocrinol Metab. 2000;85(8):2664–9.
Wolffenbuttel KP, Hersmus R, Stoop H, et al. Gonadal dysgenesis in disorders of sex development: diagnosis and surgical management. J Pediatr Urol. 2016;12(6):411–6.
Wong WI, Pasterski V, Hindmarsh PC, et al. Are there parental socialization effects on the sex-typed behavior of individuals with congenital adrenal hyperplasia? Arch Sex Behav. 2013;42(3):381–91.
Yang CC, Cao YY, Guan QY, et al. Influence of PDE5 inhibitor on MRI measurement of clitoral volume response in women with FSAD: a feasibility study of a potential technique for evaluating drug response. Int J Impot Res. 2008;20(1):105–10.
Zainuddin AA, Grover SR, Shamsuddin K, et al. Research on quality of life in female patients with congenital adrenal hyperplasia and issues in developing nations. J Pediatr Adolesc Gynecol. 2013; 26(6):296–304.
Zainuddin AA, Manickam MA, Baharudin A, et al. Self-perception of body weight status and weight control practices among adolescents in Malaysia. Asia Pac J Public Health. 2014;26(5 Suppl):18S–26S.
Zhen G, Bowen G, Feng X, et al. Effects of feminizing reconstructive surgery on sexual function and genital sensitivity in patients with female pseudohermaphroditism versus healthy control. Int Urol Nephrol. 2016;48(8):1281–5.
Zucker KJ, Bradley SJ, Oliver G, et al. Psychosexual development of women with congenital adrenal hyperplasia. Horm Behav. 1996;30(4):300–18.

25 Complete Androgen Insensitivity Syndrome: A Guide for Parents and Patients

Chloe A. Hanna

25.1 Introduction

Some medical conditions are easy to talk about and some are more challenging. A condition like androgen insensitivity syndrome (AIS), which affects the development of the genitals and reproductive system, raises some very uncomfortable issues about gender identity that are difficult to put into words. How is it that a woman can be born without a womb and with testes? For generations, women with AIS, and their parents, have struggled to understand this apparent contradiction. Many would have had no idea that there were others with the same condition, unless the condition was 'in the family'. Even then, discussion about a subject relating to genital development and sexual feelings may have been taboo.

We are now in an age when sexual matters are openly discussed in the community and media. This freedom is presenting opportunities for the community at large to be given some information about the existence and nature of AIS. The community will become more understanding and accepting of unusual medical conditions when they are better informed about them and the problems they cause. The same applies to individuals with AIS. It is a difficult condition to accept, but women will be helped if they have access to both good information about it and adequate opportunities to discuss the complex feelings that are bound to arise as this information is being absorbed.

25.2 How AIS Was First Recognised

The first medical report on AIS was published in 1953 by J.M. Morris, an American gynaecologist. His patient was a woman who had never menstruated. She had well-developed breasts and the external genitals of a normal woman, but she had only very sparse pubic hair and a swelling in each groin. An operation was performed, and in each of the swellings was a testis. The woman had no uterus and no ovaries. It is now known that women with AIS have the XY chromosome pattern usually associated with the male gender, and the Y chromosome causes testes to develop. In addition, they have a relatively short vagina. Because there is no uterus, there is also no cervix, and so the vagina ends as a pouch with no internal connections.

C. A. Hanna (✉)
Department of Gynaecology, The Royal Children's Hospital, Melbourne, VIC, Australia

Murdoch Children's Research Institute, Melbourne, VIC, Australia
e-mail: chloe.hanna@rch.org.au

J. M. Hutson et al. (eds.), *Disorders|Differences of Sex Development*,
https://doi.org/10.1007/978-981-13-7864-5_25

25.3 The Nature of AIS

AIS is just one of a number of medical conditions that affect the development of the reproductive and genital organs. It is caused by an alteration in a gene (a physical particle containing genetic information that is found in every cell in the body). This alteration in the gene blocks the body's response to masculinising hormones (androgen) during foetal development and after birth. In other words, it makes the body *insensitive* to *androgen*, and masculine development that would occur in the presence of a normal gene is impossible. The whole *syndrome* (the combination of physical changes that are characteristic of AIS) results from this alteration in a single gene. The body can respond to feminising hormone (oestrogen) but not androgen.

There are two forms of AIS: *complete* AIS (CAIS) and *partial* AIS (PAIS) although this can be explained as a spectrum. CAIS is a condition in which the external genitals have a typical female appearance, but the internal female reproductive organs are missing. PAIS is a variant of AIS in which affected children are born with masculinised genitalia. The extent of this is variable: some babies have a slightly enlarged clitoris and a smaller than usual cleft between the labia, while others may have an almost fully formed penis and scrotum. Some children with PAIS are raised as girls, others as boys. The presence of testes and the absence of a uterus is characteristic of both CAIS and PAIS.

The issues associated with CAIS are in many ways different from those of PAIS. In CAIS, the sex at birth is assumed female, whereas the sex of a newborn infant with PAIS may be unclear and a decision must be made about whether to raise the child as a girl or a boy. Therefore, to avoid confusion, this chapter will only consider CAIS, and PAIS will not be discussed, although there is a lot of information about it elsewhere in this book, particularly Chap. 7.

There are many variations in which the development of the external and internal genital and reproductive organs is incomplete or in which both male and female organs are found together. One in every 4500 newborn babies has external genitals that differ significantly from the standard male and female appearance. Most people would assume that such conditions are rare because they do not read about them in the newspapers, but they are not.

In common parlance, much is made of the difference between the sexes. How different are they really? According to Eastern philosophy, the female and male attributes *Yin* and *Yang* are considered to coexist in perfect balance and harmony. Most people have some qualities that may be regarded as feminine and some that are masculine. In bodily structure and function, there are more similarities than differences between females and males. For example, all women produce masculinising hormone (androgen) and all men produce feminising hormone (oestrogen). In the development of the human foetus, there is a stage when the internal and external genitalia of females and males appear identical. This means that all differences between the sexes develop from a common starting point, a completely neutral stage. From there, development may proceed either along female or male lines. The genetic and hormonal control of female and male sexual development in the foetus is well understood, and much more is known about it than about how most other aspects of development are controlled. This detailed knowledge provides a solid framework on which to build a clear understanding of AIS.

25.4 Hormones

Hormones are the chemical messengers in the body. They are produced in one place by a hormone-producing gland and act somewhere else in the body. Insulin, for example, is made in the pancreas and acts in the liver and the muscles to regulate the level of glucose in the bloodstream. Growth hormone is made in the pituitary gland near the brain and acts to promote bone growth in children.

25.4.1 Androgen

Androgen is a masculinising hormone that in males is responsible for the growth of the penis, development of facial and body hair, growth of the muscles and skeleton and deepening of the voice. Both males and females have androgen. In males, and in females with AIS, it comes from two sources: the testes and the adrenal glands (a pair of organs that lie above the kidneys, on the back wall of the abdomen). Nearly all of the androgen in females with the XX chromosome pattern comes from the adrenal glands with only a small contribution from the ovaries.

25.4.2 Androgen and Masculine Sexual Development

When babies begin their development in the womb, it is impossible to distinguish male genitalia from female genitalia. Figure 25.1 shows what these 'neutral' genitalia of both male and female look like. Note that in both sexes there is a midline cleft, with a button-like swelling at the top representing the future penis or clitoris.

Figure 25.2 shows how the 'neutral' genitalia develop into typical female genitalia. Typically, female foetuses do not produce high levels of androgen and the clitoris remains compact and the cleft becomes the entrance to the vagina.

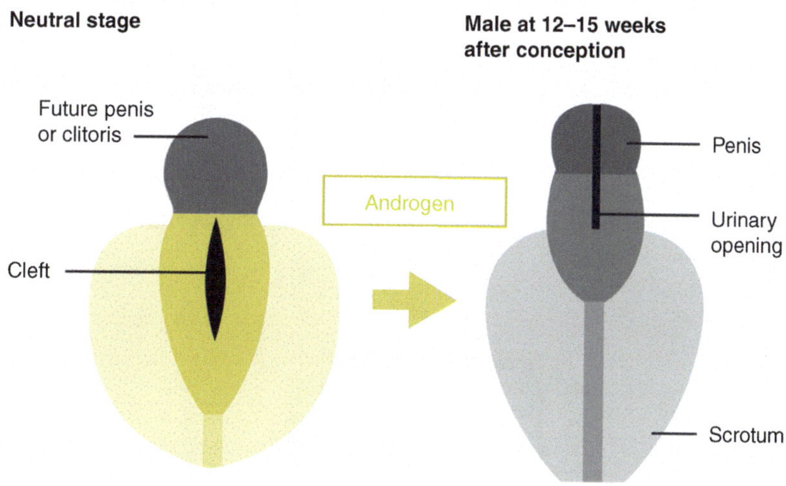

Fig. 25.1 Shows what happens in boys at 12–15 weeks after conception, as their testes start producing androgen. The button grows into a penis and the cleft closes over, starting from the bottom. This causes the urinary opening to move progressively towards the tip of the penis, and the scrotum to form

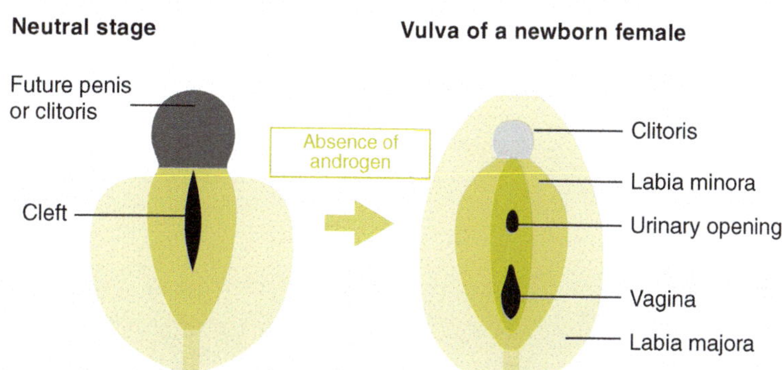

Fig. 25.2 Genital developement female

In CAIS, the testes produce androgen, but the skin covering the genital structures, and the other genital tissues, are unable to respond in the expected way, which is to develop into a boy. It is as though the androgen was not produced at all. The external genitalia develop as in typical females because the natural direction of development in the foetus is to become female. Masculine changes only occur in response to androgen.

25.4.3 The Internal Reproductive Organs

At the beginning of foetal development, males and females have identical internal reproductive organs (Fig. 25.3). In both sexes, there is a pair of tubes on the back wall of the abdomen that are capable of developing into the uterus, fallopian tubes and the upper part of the vagina. These organs do not develop in males because the foetal testes produce a hormone known as anti-Müllerian hormone, or AMH that blocks this process.

The same things happen in females with CAIS: their testes produce AMH which prevents development of the uterus, fallopian tubes and the upper part of the vagina.

The length of the vagina is variable between women with CAIS, for reasons that are still unclear. Even sisters who appear to have the same external features of CAIS may have quite different degrees of vaginal development.

25.4.4 Androgen Receptor

In a foetus with CAIS, androgen does not have the usual masculinising effect on genital development. The reason is that its body cells lack a special anchoring substance called *androgen receptor*, and without androgen receptor, the cells cannot respond to androgen, regardless of how much is present. It is a bit like a radio

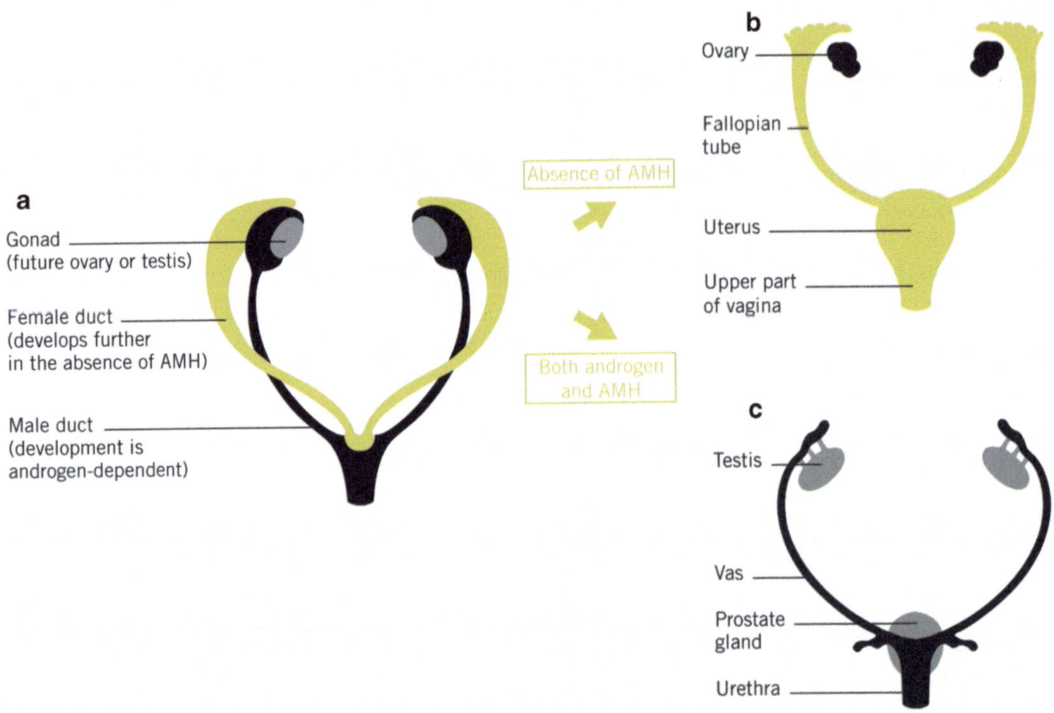

Fig. 25.3 Development of the internal reproductive organs in the female and male (**a**) neutral stage in both males and females (**b**) female organs in the absence of AMH (**c**) male organs develop when both androgen and AMH are produced by the testes

receiver that cannot be tuned to the frequency that is being transmitted. The testes can produce androgen (testosterone), but the cells don't recognise that it is there and so it doesn't have its usual effects. The oestrogen receptor is completely functional and as oestrogen is produced from testosterone, women with CAIS develop breasts and a feminine body shape.

Some females with CAIS have no androgen receptor at all, while in others, it is abnormal and does not function as a receptor. A foetus with a small amount of *active* receptor (less than normal) will begin to develop as a boy, but the process will not be completed, therefore the baby will have the features of PAIS.

25.5 The Genetic Basis of AIS

25.5.1 Chromosomes and Genes

Every new human being results from the fertilisation of an egg by a sperm. The characteristics of the father are contained in each individual sperm, and those of the mother in each of her eggs.

The sperm and egg cells contain about 30,000 tiny particles called genes. Each gene represents some characteristic of the parent that the child inherits.

When an egg has been fertilised by a sperm, the father's genes are added to the mother's, and the fertilised egg (the new human being) thus has two sets of genes. There is, for example, a gene from the mother and a gene from the father for the colour of the eyes. In fact, there is a pair of genes for every separate characteristic. The genes from the mother and father are nearly always paired, and these pairs are reproduced in every cell of the new person.

Genes are linked together on structures called chromosomes. Every cell in the body contains exactly 46 chromosomes. Typically we have twenty two pairs of autosomal chromosomes and two sex chromosomes, which may be either X or Y. Females typically have two X chromosomes, while males typically have one X and one Y chromosome. The Y chromosome contains the gene that causes testes to develop (Fig. 25.4).

25.5.2 The Androgen Receptor Gene

Females with CAIS have an X and a Y chromosome. The Y chromosome is completely normal, therefore testes develop. The X chromosome is also normal, except that one of its thousands of genes has altered. This alteration is in the androgen receptor gene. A female will have two androgen receptor genes, one inherited from her mother and one from her father. If one of these is the altered androgen receptor gene that causes CAIS, the normal gene on the other X chromosome will be sufficient to cause her to develop as a normal female. If, however, this woman has a child who is XY and who inherits the X chromosome bearing the altered gene, the altered gene will not be balanced by a functional gene and the child will be a female with CAIS. It should also be noted that in one-third of girls with CAIS, it is caused by a spontaneous genetic change in the newly-formed foetus at the time of conception, rather than being inherited.

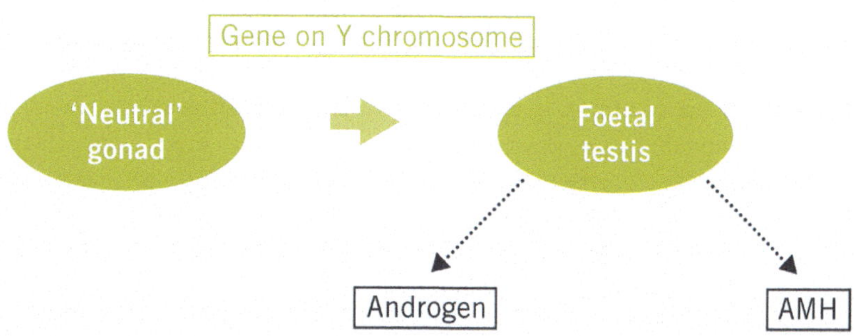

Fig. 25.4 Triggered by a gene on the Y chromosome, the 'neutral' gonad becomes a testis. It later produces two hormones, androgen and AMH

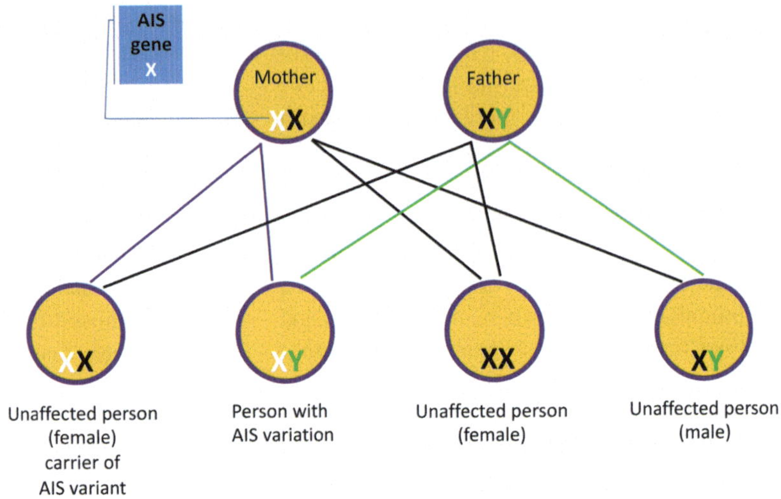

Fig. 25.5 Genetic diagram showing how a mother who carries the CAIS gene on one of her chromosomes can pass it on to her children. The risk of having a child with CAIS is one in four for every pregnancy

25.5.3 The Inheritance of AIS

The following diagram shows the different chromosome combinations that can result when a mother who carries the CAIS gene on one of her X chromosomes has children (Fig. 25.5).

A couple who have a child with CAIS can use the genetic diagram above to predict the odds of having other affected children. The way the parents' genes were distributed at the time of a particular conception is completely independent of what will happen during the conception of a future child, just as each throw of dice is independent of every other throw. Therefore, the risk of having another child with CAIS is one in four for *every* pregnancy, assuming the mother to be a carrier.

25.6 The Diagnosis of CAIS

The physical features that initially suggest the possibility of CAIS differ from person to person, and these differences influence the age at which diagnosis of the condition is usually diagnosed. The most common feature is a bulge (a hernia) in the groin area in an otherwise typical baby or little girl. When it is operated on, the hernia is found to contain a testis. If hernias go unnoticed or are not present, it may not be known that there is anything wrong until she is a teenager, when she has not begun to menstruate and neither pubic nor underarm hair has appeared, although her breast development will be normal.

To confirm the diagnosis, a blood test is done to identify the XY chromosome pattern. The ability of the testes to produce androgen can be measured in blood samples collected before and 72 h after an injection of a hormone called human chorionic gonadotrophin (hCG), which stimulates the testes. This proves that testes, rather than ovaries, are present. The hCG test is also useful for distinguishing CAIS from other medical conditions in which an XY female has testes, but they cannot produce androgen. An ultrasound examination will establish that there is no uterus.

25.7 Hormonal Changes During Childhood and Adolescence

During childhood, the testes are dormant. When the girl is about 11–12 years, they are stimulated to develop by hormones made in the pituitary gland, a part of the brain. The testes gradually enlarge and the level of androgen they produce progressively rises to adult male levels. At the same time, however, the body converts some of the androgen to oestrogen, and this causes breast development and widening of the hips.

The conversion of androgen to oestrogen is a normal process in the body and is not confined to girls with CAIS. Many healthy adolescent boys experience transient breast enlargement for the same reason. Boys, however, are fully responsive to androgen and this seems to inhibit further breast development.

Unlike many teenagers, girls with CAIS have very good skin with no acne (pimples). Acne occurs when oil-producing glands in the skin are stimulated by androgen, but this is impossible when the girl has AIS.

25.8 Surgery for Individuals with AIS

25.8.1 Testes

Testes that remain in the abdominal cavity, particularly those that are being overstimulated by the pituitary gland, are prone to develop cancer although the risk is very low before puberty. In adulthood there are varying estimates for the risk of a cancer developing in gonadal tissue, a recent review of the literature found there to be to be about a 6% risk in early adulthood.

As our knowledge in this area is evolving, medical specialists can provide up-to-date information to an individual girl / woman / person about the risk of developing a cancer.

The risk of malignant change depends on factors such as the position of the testes (risk is highest in abdominal testes) and age (increases as one gets older) and so differs for each person. Monitoring the gonads using imaging technology such as ultrasound is an alternative to having a gonadectomy.

The decision to have a gonadectomy or to plan surveillance for their testes should be made by the young person with AIS, with support from their family and medical team.

The surgery would take place after the young woman had been fully informed about her medical condition and implications of surgical intervention, and after she had been given the opportunity to discuss the feelings that arise under these circumstances. It is important to note that for girls and women with CAIS there are a number of potential benefits to having one's testes left in place as the production of testosterone which is converted in the body into oestrogen can occur in a more natural / physiological manner than can be attained with use of medications to replace these hormones.

25.8.2 The Vagina

The vagina in people with AIS may be a little shorter than average – but vaginas are very stretchy structures, so this usually does not cause significant issues. The majority of women with CAIS have satisfying sexual relationships. For most women who would like to have penetrative sex, the vagina can stretch with sexual activity or regular dilator use. Surgery is only rarely considered, and person led.

25.9 Lack of Pubic and Underarm Hair

The hair that XX women have in the genital and underarm areas is present because of the action of androgen produced in the adrenal glands and ovaries. Women with CAIS usually have either no hair at all in these areas or very sparse hair. This lack of pubic hair is a physical characteristic that cannot be altered by medical treatment. The amount of pubic hair that women generally have is very variable, and some women are relatively hairless. It has been reported that the mothers of women with CAIS have somewhat less pubic hair than women who do not carry the CAIS gene, so it can honestly be said that a lack of pubic hair is 'in the family'. In some cultures and with different fashions, having minimal pubic hair is considered normal and hair may be actively removed.

25.10 Counselling and Support

Better ways of understanding and working through the possible social and psychological effects of AIS are currently being developed. Nevertheless, parents are anxious to maintain confidentiality, and affected women may feel uncertain about how others will respond to them. Any lack of community understanding is likely to be due to ignorance rather than prejudice.

25.10.1 Parents of Newly Diagnosed Children

A medical diagnosis that affects the genital and reproductive organs is a particular challenge to understand, discuss and come to terms with in a helpful way. Since most families have never heard of anyone else with this kind of medical condition, they usually ask their doctors for help in finding words and ideas. At the same time, they must find ways of dealing with their own powerful emotions, which can include confusion, sadness and anger. 'Why me?' and 'Why my daughter?' are natural reactions.

Ideally, AIS should be correctly and promptly diagnosed, and an expert should be available immediately to provide counselling for the parents. This, however, is not always the case and parents may encounter hesitation and delays along the way. Not surprisingly, this generates confusion and anxiety. An opportunity to discuss these feelings with a professional who is familiar with the condition is often beneficial. Counselling takes the form of assistance to put words and ideas to the many powerful emotions that may be aroused. It is inevitable that parents will have stages of vulnerability as they adjust to a diagnosis with reproductive implications, and the child's future development will need to be discussed.

25.10.2 Parents of Children and Teenagers

CAIS is a complex condition that may raise complex emotions for parents. It is important for the clinical team to provide information and support to parents and assist them to talk to their child about their CAIS diagnosis. Parents face a dilemma about how and when to tell their child about AIS. Should they provide all the information they have as early as possible, or delay telling her until in their judgment she will understand the details of AIS. Individuals with CAIS have a right to know everything, but that information should be given in stages that consider her level of development and understanding what is being said. Ultimately this should strengthen their relationship with them.

25.10.2.1 Children Aged 6–11 Years

Up to the age of 11 years, most children have little ability to think about long-term consequences, and a simple explanation about the reason for seeing the doctor will generally suffice. If parents have concerns about the questions or behaviours their child is presenting to them, they could have a discussion about her with a mental health professional interested and experienced in assisting parents and children with AIS-related issues.

25.10.2.2 Adolescents with AIS

Adolescents usually develop the ability to reason and to think in philosophical terms around the age of 12 years, although the timing of this varies from person to person. It is only at this stage that a girl with AIS will be able to understand a discussion about the complex nature of her condition, and even then, she will be quite unfamiliar with the internal workings of the body.

Adolescence is a stage associated with peer pressures to conform. It is preferable for girls with CAIS to learn about their differences compared to others *before* this pressure to conform becomes dominant. Children learn about genes and chromosomes in school at around the age of 15–16 years, and it is best for them to be informed about their own diagnosis before this time. Linking in with peer support groups can be helpful in providing support for parents to share information about AIS to their child/ren.

25.10.3 Adults

It may be challenging for many people with CAIS to accept the ways in which their variation affects their lives and relationships. All medical conditions arouse complex feelings in people and their families, and relationships may at times come under strain as different family members adjust to the issues in their own way. Because it is a genetic condition, a person with CAIS may have affected siblings, nieces or aunts who can provide mutual understanding and support.

People with AIS can have satisfying relationships. Adapting to and accepting the inability to become pregnant may be difficult for women with CAIS, in the same way as it is for anyone (about 10% of all couples). Counselling or psychological support can be beneficial in this regard. Although pregnancy is not possible, many women with CAIS choose to have children / start families in other ways such as through fostering, adoption or surrogacy.

Individuals with CAIS are found in all walks of life. Counselling services are available and a referral from the doctor to a mental health professional or social worker will be arranged on request. Many women find it very helpful to meet other people with AIS, Australia has some great peer support networks that young people and adults with AIS and their families can connect with.

25.10.4 Support Groups

It is well recognised that people who share common issues or lived experiences feel empowered and less isolated when sharing their experiences with others with similar lived experiences in forums such as peer support groups. In Australia and internationally, there are many appropriate peer support groups for individuals with DSD or intersex variations. Peer support groups offer a range of beneficial elements such as community and social networks, minimising isolation, individual empowerment, and advocacy.

Further Reading

For more information and patient resources follow the Royal Children's Hospital, Melbourne website link: https://www.rch.org.au/endo/differences-of-sex-development/

Index

J. M. Hutson et al. (eds.), *Disorders|Differences of Sex Development*,
https://doi.org/10.1007/978-981-13-7864-5

B

C